D1213092

THE PSYCHOLOGY OF ACTION

The Psychology of Action

Linking Cognition and Motivation to Behavior

Edited by
PETER M. GOLLWITZER
JOHN A. BARGH

THE GUILFORD PRESS
New York London

A Division of Guilford Publications, Inc.
72 Spring Street, New York, NY 10012

Printed in the United States of America

This book is printed on acid-free paper.

Last digit is print number: 9 8 7 6 5 4 3 2 1

Library of Congress Cataloging-in-Publication Data

The psychology of action : linking cognition and motivation to behavior / edited by Peter M. Gollwitzer, John A. Bargh.
p. cm.
Includes bibliographical references and index.
ISBN 1-57230-032-9
1. Human behavior. 2. Cognition. 3. Motivation (Psychology)
I. Gollwitzer, Peter M. II. Bargh, John A.
BF121.P827 1996
150—dc20 95-39728
CIP

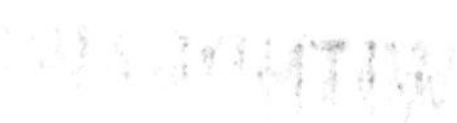

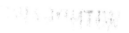

Contributors

Icek Ajzen, PhD, Department of Psychology, University of Massachusetts at Amherst, Amherst, Massachusetts

Matthew E. Ansfield, MA, Department of Psychology, University of Virginia, Charlottesville, Virginia

John A. Bargh, PhD, Department of Psychology, New York University, New York, New York

Kimberly Barndollar, MA, Department of Psychology, New York University, New York, New York

Roy F. Baumeister, PhD, Department of Psychology, Case Western Reserve University, Cleveland, Ohio

Hart Blanton, PhD, Department of Psychology, Iowa State University, Ames, Iowa

Gerd Bohner, PhD, Fakultät für Sozialwissenschaften, Universität Mannheim, Mannheim, Germany

Nancy Cantor, PhD, Department of Psychology, Princeton University, Princeton, New Jersey

Charles S. Carver, PhD, Department of Psychology, University of Miami, Coral Gables, Florida

Shelly Chaiken, PhD, Department of Psychology, New York University, New York, New York

Serena Chen, MA, Department of Psychology, New York University, New York, New York

David P. Cornell, PhD, Department of Psychology, Armstrong State College, Savannah, Georgia

Edward L. Deci, PhD, Department of Psychology, University of Rochester, Rochester, New York

Carol S. Dweck, PhD, Department of Psychology, Columbia University, New York, New York

Robert A. Emmons, PhD, Department of Psychology, University of California at Davis, Davis, California

Katherine Gannon, MA, Department of Psychology, Ohio State University, Columbus, Ohio

Roger Giner-Sorolla, MA, Department of Psychology, New York University, New York, New York

Peter M. Gollwitzer, PhD, Sozialwissenschaftliche Fakultät, Universität Konstanz, Konstanz, Germany

Bettina Hannover, PhD, Department of Psychology, Technical University of Berlin, Berlin, Germany

E. Tory Higgins, PhD, Department of Psychology, Columbia University, New York, New York

Ruth Kanfer, PhD, Department of Psychology, University of Minnesota, Minneapolis, Minnesota

Tim Kasser, PhD, Department of Psychology, University of Rochester, Rochester, New York

James Kaufman, BA, Department of Psychology, Florida Atlantic University, Boca Raton, Florida

Eric Klinger, PhD, Division of Social Sciences, University of Minnesota–Morris, Morris, Minnesota

Amy L. Kristof, BA, College of Business and Management, University of Maryland, College Park, Maryland

Arie W. Kruglanski, PhD, Department of Psychology, University of Maryland, College Park, Maryland

Edwin A. Locke, PhD, College of Business and Management, University of Maryland, College Park, Maryland

Leonard L. Martin, PhD, Institute for Behavioral Research, University of Georgia, Athens, Georgia

Walter Mischel, PhD, Department of Psychology, Columbia University, New York, New York

Steven L. Neuberg, PhD, Department of Psychology, Arizona State University, Tempe, Arizona

Gabriele Oettingen, Dr.rer.nat., Max-Planck-Institute for Human Development and Education, Berlin, Germany

Lien B. Pham, BA, Department of Psychology, University of California at Los Angeles, California

Richard M. Ryan, PhD, Department of Psychology, University of Rochester, Rochester, New York

Norbert Schwarz, Dr.phil.habil., Institute for Social Research, University of Michigan, Ann Arbor, Michigan

Kennon M. Sheldon, PhD, Department of Psychology, University of Rochester, Rochester, New York

Richard M. Sorrentino, PhD, Department of Psychology, University of Western Ontario, London, Ontario, Canada

Gisela Steins, PhD, Department of Psychology, Universität Bielefeld, Bielefeld, Germany

Fritz Strack, PhD, Department of Psychology, University of Würzburg, Germany

Shelley E. Taylor, PhD, Department of Psychology, University of California at Los Angeles, Los Angeles, California

Abraham Tesser, PhD, Institute for Behavioral Research, University of Georgia, Athens, Georgia

Robin R. Vallacher, PhD, Department of Psychology, Florida Atlantic Univeristy, Boca Raton, Florida

Gifford Weary, PhD, Department of Psychology, Ohio State University, Columbus, Ohio

Daniel M. Wegner, PhD, Department of Psychology, University of Virginia, Charlottesville, Virginia

Robert A. Wicklund, PhD, Department of Psychology, Universität Bielefeld, Bielefeld, Germany

Rex A. Wright, PhD, Department of Psychology, University of Alabama, Birmingham, Alabama

Preface

In their introduction to Volume 1 of the *Handbook of Motivation and Cognition* (1986), the editors, Richard Sorrentino and Tory Higgins, gave a vivid description of the schism separating cognitive social psychologists and social psychologists interested in motivation. Rather than studying the interaction of cognitive and motivational processes, these two groups were caught up in a battle regarding which of the two, motivation or cognition, was a better explanation of classic findings in social psychology. A fierce competition had started that culminated in attempts by the cognitive camp to find alternative cognitive explanations for so-called "motivational" phenomena (e.g., the asymmetrical attributions after success and failure), whereas the motivational camp eagerly produced data difficult to account for in purely cognitive terms (e.g., arousal's effects on the asymmetrical attributional pattern).

Sorrentino and Higgins tried to put a halt to this pseudointellectual exchange by arguing that cognition and motivation are not truly separable factors (a point they vividly illustrated with a Möbius strip on the book's cover). They advocated a synergistic perspective, acknowledging that cognition does not simply lead to motivation or motivation to cognition; rather, each is a property or facet of the other. The contributors to the two volumes of the *Handbook of Motivation and Cognition* in 1986 and 1990 were committed to this new perspective (the "warm look"), and thus successfully avoided taking a belligerent either–or, exclusively "hot" (motivational) or "cold" (cognitive) perspective in their theorizing.

There is another possible method for uniting competing camps—this one suggested by Muzafer Sherif in his studies on competition and cooperation at the Robbers Cave State Park in 1954. The Rattlers and the Eagles, two groups of 11-year-old boys at a summer camp, had developed their own group identities before they were allowed to interact. The types of interactions offered, however, were antagonistic at first: competing against each other in various games (e.g., treasure hunts) for trophies, medals, and other prizes. Sherif observed that such competition turned the well-adjusted middle-class boys into wicked, disturbed, and vicious little monsters. Members of the two groups tried to destroy each other's identity (e.g., group flags were burned), ransacked each other's cabins, and started food fights like hostile antagonists in a full-scale war.

What finally ended this uncivilized, destructive conduct most effectively was a particular request for cooperation. The two groups were given tasks that could be achieved only through cooperation between groups (i.e., Sherif set the boys superordinate goals). For instance, at the Robbers Cave State Park the experimenters arranged for the camp truck to break down, and both groups were needed to pull it up a steep hill.

Apparently, setting superordinate goals turns fruitless competition into productive collaboration. But what could possibly qualify as a superordinate task for the cognitive and the motivational camps in social psychology? We believe that social psychologists have seen this superordinate goal in the need for developing a comprehensive psychology of action. The enthusiasm with which goal concepts have been embraced in recent years by cognitive and motivational social psychologists alike seems to support our claim. Explaining when and how actions are initiated, sustained, disrupted, and resumed requires the collaboration of motivational and cognitive researchers, because it demands a multitude of theoretical perspectives: the "hot," the "cold," and the "warm."

The two of us have experienced the unifying forces of the psychology of action in our own research collaboration on the automatic control of goal-directed action (as first presented in Volume 41 of the *Nebraska Symposium on Motivation,* 1994). One of us has his roots in social cognition, the other in the psychology of motivation (the nonoverlapping contents of our bookshelves leave no doubt about this). Our theorizing on the automatic control of action has turned out to be greatly facilitated by bringing cognitive and motivational perspectives together; more importantly, it has allowed us to create new concepts (e.g., auto-motives, implementation intentions) that transcend the traditional schism between cognition and motivation.

As our research collaboration has been and continues to be generously supported by the Max Planck Society and the Humboldt Society, we thought of sharing this support and the positive experiences of our collaboration with our colleagues in social psychology. Accordingly, we organized a conference in July 1993 around the general theme of linking cognition and motivation to action, and invited social psychologists whose major affinities were with either the motivation or cognition camps, along with proponents of the "warm look." It was held at Ringberg Castle, on a Bavarian mountainside overlooking the Tegernsee. For 4 days we listened to 28 talks, each focused on the unique research program currently conducted by the speaker.

It became quickly apparent that creating a psychology of action that links motivation and cognition to behavior qualifies as a great superordinate goal—one that puts an end to the traditional, unproductive juxtaposing of cognition and motivation. The chapters in the present book, based on these talks, also carry this message. All of the central issues of a psychology of action are covered: Where do action goals come from (see Parts I and II)? When and how do people prepare their actions (see Part III)? How do people control their ongoing goal pursuits (for effortful and automatic control, see Parts

IV and V, respectively)? How do goals affect people's social interactions (Part VI)?

At the conference, a discussant spoke at the end of each day of presentations. The discussant's task was to provide critical reflections on what had been said during the day, identifying common themes and issues in the various talks. These discussions are presented in Part VII of the book. We have found these three concluding chapters particularly valuable, as they relate the unique research programs of various researchers to one another as well as to the discussant's own unique perspective.

Overviews of each of the chapters appear at the beginning of each part of the book; we have prepared these in order to help the reader connect the various parts conceptually. In addition, each transition relates the individual contributions within an upcoming part and provides a brief summary of each contribution. We distributed prepublication versions of these chapters to advanced undergraduates and graduate students, and have been informed by their feedback. As the chapters are highly concise formulations of complete research programs, they effectively familiarize the novice with important theories in the psychology of action; still, they provide enough new findings and innovative ideas to enrich the knowledge of graduate students. The book is ideally suited to elicit in-depth discussions, if the various contributions within a part are read in comparison to one another.

We would like to close these introductory remarks by expressing our appreciation of the support we received from others. Thanks are due first to the contributors to this book. We enjoyed their company during the conference; we were impressed with the quality of their first drafts; and we were even more impressed with their responsiveness to our many nagging wishes for revising initial drafts. We do not take such responsiveness for granted, and therefore we are particularly thankful for these additional efforts.

Thanks are also due to those contributors who shared at the conference in our efforts to find the perfect title for the book. Although we are very pleased with the eventual winner, it was a close competition. Among the final contenders were these:

Action at Ringberg
Wills and Deeds Made Easy
For Whom the Ring Bergs
Cognitions Are a Goal's Best Friend
Needs and Deeds: Some New Leads
Why the Action Is
Last Tango in Cognition: The Ringberg Conference
Jurassic Pork
Goals Just Want to Have Fun
The Ringberg Conference: Can You Prove It Didn't Happen?

and last, but not least:

Four Days at Ringberg: Four Days at Ringberg

Special thanks are due to the Max Planck Society, the Humboldt Society, and the Max-Planck-Institute for Psychological Research, which shared the costs of the conference; and to The Guilford Press, particularly our editor, Seymour Weingarten. Seymour's support for the publication of this book—in particular, his great patience in waiting for the final product—was of great value. We also thank the many people who helped in organizing the international conference: our colleagues Gordon Moskowitz, Ute Bayer, and Kerstin Azzazzi; the administrative staff of the Max-Planck-Institute for Psychological Research in Munich; and the staff of the Ringberg Castle, the conference center of the Max Planck Society. Listening to 28 state-of-the-art lectures in 4 days was hard work. Still, we enjoyed every minute of it and we will always enjoy browsing through the book, its final outcome.

Peter M. Gollwitzer
John A. Bargh

Contents

Part I. Sources and Contents of Action Goals 1

1. **All Goals Are Not Created Equal: An Organismic Perspective on the Nature of Goals and Their Regulation** 7
   Richard M. Ryan, Kennon M. Sheldon, Tim Kasser, and Edward L. Deci

2. **Self-Regulation and Ego Threat: Motivated Cognition, Self Deception, and Destructive Goal Setting** 27
   Roy F. Baumeister

3. **On the Substitutability of Self-Protective Mechanisms** 48
   Abraham Tesser, Leonard L. Martin, and David P. Cornell

4. **Implicit Theories as Organizers of Goals and Behavior** 69
   Carol S. Dweck

5. **Ideals, Oughts, and Regulatory Focus: Affect and Motivation from Distinct Pains and Pleasures** 91
   E. Tory Higgins

Part II. Affective Influences on Action Goals 115

6. **Feelings and Their Motivational Implications: Moods and the Action Sequence** 119
   Norbert Schwarz and Gerd Bohner

7. **Depression, Control Motivation, and Person Perception** 146
   Gifford Weary and Katherine Gannon

8. **Emotional Influences on Cognitive Processing, with Implications for Theories of Both** 168
   Eric Klinger

Part III. Preparing to Act
Section A. Mental Construction of the Goal 193

9. **From Good Intentions to Willpower** 197
   Walter Mischel

10. Mental Stimulation, Motivation, and Action 219
Shelley E. Taylor and Lien B. Pham

11. Positive Fantasy and Motivation 236
Gabriele Oettingen

12. Dynamics of Action Identification: Volatility and Structure in the Mental Representation of Behavior 260
Robin R. Vallacher and James Kaufman

Section B. Planning and Coordinating Action 283

13. The Volitional Benefits of Planning 287
Peter M. Gollwitzer

14. Striving and Feeling: Personal Goals and Subjective Well-Being 313
Robert A. Emmons

15. Effortful Pursuit of Personal Goals in Daily Life 338
Nancy Cantor and Hart Blanton

Part IV. Effortful Control of Action 361

16. Volitional Choices in the Goal Achievement Process 365
Edwin A. Locke and Amy L. Kristof

17. The Directive Influence of Attitudes on Behavior 385
Icek Ajzen

18. Self-Regulatory and Other Non-Ability Determinants of Skill Acquisition 404
Ruth Kanfer

19. Brehm's Theory of Motivation as a Model of Effort and Cardiovascular Response 424
Rex A. Wright

Part V. Nonconscious Control of Action 455

20. Automaticity in Action: The Unconscious as Repository of Chronic Goals and Motives 457
John A. Bargh and Kimberly Barndollar

21. The Feeling of Doing 482
Matthew E. Ansfield and Daniel M. Wegner

Part VI. Goal Influences on Social Interaction 507

22. Person Perception under Pressure: When Motivation Brings About Egocentrism 511
Robert A. Wicklund and Gisela Steins

23. Expectancy Influences in Social Interaction: The Moderating Role of Social Goals 529
Steven L. Neuberg

24. Beyond Accuracy: Defense and Impression Motives in Heuristic and Systematic Information Processing 553
Shelly Chaiken, Roger Giner-Sorolla, and Serena Chen

25. Awareness of Influence as a Precondition for Implementing Correctional Goals 579
Fritz Strack and Bettina Hannover

Part VII. Discussions 597

26. Goals as Knowledge Structures 599
Arie W. Kruglanski

27. The Role of Conscious Thought in a Theory of Motivation and Cognition: The Uncertainty Orientation Paradigm 619
Richard M. Sorrentino

28. Some Ways in Which Goals Differ and Some Implications of Those Differences 645
Charles S. Carver

Index 673

THE PSYCHOLOGY OF ACTION

PART I

Sources and Contents of Action Goals

Goals primarily are considered to be directors of action. Accordingly, research on goals focuses on how they guide our actions and how goal pursuit is regulated. Two questions, however, need to be answered first: What are the sources that give rise to goals, and what will be specified in a goal state? Our needs (e.g., the need for approval) and higher-order goals (e.g., the aim to excel in a chosen profession) produce wishes and desires that point to attractive incentives (e.g., being productive). What is recognized as an incentive depends on the perceived demands of the situation at hand (e.g., only when approval or professional success is perceived as contingent upon productivity will "being productive" qualify as an incentive). Setting an action goal, however, requires one further step: The individual needs to commit himself or herself to the execution of actions that produce the desired incentive. Again, the individual's beliefs as to what type of actions lead to the goal state will ultimately determine the contents of the action goals the individual chooses to pursue. It appears, then, that needs and higher-order goals are only the ultimate sources of action goals, whereas the individual's beliefs concerning what qualifies as an incentive and what actions lead to incentives determine the actual contents of action goals.

The chapters in Part I address from different viewpoints the issues of where goals come from and what contents become specified in goals. Ryan, Sheldon, Kasser, and Deci (Chapter 1) point to the basic psychic needs of autonomy, competence, and interpersonal relatedness as powerful sources of goals. The authors analyze how goals based on these special needs lead to different self-regulatory styles and different outcomes than goals based on extrinsic, derivative desires. The analysis of self-protective strategies and mechanisms leads Baumeister (Chapter 2), as well as Tesser, Martin, and Cornell (Chapter 3), to focus on people's need for self-esteem as another important source of goals. But it is not only people's needs or superordinate goals that determine which action goals are pursued. Dweck (Chapter 4) demonstrates that people's implicit theories on how reality works also determine the contents of goals. Different implicit theories about intelligence or moral character foster particular interpretations of events, and thus lead to particular goals followed by particular actions. Similarly, Higgins (Chapter 5) points out that positive as well as negative incentives are framed differently, depending on a person's outcome focus (on positive or negative outcomes). A positive outcome focus leads to conceiving of positive incentives in terms of the presence of positive outcomes, and of negative incentives in terms of the absence of positive outcomes. A negative outcome focus, on the other hand, defines negative incentives in terms of the presence of negative outcomes and positive incentives in terms of the absence of negative outcomes. Consequently, a person's goal pursuits differ according to his or her predilection for a positive or negative outcome focus.

Ryan et al. raise the question of why people pursue particular goals. The answer relates to whether goal pursuit is experienced as initiated or endorsed by one's core self or by pressures and forces felt to be external to the self. Ryan et al. discuss how goal pursuit that is originally controlled by external reasons may become increasingly internalized and integrated. They also point to the specific features of socialization contexts that favor this process (i.e., autonomy support and high interpersonal involvement). Empirical evidence is presented that links greater creativity, more cognitive flexibility, a more positive emotional tone, and better physical and psychological well-being with goal pursuits that are controlled by internal reasons rather than external reasons. This observed difference seems to hold true not only for academic goals, but also for interpersonal and health-related goals. In addition, Ryan et al. present recent research that contrasts goals serving the psychological needs for autonomy, competence, and interpersonal relatedness with goals of money, fame, status, and attractiveness (so-called "extrinsic" goals). It turns out that various indicators of psychological and physical well-being correlate positively with the former type of goals, and negatively with the latter. Most interestingly, the negative effects of external goals are stronger with individuals who report strong as opposed to weak feelings of self-efficacy. This finding reminds us that the analysis of people's goal pursuits should never forgo the contents of the goals under scrutiny, as "all goals are not created equal."

Baumeister discusses self-esteem as a basic human need. The need to maintain a positive view of oneself is seen as a powerful source of self-regulatory goals. Whenever threats to a positive self-view are encountered, multiple strategies are invoked to ward them off. This cascade of measures begins with strategies demanding little cognitive effort, and ends with more drastic, highly involving strategies in case the less effortful strategies are not successful. As a first strategy, the individual attempts to ignore the threat. Threatening negative performance evaluations from others, for instance, are processed in a cursory manner; attention is fixed on neutral distracting stimuli (so-called "defensive preoccupation"); and people may even create their own distractors (e.g., summoning up memories of pleasant experiences). In case these strategies fail and an individual must face the threat to self-esteem, a shift from avoidant defense to refutational defense occurs. These interpretational efforts include downplaying the source of the bad news; adding unrelated information that carries positive implications; blaming others for unfavorable outcomes; and, most interestingly, the self-serving temporal bracketing of the threatening experience. But the refutational defense may not be the individual's last answer to self-threats. People self-regulate not only their information processing in the service of self-defense, but also their actions. Baumeister reports data demonstrating that people with high self-esteem respond to failure experiences with invigorated goal striving (i.e., they raise their standards in an achievement task). The ideas presented by Baumeister demonstrate nicely that the psychology of the self has identified the need for self-esteem as a powerful source of self-regulatory goals. Interestingly, Baumeister analyzes these self-regulatory goals only in terms of warding off threats to self-esteem. This is in line with other research on the psychology of the self: self-handicapping, excuse making, egotistical attributions, self-completion, and downward social comparisons. So far, the role of a person's need for self-esteem as a source of self-regulatory goals has been analyzed primarily in terms of achieving effective self-defense once a threat to self-esteem has occurred. But this need not always be so. Self-esteem needs should also qualify as sources of self-regulatory goals that focus on the construction of a positive self-evaluation, rather than serving a defensive purpose.

Tesser et al. start out with an evaluation of the current status of the psychology of the self. They come to the conclusion that it is characterized best as a "self-defense zoo," because numerous different processes of protecting the self against a threat to positive evaluation are identified without an attempt at integration. The authors propose a possible integration of these different self-protection mechanisms into a unified theory. Borrowing from Lewin's idea that action goals serving the same superordinate goal or need can be substituted for one another, they propose that the various self-defense mechanisms may serve the same superordinate goal (or need) of self-esteem maintenance. A series of experiments by Tesser and Cornell supports this view. Subjects no longer employ typical self-evaluation maintenance strategies (e.g., hindering the success of a friend on a personally important task) when prior self-affirmation of values has occurred. Moreover, dissonance reduction strategies as well as efforts at self-affirmation do not occur when prior interpersonal self-evaluation maintenance strategies have been successfully employed. In closing their chapter, Tesser et al. speculate that affect may qualify as the currency of exchange between the many different action goals directed at self-defense.

Dweck stresses that the subjective reality constructed by people's implicit theories is an important determinant of goals. More specifically, two types of implicit theories (entity theories and incremental theories) are distinguished and applied to the personal attributes of intelligence and moral character. In entity theories, intelligence and moral character are seen as fixed personal attributes of a certain strength; in incremental theories, these personal attributes are seen as malleable. Dweck reports experiments demonstrating that different theories on intelligence affect both choice of achievement goals and patterns of achievement behavior. When an intellectual achievement situation is entered, people with entity theories choose the goal of judging the amount of intelligence they possess (i.e., performance goals), whereas, those with incremental theories choose the goal of developing their intelligence (i.e., learning goals). Setting one or the other type of goal turns out to have important consequences: For people with performance goals, negative outcomes signal a lack of intelligence and result in helpless reactions. People with learning goals, on the other hand, view setbacks as cues to focus on their behavioral strategies. Their reactions are oriented toward mastering the causes of the setback. Dweck also reports her new research on how implicit theories of personality and character affect the choice of goals in situations where another person's disreputable actions and transgressions raise the question of his or her moral character. In a series of very intriguing experiments, she and her colleagues have observed that entity theorists, as compared to incremental theorists, interpret information about the other person in terms of traits (e.g., mean, nasty); ignore information on psychological states (e.g., furious, enraged) and unintentionality; overemphasize the other person's physical appearance (e.g., being dressed in a respectable manner); and seem generally to encode any information about the other person in evaluative terms. This suggests that entity theorists set themselves the goal of judging the other person's relevant moral attributes, whereas incremental theorists pursue the goal of understanding the dynamics of the other person's behavior in the given situation. Again, adopting one or the other goal has behavioral consequences. When subjects are asked how they would deal with the other person's disreputable actions or transgressions, entity theorists propose punishment and retaliation, whereas incremental theorists propose education and reform.

In Higgins's theory of outcome focus, the two motivational systems of pleasure and pain have different effects on people's goal pursuits, depending on how they are framed. Pleasure can be framed as the presence of positive outcomes (positive outcome focus) or the absence of negative outcomes (negative outcome focus). Similarly, pain can be framed as the presence of negative outcomes (negative outcome focus) or the absence of positive outcomes (positive outcome focus). Achievement goals that focus on the presence or absence of positive outcomes favor task performance, whereas goals that focus on the presence or absence of negative outcomes undermine it. Higgins suggests that individuals with chronic discrepancies between their actual selves and their ideal selves (i.e., people who fall short of their ideals) are characterized by a focus on positive outcomes, whereas individuals with discrepancies between their actual selves and their ought selves (i.e., people who fall short of their duties) show a focus on negative outcomes. Empirical support comes from studies demonstrating that distinct emotions accompany the experience of falling short (sadness vs. agitation, respectively), and from recent work that points to a clear difference in goal setting (approach vs. avoidance goals, respectively). In closing his chapter, Higgins shows how adding outcome focus to the motivational systems of pain and pleasure enlightens the discussion of the popular distinction between optimists and pessimists, and adds to the understanding of the types of strategies people choose when attempting to meet their life tasks (see also Cantor & Blanton, Chapter 15, this volume).

CHAPTER 1

All Goals Are Not Created Equal

An Organismic Perspective on the Nature of Goals and Their Regulation

Richard M. Ryan
Kennon M. Sheldon
Tim Kasser
Edward L. Deci

During the past two decades, goal constructs have been increasingly emphasized in the study of motivation (Ford, 1992; Schwarzer, 1986). This trend reflects the growing recognition of the important role that goals play in the organization of human behavior, as well as the promise of goal methodologies for studying many motivational questions. However, along with the focus on goals has come a corresponding tendency to ignore some of what have traditionally been thought of as critical motivational constructs and analyses (Pervin, 1989). Thus, many theorists have suggested that the study of goals and goal-related cognition *is* the study of motivation, and that goals themselves are the instigators and directors of human action rather than being (more or less adequate) servants of deeper-lying needs and motives.

We argue that although extant goal theories have made major contributions to the understanding of *how* a motivated subject achieves conscious goals, they have given relatively little attention to the interplay of human needs and goals that underlies psychological health. Thus, while goal theories typically do examine how one can efficaciously pursue goals, they typically ignore *why* one pursues particular goals and/or the significance of *what* specific goals are pursued. Yet both of these issues are crucial for understanding the effectiveness, persistence, and experiential qualities associated with goal activity, as well as the functional impact of goal activities on personal well-being.

The "why" question concerns the source or impetus that gives rise to a goal, and its answer has direct implications for how the goal pursuit is regulated. More specifically, the answer to why people perform an action illuminates the regulatory process that underlies it, and this has a great many experiential and functional consequences. Perhaps most crucial to answering the "why" question is whether one perceives that the goal-directed behavior emanates from one self or, alternatively, is brought about by forces or pressures external to the self (Heider, 1958; Ryan & Connell, 1989). This issue pertains to the degree to which an action is autonomous or self-determined, and is examined by inquiring about the perceived locus of causality that accompanies goal selection and engagement.

The "what" question concerns the content of goals. What, for example, are the consequences of pursuing money rather than personal growth? Attractiveness rather than love? Power rather than generativity? Although many laypersons would agree that it is healthier to pursue love, personal growth, and generativity goals than money, attractiveness, and power goals, this issue of the relative costs and benefits of different kinds of goals has thus far been relatively unexplored by goal theorists.

Both of these questions (i.e., the "what" and the "why" of goals) consider the psychological and organismic *needs* being fulfilled (or not being fulfilled) by goal-directed behaviors. Historically, motivation theories have taken as a central concern the role of specific human needs in providing salience to outcomes and in giving energy to pursue them (e.g., Deci & Ryan, 1985b; Maslow, 1970; Murray, 1938; White, 1963). From this perspective, conscious goals may be evaluated as more or less adequate instruments of human needs and personal development. Thus, how different regulatory processes underlying goal pursuits and different goal contents relate to optimal health and development is the overarching focus of our inquiry. Accordingly, we review recent evidence regarding goals and their relation to needs that grows out of "self-determination theory" (Deci & Ryan, 1985b, 1991; Ryan, 1993). This theory assumes that there are three basic psychological needs: autonomy, relatedness, and competence. The remainder of this chapter explores the potential consequences associated with goal pursuits that do or do not provide satisfaction of these basic needs.

DISTINGUISHING AMONG INTENTIONAL ACTS: THE "WHY" OF BEHAVIOR

Most current theories of motivated behavior have the concept of "intention" at their core (Heider, 1958). The basic idea is that people will engage in intentional behavior (i.e., will be motivated) if they expect the behavior to attain goals or to yield desired outcomes. People are thus said to be motivated when they behave with purpose (Tolman, 1959), with the intention of attaining a goal (Lewin, 1926/1951). In such theories, motivation is treated as a unitary concept that varies only in amount or intensity, largely as a function of beliefs about one's ability to attain desired outcomes. From this general perspective, the key question becomes what factors promote motivation (i.e., intentional behavior) as opposed to lack of motivation (what Deci & Ryan, 1985b, called "amotivation"). In addressing this question, researchers have established that an internal locus of control over outcomes (Rotter, 1966), response–outcome dependence (Seligman, 1975), self-efficacy (Bandura, 1977), and a high expectancy–valence product (Vroom, 1964) are prerequisites for a high level of motivation.

In contrast to the above-mentioned theories, phenomenologically oriented approaches to motivation (e.g., deCharms, 1968; Deci & Ryan, 1985b) have gone beyond the mere distinction between motivation and amotivation to distinguish among qualitatively different types of motivated behavior by addressing the experienced locus of initiation of people's motivated behavior. Does a person pursue a goal because of pressures and forces felt to be external to the self? Or is the activity felt to be initiated or endorsed by one's core self?

Specifically, Deci and Ryan (1985b, 1991) have argued that motivated or intentional behaviors differ in the degree to which they are autonomous (i.e., self-determined) versus controlled (i.e., compelled). Autonomous behaviors are those experienced as having what deCharms (1968) called an "internal perceived locus of causality." In contrast, controlled behaviors are those pressured by some interpersonal or intrapsychic force external to the self; they thus have an "external perceived locus of causality." Although both autonomous and controlled behaviors are intentional, purposive, and motivated, they differ importantly in phenomenological character and in their effects both on the quality of behavioral engagement and on personality functioning in general.

Numerous studies in both laboratory and field settings have indicated convincingly that when people are autonomous—that is, when they perceive their intentional actions as having an internal locus of causality—they display greater creativity (e.g., Amabile, 1983), more cognitive flexibility and depth of processing (e.g., Grolnick & Ryan, 1987; McGraw & McCullers, 1979), higher self-esteem (e.g., Deci, Nezlek, & Sheinman, 1981; Ryan & Grolnick, 1986), a more positive emotional tone (e.g., Garbarino, 1975), greater satisfaction and trust (e.g., Deci, Connell, & Ryan, 1989), and better physical and psychological well-being (e.g., Langer & Rodin, 1976) than when they are controlled. The amount or level of motivation does not necessarily differ when people are autonomous versus controlled, but the type or orientation of motivation does, and this results in a different quality of functioning (Deci & Ryan, 1991; Ryan & Connell, 1989).

Intrinsic and Extrinsic Motivation

Much of the early work differentiating intentional actions in terms of their perceived locus of causality was based upon a contrast between "intrinsically motivated" and "extrinsically motivated" behaviors (Deci, 1975). Intrinsically motivated behaviors are the prototypes of autonomous or self-determined actions because they are performed out of interest and for the inherent satisfaction they yield. When intrinsically motivated, people *want* to engage in the activity; thus no external or intrapsychic prods, promises, or threats are required. Furthermore, intrinsic motivation, which takes the form of curiosity, spontaneity, and interest, is evident even from the beginning of life, as manifested in mastery strivings (White, 1959) and assimilaory tendencies (Piaget, 1967/1971). Invariably intrinsically motivated behavior has an internal perceived locus of causality.

Whereas with intrinsic motivation the reward for the activity is the spontaneous cognitions and affects inherent in the doing of the activity, with extrinsic motivation the reward is separable from the behavior itself. It is a separable consequence for which the behavior is instrumental.

Several early studies showing that extrinsic rewards could undermine intrinsic motivation (see Deci, 1975) have led some writers to infer that extrinsically motivated behaviors are non-self-determined. There is a grain of truth to this inference, and it stems from the fact that the separable consequences that are the foci of extrinsically motivated actions (e.g., rewards, praise, grades, and avoidance of punishment) are often controlled by others, such as bosses, teachers, or parents, who may use such consequences to control behavior. Thus, rewards often are associated with an external perceived locus of causality.

However, there is nothing about instrumental, extrinsically motivated activities that *necessitates* their being experienced as nonautonomous or externally caused. Many behaviors that are not intrinsically motivated (i.e., that are not rewarding or enjoyable in their own right) are volitionally initiated and valued, and are thus autonomous. For example, one may quite willingly and wholeheartedly take on an onerous administrative task—not because one sees it as interesting or fun, but because one believes it is valuable and personally important for some reason. In this instance, the task may be phenomenologically experienced as autonomous or self-caused, even though it is extrinsically motivated.

Internalization and Integration

According to self-determination theory (Deci & Ryan, 1985b, 1991; Ryan, 1993), extrinsically motivated activities can become more autonomous as a function of the fundamental developmental process we label "organismic integration." This process, which is closely akin to what has been called the tendencies toward "organization" (e.g., Piaget, 1967/1971), "hierarchical integration" (e.g., Werner, 1948), and "actualization' (Goldstein, 1939; Rogers, 1963), assumes that people are inherently oriented toward developing through the integration of new processes and structures to the self. Deci and Ryan (1991) have postulated that this tendency toward elaboration and refinement of the self is in people's nature and is motivated by their fundamental psychological needs for competence, autonomy, and relatedness. Thus, social contexts that allow satisfaction of these needs will promote the organismic integration process.

One manifestation of organismic integration is the tendency to transform heteronomous regulation into more autonomous regulation by "internalizing" (Meissner, 1981; Schafer, 1968) the regulation of extrinsically motivated behavior and the values underlying it, and then "integrating" those values and regulations with other aspects of the core self. Through this process, extrinsically motivated behaviors can become increasingly self-determined or autonomous. Self-determination theory specifies four different extrinsic regulatory processes, which vary in the degree to which they are autonomous (Ryan & Connell, 1989) and result from the organismic integration process's having been differentially effective.

"External regulation" refers to being regulated by contingencies overtly external to the person. A person's behaving so that someone will reward him or her, or so as not to be punished, is an example of external regulation. Externally regulated behaviors are intentional, but they are dependent on external contingencies and are thus considered controlled rather than autonomous. Because the regulation of these behaviors depends on external contingencies, they represent instances in which there has not been internalization of their underlying value. Thus, they would not be expected to occur unless direct external controls are in effect. Working only if one's boss or teacher is in the area exemplifies this form of motivated behavior.

"Introjected regulation" refers to the process of being directed by internal prods and pressures such as self-esteem-relevant contingencies. When a regulation has been introjected, it is internal to the person in the sense that the behavior no longer requires overtly external prompts, but the regulatory process motivating it is still external to the self. Introjected regulation, then, describes a form of internalized motivation in which actions are controlled by intrapsychic, esteem-related contingencies. Thus such actions are also said to have an external perceived locus of causality (deCharms, 1968; Ryan & Connell, 1989). A boy who works in school because he would feel guilty if he did not, or would feel "stupid" if he fell short of his parents' standards, exemplifies introjected regulation.

Although the regulation of goal-directed behavior for external or introjected reasons represents instances of low autonomy and volition, it is possible for extrinsically motivated action to become more self-determined. This is the case in "identified regulation," in which one performs extrinsically motivated actions because one has consciously accepted their value as personally important and meaningful. In the example of work behavior, identified regulation would take the form of working because one personally values the activity and its consequences.

"Integrated regulation," which is the most self-determined form of extrinsic motivation, results when particular values and actions that one has identified with have been fully reconciled with one's other values and actions, as well as with one's organismic experience. Thus integration involves congruence between one's identifications and the "whole" person. An integrated regulatory style—that is, acting with a sense of choice that accords with the whole self—is the most volitional, autonomous form of extrinsic motivation, but has to date been the least explored.

As the taxonomy above suggests, it makes a great deal of difference what type of extrinsic regulatory process is involved in one's outcome-oriented, goal-directed behavior. One can be an extrinsically motivated "pawn" insofar as one is prodded into or compliantly follows unassimilated external demands. Or one can be volitional, pursuing personally valued extrinsic ends, and in so doing can find a sense of meaning and identity. Whereas the former describes alienation, the latter reflects greater authenticity and autonomy. Both types of action can be accompanied by a sense of "self-efficacy" (Bandura, 1989)—that is, they can satisfy one's need for competence (Deci & Ryan, 1985b)—but only the latter represents true self-motivation and would satisfy one's need for autonomy.

The Consequences of Different Regulatory Styles

Various studies have demonstrated the utility of differentiating the types of extrinsic motivation and have indicated that the more autonomous regulatory styles are associated with more positive experiential and performance outcomes. For example, Ryan and Connell (1989) found that in a sample of late-elementary-school children, both introjected regulation (which is relatively controlling) and identified regulation (which is relatively autonomous) were significantly (and equally) correlated with the children's reports of how hard they tried in school and with their parents' reports of how motivated the children were. However, introjected regulation was correlated with anxiety about school and with maladaptive coping with failures, whereas identified regulation was correlated with enjoyment of school and with proactive coping with failure. In this we see clearly the importance of considering not only the amount or *level* of motivation, but also the *orientation* of that motivation. It is only when qualities of motivation are considered that many important aspects of behavior and experience can be predicted.

In another example, Ryan, Rigby, and King (1993) contrasted persons who manifested an introjected versus an identified regulatory style in their religious activities. They found that religiosity per se had no relationship to mental health; however, the identified form of motivation for religious behaviors was positively correlated with mental health outcomes, whereas the introjected form was negatively correlated with well-being. As might be expected, people who pursue religious activities out of guilt or compulsion are less healthy than those who pursue them for identified reasons.

In yet another domain of investigation, Blais, Sabourin, Boucher, and Vallerand (1990) found that whereas the identified and integrated forms of motivation for maintaining a primary "couple" relationship were positively correlated with adjustment and positive affect in the relationship, the external and introjected motivations were negatively correlated with the same outcomes. In this investigation, consideration of these different types of regulatory styles accounted for approximately 70% of the variance in relationship satisfaction.

Why a person undertakes a goal is of great practical importance to clinicians and other change agents. For example, a recent study showed that patients participating in a weight loss program for autonomous (i.e., integrated) reasons as opposed to controlled (i.e., external or introjected) reasons attended the program more regularly and showed greater maintained weight loss over a 23-month period (Williams, Grow, Friedman, Ryan, & Deci, in press). Similarly, Ryan, Plant, and O'Malley (1995) recently found that patients in an alcohol treatment program who had higher internal perceived locus of causality for participating were more likely to persist in their attendance than those who were urged or compelled to participate by external sources (e.g., courts, spouses, or doctors).

The perceived locus of causality distinction has also recently been applied to the study of goals—specifically, subjects' "personal strivings" (Emmons, 1986). Personal strivings are "relatively enduring, ideographically coherent patterns of goals that represent what an individual is typically trying to do" (Emmons & King, 1992, p. 79). Personal strivings thus represent the characteristic goals that a person strives for during his or her everyday life.

In two studies, Sheldon and Kasser (1995) used the Emmons (1986, 1989) procedure to elicit subjects' strivings, and then used the perceived locus of causality methodology introduced by Ryan and Connell (1989) to have them rate the reasons *why* they were striving for those goals. In doing so, Sheldon and Kasser were attempting to gauge the degree to which subjects were striving toward goals because the goals were personally interesting, important, and valued by them, as opposed to the subjects' feelings pressured to seek them by controlling interpersonal or intrapsychic forces. In the first study, the well-being variables of self-actualization (Jones & Crandall, 1986), vitality (Ryan & Frederick, 1994), positive affect (Watson, Tellegen, & Clark, 1988), empathy (Davis, 1980), openness to experience (Costa & McCrae, 1985), and self-esteem (Rosenberg, 1965) were measured, and results showed that these well-being indices were significantly correlated with the relative autonomy of subjects' strivings. A second study extended these findings by showing that having more autonomous reasons for striving also correlated with life satisfaction and daily well-being. Furthermore, in accordance with the assertion that an internal perceived locus of causality is associated with greater coherence among aspects of the self, striving autonomy was also found to be associated with three independent indices of self-integration. Specifically, autonomously striving subjects evidenced more coherence among different self-attributes (Harter & Monsour, 1992), reported less conflict (Emmons & King, 1988) among their strivings, and reported greater consistency between strivings and desired "possible futures." These findings thus support the view that *why* one strives for goals—specifically, the degree of autonomy represented by one's reasons for striving—has important implications both for general well-being and for the overall coherence of personality.

The Social Context and Motivational Orientations

In considering what causes differences in the relative autonomy of intentional activities, it is necessary to attend to the processes through which motivated goal behaviors are acquired, as well as to the influence of the quality of the interpersonal context within which they are adopted. Many conscious intentions and goals are internalized from the surrounding culture, and these intentions and goals can be more or less fully internalized and assimilated by the individual who carries them out. A culture may transmit many kinds of goals (e.g., spiritual, achievement, or moral ones), and it can even give people tools and skills to enact these agendas successfully. But people will still vary considerably in the extent to which such transmitted goals are taken on or internalized and integrated to the self.

Several studies have focused on the influence of the interpersonal context on self-determination with respect to culturally sanctioned activities. They have considered both the effects of the immediate context on the state of self-determination and the developmental antecedents of more trait-like self-determination. Two dimensions within the social context—referred to as "autonomy support" and "involvement" (i.e., relational support)—have been extremely useful for synthesizing a large number of studies (see Ryan, Deci, & Grolnick, 1995; Ryan & Stiller, 1991). Autonomy support occurs when significant others in a target person's context (e.g., parents, managers, coaches) take that person's perspective, provide choice, encourage self-initiation, and minimize controls; involvement is the devotion of time, attention, and resources to the target person. When socializers are both autonomy-supportive and involved, natural states of intrinsic motivation are less likely to be undermined, and the internalization and integration of extrinsically motivated behaviors will be facilitated.

A number of laboratory studies have specifically shown how conditions of autonomy support versus control affect the quality of motivation. In a context that minimizes the use of controlling rewards (e.g., Ryan, Mims, &

Koestner, 1983), reflects the target person's feelings (Koestner, Ryan, Bernieri, & Holt, 1984), avoids controlling language (Ryan, 1982), and minimizes pressure to perform or to live up to externally dictated standards (Deci, Spiegel, Ryan, Koestner, & Kaufmann, 1982; Grolnick & Ryan, 1987), people are more likely to be self-determined (i.e., to be intrinsically motivated or identified in their regulatory style) in the immediate situation, and to develop greater autonomy (i.e., greater integration in personality) over time.

Deci, Eghrari, Patrick, and Leone (1994) combined many of these contextual elements in a recent experiment in which they attempted to motivate subjects to internalize the value of an uninteresting task. They found that autonomy-supportive contexts promoted greater internalization and integration than did controlling contexts, and also resulted in self-reports of feeling free and enjoying the task more. In contrast, when internalization occurred in controlling contexts, it was only introjected and resulted in feeling pressured and not enjoying the task. In short, autonomy-supportive contexts allowed subjects to internalize and integrate more completely the extrinsically prompted activities performed in this study.

Field studies have revealed the applied significance of such findings. For example, Grolnick and Ryan (1989) examined both autonomy support and involvement in a study of achievement socialization. They interviewed a sample of parents regarding their strategies and techniques for motivating their children for schoolwork and chores around the house. They found that parents' autonomy support and involvement were associated with their children's reporting greater identification with and intrinsic motivation for achievement activities, as well as with better teacher-rated adjustment and performance in the classroom. By contrast, parents who emphasized rewards and punishments (of either tangible or emotional sorts) had children who were more likely to report external and introjected motivational orientations for achievement. As predicted, the latter children were rated by their teachers as less self-motivated and as more likely to "act out." Incidentally, they also performed less well as indicated by school grades. What is interesting about this is that controlling parents were often well-meaning. They wanted the best for their children, and they thought external control was the way to ensure it. However, it appears that in attempting to externally regulate their children's achievement-oriented activity, they unwittingly interfered with the children's tendency to internalize and accept the achievement behaviors as meaningful or valuable (see also Grolnick, Ryan, & Deci, 1991). Other field studies have supported similar models applied to other socializers, such as teachers (Deci et al., 1981; Ryan & Grolnick, 1986) and work supervisors (Deci et al., 1989).

In sum, it seems that the differentiation of motivated behavior with respect to the concept of self-determination or autonomy has been quite fruitful for predicting important outcomes, and also that the primary social-contextual variables that promote self-determination (i.e., intrinsic motivation and integration) in both the immediate context and the long-term developmental sense are autonomy support and involvement. An important aspect of this line of research is its linking heteronomous versus autonomous forms of behavioral regulation with etiological factors in the social context. It is primarily the use of controlling strategies of socialization that either forestalls internalization or promotes introjected forms of regulation. By contrast, autonomy-supportive social contexts in homes, in schools, in workplaces, and on sporting fields minimize introjection, alienation, and other hallmarks of the nonintegrated regulation of action.

THE "WHAT" OF GOALS: CONSIDERING CONTENT

In recent motivational investigations, we have begun to focus not only on how goals are regulated (i.e., *why* people pursue them), but also on the consequences of *what* goals people aspire to. That is, we are examining the well-being outcomes associated with differentially valuing some goals over others. Little attention has been given to this question, perhaps because little attention has been given to how goals relate to significant psychological and organismic needs. Indeed, social-cognitive theories (e.g., Locke & Latham, 1990) often appear to suggest that it matters only how successful one is (or perceives oneself to be) in one's goal striving, and not what the goal is. If this were so, then effective selfish greed would sit beside effective affiliation or effective generativity as equally "good for" the human organism.

One way of critically examining goal contents is to consider them in terms of the extent to which they tend to serve intrinsic psychological and organismic needs versus extrinsic, derivative desires. And this, of course, brings us to the quite knotty question of which psychological needs are intrinsic and which are not. Knotty or not, this issue is one of the most critical ones that psychological theory can tackle.

Let us first consider what the concept of "need" itself means, for in fact theorists have tended to use this term in two distinct ways. The first of these reflects a rather colloquial use of the term, in which a person has a desire or want for something. The person may say, "I need more money," or "I feel a need to achieve." Here, "need" really refers to the person's desires, wants, or conscious goals. This nontechnical usage is problematic, however, when we see that one's desires and wants may do harm to the self or organism, and thus may run against the grain of a more technical use of the term "need." In this latter usage, which applies across the biological sciences, a need is a nutriment or condition under which something grows or thrives. Thus one needs food, water, and warmth to remain healthy and, ultimately, to stay alive.

With regard to psychological growth and well-being the specific list of essential needs is perhaps more controversial. However, self-determination theory assumes that three needs are essential and quite parsimoniously account for the nurture and growth of the human psyche. These are the psychological needs for autonomy, competence, and relatedness (Deci & Ryan, 1985b, 1991; Ryan, 1993). We have argued that the psyche will be healthy and actualized only to the extent that these three needs are fulfilled, whereas it will be plagued by pathology when either inner or outer conditions thwart satisfaction of these needs (Ryan et al. 1995). Thus, from a technical point of view, one cannot tell whether goals such as "I need to achieve" or "I need more friends" represent true intrinsic psychological needs until they are further analyzed. Indeed, although any goals or aspirations can direct one's activity, some will be functionally facilitative and others functionally obstructive to psychological health, even when one is efficacious in pursuing them. Explicating this point has been the aim of our empirical analyses of goal contents.

Goal Content and Mental Health

We have specifically hypothesized that the relative value people place on goals and aspirations that are related either to intrinsic needs or to nonintrinsic wants should be indicative of their obtained psychological integration and thus predictive of their well-being. To put this differently, we assume that placing great importance on derivative, extrinsic goals will be associated with poorer mental health than placing central importance on goals that relate more directly to the needs for autonomy, competence, and relatedness. Insofar as nonintrinsic goals predominate, then we suggest that the perceived locus of causality of the goal-directed behavior is likely to be more external rather than internal, and thus that the individual will be more control-oriented (Deci & Ryan, 1985a) rather than autonomous. Indeed, we believe that the predominance of extrinsic over intrinsic goals typically represents the attempts of individuals to obtain a sense of worth through externally visible and palpable achievements and outcomes, and that such attempts reflect an absence or instability of an inner sense of worth. Thus, the more one wants or desires outcomes such as money, fame, or good looks as extrinsic goals and/or substitutes for more truly intrinsic needs of the psyche, the more insecure and destabilized one has been in the process of development (Kasser & Ryan, 1994; Ryan et al., 1995).

In initial investigations of the issue of the relative values placed on intrinsic versus extrinsic aspirations, Kasser and Ryan (1993) assessed the relative importance of four life aspirations: personal growth, satisfying relationships, contributing to one's community, and achieving wealth and financial success. The first three were assumed to reflect intrinsic needs more closely, whereas financial success was viewed as a more extrinsic need. Individual differences in control orientation (Deci & Ryan, 1985a) were also assessed, and subjects completed a self-actualization scale (Jones & Crandall,

1986) and a vitality scale (Ryan & Frederick, 1994) as indicators of general well-being. Results showed that the relative importance of each of the three intrinsic aspirations (calculated by partialing out the average aspiration score) was significantly positively related to self-actualization and vitality; however, the relative importance of financial success was negatively related to both self-actualization and vitality. In other words, the more important financial success was to a person, the less self-actualized and vital the person was. The findings were largely replicated using an alternative, rank-order measure of values as well. These results are among the first to indicate that the content of one's long-term goals may be related to one's general well-being. Furthermore, as predicted, subjects' high weightings of financial success relative to the intrinsic goals were significantly correlated with being control-oriented, thus suggesting that individuals with relatively strong aspirations for material wealth tend to be controlled in their general regulatory style. These findings were largely replicated in a second sample made up of college students; they were also extended to reveal that the relative importance of the intrinsic aspirations for personal growth and satisfying relationships was negatively related to depression (Radloff, 1977) and anxiety (Spielberger, Gorsuch, & Lushene, 1970), whereas the relative importance of the extrinsic aspiration for financial success was positively related to depression and anxiety.

As noted above, many cognitive or goal theories have emphasized that an important dimension of goal functioning is a person's expectations regarding his or her ability to achieve those goals. To assess this dimension, Kasser and Ryan (1993) measured subjects' beliefs about the likelihood that they would achieve their aspirations. These data were analyzed according to the same regression methods used for importance ratings, and indeed the results were very similar: Feeling that one was more likely to attain intrinsic aspirations was positively associated with well-being outcomes, whereas feeling that one was more likely to attain extrinsic aspirations was negatively related to such outcomes. This finding emphasizes the importance of differentiating goals in terms of their content, and it also raises some doubt about the general applicability of self-efficacy theory with regard to the mental health consequences of feeling efficacious in striving for various goal contents (e.g., Bandura, 1977). Placing relatively great importance on extrinsic goals and having strong efficacy expectations with regard to them turned out to be associated with poorer well-being.

In a third study in this series (Kasser & Ryan, 1993), 140 subjects aged 18 from backgrounds of mixed socioeconomic status were examined; half of them were at risk for psychopathology by virtue of their mothers' having been diagnosed with a psychiatric disorder. Well-being was assessed through structured interviews by two clinical psychologists, yielding assessments of global social functioning (Shaffer et al., 1983), conduct disorder (Herjanic & Reich, 1982), and social productivity (Ikle, Lipp, Butters, & Ciarlo, 1983). The results extended those of the first two studies. Whereas the relative importance of the intrinsic aspirations related positively to global social functioning and social productivity and negatively to conduct disorder, the opposite was true for the relative importance of financial success. Also as in the previous studies, placing high importance on material success relative to intrinsic aspirations, and rating the likelihood of such success as high, were deleterious to well-being.

The three studies thus far reviewed contrasted three aspirations assumed to relate closely to intrinsic needs (namely, personal growth, satisfying relationships, and community contributions) with only one "extrinsic" aspiration (namely, financial success). A more recent study (Kasser & Ryan, in press) included these same four aspirations but added two other extrinsic aspirations—namely, fame (social recognition) and physical attractiveness (looks)—as well as one additional aspiration (physical health) that was assumed from an organismic perspective to be more intrinsic. Two new samples were assessed: one college sample, and one adult sample drawn from a heterogeneous urban neighborhood.

As an important first step in these investigations, Kasser and Ryan (in press) subjected the ratings of aspiration importance to factor-analytic procedures. The results supported the intrinsic and extrinsic classifications of goal contents. Specifically, both importance and likelihood ratings of the various goals, when subjected to higher-order factor analyses, produced two factors: one made up of personal growth, affiliation, community contribution, and physical health variables, and a second consisting of the presumably extrinsic goals of money, fame, and attractiveness.

In two samples, a number of well-being indicators were assessed, including self-actualization, vitality, depression, anxiety, narcissism, positive affect, negative affect, and physical symptoms. The analytic strategy was the same as in the earlier studies, and the results were comparable. In brief, every one of the significant partial correlations between intrinsic aspirations and indicators of well-being showed a positive linkage, whereas every one of the significant correlations between extrinsic aspirations and indicators of well-being showed a negative linkage. These studies therefore replicated the earlier ones; however, they also extended them by showing how extrinsic aspirations such as fame, attractiveness, and money tend to have similar properties, and that when such aspirations are highly valued by the individual they can be associated with quite deleterious well-being outcomes.

Within U.S. culture, individuals are constantly exposed to messages suggesting that "successful" people are those who have acquired wealth, fame, or beauty. Indeed, this triad of values constitutes a crass version of the "American dream" (Kasser & Ryan, 1993). But our analyses have suggested that an inflated focus on such extrinsic outcomes, relative to intrinsic goals, may be less of a dream than a nightmare. Those chasing such dreams are at risk for more psychological difficulties and distress, even when they believe strongly that they can achieve such goals.

Why Do Some People Focus on Extrinsic Goals?

Just as we can ask what kinds of environments promote controlled (as opposed to autonomous) self-regulation, we can also ask what kinds of environments promote the adoption of extrinsic as opposed to intrinsic goals. Kasser, Ryan, Zax, and Sameroff (in press) examined the antecedents of placing high importance on financial success (relative to intrinsic goals) in two samples. In the first, college students reported their perceptions of their parents in terms of autonomy support, involvement, and warmth. These perceptions were then correlated with aspirational indices. Results indicated that the relative importance of intrinsic aspirations was positively predicted by parental autonomy support, involvement, and warmth, whereas the importance of the extrinsic aspiration for wealth was negatively associated with these parenting variables. In other words, college students who perceived their parents as controlling, uninvolved, and cold were more likely to place high importance on accumulation of material wealth, relative to the intrinsic goals such as personal growth and community participation.

The second study drew on a longitudinal data bank of the "at-risk" teenage sample assessed by Kasser and Ryan (1993). Both the teenagers' perceptions of parenting style and maternal self-reports of parenting were used to predict aspirations. The results complemented those of the college sample. When mothers were high in nurturance and autonomy support (as reflected in self-reports, their children's reports, and interviews), their teenagers placed high importance on the intrinsic aspiration of personal growth. In contrast, when mothers were low in nurturance and autonomy support, their teenage children placed high value on financial success. From the two studies, it seems quite clear that warm, involved, autonomy-supportive parents tend to have children who value intrinsic outcomes such as personal growth and community involvement, whereas cold, uninvolved, controlling parents tend to have children who place high value on material acquisitions.

Goals and Needs: Are Some Goals Better than Others?

Thus far we have argued that when goals are regulated by forces experienced as external rather than internal to the self (the "why" of goal pursuit), the quality of goal-regulated action and its impact on personality and mental health are more negative. Furthermore, we have argued that conditions of socialization that are more coercive and/or "contingently regarding" of the individual are more likely to promote such heteronomous forms of goal regulation. Both of these points grow out of the belief that the regulatory style of one's goal-related motivation is largely a function of the interpersonal and cultural contexts in which socialization takes place.

We have also argued that cultural and interpersonal contexts influence *what* goals people emphasize and stress within their hierarchy of goals, and which ones are less salient or accentuated. Our data suggest that individuals whose social context is (and has been) characterized by controllingness and insecurity are most susceptible to latching on to nonintrinsic or extrinsic psychological goals. We have inferred that children growing up in an atmosphere of high control and low warmth are inhibited in their development of more autonomous self-regulation, and thus are more likely to rely on external rewards, controls, and signposts of worth than are those coming from more optimal caregiving environments. Furthermore, controlling and insecurity-promoting environments fail to provide a secure sense of one's lovability and inherent worth. It is thus probable that children exposed to such contexts focus on external, public trappings of worth in an attempt to gain needed esteem—a sense of worth that is contingent on outcomes—in order to substitute for the more basic sense of worth that more optimal caregivers might have conveyed (Deci & Ryan, 1995). The pressure to meet external criteria of worth thus both reflects an existing deficit in a person's intrinsic satisfaction and continues to guide the person away from activities that could more directly satisfy the intrinsic psychological needs that sustain growth. Of course, this preliminary formulation is just that, and there is considerable empirical territory to be explored before these theoretical inferences can be confirmed.

Beyond the practical implications of these findings lies an important lesson for goal research more generally. The lesson is that all goals are not created equal, and that strong self-efficacy with regard to attainable goals is not necessarily healthy. To understand the functional significance of goals requires analyzing them with respect to both *why* they are selected and *what* human need fulfillment will accompany their attainment. We have seen in particular that the highly advertised goals of the "American dream" can readily become substitutes for a more intrinsic sense of self-worth—an inner security of self that all the fame, money, and good looks in the world may be insufficient to produce.

CONCLUSION: GOALS AND THEIR INTERNALIZATION

The construct of "goals" refers to representations of future states that are accompanied by some desire or affect (Pervin, 1989). In this chapter we have argued that an understanding of the dynamics and functional effects of goal regulation is deepened by organismic analyses. Such analyses examine both the forces that give rise to and sustain goal behavior (as in perceived locus of causality) and the meaning of goal contents in relation to basic or intrinsic psychological needs. They begin with the recognition that much of people's goal-directed regulation of behavior is a product of internalization. People learn what to value in the context of a culture, and this learning takes place in interpersonal contexts that vary from coercive to autonomy-supportive. The nature of the socialization process, as well as the relation of the contents of socialization to individuals' intrinsic human nature, together determine both what is represented as desirable future states and how well such goals are integrated into the self. These factors in turn are predictive of a variety of qualitative outcomes, including psychological well-being.

Our view is neither wholly sociogenetic nor biogenetic. Rather, the self-determination view of goals conceptualizes them as dialectic products of innate psychological needs in interaction with both conditions and contents of the cultural milieu. And it is the outcome of this dialectic, indexed in terms of autonomy, that has far-reaching implications for the quality of individuals' lives.

ACKNOWLEDGMENTS

Preparation of this chapter and much of the work reported herein were supported by Grant No. HD19914 from the National Institute of Child Health and Human Development and Grant No. MH18922 from the National Institute of Mental Health to the Human Motivation Program, Department of Psychology, University of Rochester.

REFERENCES

Amabile, T. M. (1983). *The social psychology of creativity.* New York: Springer-Verlag.

Bandura, A. (1977). Self-efficacy: Toward a unifying theory of behavioral change. *Psychological Review, 84,* 191–215.

Bandura, A. (1989). Self-regulation of motivation and action through internal standards and goal systems. In L. Pervin (Ed.), *Goal concepts in personality and social psychology* (pp. 19–85). Hillsdale, NJ: Erlbaum.

Blais, M. R., Sabourin, S., Boucher, C., & Vallerand, R. J. (1990). Toward a motivational model of couple happiness. *Journal of Personality and Social Psychology, 59,* 1021–1031.

Costa, P. T., Jr., & McCrae, R. R. (1985). *The NEO Personality Inventory manual.* Odessa, FL: Psychological Assessment Resources.

Davis, M. H. (1980). A multidimensional approach to individual differences in empathy. *JSAS: Catalog of Selected Documents in Psychology, 10,* 85.

deCharms, R. (1968). *Personal causation: The internal affective determinants of behavior.* New York: Academic Press.

Deci, E. L. (1975). *Intrinsic motivation.* New York: Plenum.

Deci, E. L., Connell, J. P., & Ryan, R. M. (1989). Self-determination in a work organization. *Journal of Applied Psychology, 74,* 580–590.

Deci, E. L., Eghrari, H., Patrick, B. C., & Leone, D. R. (1994). Facilitating internalization: The self-determination theory perspective. *Journal of Personality, 62,* 119–142.

Deci, E. L., Nezlek, J., & Sheinman, L. (1981). Characteristics of the rewarder and intrinsic motivation of the rewardee. *Journal of Personality and Social Psychology, 40,* 1–10.

Deci, E. L., & Ryan, R. M. (1985a). The General Causality Orientations Scale: Self-determination in personality. *Journal of Research in Personality, 19,* 109–134.

Deci, E. L., & Ryan, R. M. (1985b). *Intrinsic motivation and self-determination in human behavior.* New York: Plenum.

Deci, E. L., & Ryan, R. M. (1991). A motivational approach to self: Integration in personality. In R. Dienstbier (Ed.), *Nebraska Symposium on Motivation: Vol. 38. Perspectives on motivation* (pp. 237–288). Lincoln: University of Nebraska Press.

Deci, E. L., & Ryan, R. M. (1995). Human agency: The basis for true self-esteem. In M. Kernis (Ed.), *Efficacy, agency, and self-esteem* (pp. 31–49). New York: Plenum.

Deci, E. L., Spiegel, N. H., Ryan, R. M., Koestner, R., & Kauffman, M. (1982). The effects of performance standards on teaching styles: The behavior of controlling teachers. *Journal of Educational Psychology, 74,* 852–859.

Emmons, R. A. (1986). Personal strivings: An approach to personality and subjective well-being. *Journal of Personality and Social Psychology, 51,* 1058–1068.

Emmons, R. A. (1989). The personal strivings approach to personality. In L. A. Pervin (Ed.), *Goal concepts in personality and social psychology* (pp. 87–127). Hillsdale, NJ: Erlbaum.

Emmons, R. A., & King, L. (1988). Conflict among personal strivings: Immediate and long-term implications for psychological and physical well-being. *Journal of Personality and Social Psychology, 54,* 1040–1048.

Emmons, R. A., & King, L. A. (1992). Thematic analysis, experience sampling, and personal goals. In C. P. Smith (Ed.), *Motivation and personality: Handbook of thematic content analysis* (pp. 87–126). New York: Cambridge University Press.

Ford, M. E. (1992). *Motivating humans: Goals, emotions, and personal agency beliefs.* Newbury Park, CA: Sage.

Garbarino, J. (1975). The impact of anticipated reward upon cross-aged tutoring. *Journal of Personality and Social Psycology, 32,* 421–428.

Goldstein, K. (1939). *The organism.* New York: American Book.

Grolnick, W. S., & Ryan, R. M. (1987). Autonomy in children's learning: An experimental and individual difference investigation. *Journal of Personality and Social Psychology, 52,* 890–898.

Grolnick, W. S., & Ryan, R. M. (1989). Parent styles associated with children's self-regulation and competence in school. *Journal of Educational Psychology, 81,* 143–154.

Grolnick, W. S., Ryan, R. M., & Deci, E. L. (1991). The inner resources for school achievement: Motivational mediators of children's perceptions of their parents. *Journal of Educational Psychology, 83,* 508–517.

Harter, S., & Monsour, A. (1992). Developmental analysis of conflict caused by opposing attributes in the adolescent self-portrait. *Developmental Psychology, 28,* 251–260.

Heider, F. (1958). *The psychology of interpersonal relations.* New York: Wiley.

Herjanic, B., & Reich, W. (1982). Development of a structured psychiatric interview for children: Agreement between child and parent on individual symptoms. *Journal of Abnormal Child Psychology, 10,* 307–324.

Ikle, D. N., Lipp, D. O., Butters, E. A., & Ciarlo, J. (1983). *Development and validation of the Adolescent Community Mental Health Questionnaire.* Denver: Mental Systems Evaluation Project.

Jones, A., & Crandall, R. (1986). Validation of a short index of self-actualization. *Personality and Social Psychology Bulletin, 12,* 63–73.

Kasser, T., & Ryan, R. M. (1993). A dark side of the American dream: Correlates of financial success as a central life aspiration. *Journal of Personality and Social Psychology, 65,* 410–422.

Kasser, T., & Ryan, R. M. (in press). Further examining the American dream: The differential effects of intrinsic and extrinsic goal structures. *Personality and Social Psychology Bulletin.*

Kasser, T., Ryan, R. M., Zax, M., & Sameroff, A. J. (in press). Acquiring materialistic and prosocial values: Familial and social antecedents of young adults' aspirations. *Developmental Psychology.*

Koestner, R., Ryan, R. M., Bernieri, F., & Holt, K. (1984). Setting limits on children's behavior: The differential effects of controlling versus informational styles on intrinsic motivation and creativity. *Journal of Personality, 52,* 233–248.

Langer, E. J., & Rodin, J. (1976). The effects of choice and personal responsibility for the aged: A field experiment in an institutional setting. *Journal of Personality and Social Psychology, 34,* 191–198.

Locke, E. A., & Latham, G. P. (1990). *A theory of goal setting and task performance.* Englewood Cliffs, NJ: Prentice-Hall.

Lewin, K. (1951). Intention, will, and need. In D. Rapaport (Ed. and Trans.), *Organization and pathology of thought* (pp. 95–153). New York: Columbia University Press. (Original work published 1926)

Maslow, A. H. (1970). *Motivation and personality* (2nd ed.). New York: Harper & Row.

McGraw, K. O., & McCullers, J. C. (1979). Evidence of a detrimental effect of extrinsic incentives on breaking a mental set. *Journal of Experimental Social Psychology, 15,* 285–294.

Meissner, W. W. (1981). *Internalization in psychoanalysis.* New York: International Universities Press.

Murray, H. A. (1938). *Explorations in personality.* New York: Oxford University Press.

Pervin, L. A. (Ed.). (1989). *Goal concepts in personality and social psychology.* Hillsdale, NJ: Erlbaum.

Piaget, J. (1971). *Biology and knowledge* (B. Walsh, Trans.). Chicago: University of Chicago Press. (Original work published 1967)

Radloff, L. (1977). The CES-D scale: A self-report depression scale for research in the general population. *Applied Psychological Measurement, 1,* 385–401.

Rogers, C. (1963). The actualizing tendency in relation to "motives" and to consciousness. In M. R. Jones (Ed.), *Nebraska Symposium on Motivation* (Vol. 11, pp. 1–24). Lincoln: University of Nebraska Press.

Rosenberg, M. (1965). *Society and the adolescent self-image.* Princeton, NJ: Princeton University Press.

Rotter, J. B. (1966). Generalized expectancies for internal versus external control of reinforcement. *Psychological Monographs, 80*(1, Whole No. 609).

Ryan, R. M. (1982). Control and information in the intrapersonal sphere: An extension of cognitive evaluation theory. *Journal of Personality and Social Psychology, 43,* 450–461.

Ryan, R. M. (1993). Agency and organization: Intrinsic motivation, autonomy and the self in psychological development. In J. Jacobs (Ed.), *Nebraska Symposium on Motivation: Vol. 40. Developmental perspectives on motivation* (pp. 1–56). Lincoln: University of Nebraska Press.

Ryan, R. M., & Connell, J. P. (1989). Perceived locus of causality and internalization: Examining reasons for acting in two domains. *Journal of Personality and Social Psychology, 57,* 749–761.

Ryan, R. M., Deci, E. L., & Grolnick, W. S. (1995). Autonomy, relatedness, and the self: Their relation to development and psychopathology. In D. Cicchetti & D. J. Cohen (Eds.), *Manual of developmental psychopathology* (pp. 618–655). New York: Wiley.

Ryan, R. M., & Frederick, C. M. (1994). *On energy and health: Exploring the dynamics of subjective vitality.* Unpublished manuscript, University of Rochester.

Ryan, R. M., & Grolnick, W. S. (1986). Origins and pawns in the classroom: Self-report and projective assessments of individual differences in children's perceptions. *Journal of Personality and Social Psychology, 50,* 550–558.

Ryan, R. M., Mims, V., & Koestner, R. (1983). Relation of reward contingency and interpersonal context to intrinsic motivation: A review and test using cognitive evaluation theory. *Journal of Personality and Social Psychology, 45,* 736–750.

Ryan, R. M., Plant, R. W., & O'Malley, S. (1995). Initial motivations for alcohol treatment: Relations with patient characteristics, treatment involvement, and dropout. *Addictive Behaviors, 20,* 279–297.

Ryan, R. M., Rigby, S., & King, K. (1993). Two types of religious internalization and their relations to religious orientations and mental health. *Journal of Personality and Social Psychology, 65,* 586–596.

Ryan, R. M., & Stiller, J. (1991). The social contexts of internalization: Parent and teacher influences on autonomy, motivation and learning. In P. R. Pintrich & M. L. Maehr (Eds.), *Advances in motivation and achievement: Vol. 7. Goals and self-regulatory processes* (pp. 115–149). Greenwich, CT: JAI Press.

Schafer, R. (1968). *Aspects of internalization.* New York: International Universities Press.

Schwarzer, R. (1986). Introduction. In R. Schwarzer (Ed.), *Self-related cognitions in anxiety and motivation* (pp. 1–17). Hillsdale, NJ: Erlbaum.

Seligman, M. E. P. (1975). *Helplessness: On depression, development, and death.* San Francisco: W. H. Freeman.

Shaffer, D., Gould, M. S., Brasic, J., Ambrosini, P., Fisher, P., Bird, H., Aluwahlia, S. (1983). A Children's Global Assessment Scale (CGAS). *Archives of General Psychiatry, 40,* 1228–1231.

Sheldon, K. M., & Kasser, T. (1995). Coherence and congruence: Two aspects of personality integration. *Journal of Personality and Social Psychology, 68,* 531–543.

Spielberger, C. D., Gorsuch, R. L., & Lushene, R. (1970). *Test manual for the State–Trait Anxiety Inventory.* Palo Alto, CA: Consulting Psychologists Press.

Tolman, E. C. (1959). Principles of purposive behavior. In S. Koch (Ed.), *Psychology: A study of a science* (Vol. 2, pp. 92–157). New York: McGraw-Hill.

Vroom, V. H. (1964). *Work and motivation.* New York: Wiley.

Watson, D., Tellegen, A., & Clark, L. (1988). Development and validation of brief measures of positive and negative affect: The PANAS scales. *Journal of Personality and Social Psychology, 54,* 1063–1070.

Werner, H. (1948). *Comparative psychology of mental development.* New York: International Universities Press.

White, R. W. (1959). Motivation reconsidered: The concept of competence. *Psychological Review, 66,* 297–333.

White, R. W. (1963). *Ego and reality in psychoanalytic theory.* New York: International Universities Press.

Williams, G. C., Grow, V. M., Freedman, Z., Ryan, R. M., & Deci, E. L. (in press). Motivational predictors of weight loss and weight-loss maintenance. *Journal of Personality and Social Pscyhology.*

CHAPTER 2 Self-Regulation and Ego Threat

Motivated Cognition, Self-Deception, and Destructive Goal Setting

Roy F. Baumeister

This chapter is concerned with how people defend themselves against a threatened loss of self-esteem. The desire to think well of oneself is widely regarded as one of the most fundamental and pervasive motivations in human psychological functioning. Unfortunately, events frequently conspire to thwart this desire, as misfortune, failure, rejection, and other setbacks convey unflattering implications about the self. Maintaining a favorable view of self in spite of these ego threats is thus an important challenge throughout life.

This chapter is organized as follows. First, I provide some background and context by considering the role that ego defense plays in the broader dramas of motivation and the guidance of action (i.e., self-regulation). Second, I describe some of the studies my colleagues and I have done on the cognitive responses people use to ward off unflattering implications or esteem-threatening events. Finally, I examine how defensive responses can affect the way people commit themselves to goals—sometimes with paradoxical, self-destructive results.

MOTIVATION, ACTION, AND SELF-REGULATION

How does action begin? For decades, theorists have grappled with the issue of how the intrapsychic processes of motivation, intention, and decision making manage to set behavior in motion (see Gollwitzer, 1991, 1993, for reviews). Psychologists have made great strides in understanding the mental, emotional, and motivational processes that presumably precede behavior, and they have also done well at observing and analyzing behavior. But the conceptual gap between the prebehavioral processes and the actual behavior has been difficult to bridge. This conceptual dilemma is perhaps the latest version of the Cartesian hobgoblin—namely, the dualism of mind and body. How can mere thought or mere desire cause a body at rest to begin to move?

It could be suggested that the problem has been wrongly phrased. Perhaps there is no purely "prebehavioral" phase or state. Indeed, a cursory glance at ordinary human beings will tend to show that they are all already engaged in some form of behavior (broadly defined). Perhaps, then, the function of mental, emotional, and motivational processes is not so much to initiate behavior as to steer it—that is, to intervene in ongoing behavioral processes so as to interrupt, override, or redirect them. The body is already moving, and in the process of behavior it is already relying heavily on cognition and motivation. New thoughts or wants must only override those other processes in order to influence behavior. Cognitive and motivational processes may guide action in a way that resembles changing the channel on a television set more closely than it does turning the set on in the first place.

This analysis is quite compatible with some of the more sophisticated models of action control (e.g., Gollwitzer, 1991, 1993). Although Gollwitzer has elaborated his model in terms of predecisional and preactional phases, these can be understood as occurring while other behaviors are taking place. More to the point, self-regulatory overrides are implicit in many of his discussions. Thus, in Gollwitzer's (1993) analysis, he proposes that people may formulate specific implementation intentions to override habits or chronic goals (see also Bargh, 1989, 1990), in order to initiate desired patterns of action. Gollwitzer offers the example of a person who normally attends only to professional duties while in the office, but who resolves to call from the office on the next day in order to make a personal dentist appointment (1993, p. 152). That resolve will help interrupt the person's typical behavioral sequence and override it to make the unusual action possible.

Concern with self-regulation has recently emerged as a central concern of researchers interested in motivation and action, and this may be because self-regulation theory addresses precisely the issues of overriding and steering responses that may hold the key to this Cartesian dilemma. Self-regulation theory (e.g., Carver & Scheier, 1981; Baumeister, Heatherton, & Tice, 1994) holds that there are multiple processes going on at the same time, and that some of them take precedence over others.

It is thus with self-regulation that I concern myself in this chapter. More precisely, I focus on two sets of issues relating to how people exert control over themselves, often by overriding other tendencies or responses. The first set of issues (and the first line of work) is concerned with how people manipulate their cognitive and emotional responses so as to ward off threats to their psychological well-being. The second is concerned with how people manage their performance strivings, including both setting appropriate goals and then performing up to them.

The two lines of work that I discuss share a motivational underpinning. Both are concerned with the desire for self-esteem, which is widely recognized as one of the most fundamental and pervasive motivations in human reactions (e.g., Baumeister, 1991; Darley & Goethals, 1980; Zuckerman, 1979). Nearly everyone desires to think well of himself or herself—that is, to have some basis for a positive self-assessment and sense of self-worth. When failure, rejection, or other events threaten to undermine that basis and cast the self in a negative, unfavorable light, people are threatened. I term such events (including the anticipation of such outcomes or implications) "ego threats."

The relevance of this work to the psychology of action is in the decisive fact that self-regulation is, to paraphrase this volume's subtitle, one of the essential (but neglected) factors linking motivation and cognition to action. Ego threats provide powerful blows not only to the way the person prefers to think about himself or herself, but also to the person's basic equilibrium, which is essential for functioning effectively in the world. Rational processing and functioning often seem to be temporarily impaired by an ego threat, while the person struggles to minimize the cognitive and affective impact and to defend or reassert self-esteem. As I argue, people draw on powerful motivational forces to enable them to self-regulate the cognitive and emotional impact of ego threats. And if they happen to have to make decisions or commitments during one of these episodes, their efforts to respond to the ego threat may impair their better judgment and lead to a self-destructive pattern of excessive or irrational goal setting.

DEFENSIVE RESPONSES: WARDING OFF THREATS

Most people occasionally but inevitably confront events carrying undesirable implications that threaten their self-esteem. To accept these implications dispassionately would be the easiest approach from the standpoint of cognitive effort, but to do that would often be wholly unacceptable for motivational reasons. People want to go on thinking well of themselves, which requires defusing or discrediting those threatening implications. They must override certain cognitive processes (of understanding and accepting the pejorative implications of events) in order to maintain the beliefs that suit their motivated preferences. To put it another way, they must defend their self-concepts against these threats.

These defensive processes thus reflect the interface between motivation and cognition. Simple information processing is often enough to tell people what the meaning of some event is, but when that meaning is unacceptable, the information processing may cease to be simple. Thus, it may be relatively straightforward to read about someone who experiences a series of romantic rejections and to conclude that this person is not a desirable romantic partner. To draw such a conclusion about oneself, however, is generally unacceptable, and so one must exert oneself to find alternative ways of interpreting a series of rejections.

Refusing to draw obvious but undesirable conclusions in order to cling to preferred beliefs is one major form of self-deception (see Baumeister,

1993a). Self-deception has been a controversial concept on both conceptual and empirical grounds (e.g., Gur & Sackeim, 1979). The paradox was well articulated by Sartre (1934/1953) as follows: Deception entails one party who knows something and who acts so as to prevent another party from knowing it. In self-deception, therefore, the same person both knows and is prevented from knowing the same information, which seems logically impossible. Even the simple avoidance of threatening information seems futile, because the person must watch carefully for the approach of the threat—yet as soon as the person detects the threat, it is too late to prevent himself or herself from seeing it.

Only recently have psychological studies begun to offer empirical evidence for how people manage to circumvent this logical paradox. There are two vital explanatory keys. First, it appears that the dichotomy of noticing versus not noticing something is too simple, and that in fact there appears to be a continuum ranging from minimal notice (with consequently minimal memory) to thorough, thoughtful, detailed processing (Erdelyi, 1974). Second, it appears that people are often highly skilled at reinterpreting events so as to be able to reject unwanted conclusions by convincing themselves that alternative, less threatening implications are the correct ones (Baumeister & Newman, 1994). Our research has explored both pathways to self-deception.

Avoiding Threat

Attention is clearly the first line of defense against unpleasant thoughts or implications. If people can prevent themselves from noticing something, it will not be able to threaten their self-esteem. As noted above, the notion of keeping oneself from noticing something invokes the logical paradox of the fact that one must presumably watch carefully for precisely what one wants not to see, and yet as soon as one sees it, it is already too late to look away. But this dichotomous conceptualization (i.e., noticing vs. not noticing the threat) is too rigid and simple. People will be most affected by the things they dwell on and think about for the longest times, and so by minimizing the amount of time spent attending to unpleasant events, a person can minimize any informational effects of such events. As Erdelyi (1974) argued, people will notice a great deal of information, but only a small part of it makes the transition from iconic to short-term memory; thus, the information loss in that transition is a great opportunity for defensive selectivity.

An extreme and clever form of this argument was articulated by Greenwald (1988) in his "junk mail theory of self-deception." He pointed out that people can often recognize junk mail simply by looking at the envelope, and can therefore discard it without reading the entire contents of the mail. In the same way, people can perhaps detect the approach of threatening information from preliminary, superficial indicators, and can therefore turn their attention elsewhere without having a chance to process all the specifics and details.

To model these processes in the laboratory, we confronted subjects with potentially threatening information in the form of giving them ostensible evaluations based on a personality inventory. Subjects in these studies took a personality test administered by computer. When they finished, the experimenter explained that the computer would be able to give them feedback on what kind of persons they were, based on their responses to the test. In fact, we had only two feedback profiles (one rather favorable, and one rather unfavorable and hence threatening); subjects were assigned one or the other at random.

We predicted that subjects would respond to the unfavorable evaluation by minimizing the amount of time they spent reading it and thinking about it. To measure this, we allowed the subjects to spend as much time as they wanted reading the evaluation; unbeknownst to the subjects, the computer had been recorded to keep track of how much time they spent reading the evaluation. This is a fairly standard measure of encoding (e.g., Stern, Marrs, Millar, & Cole, 1984). Our prediction was that as long as subjects believed that no one else would ever see their evaluation, they would spend less time reading the evaluation if it was bad than if it was good. This is what we found (Baumeister & Cairns, 1992).

(Actually, this pattern was found mainly among subjects classified as "repressors"; that is, it was significant across the entire sample, but the repressors were mainly responsible for the effect. Identifying subjects who are repressive by nature is a handy way of enabling us to study defensive responses, because for ethical and practical reasons we cannot expose laboratory subjects to a serious, traumatically threatening experience, and so it is necessary to look for subjects who will respond strongly to even fairly minor threats. We used the system developed by Weinberger, Schwartz, & Davidson, 1979, for identifying repressors. In this approach, people who both score high on a measure of social desirability and low on a measure of anxiety are assumed to be repressors, insofar as their denial of subjective distress is assumed to be linked to their tendency to distort their self-reports in a favorable, socially desirable fashion.)

Thus, it appears that one response to threat is to minimize the time spent attending to it, so as to prevent it from being fully encoded. And, indeed, we found that subjects did not seem to remember the threatening information very well, which indicates that they did manage to prevent it from being stored in memory.

In the laboratory it is often difficult for subjects to withdraw attention from some threatening stimulus, because a laboratory setting typically offers few alternative stimuli to seize the attention. In this respect, laboratory studies may be quite different from the situations that people encounter in everyday life, because normally people occupy stimulus-rich environments that offer ample distractions and preoccupations. In our next study (Newman & Baumeister, 1993), therefore, we offered subjects an alternative focus of attention while giving them feedback about their personalities. We predicted that when the feedback was favorable and flattering, subjects would focus their attention on it and ignore the peripheral stimuli. When the feedback was threatening, however, we predicted that subjects would focus their attention on the peripheral stimuli, as a way of preventing themselves from paying too much attention to the feedback. This strategy of self-protection could be labeled "defensive preoccupation," insofar as people fix their attention on (i.e., become preoccupied with) a neutral stimulus as a way of preventing the threat from reaching them.

Subjects in this study took the same computer-administered (bogus) personality inventory as in our previous studies, and they too were given a chance to read an ostensible evaluation of their personalities, in the form of a list of adjectives that the computer supposedly had determined as most relevant to them. In this study, subjects did not have control over the screen display of the personality feedback; the adjectives simply appeared one after another on a fixed schedule, changing every few seconds. While they were receiving the feedback, however, subjects were told that there would be a second task to perform. They had to listen to a tape recording of a list of words, and they were told to press one key on the keyboard every time they heard a word that contained the letter C. To make this task especially challenging, the list of words contained both hard and soft C's, and some of the filler words contained the letter K or S, so that the subject had to pay close attention to identify the correct words. This was the peripheral task, and we measured how well subjects performed at it.

The notion of defensive preoccupation was supported in this study. Subjects who received favorable, flattering evaluations of their personalities tended to make errors in the peripheral monitoring task, presumably because they were attending primarily to the evaluations. In contrast, subjects who received unfavorable, threatening evaluations tended to perform the peripheral task to perfection. Apparently, they withdrew their attention from the threatening feedback and directed it instead to the peripheral task.

In everyday life, defensive preoccupation may take a variety of forms. People who feel that their self-esteem is threatened may immerse themselves in watching television or movies, in listening to wild music, or in vigorous activities such as sports or even criminal or aggressive acts. We (Tice, Muraven, & Baumeister, 1993) have found that many people cope with unpleasant emotions by engaging in actions that seem well designed to have preoccupying, distracting qualities, such as strenuous exercise or shopping. Eating binges can be provoked by an attempt to escape from some threatening thoughts and feelings, as people narrow their focus of attention to the food they are consuming (Heatherton & Baumeister, 1991).

These examples suggest one further complication of the process, which is that threats to self-esteem often invoke aversive emotions, and so sometimes it may be difficult for a researcher to establish whether the person is trying to avoid the threatening information per se or to escape from the unpleasant emotional state. Most likely, however, the answer is that people use their defenses for both purposes, especially when one considers how often the two are interrelated. Both purposes involve self-regulation, and the difference is merely whether the person is engaged primarily in affect regulation (i.e., controlling emotion) or cognitive regulation (i.e., controlling information).

Recently, we have begun to explore the uses of these defensive processes to protect oneself against unpleasant emotions that come unaccompanied by threats to self-esteem. In one investigation (Boden & Baumeister, 1993), we put people in a bad mood by having them watch an upsetting, depressing film clip about how radioactive wastes were causing the deaths of giant sea turtles. (Control subjects watched an affectively neutral film.)

In this study, instead of offering people distractors such as other stimuli or peripheral tasks, we examined their capacity for generating their own distractors. We reasoned that summoning up happy memories of pleasant experiences would be an effective way of protecting oneself against unpleasant emotions. Although recalling happy memories may be more difficult than simply turning on a television set, it is a strategy that can be used in many times and places (including those in which no television set is available), and so it may be a handy means of affect regulation. The procedure of our study, therefore, was to have subjects watch either the sad or the neutral videotape and then ask them to recall a happy memory. We measured how long it took subjects to come up with a happy memory after they were instructed to do so. Now there is broad evidence for mood-congruent memory effects (e.g., Isen, 1984; Teasdale & Russell, 1983), suggesting that it is easiest for people to recall emotional episodes that fit their current emotional state. In an important sense, we were looking for the opposite effect—a mood-*incongruent* memory effect, in which a bad mood would facilitate the recall of a happy memory. Such an effect would be a fairly clear instance of affect regulation.

Mood-incongruent memory effects were found mainly among repressors in our study. In other words, subjects who habitually showed strong defensive patterns were the ones who responded to a bad mood by increasing the accessibility of happy memories. Repressors were quicker to generate a happy memory after seeing the sad, upsetting videotape than after seeing the affectively neutral videotape. (In contrast, nonrepressors were slower to generate a happy memory after seeing the sad film, consistent with mood-congruent memory effects.) The role of trait repressiveness confirms the view that this pattern of recalling happy memories is a protective reaction that is designed to defend against unpleasant emotional states.

Thus, one means of coping with ego threats is based on a simple manipulation of attention. Although people may not be able to prevent themselves completely from noticing a threatening stimulus, they can shift attention away from it rapidly, thereby minimizing its effect on them and reducing the likelihood that they will remember it. These attentional shifts are apparently facilitated by having alternative things to think about, such as a defensive preoccupation that can absorb attention in order to keep it safely away from undesirable information. Indeed, even if no external preoccupation is available, repressors seem able to summon up happy memories in order to counter the emotional effects of upsetting or distressing stimuli.

Interpretive Defenses

I have said earlier that there are two main ways to deal with threat. The preceding section has covered our work on avoidant defenses. In this section I discuss the other type of response, in which people reinterpret events so as to defuse their threatening implications. Thus, sometimes, instead of ignoring some threat, people will devote time and energy to thinking about it in order to explain it away. In the realm of attitudes, Wyer and Frey (1983) have labeled this strategy one of "refutational" defenses, in contrast to "avoidant" defenses.

Shifting from an avoidant defense to a refutational defense requires a radical about-face in terms of cognitive processing. Refutational defenses may often require careful thought, and so instead of avoiding the threatening information, one makes it the center of one's attention. Whereas the essence of defensive preoccupation, for example, is to shift attention elsewhere, refutational defenses begin with the focusing of all one's attention onto the threat.

In our first study (Baumeister & Cairns, 1992), we reasoned that the presence, involvement, and awareness of other people would be decisive factors in determining whether someone would prefer an avoidant or a refutational defense. If some threatening event is known only to oneself, it can perhaps be safely ignored. But if other people know about it, then that information may become part of one's social world, regardless of one's own attempts to ignore it. Even if a person can dismiss any undesirable implications of the event, the person may still have to deal with the fact that other people think less of him or her because they may accept the unflattering implications. Wicklund and Gollwitzer (1982) have proposed that other people's knowledge of an event lends "social reality" to that event. A socially real, publicly known fact cannot be dismissed or ignored as readily as can a fact that is known only to the self.

In the preceding section, I have described one part of the Baumeister and Cairns (1982) experiment, which showed that repressors tended to spend minimal time reading through an unflattering evaluation of their personalities. In those conditions, subjects had been told that the evaluation was completely anonymous and confidential and that no one else would ever see it. Hence they could safely or comfortably ignore the evaluation, because it lacked social reality. In another ("public evaluation") condition, however, we told subjects that their evaluation would be shown to other people—in particular, to another subject whom they had just met and with whom they expected further interactions shortly. For them, therefore, the content of the evaluation gained considerable social reality, regardless of how they might wish to ignore it. One could also say that public circumstances increase people's accountability, which in turn increases effortful processing (Tetlock, 1983). Either way, the result is that these subjects could not simply dismiss the undesirable information.[1]

Subjects who received the public evaluation did not show the avoidant response described above as typical of the private conditions. In fact, the repressors who received the public bad evaluation spent the greatest amount of time of any group in the entire study reading the evaluation. It may seem ironic that repressors would spend extra time reading an unflattering evaluation of their personality, but that was precisely what happened. The reason, apparently, was that these subjects shifted to a refutational defense. We found that these subjects spent time in thinking of counterarguments or refutations to the bad evaluation, and in planning what they might say to the other subject who was also reading their evaluation. They also spent some extra time worrying about the bad impression that the other person was probably forming of them, based on the unflattering computer evaluation (e.g., "She'll probably think I'm a total bitch," as one subject wrote during a thought-listing procedure in this condition).

It appears, then, that people do sometimes respond to ego threats by focusing on them and trying to interpret them in ways that deflect or minimize their threatening implications. Of course, simply attending to some information does not entail that one will be able to devise a nonthreatening interpretation of it. To succeed at this, people have to exert self-regulatory control over their reasoning process—that is, to steer their inferences toward predetermined goals. We (Baumeister & Newman, 1994) have reviewed and analyzed evidence about how people regulate their inference processes. We used the heuristic of the "intuitive lawyer" (contrasted with the more familiar image of the "intuitive scientist") to describe people's efforts to make the best possible case for a preselected conclusion out of a given set of evidence.

There are several strategic options available to intuitive lawyers who want to reinterpret a recent event so as to defuse threatening implications (see Baumeister & Newman, 1994, for a review). Such individuals may become especially critical of the source of evidence, arguing, for example, that the personality test was flawed and so its results are inconclusive (e.g., Frey, 1978; Lord, Ross, & Lepper, 1979; Pyszczynski, Greenberg, & Holt, 1985; Wyer & Frey, 1983). They may go back and search for more evidence in favor of their preferred conclusion, which may then eventually seem to outweigh the threatening evidence. They may invoke complex decision rules or inferential criteria that place greatest weight on the evidence favoring their preferred conclusion.

My colleagues and I have done several studies using autobiographical accounts to learn about how people reinterpret their actual experiences to defend against threats. In these studies, people are asked to describe a significant event from their own lives and in their own words. Asking them to describe something they did wrong, or some major failure or rejection they experienced, makes it possible to learn about how they explain an event that would seemingly carry threatening implications about them.

These studies suggest that people use a variety of strategies to reinterpret such potentially threatening experiences. They construct the story so as to downplay its worst features and outcomes, while placing great emphasis on external or mitigating factors (Baumeister, Stillwell, & Wotman, 1990; Baumeister & Ilko, 1995). They add seemingly unrelated information that carries more positive implications; for example, an account of a romantic rejection might convey the impression that one is not a desirable romantic partner, and so people will end an account of such a rejection by describing a subsequent successful romantic relationship, thereby seemingly proving that they are romantically desirable after all (Baumeister & Wotman, 1992). They may simply insert positive claims about themselves, to offset any unfavorable implications (Baumeister, Wotman, & Stillwell, 1993). They may note that other people shared the blame or responsibility for the unfavorable outcome (e.g., Baumeister, Stillwell, & Wotman, 1990).

A particularly interesting defensive strategy is what we have called "temporal bracketing" (see Baumeister et al., 1990). The essence of this strategy is that although people admit to having done something wrong in the past, and even accept that the event reflected unfavorably on them, they treat it as something confined to the past and hence unrelated to the present. In accounts of interpersonal conflict, we found that perpetrators tended to describe the incident as wholly in the past, in contrast to victims, whose accounts typically linked the past event to present and future circumstances. Extreme forms of temporal bracketing may be found in religious conversion or "born-again" experiences, in which people frankly acknowledge having sinned but consign all of that to the past. The implication is that it is unfair and inappropriate to use those past misdeeds to judge the persons in the present.

Summary

Thus, people use several cognitive strategies to protect their self-esteem from threatening implications. One strategy is to ignore the threat: People shift attention away from the threatening stimulus. This strategy is facilitated by having an alternate stimulus that can absorb attention (i.e., defensive preoccupation). In the absence of such a stimulus, people may sometimes rely on summoning up happy memories that are unrelated to the aversive stimulus.

The other strategy involves focusing attention on the unpleasant stimulus, in order to use interpretive strategies so as to defuse the threatening implications. People reinterpret events so as to emphasize external causes or mitigating circumstances, which presumably reduce their own responsibility for undesirable outcomes. They may mentally bracket events off in the past, so as seemingly to deny that these events are relevant to their present circumstances or self-concepts. They may also construct their narratives of events so as to add (seemingly extraneous) facts that reflect positively on themselves, so as to offset negative implications.

These strategies reflect the motivated self-regulation of cognitive processes. Above all, people want to maintain favorable views of themselves against threat; thus, they override how they would ordinarily process information, in order to guide their thinking in more agreeable ways and toward more acceptable outcomes.

SELF-MANAGEMENT: SETTING AND MEETING GOALS

Although self-regulation begins with the relatively simple and direct processes of controlling thoughts, emotions, impulses, and actions, it is also involved in the more complex processes of managing one's life. Such processes typically combine several other processes and typically link events occurring at many different points in time. The term "self-management" is sometimes used to refer to these complex processes, to distinguish them from the simpler and more circumscribed acts of self-control. Their importance has been shown by Wagner and Sternberg (1985), who found (among other things) that businessmen with better self-management skills enjoyed greater career and financial success. Such self-management skills included knowing one's own strengths and weaknesses, and devising techniques to maximize the benefits of one's strengths while minimizing the harmful impact of one's weaknesses. Apart from simple ability (and luck, in some cases), self-management may be the single most important determinant of success in life.

In our own work, my colleagues and I have studied self-management in terms of how people set and meet goals (Baumeister, Heatherton, & Tice, 1993). Two people may be the same in terms of their intelligence and other abilities, but one may achieve far greater success in life by setting goals effectively and making sure to meet them. Even gifted persons may fail to achieve satisfaction and success if they set absurdly high or trivially low goals, or if they engage in nonoptimal performance strategies such as procrastination and self-handicapping.

In some cases, setting a goal may be nothing more than thinking to oneself about what one would like to achieve. There may be no penalty for failure and no reward for success, beyond the possible affective reactions that the person may have from evaluating the outcome of his or her performance against the goal. In other cases, however, one must *commit* oneself to a goal. Such commitments may involve staking interpersonal prestige and even material resources on that goal. Commitments may also entail forgoing other possible goals or pastimes, along with the rewards that might have attended them. In short, these cases involve placing contingencies on oneself. It is with these cases (of goal commitment) that we are concerned, because they are the ones in which self-management becomes important. When rewards and punishments become contingent on goals, then the person's commitment to those goals is a matter of creating the essential structure of the person's situation.

Another way of understanding this aspect of action control is that the person chooses whether to enter into a situation or not. A situation can be understood as a contingency structure (see Baumeister & Tice, 1985b). To enter into a situation is thus to place oneself under certain contingencies. Certain actions will bring rewards; others will bring punishments. In contrast, if one avoids that situation, then those actions will not bring those outcomes. As an example, consider a man who signs up for the office tennis tournament. By committing himself to those goals—or, to put it another way, by entering into the situation of the tournament—he puts himself in a position in which good play will gain him esteem and perhaps a cash prize, although he also risks humiliating himself in front of his colleagues in case he plays poorly or loses his poise during a match. In contrast, if he refuses to enter the tournament, all those contingencies (including both the chance for humiliation and the chance for gaining esteem) will not apply. Even if he happens to play tennis well on the afternoon of the tournament, such as in a friendly game with his overweight neighbor on a local court, very little will be contingent on it. In that sense, then, formally committing oneself to a goal creates new contingency structures.

In a broad variety of events in everyday life, people exert substantial and very important control over what happens to them by exposing themselves—or not—to various possible outcomes. Often there is some opportunity to accept or refuse a challenge, which brings various contingencies with it. For example, a person may decide to apply to law school or not. Applying brings the chance that one may be able to embark on a profitable career, whereas not applying safeguards one against the risk of rejection. One may ask an attractive member of the opposite sex for a date, or may let the opportunity pass; again, a broad contingency structure is either engaged or not.

The goals and contingencies to which people commit themselves often conform to a pattern in which difficulty is strongly correlated with desirability: The more difficult goals bring the greater rewards. (When no such correlation exists, self-management would seem rather easy; one should simply select relatively easy but highly rewarding goals. Unfortunately, such options are all too rare!) Hence one may face a tradeoff between seeking a more attainable goal with a smaller reward, or seeking a more difficult goal with a higher payoff. For example, you could ask a plump, dull, and homely person for a date, and the odds would favor acceptance; your chances of rejection would be much higher if you approached a gorgeous and brilliant person, but then again if that person did accept your offer, you would probably enjoy the date more.

Faced with such choices, a person must somehow decide the highest level of aspiration that carries an acceptable probability of success. Self-management thus requires some degree of self-knowledge, to the extent of estimating how high a goal one can expect to reach with reasonable certainty. Naturally, one must expect some errors, but one can presumably know approximately how well one can do.

A further complication of the goal commitment process in everyday life is that all errors are not equal. There is an asymmetry between the dangers in setting too high as opposed to too low a goal. If one sets the goal a little too low, success may not have the maximally desirable value, but at least one does get a success. On the other hand, setting too high a goal will tend to bring failure. And failure may often be much worse than a slightly diminished success.

To pursue the example of choosing a romantic partner: If you select a potential partner who is a little less than the best possible partner you might conceivably win, you will probably succeed in attracting that person and will very likely have a good chance at a satisfactory relationship. On the other hand, if you choose a partner who is a little more desirable than the best you could possibly win, the most likely outcomes are heartbreak and loneliness. Similar analyses could be made for many decisions in work (e.g., submitting a paper to a journal, making a bid for a contract) and other spheres in life. The optimal general strategy for self-management, therefore, may be to commit oneself to goals that are a little below the upper bound of one's capabilities. Traditional wisdom has various phrases to recommend this strategy, such as "leaving a margin for error" or "being on the safe side."

Unfortunately, however, people may tend to make the opposite kind of error. Studies of self-prediction and self-knowledge have repeatedly shown persistent and pervasive patterns of overconfidence (e.g., Vallone, Griffin, Lin, & Ross, 1990). People overestimate their abilities, their degree of control over events, and their likelihood of enjoying favorable outcomes (Taylor & Brown, 1988). This implies that people would be especially likely to commit themselves to goals that are too high, thereby increasing the chances of failure.

Research has shown that patterns of apparent overconfidence are especially likely among people with high self-esteem who receive some threat to their egos. McFarlin and Blascovich (1981) showed that people high in self-esteem paradoxically made more confident predictions following a preliminary failure than following a preliminary success. A tendency to adopt unrealistically positive views of the self (Roth, Snyder, & Pace, 1986) or a tendency to want to compensate dramatically for any failure or loss of face (Baumeister, 1982) could well lead to failures at self-management for these people. On the other hand, people with high self-esteem have been shown to be often highly effective at using available cues to determine optimal levels of effort and persistence (McFarlin, 1985; Sandelands, Brockner, & Glynn, 1988), and they appear to have more thorough, detailed, and accurate self-knowledge than people with low self-esteem (Campbell, 1990; see also Baumgardner, 1990; Campbell & Lavallee, 1993). These patterns suggest that people with high self-esteem should show a superior capacity for effective self-management.

To examine how self-esteem and ego threat would affect self-management processes, we set up a laboratory simulation in which subjects would commit themselves to goals or contingencies and would then have to perform in the context they had chosen. We felt it would be impossible to draw any sort of conclusion about self-management without including the performance component. Although goal setting alone is a worthy topic of interest in its own right, one cannot easily classify any particular pattern of goal setting as maladaptive (cf. Wright & Mischel, 1982) unless one can verify that the subject was unable to meet the goals he or she set. Obviously, there is nothing wrong with setting high goals unless one fails to meet them.

In our research (Baumeister, Heatherton, & Tice, 1993), subjects were given a chance to practice a task (a video game) for about 30 minutes, as a way of establishing and gaining knowledge of their level of skill. Then they had a series of performance trials, which afforded them further opportunities to gain clear self-knowledge about their level of ability. Then, following an ego threat manipulation, they were given a chance to set their contingencies for a final performance trial. By examining how they performed on this final trial and how they had set their contingencies, we could determine how effectively they had managed themselves. The outcome measure was how much money each subject had earned (and retained) at the end of the experiment.

The procedure varied from one study to another in our investigation, although the results were generally consistent regardless of these changes. In the final, definitive study (Baumeister, Heatherton, & Tice, 1993, Experiment 3), the ego threat was administered in the form of bogus feedback on a creativity task that was presented as entirely unrelated to the experiment's main task. Subjects in the threat condition were told they had achieved one of the lowest scores at this university and that they apparently had some serious deficiency in creative realms. Other subjects were told that they had performed quite well and presumably had a bright future in creative endeavors. (This clearly was a "success" condition; in other studies, the ego threat was compared against a no-treatment control group.)

Next came the contingency-setting part of the procedure. All subjects were told that on the previous 10 performance trials at the skill task (i.e., the video game), they had surpassed a preset criterion three times, thereby earning $3.00. They were told that they could bet any part of that sum, for triple or nothing, on themselves to surpass that same criterion on the final trial. In fact, the experimenter named a criterion by choosing a round number between each subject's third-best and fourth-best score. We deliberately set up the betting situation so that there was no statistically more rational or optimal strategy. Subjects were told that they had beaten the criterion about 3 out of 10 times, suggesting that their base rate of success was about one-third, and so the triple-or-nothing bet was roughly equitable (i.e., the expected gain was about the same regardless of the bet).

The situation thus offered the subjects two ways of achieving a good outcome and one way of achieving a bad outcome. Subjects could achieve a positive oucome by making a minimum bet (25¢), in which case they could keep the rest of their $3.00 regardless of how they performed. They could achieve an even better outcome by making a high bet and then performing well, in which case they could end up with up to $9.00. They only achieved a bad outcome if they made a large bet and then performed poorly, which would cause them to lose whatever they had bet.

In the control conditions, and in the preliminary success conditions, subjects with high self-esteem did indeed manage themselves very well. Their performances tended to confirm the wisdom of their bets, and they ended up having earned a nice amount of money. In particular, they consistently finished with more money than subjects with low self-esteem, which was the bottom-line measure of self-management. Thus, under favorable conditions and in the absence of any ego threat, high self-esteem seemed to be linked to an effective capacity for committing oneself to appropriate goals (and then performing up to them).

In response to an ego threat, however, people with high self-esteem ceased to be effective; in fact, their responses could be labeled as self-destructive. The ego threat typically caused people with high self-esteem to set high goals and make large bets. Many of them made the maximum bet that was allowed. It seemed as if they sought to refute the ego-threatening implications of our manipulation by insisting that they would perform at a superior level at the next opportunity. This inflated, compensatory self-confidence was apparently motivated by a defensive desire to respond to the threat, rather than being based on a reasonable or accurate assessment of their own capabilities. In any case, it certainly proved to be misplaced and unrealistic, because their performance generally failed to live up to it, and they ended up losing their money. Many high-self-esteem subjects in the ego threat condition finished the experiment without any money at all. On average, they earned significantly less than the low-self-esteem subjects in the same (ego threat) condition.

Thus, in these studies, the responses of high-self-esteem people illustrated both highly effective and highly ineffective self-management. Under favorable conditions, these people set their goals appropriately and performed accordingly, leading to consistently favorable outcomes. The behavior is consistent with the view that people with high self-esteem know themselves very well and can select contingencies that fit their capabilities (e.g., Campbell, 1990; Sandelands et al., 1988). Indeed, their skill at self-management may help build their self-knowledge, because it may keep them working at appropriately difficult goals, enabling them to gain further and more precise knowledge about themselves. In contrast, people with low self-esteem may fail to learn more about their capabilities in life if they frequently find themselves working for unrealistically difficult or trivially easy goals.

Furthermore, the evident skill at self-management may be a factor that helps create high self-esteem in the first place, or at least that maintains it as high. Two people may have exactly the same set of talents and abilities, but the one who manages himself or herself better will end up with more (and more meaningful) success experiences. Consistently committing oneself to achievable goals seems like a promising way to furnish a solid basis for high self-esteem.

On the other hand, people with high self-esteem appeared to lose their skill at self-management when their egotism was threatened. Consistent with previous evidence (e.g., McFarlin & Blascovich, 1981), it appeared that subjects with high self-esteem responded to an ego threat by adopting an aggressively self-enhancing stance. In this condition, they seemed to feel that they would be capable of performing at a superior level, and this self-confidence apparently resulted more from their determination to disprove the threatening implications than from any accurate appraisal of their capabilities. Buoyed by this defensive optimism, they committed themselves to unrealistically challenging contingencies, and as a result their actual performance tended to fall short. The net result was thus that instead of refuting the ego threat, they compounded it by making themselves appear both incompetent and conceited. (And they lost most or all of their money!) These subjects' responses were thus doubly self-defeating. Not only did they fail to ward off the unflattering implications contained in the initial threat, but they actually made things worse for themselves. In other words, their efforts to defend themselves against the ego threat ultimately led them into outcomes that would cause even more damage to their self-esteem.

This destructive consequence of high self-esteem raises the broader question of how people can maintain high self-esteem if they routinely engage in such self-destructive patterns. Although there are multiple answers to this question, two are most important. First, I reiterate that the subjects with high self-esteem only became self-destructive and irrational in response to an ego threat; under normal conditions, they showed a superior capacity for self-management. Ego threats may be fairly unusual (although quite important) occurrences. Indeed, the general patterns shown by people with high self-esteem indicate that they go through life expecting generally to succeed at things, which is why the occasional ego-threatening setback provokes such a drastic reaction from them—because they have really not seriously considered the possibility of such a failure (e.g., Baumeister, 1993b; Blaine & Crocker, 1993). Most of the time, people with high self-esteem are quite effective at setting appropriate goals and living up to them.

Second, people with high self-esteem tend to respond to failures or setbacks by refocusing their attention on other things that they do well. In their eyes, they are good at many things, and so a failure can be easily compartmentalized (e.g., Steele, 1988). When they fail at something, they often prefer simply to avoid the entire domain after that, which seems quite feasible to them because of the many skills and capabilities they believe they have in other areas (see Baumeister & Tice, 1985a). In contrast, people with low self-esteem tend to think they cannot afford to avoid everything at which they are less than brilliant, because that would encompass almost every sphere, and so they tend to stay concerned with things at which they fail. But people with high self-esteem shift attention and effort to unrelated positive aspects of themselves in response to failure or criticism, and these shifts enable them to preserve their favorable opinions of themselves (see also Baumeister, 1982, 1993b).

CONCLUSION

I have argued that the study of self-regulation, in the sense of overriding normal or typical response sequences, holds an important key for understanding motivation and action. By examining how people cancel one response and substitute another in its place, psychology may gain valuable insight into how action occurs. Moreover, such overrides are an important sphere for the operation of motivational factors.

The desire to think well of oneself is a major and pervasive motivation, and it activates a variety of responses to ego threats. When events carry unflattering implications about the self, people resort to several defense mechanisms to avoid having to revise their self-appraisal in a negative way. Under some circumstances, they shift attention away from the threatening stimuli, often finding a defensive preoccupation in alternative tasks or happy memories. At other times, however, they are unable to ignore the threatening implications, especially if these implications gain social reality because other people are aware of them. In these cases, people engage in various interpretive strategies to render the implications less damaging to self-esteem.

Ego threats may have powerful effects on another realm of self-regulation and motivated action—namely, the process of goal commitment. High self-esteem appears to be linked to a general capacity to set and meet goals effectively, but ego threats disrupt this effective self-management and cause people to set unrealistic, excessive goals that they then fail to meet. In this way, people with high self-esteem exhibit a destructive response to ego threats, at least when these ego threats elicit a compensatory reaction during a phase of making commitments to goals.

These two effects of ego threats—they stimulate efforts to regulate thoughts and emotions, and they impair efforts to set goals and manage one's other affairs—may well be interrelated. An important conclusion of a recent review of self-regulatory failure is that the capacity for self-regulation appears to be a limited resource; thus, when people are devoting themselves to self-regulation in one sphere, there is often a tendency for self-regulatory failure to occur in another (Baumeister et al., 1994). A familiar example would be the person who abandons a diet or resumes smoking cigarettes while attempting to cope with a stressful period at work or in school. In the present context, it may be that ego threats elicit a kind of emergency self-regulatory response aimed at minimizing the impact on a person's thoughts and feelings, and this preoccupation may cause the person to neglect other, more habitual or ongoing aspects of self-regulation, such as self-management and effective goal setting.

Self-regulatory responses to ego threats thus defy any attempt to label them as simply beneficial or harmful. Ego threats can make people more thoughtful or less thoughtful, and such threats make some people more cautious while others become more reckless in committing themselves to goals. Common to all these responses, however, is the theme that ego threats invoke basic and powerful motivations that alter the way people control their own thoughts, feelings, and actions.

ACKNOWLEDGMENTS

This work was facilitated by Research Grant No. MH43826 from the National Institute of Mental Health, by an Alexander von Humboldt Foundation Fellowship, and by a James McKeen Cattell Sabbatical Fellowship.

NOTE

1. Accountability alone cannot account for the effects found in this condition, however, because accountability would presumably increase effortful processing in general, whereas in this study the opposite pattern was found when the feedback was pleasant and favorable. That is, subjects who received favorable public information did not spend more (or even as much) time thinking about it as did subjects who received favorable private information. Thus, some reference to self-deceptive motivational patterns is necessary to explain theses results.

REFERENCES

Bargh, J. A. (1989). Conditional automaticity: Varieties of automatic influence in social perception and cognition. In J. Uleman & J. Bargh (Eds.), *Unintended thought* (pp. 3–51). New York: Guilford Press.

Bargh, J. A. (1990). Auto-motives: Preconscious determinants of social interaction. In E. Higgins & R. Sorrentino (Eds.), *Handbook of motivation and cognition: Foundations of social behavior* (Vol. 2, pp. 93–130). New York: Guilford Press.

Baumeister, R. F. (1982). Self-esteem, self-presentation, and future interaction: A dilemma of reputation. *Journal of Personality, 50,* 29–45.

Baumeister, R. F. (1991). *Meanings of life.* New York: Guilford Press.

Baumeister, R. F. (1993a). Lying to yourself: The paradox of self-deception. In M. Lewis & C. Saarni (Eds.), *Lying and deception in everyday life* (pp. 166–183). New York: Guilford Press.

Baumeister, R. F. (1993b). Understanding the inner nature of low self-esteem: Uncertain, fragile, protective, and conflicted. In R. Baumeister (Ed.), *Self-esteem: The puzzle of low self-regard* (pp. 201–218). New York: Plenum.

Baumeister, R. F., & Cairns, K. J. (1992). Repression and self-presentation: When audiences interfere with self-deceptive strategies. *Journal of Personality and Social Psychology, 62,* 851–862.

Baumeister, R. F., Heatherton, T. F., & Tice, D. M. (1993). When ego threats lead to self-regulation failure: Negative consequences of high self-esteem. *Journal of Personality and Social Psychology, 64,* 141–156.

Baumeister, R. F., Heatherton, T. F., & Tice, D. M. (1994). *Losing control: How and why people fail at self-regulation.* San Diego, CA: Academic Press.

Baumeister, R. F., & Ilko, S. A. (1995). Shallow gratitude: Public and private acknowledgement of external help in accounts of success. *Basic and Applied Social Psychology, 16,* 191–209.

Baumeister, R. F., & Newman, L. S. (1994). Self-regulation of cognitive inference and decision processes. *Personality and Social Psychology Bulletin, 20,* 3–19.

Baumeister, R. F., Stillwell, A., & Wotman, S. R. (1990). Victim and perpetrator accounts of interpersonal conflict: Autobiographical narratives about anger. *Journal of Personality and Social Psychology, 59,* 994–1005.

Baumeister, R. F., & Tice, D. M. (1985a). Self-esteem and responses to success and failure: Subsequent performance and intrinsic motivation. *Journal of Personality, 53,* 450–467.

Baumeister, R. F., & Tice, D. M. (1985b) Toward a theory of situational structure. *Environment and Behavior, 17,* 147–192.

Baumeister, R. F., & Wotman, S. R. (1992). *Breaking hearts: The two sides of unrequited love.* New York: Guilford Press.

Baumeister, R. F., Wotman, S. R., & Stillwell, A. M. (1993). Unrequited love: On heartbreak, anger, guilt, scriptlessness, and humiliation. *Journal of Personality and Social Psychology, 64,* 377–394.

Baumgardner, A.H. (1990). To know oneself is to like oneself: Self-certainty and self-affect. *Journal of Personality and Social Psychology, 58,* 1062–1072.

Blaine, B., & Crocker, J. (1993). Self-esteem and self-serving biases in reactions to positive and negative events: An integrative review. In R. Baumeister (Ed.), *Self-esteem: The puzzle of low self-regard* (pp. 55–85). New York: Plenum.

Boden, J. M., & Baumeister, R. F. (1993). *Repression and affect regulation: Responding to induced bad moods with happy memories.* Unpublished manuscript, Case Western Reserve University.

Campbell, J. D. (1990). Self-esteem and the clarity of the self-concept. *Journal of Personality and Social Psychology, 59,* 538–549.

Campbell, J. D., & Lavallee, L. F. (1993). Who am I? The role of self-concept confusion in understanding the behavior of people with low self-esteem. In R. Baumeister (Ed.), *Self-esteem: The puzzle of low self-regard* (pp. 3–20). New York: Plenum.

Carver, C. S., & Scheier, M. F. (1981). *Attention and self-regulation: A control theory approach to human behavior.* New York: Springer-Verlag.

Darley, J. M., & Goethals, G. R. (1980). People's analyses of the causes of ability-linked performances. In L. Berkowitz (Ed.), *Advances in experimental social psychology* (Vol. 13, pp. 1–37). New York: Academic Press.

Erdelyi, M. H. (1974). A new look at the New Look: Perceptual defense and vigilance. *Psychological Review, 81,* 1–25.

Frey, D. (1978). Reactions to success and failure in public and private conditions. *Journal of Experimental Social Psychology, 14,* 172–179.

Gollwitzer, P. M. (1991). *Abwägen und Planen: Bewußtseinslagen in verschiedenen Handlungsphasen.* Göttingen, Germany: Hogrefe.

Gollwitzer, P. M. (1993). Goal achievement: The role of intentions. In W. Stroebe & M. Hewstone (Eds.), *European review of social psychology* (Vol. 4, pp. 141–185). Chichester, England: Wiley.

Greenwald, A. G. (1988). Self-knowledge and self-deception. In J. B. Lockard & D. Paulhus (Eds.), *Self-deception: An adaptive mechanism?* (pp. 113–131). Englewood Cliffs, NJ: Prentice-Hall.

Gur, R. C., & Sackeim, H. A. (1979). Self-deception: A concept in search of a phenomenon. *Journal of Personality and Social Psychology, 37,* 147–169.

Heatherton, T. F., & Baumeister, R. F. (1991). Binge eating as escape from self-awareness. *Psychological Bulletin, 110,* 86–108.

Isen, A. M. (1984). Toward understanding the role of affect in cognition. In R. S. Wyer & T. K. Srull (Eds.), *Handbook of social cognition* (Vol. 3, pp. 179–236). Hillsdale, NJ: Erlbaum.

Lord, C. G., Ross, L., & Lepper, M. R., (1979). Biased assimilation and attitude polarization: The effects of prior theories on subsequently considered evidence. *Journal of Personality and Social Psychology, 37,* 2098–2109.

McFarlin, D. B. (1985). Persistence in the face of failure: The impact of self-esteem and contingency information. *Personality and Social Psychology Bulletin, 11,* 152–163.

McFarlin, D. B., & Blascovich, J. (1981). Effects of self-esteem and performance feedback on future affective preferences and cognitive expectations. *Journal of Personality and Social Psychology, 40,* 521–531.

Newman, L. S., & Baumeister, R. F. (1993). *Defensive preoccupation as a response to ego threat: When bad news gets a busy signal.* Unpublished manuscript, Case Western Reserve University.

Pyszczynski, T., Greenberg, J., & Holt, K. (1985). Maintaining consistency between self-serving beliefs and available data: A bias in information evaluation. *Personality and Social Psychology Bulletin, 11,* 179–190.

Roth, D. L., Snyder, C. R., & Pace, L. M. (1986). Dimensions of favorable self-presentation. *Journal of Personality and Social Psychology, 51,* 867–874.

Sandelands, L. E., Brockner, J., & Glynn, M. A. (1988). If at first you don't succeed, try, try again: Effects of persistence–performance contingencies, ego involvement, and self-esteem on task performance. *Journal of Applied Psychology, 73,* 208–216.

Sartre, J.-P. (1953). *The existential psychoanalysis* (H. E. Barnes, Trans.) New York: Philosophical Library. (Original work published 1934)

Steele, C. M. (1988). The psychology of self-affirmation: Sustaining the integrity of the self. In L. Berkowitz (Ed.), *Advances in experimental social psychology* (Vol. 21, pp. 261–302). New York: Academic Press.

Stern, L. D., Marrs, S., Millar, M. G., & Cole, E. (1984). Processing time and the recall of inconsistent and consistent behaviors of individuals and groups. *Journal of Personality and Social Psychology, 47,* 253–262.

Taylor, S. E., & Brown, J. D. (1988). Illusion and well-being: A social psychological perspective on mental health. *Psychological Bulletin, 103,* 193–210.

Teasdale, J. D., & Russell, M. L. (1983). Differential aspects of induced mood on the recall of positive, negative, and neutral words. *British Journal of Clinical Psychology, 22,* 163–171.

Tetlock, P. E. (1983). Accountability and complexity of thought. *Journal of Personality and Social Psychology, 45,* 74–83.

Tice, D. M., Muraven, M., & Baumeister, R. F. (1993). *Common techniques of affect regulation.* Unpublished manuscript, Case Western Reserve University.

Vallone, R. P., Griffin, D. W., Lin, S., & Ross, L. (1990). Overconfident prediction of future actions and outcomes by self and others. *Journal of Personality and Social Psychology, 58,* 582–592.

Wagner, R. K., & Sternberg, R. J. (1985). Practical intelligence in real-world pursuits: The role of tacit knowledge. *Journal of Personality and Social Psychology, 49,* 436–458.

Weinberger, D. A., Schwartz, G. E. & Davidson, R. J. (1979). Low-anxious, high-anxious, and repressive coping styles: Psychometric patterns and behavioral and physiological responses to stress. *Journal of Abnormal Psychology, 88,* 369–380.

Wicklund, R. A., & Gollwitzer, P. M. (1982). *Symbolic self-completion.* Hillsdale, NJ: Erlbaum.

Wright, J., & Mischel, W. (1982). Influence of affect on cognitive social learning person variables. *Journal of Personality and Social Psychology, 43,* 901–914.

Wyer, R. S., & Frey, D. (1983). The effects of feedback about self and others on recall and judgments of feedback-relevant information. *Journal of Experimental Social Psychology, 19,* 540–559.

Zuckerman, M. (1979). Attribution of success and failure revisited, or: The motivational bias is alive and well in attribution theory. *Journal of Personality, 47,* 245–287.

CHAPTER 3

On the Substitutability of Self-Protective Mechanisms

Abraham Tesser
Leonard L. Martin
David P. Cornell

Instead of investigating the single psychological systems which correspond to simple needs and desires, we have to deal with the interrelationships of these systems . . . and with the different kinds of larger wholes built up from them. These interrelationships and larger wholes are very labile and delicate. Yet one must try to get hold of them experimentally because they are most important for understanding the underlying reality of behavior and personality differences.

—LEWIN (1935, p. 180)

Work on the psychology of the self has grown tremendously in the last couple of decades. There is work on the structure of the self (e.g., Markus, 1977; Linville, 1987) and on the role of the self in cognitive processing (e.g., Kihlstrom et al., 1988). We would like to focus on work on self-evaluation or self-esteem.[1] Although there are exceptions (e.g., Swann, 1983), the usual assumption is that people wish to maintain a positive self-evaluation. By now, there are so many different formulations about what circumstances or behaviors threaten or augment self-esteem that we are confronted with a "self-zoo." Some of the profound differences among the processes in this zoo lead us to raise the question of whether the theorists are talking about the same self-esteem or not. The answer to this question is not trivial. If each of these model processes affects the same self-esteem, then the prospect of theoretical integration seems more tractable than if each model describes circumstances and behaviors that have independent psychological effects.

Lewin's work on goal tension systems provides clues as to how to address this question. Below, we describe some of the inhabitants of the "self-zoo." Then we review some of the Lewinian work on goal tension systems and show how it provides a tool for answering the question of whether behavior described by qualitatively different models of self-esteem maintenance are affecting the same or different psychological variables. Finally, we speculate on how the various models of self may be integrated.

THE "SELF ZOO"

Social psychology has seen an explosion of work on self-defense processes. This "zoo" includes a truly wide variety of systematic conceptions of what affects the well-being of the self and how behavior can be understood as an attempt either to restore or to increase self-evaluation. For example, the self-evaluation maintenance (SEM) model (e.g., Tesser, 1988) posits two antagonistic processes: When a performance dimension is very important (i.e., relevant to one's self-definition), the self is threatened by comparison to a psychologically close other who is performing well; when a performance dimension is not particularly self-relevant, the self is augmented by basking in the reflected glory of a psychologically close other who is performing well. There is evidence that people will behave so as to change others' performance (e.g., Tesser & Smith, 1980), their own performance (Dalhoff & Tesser, in preparation), the relevance of the performance dimension to themselves (e.g., Tesser & Campbell, 1980), and the closeness to others (e.g., Pleban & Tesser, 1981) in ways predicted to maintain self-evaluation. There is additional evidence that conditions that threaten or augment self-evaluation are associated with increased arousal and with negative and positive facial affect, respectively (e.g., Tesser, Millar, & Moore, 1988). Finally, subjects tend to make internal attributions for performances that augment self-evaluation, and external attributions for performances that threaten self-evaluation (e.g., Cornell, 1990).

There are a number of other formulations and processes about the self. For example, Wicklund and Gollwitzer (1982), also strongly influenced by Lewin, see the individual as a self-symbolizing animal who generates and clings to symbols of cherished aspects of the self when those aspects are threatened. Greenberg, Pyszczynski, and Solomon (1986) suggest that the need for self-esteem may originate in the terror associated with death. Thus, we can understand behaviors as diverse as rejecting strangers and clinging to tradition as attempts at maintaining self-esteem. Baumeister (1982) and others (e.g., Arkin, 1981; Baumgardner & Brownlee, 1987) suggest that much behavior can be understood in terms of self-presentation intended to boost self-evaluation.

The work on attribution processes suggests that concern with one's self-evaluation can affect the way in which causes are assigned to outcomes. Thus, people tend to assign internal causes for their success and external causes for their failures (see Zuckerman, 1979, for a review). Indeed, they tend to reconstruct their own histories so as to exaggerate their own importance, morality, and talent (e.g., Greenwald, 1980). When there is some ambiguity about their own ability, persons will actually handicap themselves in order to keep potential failure from disambiguating a lack of ability (e.g., Berglas & Jones, 1978).

Depression may also result from processes associated with self-evaluation. Inordinate self-focus tends to produce ruminative processes, and dwelling on shortcomings and negative attributes leads in turn to depression (e.g., Martin, Tesser, & McIntosh, 1992; Pyszczynski & Greenberg, 1987). Stable, general, internal attributions of failure to the self can produce depression (e.g., Abramson, Metalsky, & Alloy, 1989). Higgins and his students (e.g., Higgins, 1987) have shown that making discrepancies between one's actual self and one's desired self salient increases depression-like dejection, whereas making discrepancies between one's actual self and one's "ought" self salient leads to agitation.

Other research programs have not been formulated in terms of self-evaluation processes, but can be understood in those terms. A number of social motives seem to be traceable to self-evaluation. For example, the need for cognitive consistency as posited by cognitive dissonance theory (e.g., Festinger, 1957) has been interpreted as a motive to maintain self-evaluation (e.g., Aronson, 1969; Greenwald & Ronis, 1978). Striving for freedom (e.g., Brehm, 1966) or control (Seligman, 1975; Kelley, 1967) is clearly qualitatively different from striving for consistency. Yet both consistency and control motives appear to reflect self-evaluation concerns (Steele, 1988).

Each of the processes described above is assumed to be a self-protective mechanism; this is just a sample. In physics, when the number of elementary particles being discovered became large and diverse, they were known collectively as the "particle zoo." Social psychology now seems to have its own "self-defense zoo." These mechanisms have qualitatively different triggers and qualitatively different responses; yet they are all called self-esteem (self-evaluation) mechanisms. It appears to be time to raise the question of what they have in common. The answer to the question of whether the many different self-protective mechanisms affect the same or different aspects of self-evaluation would seem to be a crucial one for theory construction. If each of these mechanisms affects a common, general self-evaluation, the integration of these mechanisms into a unified theory would seem more feasible than if their products were independent.

HOW TO ADDRESS THE INDEPENDENCE QUESTION: LEWIN'S CLUES

Clue 1: Goal Tension and Incompleted Tasks

Lewin's (e.g., 1935) work provides clues about how one might address the question of whether the members of the "self-zoo" are serving the "same" self-esteem. Lewin assumed that behavior is goal-driven. The first of Lewin's clues is that adopting a goal sets up a tension state, which remains until the goal is satisfied or the individual gives up the goal (i.e., "leaves the field"). If the goal is unsatisfied and the goal is not given up, the tension remains, and behavior related to the goal will continue or re-emerge.

One of Lewin's many talented students, Bluma Zeigarnik (1927), provided a nice demonstration of how this works. She had children engage in a number of different tasks (stringing beads, enumerating city names, modeling in clay, etc.). The children were allowed to complete some of the tasks, but they were interrupted on some of the others. The interruptions took place after the children had become involved with the tasks but before they had completed them. Then, after engaging in an unrelated activity, the children were asked to recall the tasks they had previously worked on. Zeigarnik compared memory for completed tasks with memory for incompleted tasks.

There were, of course, three potential outcomes to this comparison, and each of them would have been theoretically plausible. First, if memory is simply a cold associative process in which motives and goals play no role, then there might have been no difference. After all, Zeigarnik's subjects had approximately equal exposure to the completed and incompleted tasks. Second, subjects might have been motivated to feel good about themselves and their accomplishments, and therefore might have focused on the completed tasks and ignored or "repressed" the incompleted tasks. This would have resulted in greater memory for the completed than the incompleted tasks. Third, if (as Lewin suggested) the adoption of a goal sets up a tension state that remains when the task is interrupted, this tension should have kept the accessibility of the incompleted tasks high, and subjects should have had a better memory for the incompleted tasks than the completed tasks. This was exactly what Zeigarnik found. Indeed, a better memory for incompleted tasks has come to be known as the "Zeigarnik effect."[2]

In a more recent study, we (described in Martin et al., 1993) also pitted the hypotheses of incompleted-goal tension and passive associative processes against each other, but in a different context. This context was as follows: One of the most interesting phenomena to emerge in the last couple of years is the effect of thought suppression on thought recovery. In an interesting series of studies, Wegner and his colleagues (e.g., Wegner, Carter, Schneider, & White, 1987) have asked subjects *not* to think about something (e.g., a white bear). People find this difficult to do; the thought of a white bear keeps popping into mind. Even more interesting, when people who have been asked to suppress thoughts of a white bear are given an opportunity to express anything they want, they express more thoughts about white bears than do subjects who were never asked to suppress.

One explanation of this rebound phenomenon is that under suppression instructions, people try to distract themselves from thinking about a white bear whenever it comes up. Thus the concept of white bears becomes associated with a variety of extraneous contents (the distracting materials). When subjects are given the opportunity to think freely about anything, the large number of distractors (associates) keeps bringing white bears to mind. A different explanation can be derived from the goal tension hypothesis. In the suppression condition, subjects are given the goal of not thinking about a white bear. Since a white bear pops into mind, the goal of not thinking about a white bear has not been met; the incompleted-goal tension remains, making white-bear-related material more accessible.

Here is how we attempted to pit the association hypothesis against the goal tension hypothesis. We created three experimental conditions: "Express" subjects were told to think about anything they wanted, including a white bear, and to make a note of each bear thought by placing a check mark on a sheet. Two groups of "suppress" subjects were asked not to think of a white bear, but to tally each bear thought that they had. After the thought period, the experimenter collected the tally sheets of bear thoughts from all of the subjects. In the "express" and the "suppress/incomplete" group, the experimenter said nothing; this replicated the usual Wegner conditions. For the "suppress/complete" subjects, however, the experimenter looked at the subjects' tally sheets, and told them that even though they had had some thoughts about a white bear, they had done much better than most of the other subjects at not thinking about a white bear. This success feedback was intended to provide a subjective sense of goal attainment.

In the "express" condition, no particular goal was set and subjects were not trying to distract themselves, so we felt that there should be no particular remaining goal tension or buildup of associates to a white bear. According to the association hypothesis, subjects in both "suppress" conditions should be trying to distract themselves from thoughts of a white bear and building up associations. Therefore, the white bear should be equally more accessible in the two "suppress" conditions than in the "express" condition. The goal tension hypothesis would predict something else: If the rebound effect is attributable to incompleted-goal tension, then white bear thoughts should be more accessible to "suppress/incomplete" subjects (who did not meet the goal of not thinking about a white bear) than to "express" subjects (who had no particular goal) or "suppress/complete" subjects (who were told they were successful in meeting the goal). To measure accessibility we exposed subjects to partially completed words related to "white bear" (e.g., "iceberg," "polar bear") and measured speed of identification. The pattern of means conformed to the goal tension hypothesis rather than the association hypothesis.[3]

Clue 2: Task Substitution and Goal Completion

Zeigarnik's (1927) work and the work of a number of people who followed her provided evidence for the notion that goals, once adopted, have a kind of psychological autonomy in directing behavior until they are completed. Indeed, some of the other chapters in this volume provide strong evidence for this autonomy in demonstrating that goals can be primed without awareness (Bargh & Barndollar, Chapter 20), can guide behavior automatically (Gollwitzer, Chapter 13), and can instigate automatic ironic processes that monitor their progress (Ansfield & Wegner, Chapter 21). Lewin would certainly have been delighted with this progress. He was influenced by the writings of Freud, and these developments speak to the question of the extent to which behavior can be guided by forces outside awareness (see Sorrentino, Chapter 27). Awareness was a central concern of Freud's, and is one to which we return later.

Lewin and his students were influenced by another concern of Freud's—"sublimation," or the idea that a particular need or goal can be satisfied by a number of very different behaviors that have very little similarity on the surface. According to Lewin (1935),

> Freud uses the concept of substitution extensively to explain both normal and abnormal behavior. Moreover, sublimation, which is closely related to substitution, is according to him an important foundation of our whole cultural life. We find substitution in very different forms. There is, for instance, the man who dreams of a palace and brings a few pieces of marble into his kitchen. There is the man who cannot buy a piano, but who collects piano catalogs. Again we find the delinquent boy who knows that he will not be allowed to leave his reform school but who asks for a traveling bag as a birthday present. And the little boy who threatens and scolds the larger boy whom he cannot beat on the playground. These and a hundred other examples make us realize how important and far reaching the problem of substitution is in regard to psychological needs as well as with reference to bodily needs. (p. 82)

Goals also have the property of "equifinality." That is, a goal does not dictate behavior, but rather a consummatory state. For example, if we are hungry and adopt the goal to eat food, a number of different instrumental behaviors will do. We can cook something at home and consume it; we can go to a fast-food restaurant and eat; we can go to a fine restaurant and dine; we can convince a friend or parent to invite us over for dinner; and so forth. Any one of these activities will satisfy the goal, and hence all of them are substitutable for one another. In this case, the substitution of one for the other is relatively straightforward. However, the surface similarity of activities is not always a very good means of determining whether one activity can substitute for another:

> We know, for example, from the work of Fajans, that a doll may be a real substitute for a child who has been unable to reach a piece of candy. Or the child may accept his mother's sympathy as an equally genuine substitution. On the other hand, we shall see that two actions can be very similar, without one serving as a substitute for the other. In regard to examples from psychoanalysis it is important that the similarity of two facts is not sufficient evidence for the statement that one is a substitute for the other. Whether a substitute is present or not cannot be decided from the *external* appearance of the events. It is necessary in each individual case to see whether the two facts have a certain *dynamic* connection. (Lewin, 1935, p. 182)

Ovsiankina (1928), another student of Lewin's, set the stage for the experimental study of task substitution. Although Zeigarnik had shown the motivational importance of incomplete goals, her demonstration raised concerns about differential rehearsal and memory confounds, as well as explicit experimenter demands that the subjects remember both completed and uncompleted tasks (see Weiner, 1972, and Heckhausen, 1989/1991, for reviews). Ovsiankina reasoned that if a tension is associated with an incomplete task, then that task should be spontaneously resumed after an interruption. Surreptitious observation of subjects who were interrupted in a variety of activities showed that when the experimenter left the room, the interrupted activities were more likely to be pursued than the noninterrupted activities.

It was a short step to vary the nature of the interruption; that is, a goal-directed individual could be interrupted with different tasks. If the intervening task satisfied the goal being pursued, then the goal tension would be reduced, and the original task would be less likely to be resumed. A task that satisfied the original goal was said to be substitutable for the original task.

Lewin and his students and colleagues set about studying the properties of substitutability. Lissner (1933) had children work on a variety of tasks, including making clay figures and solving mosaic problems. She found that both similarity and difficulty increased substitutability. For example, if a child was making a clay house and was interrupted by being asked to make a clay snake (very easy) or a clay horse (more difficult), the child was more likely to go back to the house after completing the snake than after completing the horse.

Mahler (1933) was concerned with the "level of reality" of substitute activities. After interrupting an initial task, she varied whether the subject was given an opportunity to simply think about the task, talk about its completion, or actually complete the task.[4] These manipulations varied in the extent to which they involved "reality." Using task resumption as an index of substitutability, she found that simply thinking resulted in the most resumption and actual completion the least resumption of the original task, with talk about completion in the middle. Thus, the greater the reality of a substitute task, the more it reduces the tension associated with an interrupted goal. It is noteworthy that even if subjects were able to solve problems in their heads, the reality of communicating that solution had an added effect on the reduction of Zeigarnik tension.

The valence of a particular activity also makes a difference in both the extent to which it can be substituted for and the extent to which it can serve as a substitute. Henle (1944) had children rate the attractiveness of various tasks (a jigsaw puzzle, pencil maze, anagram, letter cancelation, clay modeling, etc.). In her first experiment, she interrupted subjects who were working on a task that they had rated at a middle level of attractiveness to work on a task they had rated as more attractive. Forty-one percent subsequently resumed working on the first task. In her second experiment, she interrupted a more attractive task with a task of middle-level attractiveness and got a resumption rate of 81%. In short, the more attractive the substitute relative to the original task, the greater the substitutability.

Perhaps the most relevant feature of a goal's substitutability for present purposes is its level. Think of goals as being hierarchically organized (e.g., Carver & Scheier, 1981; Vallacher & Wegner, 1987; Martin & Tesser, 1989). People have high-level goals (e.g., being a good person), and low-level goals (e.g., buying a box of Girl Scout cookies). One goal is higher than another if the second goal must be met in order to reach the first goal. Vallacher and Wegner (1987) suggest that lower-order goals can be elicited by asking "how" questions ("How do you accomplish *X*?") and that higher-order goals can be elicited by asking "why" questions ("Why are you trying to accomplish *X*?"). Henle (1944) gave subjects some clay and asked them either to "be creative" or to make a horse. We suggest that the goal to be creative is at a higher level than the goal to make a clay horse. She then interrupted her subjects and asked them to build a house of blocks. Her task resumption data suggested that the substitution was more effective for the higher-order goal than for the lower-order goal.

Another integration of this aspect of the substitutability literature comes from Wicklund and Gollwitzer (1982). Whereas Lewin's interpretation of task resumption is couched in terms of completion of the original task, Wicklund and Gollwitzer suggest that only tasks that recruit ego involvement are candidates for substitutability. Moreover, the crucial feature of a task that makes it substitutable for another is that it has implications for the ego or self-esteem. This formulation integrates Lissner's (1933) observation that more difficult tasks have greater substitutability: Completing more difficult tasks has a more positive effect on self-esteem than completing less difficult tasks. It also accounts for Henle's (1944) observations concerning creativity.

TOWARD A MORE HOLISTIC UNDERSTANDING OF SELF-ESTEEM MAINTENANCE

Regardless of the interpretation, there appears to be ample evidence for the proposition that goals related to self-esteem may be substitutable for one another. Currently there are numerous theories about how we go about maintaining self-esteem. Each theory has its own set of antecedents (the things that threaten or augment self-esteem) and its own set of consequences (what people do to restore or increase self-esteem). According to Lewin (1935), "Instead of investigating the single psychological systems which correspond to simple needs and desires, we have to deal with the interrelationships of these systems . . . and with the different kinds of larger wholes built up from them" (p. 180). Presently, research on self-esteem is of the single-psychological-system type. What we hope to do in the remainder of this chapter is to move toward understanding the interrelationships among these systems and the more integrated whole. That was Lewin's goal. We have adopted it, and the spirit of the logic of task substitutability, to help move us toward that goal.

A simple expansion of the Lewin/Ovsiankina logic allows for the use of substitute activities to teach us more about goal systems and goal dynamics. If we think of the maintenance of self esteem as a goal, then we have a mechanism for addressing the question of one versus many self-esteems. The logic is simple. If each of these defense mechanisms are satisfying the *same* higher-order goal of self-esteem maintenance, then engaging in one such mechanism should substitute for engaging in another. Thus, individuals who have just basked in the reflected glory of a relative's good performance should be less likely to change their attitudes in a dissonance situation than people who have not had the opportunity to bask in reflected glory. On the other hand, if these mechanisms are satisfying *different* goals, then engaging in one should not affect the propensity to engage in the second; that is, basking in reflected glory should not affect dissonance reduction. Although there is no shortage of work on each of the defense mechanisms taken by themselves, until recently there was little in the way of combining them to see whether there is substitutability.

On the Substitutability of Members of the "Self Zoo"

One of the most influential theories in social psychology is the theory of cognitive dissonance. As noted earlier, several prominent theorists (e.g., Aronson, 1969; Greenwald & Ronis, 1978) have suggested that this theory can be construed in terms of self-evaluation maintenance. In a series of elegant studies, Steele and Liu (1981, 1983) have convincingly shown that self-affirmation has substitute value for dissonance reduction. In one study (Steele & Liu, 1983), for example, the student subjects were given either high choice or low choice to write an essay that was discrepant with their attitudes (i.e., they wrote in favor of a tuition increase). After completing this essay, the subjects filled out a questionnaire covering political/economic values. For half the subjects this was an important value orientation, and filling out the scale allowed them to reaffirm that value; for the remaining subjects it was an irrelevant value orientation. Finally, attitudes toward a tuition increase were measured. The typical dissonance effect would be greater attitude change in the direction of the essay with greater choice. However, this effect was found only for the subjects who did not have an opportunity to affirm their self-values. Dissonance reduction did not manifest itself if subjects had an intervening opportunity to reaffirm an important self-value.

Steele (Liu & Steele, 1986) has also shown that self-affirmation is substitutable for learned helplessness. Pittman and his colleagues (Pittman & Pittman, 1980; Pittman & D'Agostino, 1985) have shown that helplessness training (e.g., Seligman, 1975) leads to increases in making causal attributions, presumably in order to regain control. Liu and Steele (1986) were able to eliminate those increases in attribution due to learned helplessness by having subjects affirm an important aspect of self. Again, although learned helplessness and self-affirmation seem to be quite different in appearance, self-affirmation seems to reduce the consequences of learned helplessness.

Steele's work substitutes self-affirmation for dissonance reduction and for attribution making in connection with learned helplessness. All of these are intrapersonal processes. The self-evaluation processes with which we have been concerned over the years (i.e., reflection and comparison processes) are distinctly *inter*personal processes. Thus, we wondered whether self-affirmation can substitute for interpersonal self-evaluation processes such as those exemplified by the SEM model.

In order to address this question, we (Tesser & Cornell, 1991, Study 1) replicated a study by Tesser and Smith (1980). In the original study, subjects were given an opportunity to provide clues to affect the performance of a friend (close other) or a stranger (distant other) on a word task. Since easy clues facilitate another's performance, and difficult clues inhibit another's performance clue difficulty served as our dependent variable. The SEM model suggests that when a task is low in personal relevance, people tend to bask in the reflected glory of the good performance of a close other. So they should want their friends to do very well on such tasks. Consistent with the SEM model, when the task was described as unimportant (low in relevance) friends were given easier clues than strangers. The model also suggests that when the task is high in personal relevance, the performance of a close other can be threatening to self-evaluation. Here people should *not* want a friend to outperform them. Accordingly, we found that when the task was described as important (high in relevance), strangers were given easier clues than friends.

In the replication, half of the participants were given an opportunity to affirm themselves and half were not. If the substitutability of affirmation generalizes, then the SEM pattern should re-emerge when subjects have not previously affirmed themselves and should disappear (or become attenuated) when subjects have affirmed themselves. As can be seen in Figure 3.1, The latter is precisely what happened.

The panel on the left shows the findings of the replication without self-affirmation. (Recall that difficult clues are less helpful than easy clues.) As predicted by our SEM model and as found by Tesser and Smith (1980), there

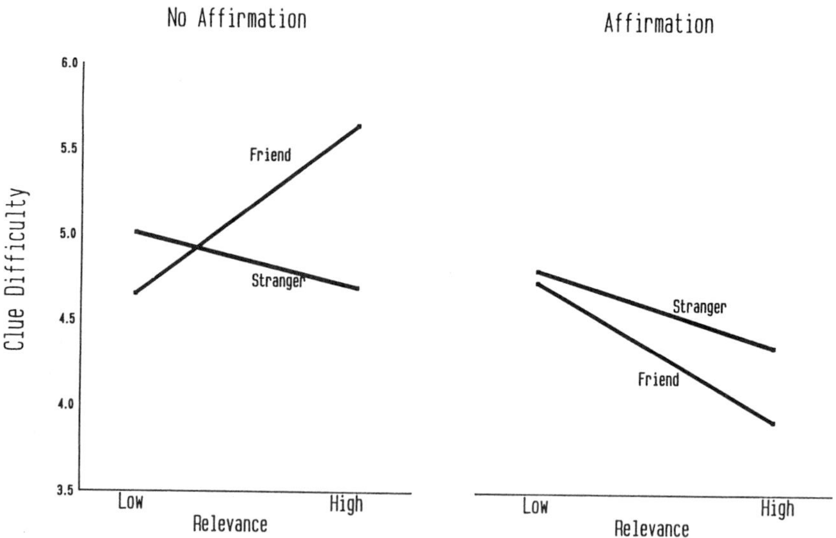

FIGURE 3.1. Difficulty of clues given to a friend and a stranger as a function of self-affirmation and self-relevance. From Tesser and Cornell (1991). Copyright 1991 by Academic Press. Reprinted by permission.

was an interaction between closeness of another and personal relevance of the task. Subjects gave easier clues to a stranger than to a friend when relevance to self was high, and this difference reversed itself when relevance was low. The picture was quite different after subjects had had an opportunity to affirm themselves (the right panel). After self-affirmation, the interaction disappeared and there were no differences among conditions.[5] It appears, then, that self-affirmation can substitute for interpersonal self protection strategies.

So far, we have seen that self-affirmation is a relatively general substitute for many self-esteem processes. If our generalization of Henle's (1944) work is correct, and there are many substitutes for higher-order goals such as maintaining self-esteem, then it should be the case that almost *any* self-evaluation maintenance process should be substitutable for almost any other. That is, there should be nothing special about self-affirmation with regard to substitutability. This can be demonstrated in two ways: (1) by showing that processes other than self-affirmation can function as substitutes (e.g., SEM processes can substitute for dissonance processes); and (2) by showing that self-affirmation can be affected by other processes (e.g., engaging in SEM processes can affect the propensity to engage in self-affirmation). We have evidence in support of both of these possibilities.

Self-Affirmation Is Not the Only Substitute

We (Tesser & Cornell, 1991, Studies 2 and 3) addressed the first possibility by manipulating circumstances that, according to the SEM model, ought to increase or decrease self-evaluation. We then observed the extent to which persons engaged in unrelated dissonance reduction strategies. Specifically, subjects were first asked to write a control essay or essays that made various SEM configurations salient: reflection (close other outperformed self on low-relevance dimension), positive comparison (self outperformed close other on high-relevance dimension), and negative comparison (close other outperformed self on high-relevance dimension). Then they were given either high or low choice to write an essay that was inconsistent with their attitudes.

As can be seen in Figure 3.2, the dissonance effect manifested itself clearly in the control essay conditions. Subjects became more favorable to the dissonant topic (a tuition increase) in the high-choice compared to the low-choice condition. More interesting for present purposes was the finding that engaging in the SEM processes had some substitute value for dissonance reduction. The augmentation of self-evaluation associated with writing about the reflection process or about positive comparison reduced the amount of dissonance, whereas a threat to self-evaluation associated with writing about negative comparison did not. In short, the SEM processes, just like self-affirmation, were able to substitute for dissonance processes.

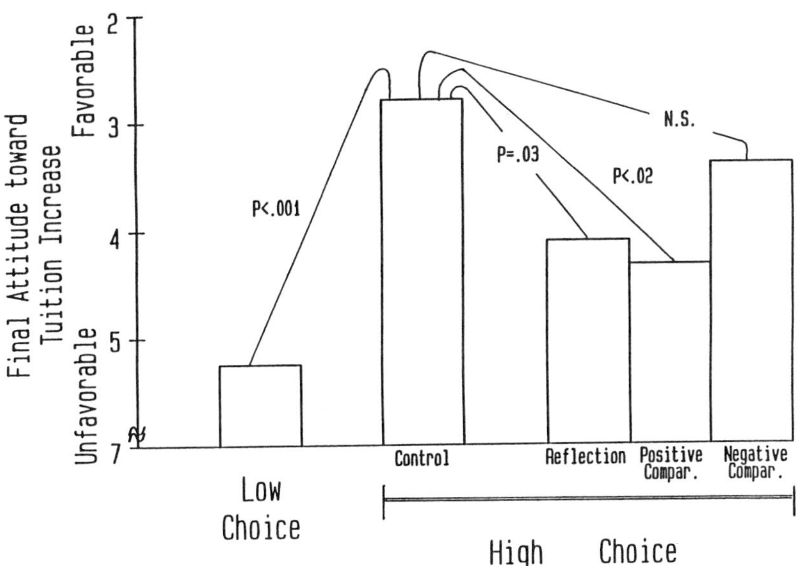

FIGURE 3.2. Attitude change as a function of choice and the priming of selected self-evaluation maintenance situations. From Tesser and Cornell (1991). Copyright 1991 by Academic Press. Reprinted by permission.

Self-Affirmation Can Be Affected by Other Processes

Can engaging in another self-defense-related behavior affect self-affirmation? For example, can engaging in SEM processes affect the tendency to engage in self-affirmation? If it can, then the idea of mutual substitutability of self-defense processes becomes more plausible, as does the notion that each of these mechanisms is serving the same higher-order goal. We (Cornell & Tesser, 1994) pursued this question as follows.

When subjects arrived, they were told that they were participating in an experiment on writing styles and that they would each have to write two short essays. The topics for the first essay were similar to those used in the Tesser and Cornell (1991) research. In the control condition, they wrote about their summer vacation. In the reflection condition, they wrote as vividly as they could about a time when someone close to them outperformed them on a task or activity for which it was not important for them personally to do well. In the positive-comparison condition, they wrote about a time when they outperformed a person who was close to them on a task or activity for which it was important for them to do well personally. Finally, in the negative-comparison condition, they wrote about a time they were outperformed by someone close to them on an activity or task on which it was personally important for them to do well. All of the subjects were encouraged to try to get back to the experience they were writing about and to try to relive their feelings at the time.

After the first essay was written, subjects were shown a list of values. Each focused on the value that was personally most important, and each wrote an essay indicating why the value was important to him or her. To our knowledge, self-affirmation has not been treated as a dependent variable, so we devised a measure. Several judges rated the essays for a number of self-related variables (e.g., the extent to which they were personal, the extent to which they were self-disclosing, level of value expressiveness, level of modesty, and positivity of self-presentation). These ratings were factor-analyzed. Scores on the first factor were taken as an index of engagement in self-affirmation.

Just as self-affirmation can turn dissonance reduction and SEM behavior on and off, other processes should be able to turn self-affirmation on and off. Therefore, we predicted and found that the positive self-experiences (reflection and positive comparison) resulted in less self-affirmation than did negative comparison. However, the former conditions did not result in less self-affirmation, but the latter condition did result in greater self-affirmation than that of controls. In sum, SEM processes can affect self-affirmation. Although there may be a variety of animals in the "self-defense zoo," their behaviors seem to be substitutable for one another. From this we infer that indeed they are all serving a single, higher-order goal, which appears to be self-esteem.

Toward an Understanding of the Interchangeability of Self-Oriented Processes

If we take seriously the notion that a number of different self-oriented processes are substitutable for one another, then we must wonder what it is about each that is being substituted. Just what is it about these ostensibly different processes that allows the kind of tradeoffs we have observed? Lewin's answer would have been couched in structural terms. We guess that he would have responded in terms of boundaries and their relative permeabilities.

Let us pursue this line of thought for a moment. Lewin thought of personality as made up of regions in a topological space. These regions may be characterized in terms of their complexity or number and in terms of the permeability of their boundaries. A goal state is associated with tension in the appropriate region. Since the system tends toward equilibration, the tension in the particular region must be reduced to that of the surrounding regions. If the region under tension is near the motor region, the tension is transferred to the motor system and the appropriate action is taken. If action is not possible but the boundaries are permeable, the tension will be transferred to neighboring regions, and substitute activities (those associated with neighboring regions) can bring the system into equilibration. If the boundary is not permeable, then the individual will remain in disequilibrium until he or she performs the appropriate behavior or leaves the field (i.e., gives up the goal).

Much of Lewin's thinking on structure was associated with his work on the feeble-minded. He found, for example, that feeble-minded children would continue doing exactly the same simple drawing for long periods of time without becoming satiated whereas normal children would vary their drawings over that time. He also found that there was virtually zero nonresumption of original activities by feeble-minded children, regardless of substitute activity. Thus, the tension associated with goals would not easily equilibriate. The way Lewin made sense of these observations was to assume that the feeble-minded have few regions (less complexity) and very little permeability among the boundaries.

Some contemporary work has taken a structural approach to adjustment. Most notably, the work of Linville (e.g., 1985, 1987) suggests that the more complex an individual's self-structure, the less emotionally volatile he or she tends to be. More complex individuals tend to be less upset by setbacks and less elated by successes than do less complex individuals. If we equate emotion with tension, then, from a Lewinian perspective, this might be understood in terms of emotion's achieving equilibrium by permeating many neighboring regions. The possibility for this is greater in a complex structure (more neighbors, greater permeability) than in a simple structure. However, Linville explicitly argues against this hypothesis. Her measure of complexity is based on the number of independent regions, and she suggests that the possibility of emotional "spillover" is reduced in more complex structures.

The work of both Lewin and Linville suggests that a structural explanation of the substitutability of self-evaluation maintenance processes may be worth pursuing. Indeed, one can think of instances where it appears implausable that self-esteem processes would be interchangeable unless they came from something like the same region. Suppose, for example, that an individual is so totally committed to becoming a lawyer that being a successful lawyer is at the center of his or her self-esteem concerns. It may be difficult to see how reducing dissonance in an irrelevant area will reduce striving to symbolize the lawyer identity (Wicklund & Gollwitzer, 1982). Perhaps, the single-minded pursuit of being a lawyer represents a compartmentalized self-structure with few neighbors and impermeable boundaries. In spite of the promise of this tack, our own research has taken a different turn. Our theorizing has focused on affect.

The Affect Hypothesis

At this time, our favorite candidate for understanding the substitution of self processes is affect. We know that dissonance arousal is associated with affect (e.g., Fazio & Cooper, 1983), and we know that SEM processes are associated with affect (e.g., Tesser et al., 1988). We also know that dissonance processes (Cooper & Fazio, 1984) and that SEM processes are mediated by affact (e.g., Achee, Tesser, & Pilkington, 1994; Tesser, Pilkington, & McIntosh, 1989). That is, dissonance reduction and SEM behaviors do not manifest themselves in the absence of affect. We know too that affect is often missattributed (e.g., Schachter, 1964; Zillman, 1983). Finally, in a partial replication of the Tesser and Cornell (1991) research, Simon, Greenberg, and Brehm (1992, Study 2) have shown that positive mood appears to reduce dissonance reduction.

Perhaps positive affect, such as that accompanying the successful completion of one of these self processes, signals well-being to the organism and leads to less vigilance (Mandler, 1975) and more benign interpretations (Isen, 1987) of subsequent events, thus decreasing self-defensive behavior with respect to the second process. Or, perhaps the positive excitation is missattributed (transfers) from the previous success and reduces the level of negative affect necessary to trigger self-defensive behavior. Regardless of the specifics, this line of thinking suggests that the role of affect in regulating behavior may be more general than previously recognized.

In spite of the intuitive appeal of the idea that affect is the medium of communication among various self-defense and augmentation processes, several lines of work argue against this notion. First, in his seminal chapter, Steele (1988) rejects this idea because self-reports of affect in some of his studies show no relationship to self-defense processes. More recently, Steele,

Spencer, and Lynch (1994, Study 3) specifically manipulated mood before putting subjects in a dissonant situation. If mood is the crucial component of self-affirmation, then positive-mood subjects should show less dissonance reduction than negative-mood subjects. Although there was good evidence that the moods were quite different in the two conditions, there were no differences with respect to dissonance reduction.

Steele has manipulated affect and found no effect on dissonance reduction. Greenberg, Pyszczynski, Solomon, and their colleagues have shown the other side of this nonrelationship—that is, evidence of change in qualitatively different systems without self-rated covariation in mood. One set of studies showed that reminding people of their mortality increases attraction to culturally similar people and decreases attraction to culturally dissimilar people. Mood did not show any evidence of mediating these effects across three studies (Greenberg et al., 1990). In a more recent set of studies, self-esteem was manipulated via personality feedback and was shown to buffer the experience of anxiety arising from making one's own mortality salient. Again, self-rated affect seemed to play no mediational role (Greenberg et al., 1992).

There is a resolution. The paradigms in which affect has consistently been related to SEM functioning and dissonance reduction are missattribution paradigms. For these paradigms to work, subjects must be unaware either of their arousal or of the source of the arousal. Recently in social psychology, a good deal of attention has been given to priming effects on judgment and the effects of feelings on judgment. Recent reviews by Bargh (1992), Clore (1992), Martin and Achee (1992), and Schwarz and Bless (1992) make it clear that priming is most effective when the individual is unaware of the prime, and that the impact of "irrelevant" feelings on a particular judgment is greatest when the individual is unaware of the locus of the feelings. More to the point is a paper by Murphy and Zajonc (1993). In their work, positive and negative affect were primed without awareness (smiling and frowning faces shown at 8 milliseconds). These feelings tended to be attached to whatever supraliminal stimulus was contiguous. However, when these affective primes were presented at supraliminal speeds, the feelings associated with them were not attached to contiguous stimuli.

This work on the impact of feelings of unknown origin suggests that the medium of communication among self-defense mechanisms may still be affect, but affect whose origin is unknown. This would explain why self-ratings of affect and overt manipulations of affect fail to relate to the communication among self processes. What is needed is research showing that affect of unknown origin has an effect on the propensity to engage self-regulatory mechanisms, whereas affect of clear origin does not.

On the Importance of Other Self-Defense Mechanisms

We believe that affect is crucial to the unfolding of all self-defense mechanisms. If that is the case, why bother studying individual self-defense mechanisms? Why not simply study affect? After all, the self-defense mechanisms appear to be substitutable one for the other, and affect is the important mediator. We strongly disagree with this response, however.

The study of different defense mechansims tells us something fundamental about the psychological situations that generate affect. The psychological situations that the organism actually confronts are paramount. Knowing that affect is important is incomplete without knowing, for example, that inconsistencies as described by dissonance theorists produce affect. Knowledge of the psychological antecedents of and behavioral responses to threat is crucial to any complete psychology. An analogy to biology may be helpful here. Growth is not possible without protein; yet understanding the production of protein is not possible without an understanding of all digestive processes (not only the digestion of protein, but that of carbohydrates, fats, etc.). In sum, even if it turns out that affect is an important integrative principle, knowledge of individual self-defense mechanisms will remain critical.

CONCLUSION

Lewin's psychology of goal tensions appears to be useful even to today's concerns in social psychology. The present scene seems laden with a "zoo" of self-defense mechanisms. By following the lead of Lewin and his students (e.g., Zeigarnik and Ovianskina), we have found evidence that these various self-defense mechanisms seem to be subserving a common, higher-order goal, self-esteem. Affect, particularly affect of which the individual is unaware, may play an important role in the intercommunication of the various mechanisms.

ACKNOWLEDGMENTS

Work on this chapter was supported by Grant No. 10211RR274100 from the National Science Foundation and Grant No. BSR R01 MH41487 from the National Institute of Mental Health.

NOTES

1. For the purpose of this chapter, we use the term "self-evaluation" and "self-esteem" interchangeably. Elsewhere (e.g., Tesser, 1988), we have distinguished these two terms by suggesting that "self-esteem" generally refers to chronic individual differences in feelings about the self, and that "self-evaluation" generally refers to acute, situationally induced differences in such feelings. In the current discussion, we use both terms to refer to situationally induced changes in feelings about the self.

2. Subsequent work has found only mixed support for the Zeigarnik effect (see discussions by Heckhausen, 1989/1991, and Weiner, 1972, for example). Our work and our review of the literature (Martin & Tesser, in press) suggest that if interrup-

tion is construed as failure, then persons tend to repress the failure immediately, but the Zeigarnik tension tends subsequently to make the interrupted goals more available than the completed goal.

3. Although this study provides evidence for the goal tension hypothesis, it does not rule out a role for associative processes in the rebound process, nor does it directly address the question of an ironic monitoring process. (See Ansfield & Wegner, Chapter 21, this volume.)

4. Although Mahler's tasks were problem-solving in nature, they bring to mind some of the Freudian notions of the purpose of primary-process thinking. Freud suggested that primary-process thinking is in the service of wish (goal) fulfillment. Mahler was testing to see whether thought alone could reduce goal tension.

5. It is particularly noteworthy that the biggest change due to self-affirmation was in how the friend was treated in the high-relevance condition. Rather than "defensively" giving the friend difficult clues, subjects were now giving him more helpful, easy clues. It is as if the self-affirmation experience permits people to act nondefensively toward those who are close to them.

REFERENCES

Abramson, L. Y. , Metalsky, G. I., & Alloy, L. B. (1989). Helplessness depression: A theory based sub-type of depression. *Psychological Review, 96,* 358–372.

Achee, J., Tesser, A., & Pilkington, C. (1994). Social perception: A test of the role of arousal in self-evaluation maintenance processes. *European Journal of Social Psychology, 24,* 147–159.

Arkin, R. M. (1981). Self-presentation styles. In J. T. Tedeschi (Ed.), *Impression management theory and social psychological research* (pp. 311–333). New York: Academic Press.

Aronson, E. (1969). The theory of cognitive dissonance: A current perspective. In L. Berkowitz (Ed.), *Advances in experimental social psychology* (Vol. 4, pp. 2–32). New York: Academic Press.

Bargh, J. A. (1992). Why subliminality might not matter to social psychology: Awareness of the stimulus versus awareness of its influence. In R.F. Bornstein & T. S. Pittman (Eds.), *Perception without awareness* (pp. 236–255). New York: Guilford Press.

Baumeister, R. F. (1982). A self presentational view of social phenomena. *Psychological Bulletin, 91,* 3–26.

Baumgardner, A. H., & Brownlee, E. A. (1987). Strategic failure in social interaction: Evidence for expectancy disconfirmation processes. *Journal of Personality and Social Psychology, 52,* 525–535.

Berglas, S., & Jones, E. E. (1978). Drug choice as a self-handicapping strategy in response to noncontingent success. *Journal of Personality and Social Psychology, 36,* 405–517.

Brehm, J. W. (Ed.). (1966). *A theory of psychological reactance.* New York: Academic Press.

Carver, C. S., & Scheier, M. F. (1981). *Attention and self-regulation: A control-theory approach to human behavior.* New York: Springer-Verlag.

Clore, G. L. (1992). Cognitive phenomonology: Feelings and the construction of judgement. In L. L. Martin & A. Tesser (Eds.), *The construction of social judgments* (pp. 133–164). Hillsdale, NJ: Erlbaum.

Cooper, J., & Fazio, R. H. (1984). A new look at dissonance theory. In L. Berkowitz

(Ed.), *Advances in experimental social psychology* (Vol. 17, pp. 229–267). New York: Academic Press.

Cornell, D. (1990). *Attribution, task performance and self-evaluation maintenance.* Unpublished master's thesis. University of Georgia.

Cornell, D. P., & Tesser, A. (1994). *On the confluence of self-processes: II. SEM affects self-affirmation.* Unpublished manuscript, University of Georgia.

Dalhoff, R., & Tesser, A. (in preparation). *Social determinants of task effect.* Athens, GA: University of Georgia.

Fazio, R., & Cooper, R. (1983). Arousal in the dissonance process. In J. T. Cacioppo & R. E. Petty (Eds.), *Social psychophysiology: A sourcebook* (pp. 122–152). New York: Guilford Press.

Festinger, L. (1957). *A theory of cognitive dissonance.* Stanford, CA: Stanford University Press.

Greenberg, J., Pyszczynski, T., & Solomon, S. (1986). The causes and consequences of a need for self-esteem: A terror management theory. In R. F. Baumeister (Ed.), *Public self and private self* (pp. 189–212). New York: Springer-Verlag.

Greenberg, J., Pyszczynski, T., Solomon, S., Rosenblatt, A., Veeder, M., Kirkland, S., & Lyon, S. (1990). Evidence for terror management theory: II. The effects of mortality salience on reactions to those who threaten or bolster the cultural worldview. *Journal of Personality and Social Psychology, 58,* 308–318.

Greenberg, J., Solomon, S., Pyszczynski, T., Rosenblatt, A., Burling, J., Lyon, D., Simon, L., & Pinel, E. (1992). Why do people need self esteem? Converging evidence that self esteem serves an anxiety buffering function. *Journal of Personality and Social Psychology, 63,* 913–922.

Greenwald, A. G. (1980). The totalitarian ego: Fabrication and revision of personal history. *American Psychologist, 35,* 603–618.

Greenwald, A. G., & Ronis, D. L. (1978). Twenty years of cognitive dissonance: Case study of the evolution of a theory. *Psychological Review, 85,* 53–57.

Heckhausen, H. (1991). *Motivation and action* (P. K. Leppman, Trans.). New York: Springer-Verlag. (Original work published 1989)

Henle, M. (1944). The influence of valence on substitution. *Journal of Psychology, 17,* 11–19.

Higgins, E. T. (1987). Self-discrepancy: A theory relating self and affect. *Psychological Review, 94*(3), 319–340.

Isen, A. M. (1987). Positive affect, cognitive processes, and social behavior. In L. Berkowitz (Ed.), *Advances in experimental social psychology* (Vol. 20, pp. 203–253). New York: Academic Press.

Kelley, H. H. (1967). Attribution theory in social psychology. In D. Levine (Ed.), *Nebraska Symposium on Motivation* (Vol. 15, pp. 192–238). Lincoln: University of Nebraska Press.

Kihlstrom, J. F., Cantor, N., Albright, J. S., Chew, B. R., Klein, S. B., & Niedenthal, P. M. (1988). Information processing and the study of the self. In L. Berkowitz (Ed.), *Advances in experimental social psychology* (Vol. 21, pp. 145–178). New York: Academic Press.

Lewin, K. (1935). *A dynamic theory of personality: Selected papers* (D. E. Adams & K. E. Zener, Trans.). New York: McGraw Hill.

Linville, P. W. (1985). Self-complexity and affective extremity: Don't put all of your eggs in one basket. *Social Cognition, 3,* 94–120.

Linville, P. W. (1987). Self-complexity as a cognitive buffer against stress-related illness and depression. *Journal of Personality and Social Psychology, 52*(4), 663–676.

Lissner, K. (1933). Die entspannung von Bedurfnissen durch Ersatzhandlungen. *Psychologische Forschung, 18,* 218–250.

Liu, T. J., & Steele, C. M. (1986). Attributional analysis as self-affirmation. *Journal of Personality and Social Psychology, 51,* 531–540.

Mahler, V. (1933). Ersatzhandlungen verschiedenen Realitatsgrades. *Psychologische Forschung, 18,* 26–89.

Mandler, G. (1975). *Mind and emotion.* New York: Wiley.

Markus, H. (1977). Self-schemata and processing information about the self. *Journal of Personality and Social Psychology, 35,* 63–78.

Martin, L. L., & Achee, J. W. (1992). Beyond accessibility: The role of processing objectives in judgment. In L. L. Martin & A. Tesser (Eds.) *The construction of social judgments* (pp. 195–216). Hillsdale, NJ: Erlbaum.

Martin, L. L., & Tesser, A. (1989). Toward a motivational and structural theory of ruminative thought. In J. S. Uleman & J. A. Bargh (Eds.), *Unintended thought: Limits of awareness, intention, and control* (pp. 306–326). New York: Guilford Press.

Martin, L. L., & Tesser, A. (in press). Some ruminative thoughs. In R. S. Wyer (Ed.), *Advances in social cognition.* Hillsdale, NJ: Erlbaum.

Martin, L. L., Tesser, A., & McIntosh, W. D. (1993). Wanting but not having: The effects of unattained goals on thoughts and feelings. In D. M. Wegner & J. W. Pennebaker (Eds.), *The handbook of mental control* (pp. 552–572). New York: Prentice Hall.

Murphy, S. T., & Zajonc, R. B. (1993). Affect, cognition, and awareness: Affective priming with optimal and suboptimal stimulus exposures. *Journal of Personality and Social Psychology, 64,* 723–739.

Ovsiankina, M. (1928). Die Wiederaufnahme unterbrochener Handlugen. *Psychologische Forschung, 11,* 302–379.

Pittman, T. S., & D'Agostino, P. R. (1985). Motivation and attribution: The effects of control deprivation and subsequent information processing. In J. Harvey & G. Weary (Eds.), *Current perspectives on attribution research* (Vol. 1, pp. 117–141). New York: Academic Press.

Pittman, T. S., & Pittman, N. L. (1980). Deprivation of control and the attribution process. *Journal of Personality and Social Psychology, 39,* 377–389.

Pleban, R., & Tesser, A. (1981). The effects of relevance and quality of another's performance on interpersonal closeness. *Social Psychology Quarterly, 44,* 278–285.

Pyszczynski, T., & Greenberg, J. (1987). Self-regulatory perseveration and the depressive self-focusing style: A self-awareness theory of reactive depression. *Psychological Bulletin, 102,* 122–138.

Schachter, S. (1964). The interaction of cognitive and physiological determinants of emotional state. In L. Berkowitz (Ed.), *Advances in experimental social psychology* (Vol. 1, pp. 49–79). New York: Academic Press.

Schwarz, N., & Bless, H. (1992). Constructing reality and its alternatives: An inclusion/exclusion model of assimilation and contrast effects in social judgment. In L. L. Martin & A. Tesser (Eds.), *The construction of social judgments* (pp. 217–245). Hillsdale, NJ: Erlbaum.

Seligman, M. E. P. (1975). *Helplessness: On depression, development, and death.* San Francisco: W. H. Freeman.

Simon, L., Greenberg, J., & Brehm, J. (1992). *In defense of Festinger's original cognitive dissonance theory: Conceptual and empirical challenges to alternative formulations.* Unpublished manuscript, University of Arizona.

Steele, C. M. (1988). The psychology of self-affirmation: Sustaining the integrity of self. In L. Berkowitz (Ed.), *Advances in experimental social psychology* (Vol. 21, pp. 261–302). New York: Academic Press.

Steele, C. M., & Liu, T. J. (1981). Making the dissonance act unreflective of the self: Dissonance avoidance and the expectancy of a value affirming response. *Personality and Social Psychology Bulletin, 45,* 5–19.

Steele, C. M., & Liu, T. J. (1983). Dissonance processes as self-affirmation. *Journal of Personality and Social Psychology. 45,* 5–19.

Steele, C. M., Spencer, S. J., & Lynch, M. (1994). Self-image resilience and dissonance: The role of affirmational resources. *Journal of Personality and Social Psychology, 64,* 885–896.

Swann, W. B. (1983). Self-verification: Bringing social reality into harmony with the self. In J. Suls & A. G. Greenwald (Eds.), *Psychological perspectives on the self* (Vol. 2, pp. 33–66). Hillsdale, NJ: Erlbaum.

Tesser, A. (1988). Toward a self-evaluation maintenance model of social behavior. In L. Berkowitz (Ed.), *Advances in experimental social psychology* (Vol. 21, pp. 181–227). New York: Academic Press.

Tesser, A., & Campbell, J. (1980). Self-definition: The impact of the relative performance and similarity of others. *Social Psychology Quarterly, 43,* 341–347.

Tesser, A., & Cornell, D. P. (1991). On the confluence of self-processes. *Journal of Experimental Social Psychology, 27,* 501–526.

Tesser, A., Millar, M., & Moore, J. (1988). Some affective consequences of social comparison and reflection processes: The pain and pleasure of being close. *Journal of Personality and Social Psychology, 54,* 49–61.

Tesser, A., Pilkington, C., & McIntosh, W. (1989). Self-evaluation maintenance and the mediational role of emotion: The perception of friends and strangers. *Journal of Personality and Social Psychology, 57,* 442–456.

Tesser, A., & Smith, J. (1980). Some effects of friendship and task relevance on helping: You don't always help the one you like. *Journal of Experimental Social Psychology, 16,* 582–590.

Vallacher, R. R., & Wegner, D. M. (1987). What do people think they're doing? Action identification and human behavior. *Psychological Review, 94,* 3–15.

Wegner, D. M., Schneider, D. J., Carter, S. R., & White, T. L. (1987). Paradoxical effects of thought suppression. *Journal of Personality and Social Psychology, 47,* 237–252.

Weiner, B. (1972). *Theories of motivation.* Chicago: Rand McNally.

Wicklund, R. A., & Gollwitzer, P. M. (1982). *Symbolic self-completion.* Hillsdale, NJ: Erlbaum.

Zeigarnik, B. (1927). Das Behalten erledigter und unerledigter Handlugen. *Psychologische Forshung, 9,* 1–85.

Zillman, D. (1983). Transfer of excitation in emotional behavior. In J. T. Cacioppo & R. E. Petty (Eds.), *Social psychophysiology: A sourcebook* (pp. 215–240). New York: Guilford Press.

Zuckerman, M. (1979). Attribution of success and failure revisited, or: The motivational bias is alive and well in attribution theory. *Journal of Personality, 47,* 245–287.

CHAPTER 4

Implicit Theories as Organizers of Goals and Behavior

Carol S. Dweck

The study of motivation is the study of people's goals and of the processes that guide the choice and pursuit of those goals. In this chapter, I show how "implicit theories"—people's basic assumptions about themselves and their world—guide the choice and pursuit of goals. I argue that these implicit theories create a meaning system or conceptual framework that influences which goals are salient and important to the individual.

The implicit theories that my colleagues and I have focused on in our research are beliefs about the malleability of human attributes, such as intelligence, personality, or moral character. We have found that believing that an attribute is a fixed entity (i.e., holding an entity theory) is consistently associated with different goals and behavior than is believing that an attribute is a dynamic, malleable quality. The study of implicit theories has a long and venerable history in psychology (Heider, 1958; Kelly, 1955) and is enjoying renewed interest (Epstein, 1989; Medin, 1989; Murphy & Medin, 1985; Ross, 1989). However, only recently have investigators identified specific theories that are central to people's belief systems and begun to spell out their consequences for motivation and behavior (see Epstein, 1989; Ross, 1989; Wittenbrink, Gist, & Hilton, 1993). This is precisely what we are attempting to do.

Our basic model is presented in Table 4.1. Essentially, it is proposed that a belief in a fixed trait orients an individual toward the goal of measuring, judging, or evaluating the trait. That is, when one holds an entity theory, the way one strives to know oneself and others is by diagnosing people's fixed attributes. In contrast, a belief in a more dynamic, malleable attribute—one that can be cultivated and changed—is proposed to orient the individual toward the goals of developing that attribute and of understanding the dynamics behind human behavior in that domain.

What impact will these theories and goals have on actions? It is important to note that we have studied people's reactions to negative outcomes and behaviors, and so I focus on that here. Moreover, for illustrative pur-

TABLE 4.1. Overview of Model

Theory	Goal	Reaction (given negative outcome or behavior)
Entity (attribute is fixed)	To evaluate, judge attribute	Global judgment → helplessness; punishment
Incremental (attribute is malleable)	To develop attribute, to understand dynamics	Process analysis → mastery orientation; education, rehabilitation

poses I focus on individuals' implicit theories about their own intelligence and about other people's moral characters as I examine the effects of theories on goals and actions.

In overview, the model proposes that when individuals hold an entity theory of their intelligence and are oriented toward the goal of judging their intelligence, they are likely to view negative outcomes as reflections of their intelligence and will be vulnerable to a "helpless" reaction. In contrast, when individuals hold an incremental theory of their intelligence and are oriented toward developing their intelligence, they will be more likely to view setbacks as cues to focus on their effort or strategy (process analysis) and will be more likely to display a more mastery-oriented reaction. Thus, in the domain of intelligence, I argue that the different theories create frameworks that foster different goals, impart different meanings to failure outcomes, and thus promote different reactions.

With regard to theories about others' character, the model proposes that when individuals hold an entity theory and are oriented toward evaluating character from people's behavior, they are likely to view negative behavior (1) as reflecting global negative character traits (e.g., "dishonest" or "evil") and (2) as calling for punishment. In contrast, when individuals who hold an incremental theory of character (and are oriented toward behavior analysis and attribute development) observe a negative behavior and analyze the reasons for it, their reaction is likely to be a desire to educate or rehabilitate the wrongdoer. Thus, here, too, I argue that one's implicit theory creates a meaning system within which goals are adopted and events are interpreted and reacted to.

Before I turn to the research that provides support for the model, it is important to note several things about our implicit-theory construct and measures.

MEASUREMENT OF IMPLICIT THEORIES

First, it should be emphasized that implicit theories can be domain-specific. That is, people may have different theories about different attributes; they may believe, for example, that intelligence is fixed but moral character is malleable. Moreover, it is the theory in a particular domain that predicts goals and reactions in that domain. Thus, for an individual who has an entity theory of intelligence but an incremental theory of moral character, the entity theory will provide the framework for motivation and reactions in the intellectual domain, while the incremental theory will provide the framework that structures issues relating to moral character.

In line with the domain-specific nature of implicit-theories, individuals' entity versus incremental theories about different attributes are assessed by separate implicit theory measures. For example, an entity versus incremental theory of intelligence is assessed by items such as "You have a certain amount of intelligence and you really can't do much to change it," and "Your intelligence is something about you that you can't change very much." An entity versus incremental theory of moral character is assessed by items such as "A person's moral character is something very basic about them and it can't be changed very much," and "Whether a person is responsible and sincere or not is deeply ingrained in their personality. It cannot be changed very much." (Note that the implicit theory of intelligence and the implicit theory of moral character form clear, independent factors in a factor analysis, further supporting the domain specificity of the theories.) The respondents are asked to indicate their agreement with each item on a 6-point scale ranging from 1 ("strongly agree"), to 2 ("agree"), 3 ("mostly agree"), . . . and 6 ("strongly disagree"). Then their scores on items measuring implicit theory *in the same domain* are averaged to form an overall implicit-theory score for that domain, with a lower score indicating a stronger endorsement of an entity theory. In each domain in our research, typically about 42.5% of the respondents agree consistently with an entity theory (an average implicit-theory score of 3.0 or below), and about the same percentage of respondents agree consistently with an incremental theory. The remaining 15% of the respondents have unclear theories, and they are excluded from our analyses. Because only 15% of the participants are excluded, the two theory groups do not represent extreme groups.

Extensive data attesting to the reliability and validity of the implicit-theory measures are summarized elsewhere (Dweck, Chiu, & Hong, 1995). Very briefly, both the implicit theory of intelligence measure and the implicit theory of morality measure have high internal reliability (across studies, α ranged from .94 to .98 for the implicit theory of intelligence, and .85 to .94 for the implicit theory of morality). The test–retest reliability of the measures over a 2-week interval was .80 for the measure of the intelligence theory, and .80 for the measure of the morality theory. With respect to the theory measures' validity, both the implicit-theory measure of intelligence and that of morality are independent of the respondents' sex, age, political affiliation, and religion. Moreover, they do not correlate with measures of self-presentation concerns (the Snyder [1974] Self-Monitoring Scale and the Paulhus [1984] Social Desirability Scale), cognitive ability (as indexed by Scholastic Aptitude Test scores), self-esteem (Coopersmith, 1967), optimism or confidence in other people and the world (Chiu & Dweck, 1994), social/political attitudes such as authoritarianism (Altemeyer, 1981), and political conservatism or liberalism (Kerlinger, 1984). In summary, the implicit-theory measures appear to be reliable and valid measures of the constructs.

It is important to note that neither theory is the "correct" one. We view these theories simply as different ways of constructing reality, each with its potential costs and benefits. For example, an entity theory, with its emphasis on stable traits that can be readily assessed, constructs for its adherents a parsimonious and knowable reality. However, the simplicity of an entity theory can sometimes lead too quickly to global trait judgments and helpless coping styles. In contrast, a incremental theory, with its emphasis on more specific process analysis, offers its adherents a more complex and less knowable reality. It is a theory that can foster effective persistence in the face of obstacles, but the possibility of change inherent in the theory means that the reality can never be known with any finality. Thus, the goal of our research is not to evaluate the correctness of the two theories, but to demonstrate that holding one view or the other has potentially important consequences.

IMPLICIT THEORIES OF INTELLIGENCE: RELATION TO GOALS AND BEHAVIOR

Our research on how implicit theories of intelligence predict achievement goals and patterns of behavior in the face of failure has been reviewed extensively elsewhere (Dweck, 1991; Dweck & Leggett, 1988). Here, I review the key studies from the past that tested the model, as well as some of the new studies that are particularly germane to the issues at hand.

Mary Bandura and I (Bandura & Dweck, 1985) set out to test the hypothesis that holding a fixed, or entity, theory of intelligence would predict a preference for "performance" goals (goals concerned with judgments of ability—gaining favorable judgments and avoiding unfavorable ones), whereas holding a malleable, or incremental, theory would predict a preference for "learning" goals (goals concerned with developing one's ability). In this study of fifth-grade children, and later in a study of eighth-grade children with Ellen Leggett (see Dweck & Leggett, 1988), we measured students' theories of intelligence and then gave them a choice of learning or performance goals to pursue. Choosing to pursue a learning goal involved choosing to work on a task that was described as hard, new, and different, and as involving the risk of poor performance, but as providing an opportunity to learn some potentially important new skills. Choosing to pursue a performance goal involved choosing either (1) a task that was described as being something the child was good at and would show he or she was smart, or (2) a task that was said to be easy enough to ensure error-free performance. Thus the learning goal tasks provided students with the chance to develop an ability, whereas the performance goal tasks focused on gaining a positive judgment of their ability or avoiding a negative judgment. In both studies we found a clear, significant relation between the theory of intelligence the students endorsed and the goal they chose to pursue on an upcoming achievement task.

In the study by Dweck and Leggett (1988), for example, over 80% of the children classified as entity theorists selected performance goal tasks (tasks that would lead to favorable judgments), with a full 50% of the entity theorists choosing a task that was so easy that it eliminated any risk of a negative judgment. In contrast, the majority (over 60%) of the children classified as incremental theorists selected the learning goal task (one that they could learn from, but would not necessarily do well on). Fewer than 10% of the incremental theorists chose the easy task.

These studies thus showed that among children of equal ability, those who believed that their intelligence was a fixed trait were highly concerned with documenting the adequacy of that trait, whereas those who believed that their intelligence was a malleable quality were more concerned with taking on challenges that would develop that quality.

Our research has also shown that implicit theories predict helpless and mastery-oriented reactions to failure. But first, let us back up a moment and discuss how the motivational patterns we have been investigating relate to students' actual academic achievement. Interestingly, in grade school, they mostly do not. Many of the very brightest students hold an entity theory, prefer performance goals, and tend to display helpless responses in our experimental situations. However, this may pose no liability in grade school, because challenges and obstacles may generally be at a minimum. By the same token, the incremental theory, learning goals, and mastery-oriented pattern may not confer an advantage in grade school, since challenge seeking and long-term persistence may not yet be rewarded or required.

However, we made the clear prediction that when the academic work became more challenging, and persistence in the face of failure became necessary, then the implicit theories would begin to predict actual academic achievement. This heightened challenge is precisely what occurs in junior high school: The material becomes more difficult, the grading becomes more stringent, and the instruction often becomes less personalized.

To test our hypothesis, we (Henderson & Dweck, 1990) followed seventh-grade students through their transition to junior high school. At the beginning of seventh grade, we measured their theories of intelligence and their confidence in their intelligence. We had their grades and achievement test scores from sixth grade, and we had the grades they later earned on their seventh-grade report cards. The question, again, was whether children's theories of intelligence would predict their gains and losses in academic achievement over this challenging transition.

As we predicted, when they faced the difficulties of this new setting, entity theorists showed clear losses in their academic standing, whereas incremental theorists showed clear gains. Basically, among the entity theorists, those who had been low achievers in sixth grade remained low achievers in seventh grade, and many of those who had previously been high achievers now joined the ranks of the lower achievers. In contrast, among the incremental theorists, those who had been high achievers in sixth grade were still high achievers in seventh grade, and many of those who had been relatively low in achievement were now among the higher achievers. Interestingly, students' confidence in their intelligence, unlike their theories about their intelligence, did not predict their achievement over this challenging transition (see also Hong, Chiu, & Dweck, 1995.)

Entity theorists also reported being more apprehensive about their schoolwork than incremental theorists, and were more likely to believe that failures reflected on their ability. Entity theorists thus showed the negative ability inferences, the negative affect, and the performance decline characteristic of the helpless pattern. In summary, believing in fixed intelligence did not appear to stand students in good stead when they encountered a sustained academic challenge. In contrast, children who believed in acquirable intelligence appeared to thrive in an environment that presented challenging learning opportunities.[1]

In a study of college students, we (Zhao & Dweck, 1994) gave subjects with entity and incremental theories of intelligence actual and hypothetical failures to respond to. Entity theorists showed more negative responses to both. For example, for the hypothetical failures, subjects were given three scenarios vividly describing academic setbacks. Following each, they were asked to describe what they would think, how they would feel, and what they would do. Entity theorists' responses contained significantly more global, negative inferences about themselves and their intelligence ("I would think I was a loser," "a failure," "stupid") than did incremental theorists' responses. Entity theorists also significantly more often reported extreme negative affect ("I would feel devastated") and significantly less often reported that they would use constructive problem-solving strategies. In contrast, incremental theorists' responses were consistently more mastery-oriented in their emphasis on direct confrontation of the situation through effort and problem solving.

In several studies, we have manipulated students' theories of intelligence (Bergen, 1991; Dweck, Tenney, & Dinces, reported in Dweck & Leggett, 1988) and documented their impact on goal choice and behavior. These studies showed, first, that people's theories are not fixed traits; they are beliefs that, like most beliefs, are subject to influence. The studies also suggested that the theories of intelligence can have a direct causal effect on goals and behaviors in situations that involve intellectual achievement.

To review, we have shown that holding an entity theory of intelligence predicts (1) a concern with judgment—that is, with documenting the adequacy of one's intelligence through the pursuit of performance goals, and (2) a vulnerability to the helpless response pattern in the face of negative outcomes. In contrast, holding an incremental theory of intelligence predicts

(1) a concern with developing one's abilities through the pursuit of learning goals, and (2) a mastery-oriented response to challenge and obstacles.

IMPLICIT THEORIES OF PERSONALITY AND CHARACTER

I now turn to an examination of how implicit theories predict the goals and actions people pursue as they deal with other people—as they form impressions of them, make decisions about them, and act on those decisions. Thus I turn to implicit theories about others, particularly theories about their personality and moral character, for these are major dimensions on which people base their impressions.

Much of our research in this area has involved asking people to react to negative behavior on the part of others. This is because we are especially interested in negative labeling and the actions that follow from it, but we have also begun to look at reactions to positive behavior, and I report these findings as well.

In most of the studies I describe, the research participants are presented with information about a "target" person (e.g., in the form of a narrated slide show, a written description, or a photograph). This information is, of course, quite preliminary, but it is ideal for studying a number of things—how quickly people think they can make confident judgments about others, what information they think is relevant for rendering those judgments, for how long they expect these judgments to be valid, and what decisions they feel comfortable basing on this information. In most cases, the "behaviors" or "reactions" we have studied are the actions our research participants say should be taken or say they would engage in, given the target person's behavior.

In all of the studies, we first classify participants with respect to their implicit theories—most typically in these studies, their theory about the malleability of moral character. As noted at the outset, we have hypothesized that entity theorists, believing in static traits, should view the goal of impression formation as being to make judgments of those traits. In this framework, I have suggested, to come to know someone is to form an evaluation of his or her major attributes.

In contrast, it was hypothesized that incremental theorists, believing in a more dynamic and malleable human reality, should seek to understand people in a way that fit with this view of reality. I have suggested that instead of trying to measure traits, they should try to understand the dynamics of people's behavior—what people's beliefs, motives, feelings, and the like must have been to lead them to behave in the way they did.

Trait versus State Social Judgments

The idea that the entity theory would be accompanied by a focus on trait judgments, whereas the incremental theory would be accompanied by a relatively greater emphasis on understanding the dynamics of behavior, was tested in several ways. First, we looked at the kinds of inferences people with different theories made from a behavior—whether they made inferences about a rather global trait, or instead about a mediating psychological process or state. To begin to explore this question, Hong (1994) presented college students with descriptions of 24 simple episodes in which a person performed a positive or negative behavior—for example, "Alexis stole the bread from the bakery shop." After each of these episodes, participants were asked to make causal attributions for the behavior by completing the sentence "This probably occurred because. . . . "

Participants' responses were coded to determine the number of global traits and the number of psychological states they generated. For instance, if in response to "Alexis stole the bread from the bakery shop," they said that it probably occurred because Alexis was a thief or a dishonest person, then these responses were categorized as "trait" responses. If, instead, they said that it probably happened because Alexis was hungry or desperate, then these were coded as "state" responses (as were all responses that referred to the person's goals, needs, emotions, or construals of the situation).

The findings showed that in explaining people's actions, entity theorists offered appreciably and significantly more trait responses than did incremental theorists. Although both groups offered many state responses, only the incremental theorists generated significantly more state responses than trait responses. Thus, very clear differences emerged between entity and incremental theorists in their relative emphasis on traits and states as descriptions and explanations. This was true for both positive and negative actions, suggesting that the entity theorists are not simply more negative, but rather readily draw global positive inferences as well.

Given this initial evidence that people with different theories do in fact differ in the ways that they characterize people and understand their behavior, we next asked whether these are differences that arise rather spontaneously at the time that they first encode social information. That is, are these differences so basic to the way that entity versus incremental theorists organize and understand their social world that they actually take in social information in these different ways?

To address this question, Hong (1994) presented research participants with social information: pictures of faces expressing positive or negative emotions (on a computer screen), followed by a trait or state (i.e., emotion) word. For example, a picture of an angry face might be followed by the trait word "mean" or "violent" or by the state word "furious" or "enraged"; a happy face might be followed by the trait word "friendly" or "amiable" or by the state word "happy" or "pleased." (Both the trait and the state words had been generated by participants in a pilot study in response to the faces.) It was reasoned that people who encoded the faces in terms of traits should show facilitation in their response to the trait words. Since these were emotion faces, everyone was expected to encode in terms of emotions to some extent. It was therefore predicted that group differences would lie primarily in responses to trait words.

The faces were selected from Ekman and Friesen's (1975) standard emotion faces. It was decided to present faces as the social information in this study, as opposed to the descriptive sentences used in the previously described study, because stimuli involving actions create an interpretation problem (Bassili, 1989; Newman & Uleman, 1993). If, for example, a depiction of an action is followed with the word "violent," does this word refer to a trait of the actor, or is it simply a description of the act? Participants, regardless of their implicit theory, may quickly recognize and respond to the word "violent," but we would not know which sense of the word they were responding to. The facial stimuli do not pose this problem (see Trope, 1986, for a similar use of emotion faces, as social stimuli).

The procedure, more fully, was as follows. Participants, seated in front of a computer, were first shown each of the five faces for 10 seconds, to familiarize them with the faces and to permit them to form an impression. Each face was then presented again and was followed rapidly by a trait word, state words, or neutral word (matched with the trait and state word for length and frequency). Sometimes the words appeared in their normal form, and sometimes the letters were scrambled. The task for the participants was to judge, as quickly as they could, whether the string of letters they saw was a word or a nonword.

The results showed a striking difference between entity and incremental theorists in their responses to trait words. The measure of how much the emotion face facilitated responses to the trait and state words consisted of how much more quickly participants responded to trait or state words preceded by the relevant face than they responded to the matched neutral words (preceded by that same face). It was found that entity theorists showed far more facilitation to the trait words than incremental theorists showed, suggesting that they had indeed encoded the social information in terms of traits. Although both groups showed appreciable facilitation of the state/emotion words, incremental theorists showed far more facilitation (nearly twice as much) to the state words than to the trait terms; this suggested that emotion words were more familiar or meaningful to them, given the way they had encoded the information.

In summary, the results from this study provided strong support for the idea that entity and incremental theorists focus differentially on trait versus psychological process information as they form impressions, with entity theorists appearing to make spontaneous judgments of underlying traits, and incremental theorists focusing relatively more on specific psychological states.

Thus far we have shown that when confronted with information about a person, entity and incremental theorists differ in the way they understand it (e.g., what it implies about the person and why it happened). Moreover, these differences in understanding appear to happen rather quickly and spontaneously. But subjects in these studies were presented with information out of context; they were told nothing about the situation in which the action occurred or the intention of the person performing the action. Would the differences between the entity and incremental theorists disappear if this kind of information were to be introduced? In particular, would the tendency of entity theorists to render trait inferences be diminished if they were told more about the situational pressures acting on the person or if they learned that the intentions of the person were benign? The studies described next were designed to illuminate this issue.

Providing Contextual Information

In the first study (Sorich & Dweck, 1994), college students were given two scenarios in which they read about a person performing an undesirable action, but were also told about the person's psychological state and about the situational pressures acting on him or her. For example, they read about a student who was distraught about performing poorly in an important course, who came across a copy of an upcoming exam, and who succumbed to the temptation to look at it. Participants then rated the causes of the target's actions on a number of dimensions, including negative traits (e.g., dishonesty or selfishness). Our findings showed that across scenarios, entity theorists rated the negative traits as significantly more important causes of the actions than did the incremental theorists. That is, even when clear information was presented about the target person's situation and psychological state, entity theorists still were more likely to focus on traits. I return to this study later to examine what consequences the participants thought should befall the wrongdoers.

A study with children (fourth- and fifth-graders) yielded similar findings (Erdley & Dweck, 1993). In this study, children were presented with a narrated slide show portraying a new boy in school. The boy had recently moved to town and was entering the class in the middle of the year. Thus he was particularly nervous and eager to make a good impression on his new classmates. However, in the service of making a good impression, he committed a number of transgressions. For example, embarrassed that he did not know how to solve the math problems in the assignment, he tried to copy his neighbor's work. Before each transgression, the boy displayed his discomfort and ruminated about what to do. That is, his motives and his psychological state were made very clear, as was the fact that his actions really never harmed anyone.

Children rated the boy on a number of characteristics, including the global traits "bad," "mean," and "nasty." As we predicted, after children observed the transgressions, entity theorists rated the boy far more negatively on these global traits than did incremental theorists. Is it just that entity theorists are more negative or extreme in their judgments of people? Other findings from this study indicate that they are not. Children in the study were also asked to rate the boy in the slide show on very specific characteristics—ones directly related to the behaviors he displayed. Our results showed that on these more specific characteristics, incremental theorists were just as negative and extreme as entity theorists. Both groups rated the boy as having exhibited these characteristics to a great degree. Thus it is not the case that incremental theorists simply view negative behavior in a positive light or are reluctant to voice disapproval of a negative act. Nor is it the case that incremental theorists do not use traits. Rather, it appears that incremental theorists tend to remain more anchored than entity theorists to the specific behaviors they observe in drawing their inferences, and are less drawn to more global conclusions about the person.

In summary, then, providing more information about situational pressures or psychological states does not seem to eliminate the differences between entity and incremental theorists in their trait explanations or trait inferences. Of course, we would expect that these differences might be eliminated if situational pressures became very strong, so that people thought that virtually anyone in that situation would act that way (Jones & Thibaut, 1958). The difference between entity and incremental theorists might also be attenuated if the behaviors were so distinctive that they appeared to speak strongly and exclusively to the character of the person (Kelley & Michela, 1980). In fact, a variety of studies have shown that trait inferences become less frequent as the behavior becomes more universal and more frequent as the behavior becomes more distinctive (for reviews, see Bierhoff, 1989, and Kelley & Michela, 1980). We next asked about the effects of providing information about a person's intention. In all of the studies presented thus far, our participants judged people who consciously and intentionally performed an action. They may have felt pressured or they may have felt some reluctance in some cases, but nonetheless they willingly committed the act. Therefore we conducted several studies to explore how entity and incremental theorists would judge people who performed an action unintentionally—that is, accidentally.

Providing Intention Information

In these studies (Chiu, Parker, Hong, & Dweck, 1994), our participants read scenarios in which similar actions were performed intentionally versus accidentally. For example, they read about a jealous student who tried to sabotage a classmate's chemistry work by mixing the wrong chemicals together. They also read about a student who accidentally mixed the wrong chemicals, thereby putting his classmate's work in jeopardy. After each scenario, we asked our participants to generate personality adjectives that described the person in the story, and to rate him or her on a number of trait dimensions, such as "kind–cruel," "benevolent–malicious," and "responsible–irresponsible."

Our results showed that, as expected, when the person performing the act had a negative intention, entity theorists generated more negative character traits (e.g., "evil" or "heartless") than did incremental theorists. (When we portrayed the person as having a positive intention, entity theorists ascribed more positive traits to him or her.) Entity theorists also rated the person more extremely on the traits we presented to them. Thus, when the actions were intentional, entity theorists, in line with our previous findings, saw the actions as indicative of the badness or goodness of the person's moral character.

What happened when the actions were unintentional? We still found a significant difference between entity and incremental theorists in their trait inferences, with entity theorists again generating more traits to describe the person and making more extreme trait ratings. However, these traits referred primarily to the social competence and responsibility of the person (e.g., "jerk," "clumsy idiot," or "complete nerd"), rather than to his or her general goodness. These findings show that depicting actions as accidental rather than intentional does not at all eliminate the difference between entity and incremental theorists in their tendency to make trait inferences. It simply leads entity theorists to make inferences about different traits. That is, someone who intentionally creates the potential for harm is evil, but someone who does it unintentionally is socially incompetent or irresponsible.

How Readily Are Trait Judgments Made?

In the studies described so far, we gave people very sparse and preliminary information about the persons they were supposed to judge. Usually this information consisted of a single action or several actions, with, at most, some information about each situation and the person's motives and feelings. How sparse can this information be and still provide a basis for trait judgments? I have already described one study in which we provided nothing more than facial expressions, and still found evidence for different patterns of judgment. In another set of studies (Gervey, Chiu, Hong, & Dweck, 1993), which I describe in more detail later, people were simply given a written physical description embedded in a much larger passage. Here we were interested in whether people (particularly entity theorists) would use the physical description as a basis for moral judgments, and as a basis for the decision we asked them to make: whether the person was guilty of murder. In these studies, our participants read a summary transcript of a murder trial in which the defendant was described by a witness as having been dressed and groomed in a "respectable" manner (a business suit, clean-shaven) or in a less respectable manner (a leather jacket with zippers, a beard) on the day of the crime. We found that these physical descriptions had a clear and significant impact on the morality ratings of the entity theorists. Entity theorists consistently rated the respectably groomed defendant as more moral than his less respectably groomed counterpart. In contrast, these descriptions had no effect on the morality ratings incremental theorists made of the defendants. Moreover, as I describe later, the descriptions also had a clear impact on the entity theorists' verdicts.

All of these findings imply that entity theorists find it rather easy to judge people's moral character. In each case, very simple information about a person's actions or demeanor was sufficient to produce moral judgments. These findings led us to wonder whether, if asked, entity theorists would in fact say that it was easy to judge people's moral character. Therefore, as part of a larger study (Sorich & Dweck, 1994), we directly asked entity and incremental theorists this question. Specifically, we asked college students to indicate their degree of disagreement with the following statements: "Each person has a basic character, and you can tell what kind of person someone is even by details of their behavior or appearance," "A single act often tells you a lot about a person's fundamental character," and "It's fairly easy to tell what kind of a person someone is by observing them on one or two occasions." The results showed a significant difference between entity and incremental theorists in their tendency to agree with these statements, with entity theorists falling on the "agree" side of the scale and incremental theorists falling on the "disagree" side.

Our findings, then, are consistent in suggesting that those who believe in fixed traits believe that these traits are easily known from their external manifestations. Incremental theorists, believing in a more dynamic reality, do not tend to view small samples of behavior observed in a limited context at a given moment in time as diagnostic of a person's underlying character. For them, moral character is likely to be something that one comes to know by observing someone in many contexts over a long period of time. Moreover, since in their view people can change, it is difficult in most cases to make a final diagnosis of someone's character.

Encoding Information

So far I have dealt with the kinds of impressions people form—whether they attempt to diagnose global traits or to understand the dynamics of behavior. If entity and incremental theorists have these different goals as they seek to know people, we wondered whether they actually take in information in different ways—whether they encode information in ways that are consonant with these goals and that further these goals. Specifically, if entity theorists are seeking to make global trait judgments (Is this person good or bad? Competent or incompetent?), will they code incoming information in highly evaluative ways so that they can readily weigh that information and arrive at a trait judgment? In contrast, if incremental theorists are seeking to understand the dynamics of behavior, will they code the same information in a less evaluative, more neutral way, so that they can reconfigure and reinterpret this information as new evidence accrues?

To test this hypothesis, we (Hong, Chiu, Dweck, & Sacks, 1994) gave entity and incremental theorists (college students) information about an aspiring pilot who was attending a pilot-training school. The information we gave them consisted of the trainee's scores on the 20 scales of a pilot aptitude test. There was a range of scores, and the average score was about average for a pilot trainee. How did we know whether our participants attached clear evaluations to the scores? Previous researchers (Bargh, Chaiken, Govender, & Pratto, 1992; cf. Fazio, Sanbonmatsu, Powell, & Kardes, 1986) have found that when people have evaluated something positively (e.g., ice cream) or negatively (e.g., rats), these items will have an effect on how they react to what they see next. For example, if the word "ice cream" on a computer screen is followed by another positive word ("lovely"), then people will recognize and respond more quickly to "lovely" than they would have ordinarily. On the other hand, if "ice cream" is followed by a negative word ("gruesome"), then people will recognize and respond more slowly to "gruesome" then they ordinarily would have. In the same vein, a negative object ("rats") will speed up people's responses to negative words and will slow their responses to positive ones. We reasoned that if our participants had attached clear evaluations to the trainee's scores, then the scores should work in the same way as "ice cream" or "rats," facilitating or retarding responding to positive and negative words that followed them.

This was precisely what happened for entity theorists: High and low scores worked just like positive and negative objects. Specifically, a while after subjects were exposed to the test scores, they were asked to work on a task in which an attitude object (e.g., "ice cream" or "rats") or a test score (a high or low score earned by the pilot trained on the aptitude test) was presented briefly, followed by a positive or negative adjective (e.g., "lovely" or "gruesome"). The subjects' task was to decide as quickly as possible whether the adjective presented was positive or negative. As predicted, high scores helped entity theorists to recognize and respond to positive words and hindered their responding to negative ones. The scores produced no such effects for incremental theorists. That is, although incremental theorists clearly recognized which scores were high and which were low, they did not attach strong personal evaluations to them.

According to these findings, then, entity theorists indeed appear to attach evaluative labels to new information in the same way that they attach evaluative labels to liked and disliked objects. These results provide support for our idea that entity theorists encode information in ways that prepare them to make trait inferences, whereas incremental theorists encode the same information in ways that keep it more neutral and perhaps more amenable to reconsideration.

We have shown that people with different theories tend to characterize people in different ways. They form different kinds of judgments, and even encode new information in ways that may set up the different judgments. Do these differences extend beyond judgments? That is, do entity theorists and incremental theorists make different decisions or favor different courses of action vis-à-vis the people they have observed?

Differences in Recommended Consequences for Wrongdoing

In a series of studies, we have shown that when entity theorists have observed wrongdoing and made negative judgments, they typically favor clear punitive actions toward the person. We did not necessarily expect these findings. It could have been that entity theorists, believing that one's character is not in one's control, would take a more lenient stance toward transgressions. However, they might believe that the transgressor, a "bad" person, deserves punishment. Or they might also believe that regardless of their underlying traits, people have an obligation to control their behavior, and should be punished when they do not. That is, they might believe that although character is fixed, the expression of that character in behavior can be regulated and that people have the obligation to do so. Nevertheless, it has been clear in each of our studies that entity theorists strongly believe in retribution.

In contrast, incremental theorists, who may be just as disapproving of the transgression, tend to favor measures for educating the wrongdoers—for example, teaching them why something is wrong, or giving them the means to cope with the situation in more appropriate ways. In other words, incremental theorists (who focus more on such things as people's beliefs, values, feelings, or skills as causes of their behavior) favor interventions that address these causes and thereby encourage more desirable behavior. I turn now to the research that has yielded these findings.

The first study that suggested this difference between entity and incremental theorists was the Erdley and Dweck (1993) study with children. You will recall that children watched a narrated slide show depicting a new boy in school who committed a number of transgressions. After watching the slide show, children answered a number of questions about the boy. One question referred to the amount of punishment they thought he deserved. It read: "Suppose the teacher found out about what John did and decided to punish him. How much punishment do you think he deserves?" Children indicated their decisions on a scale that ranged from "a little" to "a lot." Entity theorists recommended significantly more punishment than did incremental theorists (their recommendations fell near the end of the scale labeled "a lot," whereas the recommendations of incremental theorists fell in the middle of the scale labeled "a medium amount").

Another study described earlier (Sorich & Dweck, 1994) yielded further evidence for a difference between entity and incremental theorists in how they believe transgressions should be treated. In this study, our research participants read scenarios that depicted wrongdoing. In one case, a distraught student who was doing poorly in a course looked through a copy of an upcoming exam that was lying unattended. In another, a young man who was unhappy with his social life asked his friend's girlfriend for a date. As noted earlier, entity theorists were significantly more likely than incremental theorists to endorse global traits (e.g., "dishonest") as the causes of these behaviors. What is relevant here is that entity and incremental theorists also thought different things should happen to the transgressors. Entity theorists, compared to incremental theorists, more strongly endorsed the options that recommended punishment—for example, that the student be suspended or that the poacher's reputation be smeared. In contrast, incremental theorists showed a significantly greater preference than the entity theorists for options that recommended remediation or education of the wrongdoers—for example, confronting the transgressors and showing them why what they did was wrong.

As part of a larger study, we (Chiu & Dweck, 1994) gave college students scenarios depicting transgressions, and had them report what they would do or how they would act toward each transgressor if they were in that situation. In one scenario, students were asked to imagine that they were in a course in which the professor announced at the beginning of the semester how many points students would have to accumulate over the semester to earn final grades of A, B, or C. According to the scenario, the student, already having enough points for an A before the final, decides to spend more time studying for another course. Later, when too many students have earned A's, the professor decides to raise the cutoffs, and the student is now left with a B.

Entity theorists, far more often than incremental theorists, reported that they would try to retaliate—to punish the professor for going back on his word. Whereas over 20% of entity theorists spontaneously reported that they would take such an action, none of the incremental theorists offered this response. In contrast, incremental theorists, more often than entity theorists, reported that they would try to educate the professor, explaining to him the moral principle he had violated. Whereas over a third of the incremental theorists spontaneously generated this response, none of the entity theorists did so.

We also gave participants scenarios in which children did not obey adults or do the jobs that they were assigned to them. The most frequent response from the entity theorists (but a rare one from incremental theorists) was that they would punish the children for not acting the way they should. The most frequent response from incremental theorists (but one given by extremely few entity theorists) was that they would try to understand why the children had been unable or unwilling to do the job, and/or would provide the necessary encouragement or information for them to do the job in the future. Thus, once again, entity and incremental theorists showed a difference in their preference for punishment versus instruction.

In another recent study, we (Loeb & Dweck, 1994) gave college students vivid scenarios that portrayed incidents of victimization and asked them to imagine that the incidents had happened to them. In one, their long-term partner left them with no explanation. In another, they were in the library studying for a very important test and momentarily left their study notes unattended, when several students rushed by and stole their notes. In the third scenario, a medical laboratory failed to provide test results in a timely fashion, leaving them with some irreversible physical damage that could otherwise have been prevented.

After each scenario, the participants responded to a series of specific questions about the reactions they would have and the actions and the coping strategies they would pursue. Entity and incremental theorists showed dramatically different reactions to the incidents. As we will see, entity theorists appeared to feel extremely victimized and sought punishment and retaliation. In contrast, incremental theorists, although also quite upset, focused more than entity theorists on understanding and educating the perpetrators, as well as on addressing their own problems and getting on with their lives.

In terms of the specific reactions they endorsed, entity theorists felt much more strongly than incremental theorists that they would make strong and lasting negative judgments of the perpetrators. That is, they expressed significantly stronger agreement with such statements as "I would have strong and lasting negative thoughts about [the perpetrator], e.g., that he is a jerk or is evil." In the same vein, they reported more than incremental theorists that they would have strong, enduring negative feelings toward the perpetrators. However, more strikingly, they more strongly endorsed a desire to retaliate and harm, indicating greater agreement with such statements as "Frankly, I would try to hurt [the perpetrator] when the opportunity comes along," or "I would seriously consider aggression toward [the perpetrator]." And, when asked what the overall goal of their reaction would be, entity theorists, far more strongly than incremental theorists, endorsed the goal of punishing the perpetrators for the suffering and loss that they caused. Interestingly, this was the goal that received the lowest degree of endorsement from incremental theorists.

Incremental theorists, in contrast, reported that they would try to understand and forgive the perpetrators. That is, significantly more than entity theorists, they agreed with statements saying that they would feel sorry for the perpetrators, they would think there were strong situational reasons for what the perpetrators did, and they would try to understand and forgive them. Incremental theorists were also more mastery-oriented, in that they more strongly endorsed items that depicted problem-solving strategies (e.g., "I would collect information and analyze the situation and possible actions," "I would work out ways of improving the situation"). Finally, when asked what the overall goal of their reaction would be, incremental theorists, significantly more than entity theorists, endorsed the goal of educating the perpetrators ("I would focus on changing and educating [the perpetrators], explaining to them the consequences of their behavior and how they can improve"). This was the goal that received the lowest degree of endorsement from entity theorists.

In summary, this study provides further support for the idea that those who believe in fixed moral character tend to render stronger negative judgments in the face of wrongdoing, and tend to focus more on punishing the wrongdoers, than do those who believe that character is a more dynamic, malleable quality. The latter, in contrast, appear to focus more on understanding and educating those who have erred.

Earlier, in the discussion of trait judgments, I briefly described studies in which we asked our participants to imagine that they were jurors in a murder trial (see Gervey et al., 1993). In three studies, they read a summary transcript of a fictitious trial, and then rendered a verdict of guilt or innocence and rated the defendant on a variety of traits. As we noted, there were different versions of the transcript. In one version, the defendant was described by a witness as having been groomed in a more "respectable" manner on the day of the crime (i.e., as being clean-shaven and wearing a business suit). In the other version, he was described as having been groomed and garbed in a less respectable manner (i.e., as having a beard, wearing an earring in one ear, and wearing a leather jacket with lots of zippers). In one of the studies, we introduced a different way of varying respectability. In this study, a witness described the defendant as either having parked his Toyota and emerged from the public library with some books, or as having parked his motorcycle and emerged from the adult bookstore with some magazines.

As we reported earlier, the respectability information had a major impact on the moral judgments that the entity theorists made, but they had no impact on those of the incremental theorists. That is, entity theorists were far more likely than incremental theorists to see the defendant's exterior as a mirror of his interior. But the more important question was whether they were willing to base their verdict on the respectability information. In all three studies, entity theorists rendered dramatically different verdicts for the more respectable and less respectable defendants. Regardless of the actual evidence, they were very likely to find the less respectable defendant guilty and substantially less likely to find the more respectable one guilty. In contrast, the respectability evidence had no impact on whether incremental theorists convicted or exonerated the defendant.

Participants in one of the three studies were also asked what they thought the primary purpose of imprisonment was. Entity theorists were twice as likely as incremental theorists to say that the primary function of imprisonment is punishment or retribution. Incremental theorists were far more likely than entity theorists to say that the primary function of imprisonment is rehabilitation. Thus, entity and incremental theorists have very different ideas not only about how to judge wrongdoers (or suspected wrongdoers), but also about how to deal with them, with entity theorists more oriented toward punishment and retaliation, but incremental theorists more zealous about education or reform. Incremental theorists may view entity theorists' measures as harsh and as unlikely to address the root cause of the wrongdoing (e.g., the beliefs, the goals, or the skill deficits that might have led to the errant behavior). Entity theorists, not believing in fundamental change, may well view incremental theorists' measures as naive or idealistic and as coddling the wrongdoers instead of acting decisively to punish the misdeeds.

RELATIONS BETWEEN IMPLICIT THEORIES AND OTHER INDIVIDUAL-DIFFERENCE VARIABLES

Implicit theories of intelligence and moral character are statistically independent of generalized attitudes toward the self (self-confidence, self-esteem) and toward other people (optimism about human nature). They are independent of self-presentational concerns (self-monitoring, social desirability). They are also largely independent of such attitudinal syndromes as authoritarianism, liberalism, and conservatism. Thus the effects of implicit theories on judgments and reactions are not mediated by these other beliefs or attitudes.

However, the relation between these implicit theories and other process-oriented individual differences, such as attributional style (Peterson et al., 1982), uncertainty orientation (Sorrentino, Short, & Raynor, 1984), the need for cognition (Cacioppo & Petty, 1982), the need for closure (Kruglanski, Webster, & Klem, 1993), and the personal need for structure (Neuberg & Newsom, 1993), has not yet been examined. It is important to note that there are two important differences between implicit theories and these other process-oriented variables. First, by definition, an entity versus incremental theory refers only to the belief individuals hold about the fixedness or malleability of the attribute in question. This definition does not contain a processing style component or a motivational component, although as we have seen, subscribing to either theory may lead to certain processing strategies and goals (see also Dweck, Hong, & Chiu, 1993). The construct itself, then, has little overlap with individual differences in processing style or motivational set. Second, implicit theories are domain-specific, whereas most other process-oriented individual differences are not.

Nevertheless, implicit theories may form an interesting network with these other individual-difference variables. For example, my colleagues and I would predict that implicit theories would be associated with attributional style—specifically, with making internal trait attributions in the relevant domain. The studies described above showed that an entity theory in a particular domain is consistently associated with the tendency to make internal, global, and stable attributions in that domain. However, our model views causal attributions as part of a system of beliefs that begins with implicit theories. In our model, a belief in fixed traits is what leads to a focus on such traits as causal explanations for actions and outcomes. Thus, although attributions may well be mediators of subsequent reactions (Weiner, 1985), we propose that these attributions are fostered by people's implicit theories.

Our findings also suggest that the social world of the entity theorist is perceived to be relatively stable and predictable. Entity theorists' belief in a relatively simpler reality—one that may afford rather rapid closure—suggests the possibility that, relative to incremental theorists, entity theorists may exhibit a greater need for closure, a lower uncertainty orientation, a lower need for cognition, and a greater need for structure in the relevant domain. In our model, however, these orientations are seen to stem from the belief in a fixed, readily knowable reality versus a more complex and dynamic one.

In summary, although implicit theories and other process-oriented individual-difference variables are conceptually distinct and operationally independent, they may well be related to each other in interesting ways.

CONCLUSION

I have argued that people's implicit theories create a motivational framework—orienting people toward particular goals, fostering particular interpretations of events and actions, and promoting particular reactions. I have illustrated the theories and their motivational frameworks with research on people's implicit theories of intelligence and of moral character. Both of the frameworks I have described portray a coherent (albeit distinctly different) reality. Moreover, both frameworks are prevalent and plausible, and each has distinct advantages. The entity theory is a more parsimonious one that promises ready understanding of human behavior, and the incremental theory appears to be a more flexible one that can promote more constructive problem solving.

The thesis of this chapter, then, has been that people's motivational systems must be understood within the reality that they construct. Understanding people's implicit theories may be one way to gain insight into their reality.

NOTE

1. It is interesting to note that the different foci of the entity and incremental theorists are reminiscent of the deliberative versus implemental mind-sets described by Gollwitzer, Heckhausen, and Steller (1990), in that both individuals with incremental theories and implemental mind-sets seem more optimistic and mastery-oriented than their counterparts with entity theories and deliberative mind-sets.

REFERENCES

Altemeyer, B. (1981). *Right-wing authoritarianism.* Winnipeg: University of Manitoba Press.

Bandura, M. M., & Dweck, C. S. (1985). *The relationship of conceptions of intelligence and achievement goals to achievement-related behaviors.* Unpublished manuscript, Harvard University.

Bargh, J. A., Chaiken, S., Govender, R., & Pratto, F. (1992). The generality of the automatic attitude activation effect. *Journal of Personality and Social Psychology, 62,* 893–912.

Bassili, J. N. (1989). Traits as action categories versus traits as person attributes in social cognition. In J. N. Bassili (Ed.), *On-line cognition in person perception* (pp. 61–89). Hillsdale, NJ: Erlbaum.

Bergen, R. (1991). *Beliefs about intelligence and achievement-related behaviors.* Unpublished doctoral dissertation, University of Illinois.

Bierhoff, H. (1989). *Person perception and attribution.* London: Springer-Verlag.

Cacioppo, J. T., & Petty, R. E. (1982). The need for cognition. *Journal of Personality and Social Psychology, 42,* 116–131.

Chiu, C., & Dweck, C. S. (1994). *Implicit theories and bases of morality.* Unpublished manuscript, Columbia University.

Chiu, C., Parker, C., Hong, Y., & Dweck, C. S. (1994). *Lay dispositionism and implicit theories of personality.* Manuscript submitted for publication.

Coopersmith, S. (1967). *The antecedents of self-esteem.* San Francisco: W. H. Freeman.

Dweck, C. S. (1991). Self-theories and goals: Their role in motivation, personality, and development. In R. Dienstbier (Ed.), *Nebraska Symposium on Motivation: Vol. 38. Perspectives on motivation* (pp. 199–255). Lincoln: University of Nebraska Press.

Dweck, C. S., Chiu, C., & Hong, Y. (1995). The role of implicit theories in judgments and reactions: A world from two perspectives. *Psychological Inquiry, 6,* 267–285.

Dweck, C. S., Hong, Y., & Chiu, C. (1993). Implicit theories: Individual differences in the likelihood and meaning of dispositional inference. *Personality and Social Psychology Bulletin, 19,* 644–656.

Dweck, C. S., & Leggett, E. L. (1988). A social-cognitive approach to motivation and personality. *Psychological Review, 25,* 109–116.

Ekman, P., & Friesen, W. V. (1975). *Unmasking the face: A guide to recognizing emotions from facial clues.* Englewood Cliffs, NJ: Prentice-Hall.

Epstein, S. (1989). Values from the perspective of cognitive-experiential self-theory. In N. Eisenberg, J. Reykowski, & E. Staub (Eds.), *Social and moral values: Individual and social perspectives* (pp. 3–61). Hillsdale, NJ: Erlbaum.

Erdley, C. A., & Dweck, C. S. (1993). Children's implicit personality theories as predictors of their social judgments. *Child Development, 64,* 863–878.

Fazio, R. H., Sanbonmatsu, D. M., Powell, M. C., & Kardes, F. R. (1986). On the automatic activation of attitudes. *Journal of Personality and Social Psychology, 50,* 229–238.

Gervey, B. M., Chiu, C., Hong, Y., & Dweck, C. S. (1993). *Processing and utilizing information in social judgment: The role of implicit theories.* Paper presented at the Fifth Annual Convention of the American Psychological Society, Chicago.

Gollwitzer, P. M., Heckhausen, H., & Steller, B. (1990). Deliberative and implemental mind-sets: Cognitive tuning toward congruous thoughts and information. *Journal of Personality and Social Psychology, 59,* 1119–1127.

Heider, F. (1958). *The psychology of interpersonal relations.* New York: Wiley.

Henderson, V., & Dweck, C. S. (1990). Adolescence and achievement. In S. Feldman & G. Elliott (Eds.), *At the threshold: Adolescent development* (pp. 308–329). Cambridge, MA: Harvard University Press.

Hong, Y. (1994). *Predicting trait versus process inferences: The role of implicit theories.* Unpublished doctoral dissertation, Columbia University.

Hong, Y., Chiu, C., & Dweck, C. S. (1995). Implicit theories of intelligence: Reconsidering the role of confidence in achievement motivation. In M. Kernis (Ed.), *Efficacy, agency and self- esteem* (pp. 197–216). New York: Plenum.

Hong, Y., Chiu, C., Dweck, C. S., & Sacks, R. (1994). *Implicit theories and evaluative processes in person cognition.* Unpublished manuscript, Columbia University.

Jones, E. E., & Thibaut, J. W. (1958). Interaction goals as bases of inference in interpersonal perception. In R. Tagiuri & L. Petrullo (Eds.), *Person perception and interpersonal behavior* (pp. 151–178). Stanford, CA: Stanford University Press.

Kelley, H. H., & Michela, J. L. (1980). Attribution theory and research. *Annual Review of Psychology, 31,* 457–501.

Kelly, G. A. (1955). *The psychology of personal constructs.* New York: Norton.

Kerlinger, F. N. (1984). *Liberalism and conservatism: The nature and structure of social attitudes.* Hillsdale, NJ: Erlbaum.

Kruglanski, A. W., Webster, D. M., & Klem, A. (1993). Motivational resistance and openness to persuasion in the presence and absence of prior information. *Journal of Personality and Social Psychology, 65,* 861–876.

Loeb, I., & Dweck, C. S. (1994). *Beliefs about human nature as predictors of reactions to victimization.* Paper presented at the Sixth Annual Convention of the American Psychological Society, Washington, DC.

Medin, D. L. (1989). Concepts and conceptual structure. *American Psychologist, 44,* 1469–1481.

Murphy, G. L., & Medin, D. L. (1985). The role of theories in conceptual coherence. *Psychological Review, 92,* 289–316.

Neuberg, S. L., & Newsom, J. T. (1993). Personal need for structure: Individual differences in the desire for simple structure. *Journal of Personality and Social Psychology, 65,* 113–131.

Newman, L. S., & Uleman, J. S. (1993). When are you what you did? Behavior identification and dispositional inference in person memory, attribution, and social judgment. *Personality and Social Psychology Bulletin, 19,* 513–525.

Paulhus, D. L. (1984). Two-component models of socially desirable responding. *Journal of Personality and Social Psychology, 46,* 598–609.

Peterson, R. E., Semmel, A., von Baeyer, C., Abramson, L. Y., Metalsky, G. I., & Seligman, M. E. P. (1982). The Attributional Style Questionnaire. *Cognitive Therapy and Research, 6,* 287–300.

Ross, M. (1989). Relation of implicit theories to the construction of personal histories. *Psychological Review, 96,* 341–357.

Snyder, M. (1974). The self-monitoring of expressive behavior. *Journal of Personality and Social Psychology, 30,* 526–537.

Sorich, L., & Dweck, C. S. (1994). *Implicit theories as predictors of attributions for and response to wrongdoing* [Unpublished raw data]. Columbia University.

Sorrentino, R. M., Short, A. C., & Raynor, J. O. (1984). Uncertainty orientation: Implications for affective and cognitive views of achievement behavior. *Journal of Personality and Social Psychology, 46,* 189–206.

Trope, Y. (1986). Identification and inferential processes in dispositional attribution. *Psychological Review, 93,* 239–257.

Weiner, B. (1985). An attributional theory of achievement motivation and emotion. *Psychological Review, 92,* 548–573.

Wittenbrink, B., Gist, P. L., & Hilton, J. L. (1993). *The perceiver as alchemist: Conceptualizing stereotypes as theories.* Paper presented at the Fifth Annual Convention of the American Psychological Society, Chicago.

Zhao, W., & Dweck, C. S. (1994). *Implicit theories and vulnerability to depression-like responses.* Unpublished manuscript, Columbia University.

CHAPTER 5

Ideals, Oughts, and Regulatory Focus

Affect and Motivation from Distinct Pains and Pleasures

E. Tory Higgins

In one way or another, motivational theories have typically distinguished between a motivational system that concerns positive or pleasurable experiences and a motivational system that concerns negative or painful experiences. Conditioning theories distinguish between reward and punishment. Incentive theories distinguish between opportunity and threat. Attitude theories distinguish between like and dislike. Consistency theories distinguish between consonance or balance and dissonance or imbalance. Cognitive therapy theories distinguish between rational or functional beliefs and irrational or dysfunctional beliefs. Theories of mood effects distinguish between good and bad moods. And so on.

It is not my purpose to dispute the importance of pain versus pleasure—that is, "valence" in Lewin's (1951) terms—as a motivational distinction. Indeed, my position is that valence is such a critical motivational variable that it would be unreasonable if only one system were involved in regulating it. One would expect that alternative systems to regulate pain and pleasure would exist. If so, it could be that many important motivational phenomena reflect not only the distinction between experiencing pain versus pleasure, but also the different systems involved in regulating distinct kinds of pains and pleasures.

I propose that different systems of regulating pains and pleasures can be distinguished in terms of the variable of "regulatory focus." In his classic book *Learning Theory and Behavior,* Mowrer (1960) distinguished between two positive or pleasurable psychological situations, the presence of positive outcomes and the absence of negative outcomes, and between two negative or painful psychological situations, the absence of positive outcomes and the presence of negative outcomes. Mowrer (1960) and others (e.g., Higgins, 1987; Roseman, 1984; Stein & Jewett, 1982) have related these distinct psychological situations to distinct emotions. These distinct emotions are organized in Table 5.1 as a function of the valence of the experience and the outcome focus of the experience.

It is clear from Table 5.1 that two distinct systems for regulating pain and pleasure can be distinguished in terms of the variable of regulatory focus. First, there is a positive outcome focus regulatory system, which involves maximizing the presence of positive outcomes (pleasure) and minimizing the absence of positive outcomes (pain). Second, there is a negative outcome focus regulatory system, which involves maximizing the absence of negative outcomes (pleasure) and minimizing the presence of negative outcomes (pain).

In terms of Bowlby's (1969, 1973) classic account of people's fundamental survival needs, the positive-outcome-focus system is responsive to people's nurturance needs, and the negative-outcome focus system is responsive to people's security needs. Both systems for regulating pain and pleasure are adaptive, and thus all people possess both systems. Nevertheless, different socialization experiences may make one system predominate in self-regulation.

Self-discrepancy theory (see Higgins, 1989, 1991) postulates that the psychological significance of matches (i.e., congruence) and mismatches (i.e., discrepancy) between an individual's actual self (or self-concept) and his or her desired self derives from distinct developmental histories of caretaker–child interactions. Parents (as the usual caretakers) who hope or wish that their child will possess certain types of valued attributes orient to their child in terms of positive outcomes. When the child matches their hopes, wishes, or aspirations, the parents respond so as to produce positive outcomes for the child (e.g., hugging or kissing). When the child is discrepant from their hopes or wishes, the parents respond so as to remove positive outcomes for the child (e.g., love withdrawal). Over time, the child develops a representation of the parents' hopes or wishes for him or her as a self-regulatory guide. According to self-discrepancy theory, the child begins to self-regulate in terms of this "ideal self-guide," which orients him or her toward positive outcomes—to maximize the presence of positive outcomes (as a type of positive event) and to minimize the absence of positive outcomes (as a type of negative event).

In contrast, parents who believe that it is their child's duty, obligation, or responsibility to possess certain types of valued attributes orient to their child in terms of negative outcomes. When the child behaves in a manner that mismatches their demands or prescriptions, the parents respond so as to produce negative outcomes for the child (e.g., sanctions or punishment). When the child behaves in a manner that matches their demands or prescriptions, the parents respond so as to remove the threat of negative outcomes for the child (e.g., reassurance). Over time, the child begins to self-regulate

TABLE 5.1. Types of Psychological Situations and Emotions as a Function of Outcome Focus and Overall Valence of Experience

Outcome focus	Positive valence	Negative valence
Positive focus	Presence of positive; happy, satisfied	Absence of positive; sad, dissatisfied
Negative focus	Absence of negative; calm, relieved	Presence of negative; tense, nervous

in terms of an "ought self-guide," which orients him or her toward negative outcomes—to maximize the absence of negative outcomes (as a type of positive event) and to minimize the presence of negative outcomes (as a type of negative event).

IDEALS VERSUS OUGHTS AND DISTINCT EMOTIONAL VULNERABILITIES

According to self-discrepancy theory, then, self-regulation in relation to ideal self-guides involves a focus on positive outcomes, whereas self-regulation in relation to ought self-guides involves a focus on negative outcomes. If so, then activating actual–ideal self-discrepancies should produce dejection-related emotions reflecting the absence of positive outcomes, such as feeling sad and disappointed, whereas activating actual–ought self-discrepancies should produce agitation-related emotions reflecting the presence of negative outcomes, such as feeling nervous and tense. The results of an early study (Higgins, Bond, Klein, & Strauman, 1986, Study 2) support this prediction.

Two groups of undergraduates were recruited for the experiment—subjects who had *both* an actual–ideal *and* an actual–ought discrepancy, and subjects who had neither type of self-discrepancy. The ostensible purpose of the study was to obtain the self-reflections of a youth sample for a lifespan developmental study. In the ideal-priming condition, the subjects were asked to describe the kind of person that they and their parents would ideally like them to be, and to discuss whether there had been any change over the years in these hopes and aims for them. In the ought-priming condition, the subjects were asked to describe the kind of person that they and their parents believed they ought to be, and to discuss whether there had been any change over the years in these beliefs about their obligations. Both before and after this priming manipulation, subjects filled out a mood questionnaire that included both dejection-related and agitation-related emotions, and were asked to rate the extent to which they now were feeling each emotion.

As predicted, subjects high in both actual–ideal and actual–ought self-discrepancies experienced an increase in the kind of discomfort associated with the type of self-discrepancy that was recently activated by priming—an increase in dejection-related emotions when the ideal self was primed, and an increase in agitation-related emotions when the ought self was primed (see Table 5.2). In contrast, subjects who were low in both types of self-discrepancies experienced, if anything, the opposite pattern—a slight decrease in dejection-related emotions in the ideal-priming condition, and a slight decrease in agitation-related emotions in the ought-priming condition (see Table 5.2). This slight reversal for subjects who were low in both types of self-discrepancies was probably attributable to the priming manipulation activating these subjects' matches (either actual self-matches to the ideal self or actual self-matches to the ought self), which would produce the positive emotions associated with whichever type of match had been primed.

In another study, we (Strauman & Higgins, 1987) tested whether ideal self-regulation and ought self-regulation involve distinct regulatory systems in an even more stringent manner. Two groups of undergraduates were selected on the basis of their self-discrepancies as measured weeks earlier—subjects who had predominant actual–ideal discrepancies and subjects who had predominant actual–ought discrepancies. A covert, idiographic priming technique was used to activate self-attributes in a task supposedly investigating the "physiological effects of thinking about other people." Subjects were given phrases of the form, "An *X* person______" (where *X* was a trait adjective such as "friendly" or "intelligent"), and were asked to complete each sentence as quickly as possible. For each sentence, each subject's total verbalization time and skin conductance amplitude were recorded. Subjects also reported their mood on scales measuring dejection-related and agitation-related emotions at both the beginning and end of the session.

Subjects were randomly assigned to one of the following priming conditions: (1) "nonmatching" priming, where the trait adjectives were attributes in a subject's self-guide but the attributes did not appear in the subject's actual self; (2) "mismatching" priming, where the trait adjectives were attributes in a subject's self-guide and the subject's actual self was discrepant from the self-guide for those attributes; and (3) "yoked (mismatching)" priming, where the trait adjectives were attributes that did not appear in either a subject's self-guide or actual self, but were the *same* attributes that were used for some other subject in the "mismatching" priming condition. In the "mis-

TABLE 5.2. Mean Change in Dejection-Related Emotions and Agitation-Related Emotions as a Function of Level of Self-Discrepancies and Type of Priming

Level of actual–ideal and actual–ought discrepancies	Ideal priming		Ought priming	
	Dejection	Agitation	Dejection	Agitation
High in both discrepancies	3.2	−0.8	0.9	5.1
Low in both discrepancies	−1.2	0.9	0.3	−2.6

Note. The more positive the number, the greater the increase in discomfort. From Higgins, Bond, Klein, and Strauman (1986, p. 13). Copyright 1986 by the American Psychological Association. Reprinted by permission.

matching" priming condition *only*, as predicted, a dejection-related syndrome (i.e., increased dejected mood, lowered standardized skin conductance amplitude, decreased total verbalization time) was produced in the subjects with predominant actual–ideal discrepancies, whereas an agitation-related syndrome (i.e., increased agitated mood, raised standardized skin conductance amplitude, increased total verbalization time) was produced in the subjects with predominant actual–ought discrepancies.

SOCIALIZATION, IDEALS VERSUS OUGHTS, AND DISTINCT REGULATORY DISORDERS

The results of the studies described above, as well as of other studies (for reviews, see Higgins, 1987, 1989), clearly demonstrate that regulation in relation to ideal versus ought self-guides involves different regulatory systems and produces distinct emotional syndromes. These studies, however, provide only indirect support for the proposal that the regulation in relation to ideal self-guides involves a focus on positive outcomes, whereas regulation in relation to ought self-guides involves a focus on negative outcomes. The indirect support is that the emotions produced when the ideal system is activated are those associated with a positive-outcome focus, whereas the emotions produced when the ought system is activated are those associated with a negative-outcome focus. Additional indirect support for the proposal has been provided by studies based on the developmental assumptions underlying the proposal.

As discussed earlier, the developmental etiology of a dominant ought self-regulatory system is hypothesized to involve parents (or other catetakers) who respond to their child in terms of their sense of the child's duties and responsibilities, and cause their child to experience the absence or presence of negative outcomes. In contrast, the developmental etiology of a dominant ideal self-regulatory system is hypothesized to involve parents (or other caretakers) who respond to their child in terms of their hopes and aspirations for the child, and cause their child to experience the presence or absence of positive outcomes.

Patients with anorexia nervosa have been described in the literature as growing up to be obedient, well-behaved, conscientious, and quiet. They have also been described as being perfectionistic and as working to live up to the demands of others (e.g., Bruch, 1973; Bliss & Branch, 1960). Such self-regulatory orientations suggest that vulnerability to anorexia-related symptoms may be associated with acquiring strong ought self-guides. Moreover, the characteristics of anorexic patients include morbid and persistent fears and self-punitive behaviors (Strober, 1986). Thus, according to the developmental assumptions of self-discrepancy theory, anorexia-related symptoms should be associated with actual–ought discrepancies. In contrast, descriptions of patients with bulimia nervosa suggest that, if anything, bulimia-related symptoms should be associated with acquiring strong ideal self-guides and possessing actual–ideal discrepancies. Bulimics are described as feeling a lack of control over obtaining their goals and as having failed to meet their potential (American Psychiatric Association, 1994). Moreover, several authors report a relationship between bulimia and chronic depressive affect (Carroll et al., 1981; Hudson, Pope, Jonas, & Yurgelum-Todd, 1983; Walsh et al., 1982). Both of these developmentally-based predictions relating predominant type of self-regulatory system to type of eating disorder have been confirmed (see Higgins, Vookles, & Tykocinski, 1992).

IDEALS VERSUS OUGHTS AND DISTINCT PROCESSING SENSITIVITIES

Although the studies reviewed thus far provide converging evidence for the proposal that self-regulation in relation to ideal self-guides involves a focus on positive outcomes, whereas self-regulation in relation to ought self-guides involves a focus on negative outcomes, none of them provide direct support for the proposal. The study described in this section was designed to provide such support.

In a classic approach to relating personality and cognition, George Kelly (1955) proposed that each individual possesses "personal constructs" through which he or she views the world of events. Accordingly, events should be remembered better by people whose personal constructs are related to them than by people whose personal constructs are unrelated to them. And this should be true not only for events in which they are involved (i.e., autobiographical memory), but also for events in which others are involved (i.e., biographical memory). The positive-outcome focus associated with regulation in relation to an ideal self-guide can produce experiences of both positive overall valence (the presence of positive outcomes) and negative overall valence (the absence of positive outcomes). Similarly, the negative-outcome focus associated with regulation in relation to an ought self-guide can produce experiences of both positive overall valence (the absence of negative outcomes) and negative overall valence (the presence of negative outcomes).

According to self-discrepancy theory, then, the effects of chronic self-discrepancies on memory should involve differences between events in outcome focus rather than differences between events in overall valence. Therefore, we (Higgins & Tykocinski, 1992) predicted that when people read descriptions of events in another person's life, those events that reflected the presence and absence of positive outcomes would be remembered better by persons with predominant actual–ideal discrepancies than by persons with predominant actual–ought discrepancies, whereas the reverse would be true for those events that reflected the absence and presence of negative outcomes. Given the emphasis in the literature on memory for events varying in overall valence, such as the literature on mood and memory (e.g., Gilligan & Bower, 1984; Isen, 1984), this was a rather novel prediction.

This prediction was tested by selecting subjects who either were relatively high in actual–ideal discrepancy and relatively low in actual–ought discrepancy (i.e., persons with predominant actual–ideal discrepancy) or were relatively high in actual–ought discrepancy and relatively low in actual–ideal discrepancy (i.e., persons with predominant actual–ought discrepancy). A few weeks after the selection procedure, all subjects were given the same essay to read about several days in the life of a target person. Ten minutes after reading the essay (following a nonverbal filler task), the subjects were asked to reproduce the essay word for word.

In the essay, the different types of psychological situations described earlier were represented by different events that the target person experienced. The target person's experiences were circumstantial and not personality-related. The different types of psychological situations were represented in each day of the target person's life as follows:

1. The presence of positive outcomes (positive-outcome focus, positive overall valence): for example, "I found a $20 bill on the pavement of Canal Street near the paint store."
2. The absence of positive outcomes (positive-outcome focus, negative overall valence): for example, "I've been wanting to see this movie at the 8th Street Theater for some time, so this evening I went there straight after school to find out that it's not showing any more."
3. The presence of negative outcomes (negative-outcome focus, negative overall valence): for example, "I was stuck in the subway for 35 minutes with at least 15 sweating passengers breathing down my neck."
4. The absence of negative outcomes (negative-outcome focus, positive overall valence): for example, "This is usually my worst school day. Awful schedule, class after class with no break. But today is Election Day—no school!"

By using these materials, we could test whether a self-discrepancy involving a distinct regulatory focus produces sensitivity to events reflecting that focus, *despite there being no overlap between the self-discrepancy and the events in either their specific content or topic.*

Because self-discrepancies can influence mood (see Higgins, 1987, 1989) and mood can influence memory (see Gilligan & Bower, 1984; Isen, 1984), this study was designed both to control and to check for any possible effects of mood on memory. Previous studies of self-discrepancies have found that exposure to trait-related input can prime self-discrepancies and change subjects' mood (see Higgins, 1989). The essay used as input in this study minimized such priming by containing events that did not relate to personality traits. Rather, the events were clearly circumstantial factors, such as finding money by chance or getting stuck in a crowded subway. In addition to attempting to control for mood in this way, subjects' mood was also measured both before and after they read the essay, in order to be able to check whether individual differences in mood contributed to the findings.

A type of predominant self-discrepancy (actual–ideal vs. actual–ought) × outcome focus of event (positive vs. negative) × overall valence of event (positive vs. negative) analysis of variance was performed on the number of target events recalled. As shown in Table 5.3, the subjects remembered the events with negative overall valence better than those with positive overall valence, but they remembered the positive-outcome-focus events better than the negative-outcome-focus events; this is interesting because it highlights the distinction between overall valence and regulatory focus. But most importantly, this analysis revealed, as predicted, a significant interaction between type of predominant self-discrepancy and outcome focus of event. As shown in Table 5.3, this interaction reflected the fact that, as predicted, subjects with predominant actual–ideal discrepancies tended to remember target events representing the presence and absence of positive outcomes better than did subjects with predominant actual–ought discrepancies, whereas subjects with predominant actual–ought discrepancies tended to remember target events representing the absence and presence of negative outcomes better than did subjects with predominant actual–ideal discepancies. No other interactions were significant. Thus, subjects with the two types of self-discrepancies were differentially sensitive to the target events as a function of the events' outcome focus, but *not* as a function of the events' overall valence.

This above 2 × 2 × 2 analysis of variance was performed again three times—once with pre-essay mood as the covariate, once with post-essay mood as the covariate, and once with change in mood as the covariate. The interaction between type of predominant self-discrepancy and outcome focus of event, described earlier, remained significant in every case. Thus, the obtained interaction was independent of any differences in mood.

REGULATORY FOCUS AND DISTINCT STRATEGIC CONCERNS

The results of the Higgins and Tykocinski (1992) study provide more direct evidence that the ideal self-regulatory system involves a focus on positive outcomes, whereas the ought self-regulatory system involves a focus on negative outcomes. The studies described below considered further implications of such distinct regulatory systems, particulary implications for self-regulatory strategies and tactics.

Two basic distinctions regarding self-regulation have been made in the literature—one involving the valence of the end-state that functions as the reference value for the movement (positive vs. negative), and one involving the direction of the motivated movement (approach vs. avoidance). In regard to valence, the self-regulatory system can have either a desired end-state functioning as the standard (i.e., a positive reference value), or an undesired end-

TABLE 5.3. Mean Recall of Events Reflecting Different Types of Psychological Situations as a Function of Outcome Focus of Event, Overall Valence of Event, and Subjects' Type of Predominant Self-Discrepancy

	Positive-outcome focus		Negative-outcome focus	
Self-discrepancy	Positive valence (PP)	Negative valence (AP)	Positive valence (AN)	Negative valence (PN)
Actual–ideal	2.7	3.5	2.2	2.3
Actual–ought	2.3	2.8	2.4	2.6

Note. PP, presence of positive outcomes; AP, absence of positive outcomes; AN, absence of negative outcomes; PN, presence of negative outcomes. From Higgins and Tykocinski (1992, p. 531).

state functioning as the standard (i.e., a negative reference value). Both positive and negative reference values have been described in the literature (see Carver & Scheier, 1990). Various theories of the self have described positive selves as reference values in self-regulation, such as the type of person individuals would like to be (e.g., Cooley, 1902/1964; Higgins, 1987; James, 1890/1948; Markus & Nurius, 1986; Rogers, 1961; Schlenker & Weigold, 1989) or the type of person they believe they should be (e.g., Freud, 1923/1961; Higgins, 1987; James, 1890/1948; Schlenker & Weigold, 1989). Self theories have also described negative selves as reference values in self-regulation, such as Erikson's (1963) "evil identity," Sullivan's (1953) "bad me," and Markus and Nurius's (1986) "feared self."

In regard to the direction of the motivated movement, the literature distinguishes between approaching a positive self-state and avoiding a negative self-state. Carver and Scheier (1990) propose that when a self-regulatory system has a desired end-state as a reference value, the system is discrepancy-reducing and involves attempts to move the currently perceived actual self-state as close as possible to the desired reference point. And when a self-regulatory system has an undesired end-state as a reference value, the system is discrepancy-amplifying and involves attempts to move the currently perceived actual self-state as far away as possible from the undesired reference point. Carver and Scheier (1990) refer to the former, discrepancy-reducing system as an "approach system" and the latter, discrepancy-amplifying system as an "avoidance system." In this case, the approach or avoidance concerns the direction of the movement in relation to a desired or an undesired end-state, respectively.

In a discrepancy-reducing system, a person is motivated to move the actual self as close as possible to the desired end-state. There are two alternative means to reduce the discrepancy between the actual self and a desired end-state as reference point: to approach self-states that match the desired end-state, or to avoid self-states that mismatch the desired end-state. For example, a person who wants to get a good grade on a quiz (a desired end-state) could either study hard at the library the day before the quiz (approaching a match to the desired end-state) or turn down an invitation to go out drinking with friends the night before the quiz (avoiding a mismatch to the desired end state).

In a discrepancy-amplifying system, a person is motivated to move the actual self as far away as possible from the undesired end-state. Again, there are two alternative means to amplify the discrepancy between the actual self and an undesired end-state as reference point: to approach self-states that mismatch the undesired end-state or to avoid self-states that match the undesired end-state. For example, a person who dislikes interpersonal conflict (an undesired end-state) could either arrange a meeting with his or her apartment-mates to work out a schedule for cleaning the apartment (approaching a mismatch to the undesired end-state) or leave the apartment when his or her two apartment-mates start to argue (avoiding a match to the undesired end-state).

Thus, by considering the alternative means for accomplishing discrepancy reduction in relation to desired end-states and discrepancy amplification in relation to undesired end-states, four different forms of self-regulation can be identified. Table 5.4 summarizes how "valence of end-state as reference point" combines with "direction of means" to produce the four different regulatory forms. One might expect that a focus on positive outcomes would be associated with a predilection for self-regulatory forms involving approach, whereas a focus on negative outcomes would be associated with a predilection for self-regulatory forms involving avoidance. This would also be reasonable if, as suggested earlier, the positive-outcome-focus system is responsive to nurturance-like needs (e.g., obtaining nourishment) and the negative-outcome-focus system is responsive to survival-like needs (e.g., escaping danger). Given that ideal self-regulation is a positive-outcome-focus system and ought self-regulation is a negative-outcome-focus system, it should follow that regulation in relation to ideal self-guides involves approach-related self-regulatory forms, whereas regulation in relation to ought self-guides involves avoidance-related self-regulatory forms. There is more than one possibility, however, for how ideal self-regulation may involve approach forms and ought self-regulation may involve avoidance forms.

From the perspective of self-discrepancy theory, which has considered only discrepancy reduction to desired end-states as reference points, ideal self-regulation may involve a predilection for approaching matches to desired end-states, whereas ought self-regulation may involve a predilection for avoiding mismatches to desired end-states (see Table 5.4). When one considers both desired and undesired end-states as reference points, a second possibility would follow from Carver and Scheier's (1990) distinction between overall directional movements. They suggest that the ideal self may be associated with desired end-states, whereas the ought self may be associated with undesired end-states. From this perspective, then, ideal self-regulation involves a concern with any means for reducing discrepancies to desired end-states—that is, a predilection for both approaching matches and avoiding mismatches

TABLE 5.4. Summary of Regulatory Forms as a Function of Valence of End-State as Reference Point and Direction of Means

	Valence of end-state as reference point	
Direction of means	Desired end-state (discrepancy-reducing)	Undesired end-state (discrepancy-amplifying)
Approach	Approaching matches to desired end-states	Approaching mismatches to undesired end-states
Avoidance	Avoiding mismatches to desired end-states	Avoiding matches to undesired end-states

to desired end-states (i.e., approach at the system level). By contrast, ought self-regulation involves a concern with any means for amplifying discrepancies to undesired end-states—that is, a predilection for both avoiding matches and approaching mismatches to undesired end-states (i.e., avoidance at the system level) (see Table 5.4). These predictions were tested in a series of studies (Higgins, Roney, Crowe, & Hymes, 1994).

The first study was designed to examine whether and how activation of ideal versus ought self-guides influences subjects' predilections for different regulatory forms. Weeks prior to the experimental session, the subjects filled out a Selves Questionnaire, which measured the attributes in their ideal and ought self-guides. The responses of each subject to this questionnaire were used to identify attributes from the ideal self-guides that were *not* listed as attributes in any ought self-guide. Two attributes were selected from among this set of "distinctive" ideal attributes. By the same procedure, two "distinctive" ought attributes were selected for each subject. At the experimental session held weeks later, the subjects filled out a Ways of Behaving Questionnaire. This questionnaire purportedly had to do with concerns in daily life. There was a set of statements in the first person expressing a way of behaving in regard to some aspect of life. Each statement began with the words "What really matters to me is to try. . . ." This initial phrase was completed by one of four types of phrases representing each of the four different regulatory forms, as follows (where *x* was the desired endpoint and *y* was the undesired endpoint of a bipolar attribute dimension):

1. ". . . to be *x*" (e.g., "to be smart")—approaching a match to a desired end-state.
2. ". . . to avoid being not *x*" (e.g., "to avoid being not smart")—avoiding a mismatch to a desired end-state.
3. ". . . to be not *y*" (e.g., "to be not stupid")—approaching a mismatch to an undesired end-state.
4. ". . . to avoid being *y*" (e.g., to avoid being stupid)—avoiding a match to an undesired end-state.

For each statement, subjects selected a number on a 6-point scale to indicate the degree to which the statement expressed what they would do.

Each of the distinct attributes selected for each subject from their responses to the Selves Questionnaire was used to generate statements representing each of the different types of strategic means. Because the attributes listed in subjects' ideals and oughts on the Selves Questionnaire were desired end-states (i.e., *x* on the dimension), Roget's Thesaurus was used to select appropriate antonyms to represent the undesired end-states (i.e., *y* on the dimension). Each regulatory form appeared four times, twice instantiated by attributes that were distinctive to a subject's ideal self-guide and twice instantiated by attributes that were distinctive to a subject's ought self-guide (which manipulated ideal vs. ought activation, respectively). We expected that activating either the ideal or the ought self-regulatory system would increase subjects' predilection for particular regulatory forms, as revealed in judging that a statement expressing the importance of these forms was "like me."

An overall type of self-guide activated (ideal vs. ought) × valence of stated end-state (desired vs. undesired) × direction of stated means (approach vs. avoidance) × statement order analysis of variance was performed on subjects' ratings of how much a statement expressing a particular regulatory form resembled them. This analysis revealed a significant interaction between type of self-guide activated and valence of stated end-state. Consistent with the prediction derived from Carver and Scheier's (1990) analysis for how ideal self-regulation would involve approach forms and ought self-regulation would involve avoidance forms, subjects judged statements expressing the importance of regulatory forms with desired end-states to be more like them when ideal self-guides were activated than when ought self-guides were activated, whereas subjects judged statements expressing the importance of regulatory forms with undesired end-states to be more like them when ought self-guides were activated than when ideal self-guides were activated.

The analysis also revealed a significant higher-order interaction among type of self-guide activated, valence of stated end-state, and direction of stated means. As shown in Table 5.5, this three-way interaction reflects the fact that there was, as predicted, a significant interaction between type of self-guide activated and direction of stated means for desired end-states, but there was no significant interaction for undesired end-states. For desired end-states, subjects judged statements expressing the importance of approaching matches to desired end-states to be more like them when ideal self-guides were activated than when ought self-guides were activated, whereas there was no difference in how subjects judged statements expressing the importance of avoiding mismatches to desired end-states as a function of which type of self-guide was activated.

The results of this study supported the prediction that ideal self-regulation would involve approach forms, but they did not support the prediction that ought self-regulation would involve avoidance forms. It could be that the phrasing for avoiding mismatches to desired end-states (e.g., " . . . to avoid being not smart") was simply too awkward. Equally important, the

TABLE 5.5. Mean Judgments of Statements as Resembling Self as a Function of Type of Self-Guide Activated, Valence of Stated End-State, and Direction of Stated Means

	Desired end-state		Undesired end-state	
Type of activation	Approach matches	Avoid mismatches	Approach mismatches	Avoid matches
Ideal self-guide	4.62	4.11	4.06	4.04
Ought self-guide	4.28	4.11	4.22	4.19

Note. From Higgins, Roney, Crowe, and Hymes (1994, p. 279). Copyright 1994 by the American Psychological Association. Adapted by permission.

manipulation of ideal versus ought self-guide activation in this study was a within-subject variable. It is possible that activating both the ideal and the ought self-regulatory systems in the same subject during the experimental session produced some competition between these systems. This could have reduced the impact of activating each system on subjects' predilection for particular regulatory forms. The paradigm used in the next study overcame this potential problem by manipulating ideal versus ought self-guide activation as a between-subjects variable.

In our next study (Higgins et al., 1994, Study 2), a between-subjects manipulation of self-guide activation was used. The manipulation was based on the technique used in Study 2 of Higgins, Bond, et al. (1986) and described earlier. Subjects were asked either to report on how their hopes and goals had changed over time (activating ideal self-guides) or to report on how their sense of duty and obligation had changed over time (activating ought self-guides). Our second 1994 study also differed from the first study in the technique used to reveal subjects' predilections for different regulatory forms. The first study had subjects make judgments of the extent to which statements expressing the importance of different regulatory forms were like them. This technique had the advantage of revealing subjects' concern with different regulatory forms rather directly. It had the disadvantage of involving conscious judgments that might be influenced more by extraneous variables, such as which speech phrase was less awkward. The technique used in the second study to reveal subjects' predilections for different regulatory forms did not require subjects to make a conscious judgment. Rather, a free-recall technique similar to that used in the Higgins and Tykocinski (1992) study was employed. Subjects read about 16 episodes that occurred over 4 days in the life of another student. Each of the four regulatory forms was exemplified by four different episodes. We expected that activating either the ideal or ought self-regulatory system would increase subjects' predilection for particular regulatory forms, which in turn would make them more sensitive to, and thus more likely to recall, those episodes that exemplified those particular forms.

In each of the episodes, the target was trying either to experience a desired end-state or not to experience an undesired end-state. In order to experience a desired end-state, the target either used means that would decrease the discrepancy to a desired end-state (approaching matches to desired end-states) or used means that would avoid increasing the discrepancy to a desired end-state (avoiding mismatches to desired end-states). In order not to experience an undesired end-state, the target either used means that would increase the discrepancy to an undesired end-state (approaching mismatches to undesired end-states) or used means that would avoid decreasing the discrepancy to an undesired outcome (avoiding matches to undesired end-states). The following are examples of episodes exemplifying each of the regulatory forms:

1. Approaching matches to desired end-states: "Because I wanted to be at school for the beginning of my 8:30 psychology class, which is usually excellent, I woke up early this morning."
2. Avoiding mismatches to desired end-states: "I wanted to take a class in photography at the community center, so I didn't register for a class in Spanish that was scheduled at the same time."
3. Approaching mismatches to undesired end-states: "I dislike eating in crowded places, so at noon I picked up a sandwich from a local deli and ate outside."
4. Avoiding matches to undesired end-states: "I didn't want to feel tired during my very long morning of classes, so I skipped the most strenuous part of my morning workout."

An overall type of self-guide activated (ideal vs. ought) × direction of stated means (approach vs. avoidance) × valence of stated end-state (desired vs. undesired) × story version × event order analysis of variance was performed on the number of episodes subjects recalled for each type of episode in the story. Table 5.6 shows subjects' recall of each type of episode in the story as a function of the type of self-guide that was activated.

The overall analysis revealed a significant interaction between type of self-guide activated and direction of stated means, reflecting the fact that there was an overall tendency for subjects to remember better episodes exemplifying an approach direction of means when ideal self-guides were activated than when ought self-guides were activated, but to remember better episodes exemplifying an avoidance direction of means when ought self-guides were activated than when ideal self-guides were activated. The specific prediction that ideal self-regulation would involve approach forms and ought self-regulation would involve avoidance forms predicted an interaction between type of self-guide activated and direction of stated means for desired end-states alone. As evident in Table 5.6. the predicted interaction was obtained. Subjects remembered episodes exemplifying approaching matches to desired end-states significantly better when ideal self-guides were activated than when ought self-guides were activated, whereas they remembered episodes exemplifying avoiding mismatches to desired end-states significantly

TABLE 5.6. Mean Number of Episodes Recalled as a Function of Type of Self-Guide Activated, Valence of Stated End-State, and Direction of Stated Means

	Desired end-state		Undesired end-state	
Type of activation	Approach matches	Avoid mismatches	Approach mismatches	Avoid matches
Ideal self-guide	1.75	1.37	1.50	1.39
Ought self-guide	1.19	1.96	1.38	1.75

Note. From Higgins et al. (1994, p. 281). Copyright 1994 by the American Psychological Association. Adapted by permission.

better when ought self-guides were activated than when ideal self-guides were activated. (It should be noted that this interaction was considerably weaker and nonsignificant for undesired end-states.)

The results of these two studies support the general prediction that follows from assuming that ideal and ought self-regulation reflect distinct systems for regulating valence—namely, that ideal self-regulation, with its positive-outcome focus, is associated with self-regulatory forms involving approach, whereas ought self-regulation, with its negative-outcome focus, is associated with self-regulatory forms involving avoidance. The significant results of both studies support the general conclusion that, either at the level of means or at the system level, a predilection for approach is greater when ideal versus ought self-guides are activated, whereas a predilection for avoidance is greater when ought versus ideal self-guides are activated.

The two studies had at least a couple of limitations, however. First, the predilections for different regulatory forms were measured after either ideal self-guides or ought self-guides were made temporarily more accessible through recent activation. Although this method had the advantage of enhancing experimental control, it did not permit stable predilections associated with chronic differences in ideal versus ought orientation to be examined. Our third study (Higgins et al., 1994, Study 3) was designed to examine this issue by selecting subjects whose predominant orientation involved either ideal self-guides (i.e., subjects with predominant actual–ideal discrepancies) or ought self-guides (i.e, subjects with predominant actual–ought discrepancies). Second, the predilections that were studied were quite general regulatory forms, such as predilections for approaching matches or for avoiding mismatches to desired end-states. Are these general predilections also revealed in specific strategies or tactics of self-regulation? Would individuals with a predominant ideal self-guide orientation versus a predominant ought self-guide orientation select different tactics for regulating an important region of their lives, such as friendship? Another aim of our third study was to begin to address this important question.

The third study consisted of three phases. The first phase elicited undergraduates' spontaneous strategies for friendship as a function of regulatory focus. The question about friendship that each subject answered was included as part of a 30-minute battery of questions on a variety of different issues. The subjects were randomly assigned to answer one of two different questions about friendship, with half of the subjects answering each question. The question framed with a positive-outcome focus was as follows: "Imagine that you are the kind of person who would like to be a good friend in your close relationships. What would your strategy be to meet this goal?" The question framed with a negative-outcome focus was as follows: "Imagine that you are the kind of person who believes you should try not to be a poor friend in your close relationships. What would your strategy be to meet this goal?"

Although a few subjects gave only one strategy, most subjects offered several strategies in response to the question they received. A rough classification system was developed to group the strategies into different types. Most of the proposed strategies fell into nine category types (75% of the strategies). Subjects in the positive-outcome-focus framing condition responded with some of these strategy types more than subjects in the negative-outcome-focus framing condition, and vice versa. Six strategy types that most differentiated subjects in the two framing conditions were selected—three strategy types that were used more by subjects in the positive-outcome-focus condition, and three that were used more by subjects in the negative-outcome-focus condition. For each of these six strategy types, one or more sentences that best captured the strategy were written, using the subjects' original words as much as possible. The strategies associated more with the positive-outcome-focus framing condition were as follows: (1) "Be generous and willing to give of yourself." (2) "Be supportive to your friends. Be emotionally supportive." (3) "Be loving and attentive." The strategies associated more with the negative-outcome-focus framing condition were as follows: (4) "Stay in touch. Don't lose contact with friends." (5) "Try to make time for your friends and not neglect them." (6) "Keep the secrets friends have told you and don't gossip about friends."

On the basis of these Phase 1 results, strategies 1–3 were selected as the "approach" strategies, and strategies 4–6 were selected as the "avoidance" strategies. The purpose of Phase 2 was to test experimentally whether the approach strategies would be selected more when friendship was framed with a positive-outcome focus versus a negative-outcome focus, whereas the avoidance strategies would be selected more when friendship was framed with a negative-outcome focus versus a positive-outcome focus. Subjects in a new sample were randomly assigned to answer one of two different questions about friendship strategies, with half of the subjects answering each question. The question framed with a positive-outcome focus was as follows: "When you think about strategies for *being a good friend* in your close relationships, which THREE of the following would you choose?" The question framed with a negative-outcome focus was as follows: "When you think about strategies for *not being a poor friend* in your close relationship, which THREE of the following would you choose?"

There was a significant difference between the two framing conditions.

Subjects in the positive-outcome-focus framing condition choose significantly more "approach" strategies than subjects in the negative-outcome-focus framing condition, and subjects in the negative-outcome-focus framing condition choose significantly more "avoidance" strategies than subjects in the positive-outcome-focus framing condition.

In Phase 3 of the study, we used the same approach and avoidance strategies found to be related to outcome focus in Phase 2. The purpose of Phase 3 was to test whether approach strategies would be spontaneously selected more by individuals with a predominant ideal versus ought self-guide orientation, whereas avoidance strategies would be selected more by individuals with a predominant ought versus ideal self-guide orientation. Again, a new sample of undergraduates was used. A median split was performed on subjects' actual–ideal discrepancy scores to classify them as either high or low in actual–ideal discrepancy, and a median split was performed on their actual–ought discrepancy scores to classify them as either high or low in actual–ought discrepancy. Subjects who were high in actual–ideal discrepancy and low in actual–ought discrepancy were classified as predominantly ideal-discrepant subjects. Subjects who were high in actual–ought discrepancy and low in actual–ideal discrepancy were classified as predominantly ought-discrepant subjects.

In the experimental session, held over 2 months after measuring subjects' self-discrepancies, each subject was asked the same *unframed* question about friendship, as follows: "When you think about strategies for *friendship,* which THREE of the following strategies would you choose?" This question was followed by the same six choices of strategies used in the Phase 2 framing study.

As predicted, a significant difference was found between the two groups. The predominantly ideal-discrepant subjects chose significantly more "approach" strategies than the predominantly ought-discrepant subjects. And the predominantly ought-discrepant subjects chose significantly more "avoidance" strategies than the predominantly ideal-discrepant subjects. To check on whether subjects' choice of strategies might be related somehow to their self-guide attributes, the content of subjects' self-guides was compared to the content of the different strategies. The results of this study were not attributable to content overlap between subjects' self-guide attributes and the presented strategies.

It is worth noting that the greater predilection of ought-oriented individuals than ideal-oriented individuals to choose avoidance strategies for friendship was particularly strong for avoidance strategy 4: "Stay in touch. Don't lose contact with friends." This strategy was chosen by 46% of the predominantly ought-discrepant individuals compared to only 13% of the predominantly ideal-discrepant individuals. The aim of this strategy is to avoid losing contact with friends; the method for attaining this aim is to stay in touch. What is significant is that this avoidance strategy involves *taking action.* Thus, it is not the case that an avoidance strategy implies inhibition, suppression, or inaction. Indeed, as in the case of animals escaping electric shock, it can require vigorous action.

REGULATORY FOCUS AND MOTIVATION AND PERFORMANCE

Together, the results of the Higgins and Tykocinski (1992) and Higgins et al. (1994) studies support the proposal that there are two distinct systems for regulating pain and pleasure—the positive-outcome-focus system (associated with nurturance and ideal self-guides) and the negative-outcome-focus system (associated with security and ought self-guides)—and that these two systems are related to distinct emotional experiences and strategic concerns. These studies investigated this proposal in terms of ideal versus ought self-guides. A couple of recent studies investigated this proposal even more directly, and apart from individual-difference considerations, by framing a performance task with either a positive-outcome focus or a negative-outcome focus (see Roney, Higgins, & Shah, in press).

Earlier, we (Higgins, Strauman, & Klein, 1986) noted a parallel between self-discrepancy theory and achievement motivation. Atkinson's work on individual differences in achievement-related motives emphasizes differences between people who are "success-oriented" and people who are "failure-threatened" (see Atkinson & Feather, 1966). According to Atkinson, when confronted with an important achievement task, success-oriented persons focus on the possibility of experiencing "pride in accomplishment," whereas failure-threatened persons in the same situation focus on how they might experience "shame due to failure." One might reconceptualize this distinction in terms of individuals or conditions where the focus is on possible positive outcomes (as in the case of success-oriented persons) versus individuals or conditions where the focus is on possible negative outcomes (as in the case of failure-threatened persons). Based on previous research on achievement motivation, we (Roney et al., in press) predicted that framing a performance task with a positive-outcome focus would produce better performance and greater persistence than would framing the same task with a negative-outcome focus.

In one study, we had undergraduates work on a set of anagrams that included both solvable and unsolvable anagrams. The subjects were given feedback on each trial about their performance. In one condition the feedback was framed with a positive-outcome focus, such as by telling subjects, "Right, you got that one," when they solved an anagram, and telling them, "You didn't get that one right," when they did not solve an anagram. In the other condition the feedback was framed with a negative-outcome focus, such as by telling subjects, "You didn't miss that one," when they solved an anagram, and telling them, "No, you missed that one," when they did not solve an anagram. The study found that the subjects in the positive-outcome-focus framing condition solved more of the solvable anagrams and persisted longer in trying to solve the unsolvable anagrams than did the subjects in the negative-outcome-focus framing condition.

In another study designed to test motivational persistence, we (Roney et al., in press) told undergraduates that they would perform two tasks. The first task was always an anagrams task that included anagrams pretested to be solvable by everyone, as well as a set of unsolvable anagrams. The subjects were told that the second task would be either a computer simulation of the popular *Wheel of Fortune* game show or a task called "unvaried repetition" that was described so as to appear very boring. The performance contingency that would permit subjects to play the fun game rather than the boring game as the second task was the same for all the subjects, but the framing of the contingency was experimentally varied. In one condition, the contingency was framed with a positive-outcome focus: Subjects were told that if they solved 22 (or more) out of the 25 anagrams they would get to play the *Wheel of Fortune* game; otherwise, they would do the "unvaried repetition" task. In the other condition the contingency was framed with a negative-outcome focus: Subjects were told that if they got 4 (or more) out of the 25 anagrams wrong, they would do the "unvaried repetition" task; otherwise, they would play the *Wheel of Fortune* game.

This study also found that the subjects in the positive-outcome-focus framing condition persisted longer in trying to solve the unsolvable anagrams than the subjects in the negative-outcome-focus framing condition. It should also be noted that in both studies there was a tendency for the negative-outcome-focus framing condition to produce greater change in agitation-related emotions than in dejection-related emotions, with the reverse being true for the positive-outcome-focus framing condition, as reflected in significant interactions between type of outcome focus framing and type of emotion change.

GENERAL DISCUSSION

My starting position in this chapter has been that pain versus pleasure, or valence, is such a critical motivational variable that it would be unreasonable if only one system were involved in regulating it. One would expect the existence of alternative systems that regulate distinct kinds of pains and pleasures. I have proposed that the variable of "regulatory focus" is one way in which different systems of regulating pains and pleasures can be distinguished. Direct and indirect evidence from many different kinds of studies has been described in support of this proposal. The results of these different studies suggest that it may be fruitful to consider emotional experiences and motivation in terms of the distinct pains and pleasures involved in the nurturance-based, positive-outcome-focus system versus the security-based, negative-outcome-focus system (see also Higgins, in press, for further discussion of regulatory focus and emotional experiences). It is important to emphasize, however, that the significance of regulatory focus as a variable does not lessen the significance of valence as a variable. Indeed, the specific combinations of these two variables are what may provide key insights into the nature of motivation and affect. A couple of examples of specific combinations may be instructive.

As one example, consider the classic distinction between optimists and pessimists, in which optimists describe a glass half filled with water as "pretty full" and pessimists describe the same glass as "pretty empty." Does this individual difference reflect a regulatory difference in valence orientation or in outcome focus? Before answering this question, one must first recognize that this half-filled glass can actually be described in terms of four specific combinations of valence and outcome focus, as shown in Table 5.7. Is an optimist a person who describes events with a positive valence (i.e., the glass is "almost full" or "not at all empty"), or a person who describes events with a positive-outcome focus (i.e., the glass is "almost full" or "not at all full")? Is a pessimist a person who describes events with a negative valence (i.e., the glass is "almost empty" or "not at all full") or a person who describes events with a negative-outcome focus (i.e., the glass is "almost empty" or "not at all empty")?

There are some interesting implications of conceptualizing optimism–pessimism as an outcome focus variable, especially when the outcome focus variable is combined with the valence of people's chronic experiences—that is, specific combinations of people's outcome focus and either chronic matches or chronic mismatches between their actual selves and their self-guides. Consider Cantor's recent research on the different ways that students use "social support" to meet their academic goals (see Cantor, 1994; Cantor & Blanton, Chapter 15, this volume). Some students turn to others to seek reassurance ("outcome-focused persons," in Cantor's terminology). Other students want others to listen to their "worst-case analyses" of why they are likely to fail on an impending task ("defensive pessimists"). Still other students want to study with their "idols" to inspire self-improvement ("persons with actual–ideal discrepancies"). Finally, some students want simply to enjoy the intrinsically positive properties of socializing before tackling the chores of studying ("mood enhancers").

Consider now the combination of outcome focus and valence of experience. Individuals with strong ought self-guides have a negative-outcome focus. Those with an actual–ought discrepancy feel nervous and tense (negative valence). They seek reassurance to prevent their anxiety from overwhelming them. Individuals with an actual–ought congruency feel calm and relaxed (positive valence). Given their negative-outcome focus, they perceive this state as a problem. If they are going to succeed on the impending task, they need to become less calm and relaxed in order to get motivated. Thus, they construct "worst case scenarios" and actively avoid reassurance. Individuals with strong ideal self-guides have a positive-outcome focus. Those with an actual–ideal discrepancy feel disappointed and dissatisfied (negative valence).

TABLE 5.7. Ways of Describing a Glass Half Filled With Water as a Function of Outcome Focus of Event and Overall Valence of Event

Outcome focus	Positive valence	Negative valence
Positive	"Almost full"	"Not at all full"
Negative	"Not at all empty"	"Almost empty"

Their goal is self-improvement, and their positive-outcome focus inclines them to use "idols" as their self-regulatory means. Individuals with an actual–ideal congruency feel happy and satisfied and want to maintain their positive mood. They use the intrinsic pleasures of socializing simply to give their mood that extra lift to face the task of studying.

As another example of how specific combinations of valence and outcome focus may underlie important affective and motivational phenomena, consider the relation between affective states and strategic responses. There is considerable evidence that the strategies involved in people's information processing, reasoning, and performance can vary as a function of whether they are feeling good or bad (see Schwarz, 1990, for a review). Clearly, there are important differences in the psychological situation of experiencing pain versus pleasure. As Schwarz (1990) points out, pain is more likely to produce a problem-solving orientation in which there is a need to take action, and it is generally worth the effort to be attentive, thorough, and accurate. This problem-solving orientation can induce strategies that generally differ from those induced by a pleasant state.

Rather than restricting attention to valence alone, however, we may find it useful to consider what strategies might be induced by specific combinations of valence and outcome focus. Pain, for instance, could involve either the absence of positive outcomes (when people feel sad or disappointed) or the presence of negative outcomes (when people feel nervous or tense). The former combination of negative valence and positive-outcome focus may induce a relatively impatient inclination toward approach, in which gratification is wanted soon through whatever resources are immediately available, even if this entails risk. The latter combination of negative valence and negative-outcome focus may induce a relatively vigilant, avoidant inclination, in which scrutiny and certainty are emphasized and risk is avoided.

In sum, future work on affect and motivation will benefit from going beyond a consideration of valence alone to considering valence in combination with outcome focus. In doing so, we can explore not only how specific combinations of valence and outcome focus relate to particular emotional and motivational states, but how these particular emotional and motivational states induce specific self-regulatory strategies that influence behavior and performance. Although it is tempting to believe that some specific combination of valence and outcome focus will be motivationally optimal, it is just as likely that the utility of different combinations will vary depending on motivational conditions (e.g., retrospective states vs. prospective states) and situational constraints (e.g., abundant vs. scarce resources). The challenge is great because there is so much to be learned. But the payoff at home, at school, and at the workplace from gaining such knowledge is equally great.

REFERENCES

American Psychiatric Association. (1994). *Diagnostic and statistical manual of mental disorders* (4th ed.). Washington, DC: Author.

Atkinson, J. W., & Feather, N. T. (Eds.). (1966). *A theory of achievement motivation.* New York: Wiley.

Bliss, E. L., & Branch, C. H. H. (Eds). (1960). *Anorexia nervosa: Its history, psychology, and biology.* New York: Hoeber.

Bowlby, J. (1969). *Attachment and loss: Vol. 1. Attachment.* New York: Basic Books.

Bowlby, J. (1973). *Attachment and loss: Vol. 2. Separation: Anxiety and anger.* New York: Basic Books.

Bruch, H. (1973). *Eating disorders: Obesity, anorexia nervosa and the person within.* New York: Basic Books.

Cantor, N. (1994). Life task problem-solving: Situational affordances and personal needs. *Personality and Social Psychology Bulletin, 20*(3), 235–243.

Carroll, B. J., Feinberg, M. F., Greden, J. F., Tarika, J., Albala, A., Haskett, R., James, N., Kronfol, Z., Lohr, N., Steiner, M., de Vigne, J., & Young, E. (1981). A specific laboratory test for the diagnosis of melancholia. *Archives of General Psychiatry, 38,* 15–22.

Carver, C. S., & Scheier, M. F. (1990). Principles of self-regulation: Action and emotion. In E. T. Higgins & R. M. Sorrentino (Eds.), *Handbook of motivation and cognition: Foundations of social behavior* (Vol. 2, pp. 3–52). New York: Guilford Press.

Cooley, C. H. (1964). *Human nature and the social order.* New York: Schocken Books. (Original work published 1902)

Erikson, E. H. (1963). *Childhood and society* (rev. ed.). New York: Norton.

Freud, S. (1961). The ego and the id. In J. Strachey (Ed. and Trans.), *Standard edition of the complete psychological works of Sigmund Freud* (Vol. 19, pp. 3–66). London: Hogarth Press. (Original work published 1923)

Higgins, E. T. (1987). Self-discrepancy: A theory relating self and affect. *Psychological Review, 94,* 319–340.

Higgins, E. T. (1989). Self-discrepancy theory: What patterns of self-beliefs cause people to suffer? In L. Berkowitz (Ed.), *Advances in experimental social psychology* (Vol. 22, pp. 93–136). New York: Academic Press.

Higgins, E. T. (1991). Development of self-regulatory and self-evaluative processes: Costs, benefits, and tradeoffs. In M. R. Gunnar & L. A. Sroufe (Eds.), *The Minnesota Symposia on Child Psychology: Vol. 23. Self processes and development* (pp. 125–165). Hillsdale, N.J.: Erlbaum.

Higgins, E. T. (in press). Emotional experiences: The pains and pleasures of distinct regulatory systems. In R. D. Kavanaugh, B. Z. Glick, & S. Fein (Eds.), *Emotion: The G. Stanley Hall Symposium.* Hillsdale, NJ: Erlbaum.

Higgins, E. T., Bond, R. N., Klein, R., & Strauman, T. (1986). Self-discrepancies and emotional vulnerability: How magnitude, accessibility, and type of discrepancy influence affect. *Journal of Personality and Social Psychology, 51,* 5–15.

Higgins, E. T., Roney, C. J. R., Crowe, E., & Hymes, C. (1994). Ideal versus ought predilections for approach and avoidance: Distinct self-regulatory systems. *Journal of Personality and Social Psychology, 66,* 276–286.

Higgins, E. T., Strauman, T., & Klein, R. (1986). Standards and the process of self-evaluation: Multiple affects from multiple stages. In R. M. Sorrentino & E. T. Higgins (Eds.), *Handbook of motivation and cognition: Foundations of social behavior* (Vol. 1, pp. 23–63). New York: Guilford Press.

Higgins, E. T., & Tykocinski, O. (1992). Self-discrepancies and biographical memory: Personality and cognition at the level of psychological situation. *Personality and Social Psychology Bulletin, 18,* 527–535.

Higgins, E. T., Vookles, J., & Tykocinski, O. (1992). Self and health: How "patterns" of self-beliefs predict types of emotional and physical problems. *Social Cognition, 10,* 125–150.

Hudson, J. L., Pope, H. C., Jonas, J. M., & Yurgelum-Todd, D. (1983). Bulimia related to affective disorder by family history and response to the dexamethasone suppression test. *American Journal of Psychiatry, 139,* 685–687.

Isen, A. M. (1984). Toward understanding the role of affect in cognition. In R. S. Wyer & T. K. Srull (Eds.), *Handbook of social cognition* (Vol. 3, pp. 179–236). Hillsdale, NJ: Erlbaum.

James, W. (1948). *Psychology.* New York: World Publishing Company. (Original work published 1890)

Kelly, G. A. (1955). *The psychology of personal constructs.* New York: Norton.

Lewin, K. (1951). *Field theory in social science.* New York: Harper.

Markus, H., & Nurius, P. (1986). Possible selves. *American Psychologist, 41,* 954–969.

Mowrer, O. H. (1960). *Learning theory and behavior.* New York: Wiley.

Rogers, C. R. (1961). *On becoming a person.* Boston: Houghton Mifflin Company.

Roney, C. J. R., Higgins, E. T., & Shah, J. (in press). Goals and framing: How outcome focus influences motivation and emotion. *Personality and Social Psychology Bulletin.*

Roseman, I. J. (1984). Cognitive determinants of emotion: A structural theory. *Review of Personality and Social Psychology, 5,* 11–36.

Schlenker, B. R., & Weigold, M. F. (1989). Goals and the self-identification process: Constructing desired identities. In L. A. Pervin (Ed.), *Goal concepts in personality and social psychology* (pp. 243–290). Hillsdale, NJ: Erlbaum.

Schwarz, N. (1990). Feelings as information: Informational and motivational functions of affective states. In E. T. Higgins & R. M. Sorrentino (Eds.), *Handbook of motivation and cognition: Foundations of social behavior* (Vol. 2, pp. 527–561). New York: Guilford Press.

Stein, N. L., & Jewett, J. L. (1982). A conceptual analysis of the meaning of negative emotions: Implications for a theory of development. In C. E. Izard (Ed.), *Measuring emotions in infants and children* (pp. 401–443). New York: Cambridge University Press.

Strauman, T. J., & Higgins, E. T. (1987). Automatic activation of self-discrepancies and emotional syndromes: When cognitive structures influence affect. *Journal of Personality and Social Psychology, 53,* 1004–1014.

Strober, M. (1986). Anorexia nervosa: History and psychological concepts. In K. Brownell & J. Foreyt (Eds.), *Handbook of eating disorders: Physiology, psychology, and treatment of obesity, anorexia, and bulimia* (pp. 231–346). New York: Basic Books.

Sullivan, H. S. (1953). *The collected works of Harry Stack Sullivan* (Vol. 1) (H. S. Perry & M. L. Gawel, Eds.). New York: Norton.

Walsh, B. T., Stewart, J. W., Wright, L., Harrison, W., Roose, S. D., & Glassman, A. H. (1982). Treatment of bulimia with monoamine oxidase inhibitors. *American Journal of Psychiatry, 139,* 1629–1630.

PART II

Affective Influences on Action Goals

Another source of action goals is the affective state of the individual. The chapters in Part II explore and discuss the causal path between affect and motivation. Both Schwarz and Bohner (Chapter 6) and Weary and Gannon (Chapter 7) present theoretical reasons and empirical evidence for the idea that negative emotional states—both temporary ones, such as being in a bad mood or having a headache, and chronic ones, such as being depressed—have motivational consequences for information processing. Klinger (Chapter 8) describes the complex and intertwined relationship among emotion, motivation, and cognition. Motivational states, which Klinger discusses in terms of the person's current concerns, are argued to produce emotional reactions to goal-relevant events and cues, and also to make the individual more attentionally (cognitively) sensitive to goal-relevant events.

Schwarz and Bohner focus on the motivational consequences of affective states. Taking the perspective that mood and emotion serve a function for cognition and action—that of signaling something basic about the current state of the world for the individual—they contend that motivations either to escape or change the current situation on the one hand (negative moods and emotions), or to stay in and enjoy the current environment on the other (positive affective states), are activated. This leads to a greater amount of effortful, systematic thought when a person is in a negative mood, and a less effortful, more heuristic form of information processing when the individual is in a good mood. Schwarz and Bohner then analyze the impact of the current affective state for each phase of the action sequence, from goal setting to engagement to postactional assessment of the outcome, and also describe how affective reactions to the progress (or lack of it) one is making toward the goal and the effort being required to attain it influence goal striving and persistence. In short, the chapter provides an insightful look at how affective and motivational systems are intertwined and influence each other.

Weary and Gannon consider the feelings of helplessness and, more specifically, loss of control over important life outcomes that are felt by depressed individuals. Considerable research has documented the certainty with which depressives believe that negative things will continue to happen to them and that they are powerless to do anything about them. Pittman's concept of control motivation suggests that when people are faced with a perceived loss of control over important outcomes, they are motivated to exert and regain control however they can. Weary and Gannon review a program of research in a variety of social-cognitive research paradigms; this research demonstrates that depressives have a chronic motive to assert control, resulting in a greater exertion of effortful cognitive processing. For instance, depressives are more likely than nondepressives to pay attention to and integrate individuating personal details about a target person (i.e., piecemeal processing) when forming an impression of him or her, and to rely less on easier-to-process category memberships or stereotypes as a basis for their opinion. Their research provides some of the best examples to date of how affective states can have social-psychological consequences, via the influence of the affective state on information-processing motivations.

Klinger provides a thoughtful analysis of the ways in which emotional, motivational, and cognitive systems influence and feed back on one another. Recognizing at the outset the centrality of motivation and successive goal commitments for all motile varieties of life, he proceeds to trace the ways in which these goal commitments cause the individual to be emotionally reactive to information relevant to those current concerns, and also to be more sensitive to and likely to cognitively process and remember such information. He describes a program of research documenting these emotional and cognitive sensitivities to current-concern-related stimuli, and, moreover, the automaticity (i.e., unintentionality and uncontrollability) of such effects. Of particular value is a section relating this body of research to parallel lines of automaticity research within social psychology, in the construct and attitude accessibility traditions, in which similar effects were observed. Although noting that crucial tests between the current-concern and accessibility accounts of such findings are virtually impossible to perform, Klinger concludes that nonmotivational models cannot account for the range of effects produced in the current-concern research.

Regarding the remarkable similarity of effects produced by construct accessibility and current-concern research, we would note that Bruner's original model of perceptual readiness, in which the notion of construct or category accessibility was introduced, posited the perceiver's current goal or purpose as the major determinant of accessibility effects. It may be, therefore, that one's current concerns or goal commitments are important determinants of construct accessibility, and that in this way current concerns produce the same quality of results in cognitive paradigms as does accessibility when measured or manipulated by other means (e.g., frequency or recency). This notion is compatible with Klinger's argument that frequency and recency determinants of accessibility may be primarily due to the relevance of the construct for the individual's current concerns—a very valuable point that suggests an important determinant of both long- and short-term accessibility influences. In our view, therefore, the two parallel bodies of research are more compatible than competing: Accessibility is the mechanism by which current goal commitments influence perceptual and cognitive processing.

CHAPTER 6

Feelings and Their Motivational Implications

Moods and the Action Sequence

Norbert Schwarz
Gerd Bohner

One of the most widely shared assumptions about moods and emotions is that they serve a signaling function. As Nico Frijda put it, "emotions exist for the sake of signaling states of the world that have to be responded to, or that no longer need response and action" (Frijda, 1988, p. 354). Similarly, researchers have long assumed that moods reflect the general state of the organism—an assumption that prompted Jacobsen (1957) to refer to moods as "barometers of the ego." In a related vein, Nowlis and Nowlis (1956, p. 352) suggested that moods are "a source of information or discriminable stimuli to the organism about the current functioning characteristics of the organism." Extending these assumptions, Wyer and Carlston (1979) suggested that individuals' affective states may serve as information in making judgments; this possibility was systematically explored by Schwarz and Clore (1983, 1988). Whereas initial tests of the feelings-as-information hypothesis focused on mood effects on evaluative judgments, subsequent research suggested that people's feelings may inform them about the nature of their current psychological situation and may influence the spontaneous adoption of a systematic or heuristic strategy of information processing, in ways to be discussed below (Schwarz, 1990; for a recent review, see Clore, Schwarz, & Conway, 1994).

In the present chapter, we explore the motivational implications of the information provided by individuals' elated or depressed mood states. In the first section, we review research suggesting that negative affective states are likely to trigger systematic, detail-oriented strategies of information processing, whereas positive affective states are likely to trigger heuristic strategies of information processing. These findings presumably indicate that cognitive processes are tuned to meet the situational requirements signaled by different affective states. Following this review, we relate the information provided by one's affective state to different stages of the action sequence; we explore the impact of moods on goal setting, estimates of attainment likelihood, and performance evaluation. This discussion suggests that the impact of affective states may be more complex than has been reflected in previous research, and that mood states may have very different effects, depending on the stage at which moods exert their influence. Although we draw on relevant experimental research whenever this is available, we note at the outset that much of our discussion of the role of moods at different stages of the action sequence reflects educated guesses on the basis of current theorizing, rather than firmly established empirical evidence.

COGNITIVE TUNING: MOODS AND STRATEGIES OF INFORMATION PROCESSING

Several recent lines of research indicate that individuals' cognitive performance on a wide variety of tasks may be profoundly influenced by the affective state they are in (see Clore et al., 1994; Fiedler, 1988; Schwarz, 1990; Schwarz & Bless, 1991; Schwarz, Bless, & Bohner, 1991; Sinclair & Mark, 1992; and Weary & Gannon, Chapter 7, this volume, for reviews). These influences can be conceptualized by assuming that affective states serve informative functions. As many authors have pointed out (e.g., Arnold, 1960; Frijda, 1988; Higgins, 1987; Ortony, Clore, & Collins, 1988), different affective states are closely linked to different psychological situations. In Frijda's words (1988, p. 349), "emotions arise in response to the meaning structures of given situations, [and] different emotions arise in response to different meaning structures." In general, "events that satisfy the individual's goals, or promise to do so, yield positive emotions; events that harm or threaten the individual's concerns lead to negative emotions" (p. 349).

We may assume, however, that the relationship between emotions and the "meaning structures" that constitute a "psychological situation" (Higgins, 1987) is likely to be bidirectional: While different psychological situations result in different emotions, the presence of a certain emotion also informs the individual about the nature of its current psychological situation (Schwarz, 1990). From this perspective, positive affective states inform people that the world is a safe place that does not threaten their current goals. Negative affective states, on the other hand, inform people that the current situation is problematic, and is characterized either by a lack of positive or a threat of negative outcomes. Hence, affective states may serve as simple but highly salient indicators of the nature of the current psychological situation. Indeed, empirical evidence indicates that different emotions are associated with different states of "action readiness," which are evident in physiological changes (e.g., Lacey & Lacey, 1970; Obrist, 1981) and overt behavior (e.g., Ekman, 1982; Izard, 1977), as well as in introspective reports (e.g., Davitz, 1969; Frijda, 1986, 1987). Accordingly, many theories of emotion hold that "emotions exist for the sake of signaling states of the world that have to be responded to, or that no longer need response and action" (Frijda, 1988, p. 354).

These considerations suggest that individuals' processing strategies may be tuned to meet the requirements of the psychological situation that is reflected in their feelings. If negative affective states inform them about a lack of positive outcomes, or a threat of negative outcomes, they may be motivated to change the current situation. Attempts to change the situation, however, initially require a careful assessment of the features of the current situation, an analysis of their causal links, and explorations of possible mechanisms of change and their potential outcomes (e.g., Bohner, Bless, Schwarz, & Strack, 1988). Accordingly, it would be highly adaptive if negative feelings increased the cognitive accessibility of procedural knowledge that is adequate for handling negative situations. Increased accessibility of this procedural knowledge, however, would also increase the likelihood that the respective procedures are applied to other tasks that people work on while in a bad mood, resulting in a generalized use of analytic reasoning procedures during bad moods (see Higgins, 1989). Moreover, people may be unlikely to take risks in a situation that is already considered problematic and gives rise to an increased control motivation (see Weary & Gannon, Chapter 7, this volume). As a result, they may avoid simple heuristics and the playful exploration of novel solutions under negative affect, relying instead on more systematic, effortful, and detail-oriented processing strategies.

On the other hand, if positive feelings inform people that their personal world is currently a safe place, they may see little need to engage in cognitive effort, *unless* this is required by other currently active goals. In pursuing these goals, they may also be willing to take some risk, given that the general situation is considered safe. Thus, simple heuristics may be preferred to more effortful, detail-oriented judgmental strategies; new procedures and possibilities may be explored; and unusual, creative associations may be elaborated. Moreover, diverse types of procedural knowledge may be equally accessible (given that no specific procedure has been activated to deal with a problematic situation), thus further increasing the potential for unusual solutions.

These conjectures predict numerous mood-induced differences in processing style, for which considerable support can be found in a diverse body of literature (see Clore et al., 1994; Schwarz, 1990; Sinclair & Mark, 1992; and Weary & Gannon, Chapter 7, this volume, for reviews). On a wide variety of tasks, individuals in an elated mood have been found to be less likely to use systematic strategies of information processing than individuals in a neutral mood, whereas individuals in a mildly depressed mood have been found to be more likely to do so.

Some Selected Evidence

To date, the impact of mood states on processing style has been most systematically explored in the domain of persuasion, in part because the cognitive dynamics underlying the processing of persuasive communications are well understood (see Eagly & Chaiken, 1993; Petty & Cacioppo, 1986a, 1986b). In general, a message that presents strong arguments is more persuasive than a message that presents weak arguments, provided that recipients are motivated and able to process the content of the message. If recipients do not engage in elaborative processing of message content, the advantage of strong over weak arguments is eliminated. To the extent that elated moods decrease systematic processing, whereas depressed moods increase systematic processing, we should therefore observe that the quality of the presented arguments has more impact on individuals in a depressed mood than on individuals in an elated mood. Several studies have confirmed this prediction (e.g., Bless, Bohner, Schwarz, & Strack, 1990; Bless, Mackie, & Schwarz, 1992; Bohner, Chaiken, & Hunyadi, 1994; Bohner, Crow, Erb, & Schwarz, 1992; Mackie & Worth, 1989; Worth & Mackie, 1987; see Schwarz, Bless, & Bohner, 1991, for a review).

Figure 6.1 shows a typical example, taken from Bless et al. (1990, Experiment 1). In this study, college students were put into a good or bad mood and were exposed to a counterattitudinal persuasive message that presented strong or weak arguments. Compared to control subjects who were not exposed to a persuasive message, subjects in an elated mood were moderately and equally persuaded by strong as well as by weak arguments, indicating that they did not engage in systematic message elaboration. In contrast, subjects in a depressed mood were strongly persuaded by strong arguments, but were not persuaded by weak arguments, indicating that they engaged in systematic message elaboration. These differences in message elaboration are also reflected in the message-related thoughts that subjects reported, as shown in Figure 6.2. Whereas recipients in a depressed mood reported more disagreeing thoughts in response to weak messages, and more agreeing thoughts in response to strong messages, elated recipients' cognitive responses showed no differences as a function of message strength.

The assumption that elated moods inhibit, whereas depressed moods facilitate, systematic information processing is further supported by research into person perception (see Sinclair & Mark, 1992, for a review). For example, Sinclair (1988) observed that subjects in an elated mood made less use of detailed performance information and showed more halo effects and lower accuracy on a performance appraisal task than subjects in a depressed mood, with subjects in a neutral mood falling in between. Similarly, subjects in an induced elated mood showed more pronounced primacy effects in impression formation than subjects in a depressed mood did (Sinclair & Mark, 1992). Moreover, subjects in induced elated moods have been found to rely more on category membership information in judging a target person, whereas

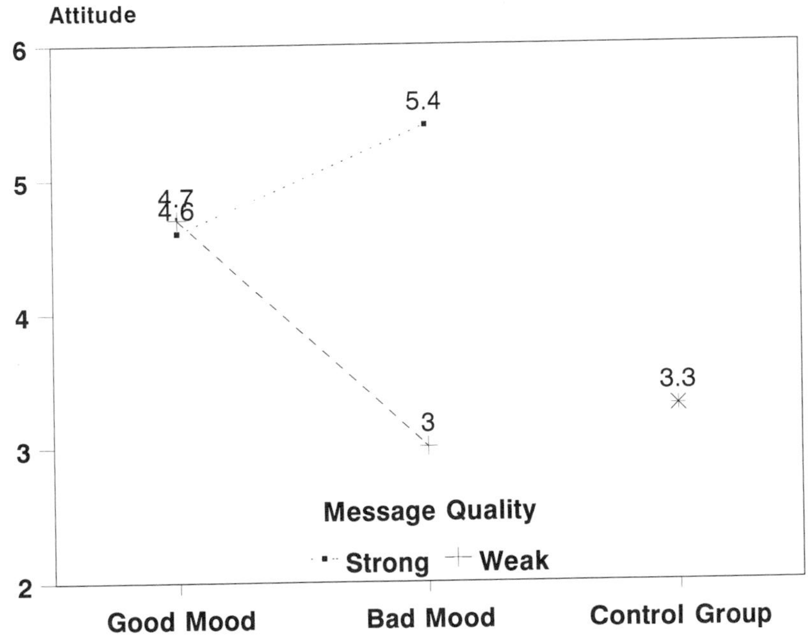

FIGURE 6.1. Attitude change as function of mood and message quality. Mean attitude reports of happy and sad subjects after exposure a strong, a weak, or no (control) message are shown. Data from Bless et al. (1990, Experiment 1).

subjects in induced depressed moods are likely to make use of a wider range of individuating information (e.g., Bless, 1992; Bodenhausen, 1993; Edwards & Weary, 1993). Given that reliance on category membership information is assumed to reflect the heuristic use of stereotypes to simplify the judgment task (Bodenhausen, 1993; Fiske & Neuberg, 1990), these findings again illustrate the impact of moods on the adoption of systematic versus heuristic processing strategies.

Finally, individuals' mood states frequently affect behavioral decisions in line with the assumptions offered here. In the domain of helping behavior, for example, individuals in a depressed mood have been found to calculate the costs and benefits of helping in deciding what to do, whereas individuals in an elated mood are likely to help regardless of these considerations (see Schaller & Cialdini, 1990, for a review). In combination, these findings indicate that individuals in a depressed mood are more likely to engage in systematic information processing than individuals in an elated mood, who are more likely to rely on heuristic strategies. As a "flip side" of these findings, however, individuals in an elated mood have also been found to be more likely to engage in the playful exploration of novel solutions, which fosters creative problem solving during good moods (see Isen, 1987, for a

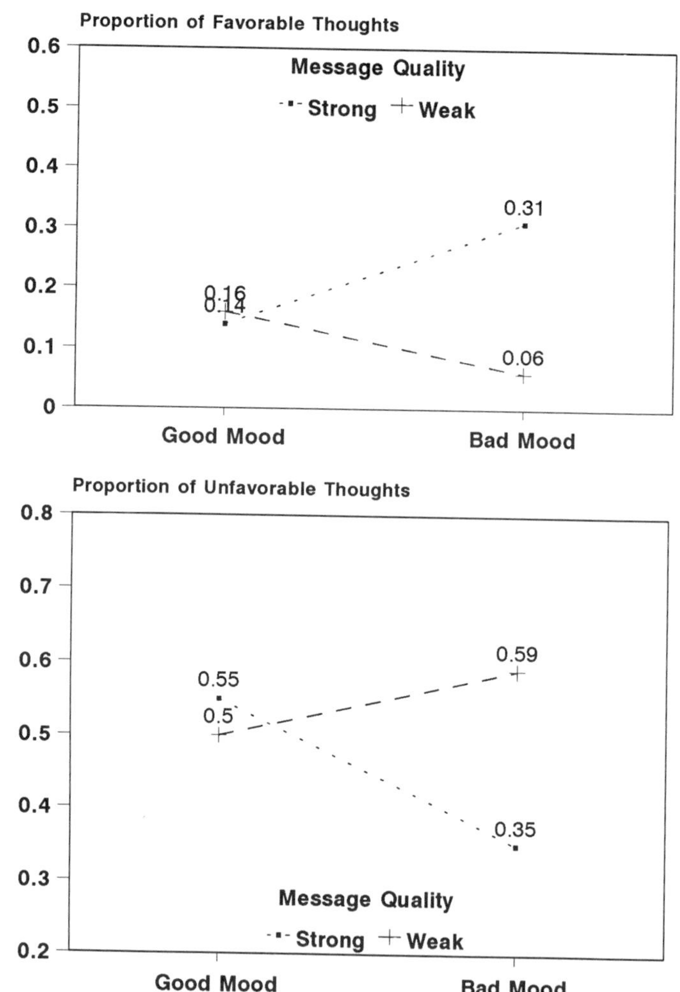

FIGURE 6.2. Cognitive responses as a function of mood and message quality. Proportion of favorable or unfavorable thoughts reported by happy or sad subjects in response to strong or weak messages are shown. Data from Bless et al. (1990, Experiment 1).

review). Clore et al. (1994) provide a more extensive discussion of different theoretical approaches to the interplay of affective states and style of reasoning, as well as a more detailed review of the available data, which is beyond the scope of this chapter. Next, we turn to some limiting conditions.

Some Limitations

Several limitations of the above-described generalizations deserve attention. First, the frequently observed increase in systematic processing during a bad mood may be limited by the extent to which handling the negative situation itself binds a considerable degree of subjects' cognitive capacity, thus restricting their capacity to work on an unrelated task (see Easterbrook, 1959, for an early review, and Ellis & Ashbrook, 1988, for a more recent discussion). Such interference effects of negative affect have primarily been observed in memory paradigms that require subjects to learn lists of words, and it is difficult to reconcile these findings with results obtained in the domains reviewed above (see Clore et al., 1994).

Second, any potential advantage of different processing styles cannot be observed if individuals are not motivated to work on a task to begin with, as is frequently the case in severe depression. Accordingly, the literature on depressive realism (see Ruehlman, West, & Pasahow, 1985; Weary & Gannon, Chapter 7, this volume) suggests that severe depression, in contrast to being in a "depressed mood," is unlikely to improve analytic performance. It is interesting to note, however, that phenomenological studies of the subjective experience of severe depression (see Tölle, 1982, for a review) indicate that the experience of "sadness" or of "being in a bad mood" is not part of the melancholic state that characterizes severe depression. Thus, the subjective experiences that accompany severe depression may be different in nature from the "normal" negative affective states considered in the present chapter. Moreover, the experiences associated with severe depression are likely to endure over extended periods of time with limited variation, and may therefore lose whatever informational value they may have had at their onset.

Third, an increased motivation to engage in systematic processing can only be observed in improved performance on a task if individuals have the appropriate procedural knowledge. In the absence of knowing the appropriate algorithm, for example, more effort or attention to detail alone is of little help. Accordingly, it is not surprising that studies on logical problem solving obtained more mixed support for the beneficial impact of depressed moods (see Clore et al., 1994, for a review) than did studies that presented tasks closer to daily life, such as evaluating another person or dealing with a persuasion attempt.

Finally, other currently active goals (see Srull & Wyer, 1986) may override the general impact of affective states. In line with this assumption, we (Bless et al., 1990, Experiment 1) observed, for example, that subjects in an elated mood could differentiate between strong and weak arguments when explicitly instructed to pay attention to argument quality. Note, however, that the informative-functions logic offered here implies that it should be easier to induce individuals in a good mood to use a systematic processing style than to induce individuals in a bad mood to use a heuristic style. If positive feelings inform people that no action is needed, overriding this message because of other action requirements poses no problem. In contrast, if negative feelings inform people about current problems, ignoring this message would not be adaptive. Accordingly, we may expect that the impact of negative feelings on processing style is more immune than the impact of positive feelings to the influence of other variables.

MOODS AND THE ACTION SEQUENCE: WHY THINGS ARE LIKELY TO BE MORE COMPLEX

Whereas the preceding review of the available evidence suggests that elated moods decrease, and depressed moods increase, the motivation to engage in systematic information processing, there is good reason to believe that the impact of mood is more complex. So far, we have assumed that people's affective states inform them about the nature of the psychological situation they are in, which in turn determines the spontaneously adopted strategy of information processing. Affective states, however, may serve as an informational basis for a variety of different judgments, ranging from the evaluation of consumer goods (e.g., Isen, Shalker, Clark, & Karp, 1978), other persons (e.g., Clore & Byrne, 1974), selected activities (Carson & Adams, 1980), and past life events (Clark & Teasdale, 1982) to reports of happiness and satisfaction with one's life as a whole (Schwarz & Clore, 1983). Throughout, individuals in an elated mood have been found to provide more positive evaluations of the respective target than have individuals in a depressed mood.

In line with the informative-functions approach adopted in the present chapter, Schwarz and Clore (1983, 1988) traced this impact of affective states on evaluative judgments to the use of one's feelings as a source of information. Specifically, they proposed that individuals may use their apparent affective reaction to the target as relevant information when making evaluative judgments. In fact, some evaluative judgments refer, by definition, to one's affective reaction to the stimulus. For example, when asked how "likeable" Mary is, individuals may interpret this question to refer to their feelings toward Mary. If so, they may not engage in detailed analyses of Mary's behaviors and traits, but may assess their own feelings toward Mary and use them as a basis for judgment. Other evaluative judgments may not refer directly to one's feelings about the target, but may pose a task that is very complex and demanding. Again, the judgmental task may be simplified by assessing one's own feelings about the target. Rather than computing a judgment on the basis of recalled features of the target, individuals may therefore ask themselves, "How do I feel about it?" In doing so, however, they may mistake feelings stemming from a pre-existing mood state for a reaction to the target stimulus, and this may result in more positive evaluations under pleasant than under unpleasant moods.

If so, the impact of affective states on evaluative judgments should depend on the respective states' perceived informational value. If individuals attribute their current feelings to a source that is irrelevant to the evaluation of the target stimulus, the informational value of their affective state should be discredited, and their feelings should not influence the evaluative judgment. In line with this hypothesis, Schwarz and Clore (1983) observed that the impact of mood on judgments of life satisfaction was eliminated when subjects attributed their current feelings either correctly (Experiment 2) or incorrectly (Experiment 1) to a transient source. For example, subjects reported higher life satisfaction and a more elated current mood in telephone interviews when they were called on sunny rather than rainy days. This difference was eliminated, however, when the interviewer mentioned the weather as part of a private aside, thus directing subjects' attention to this source of their elated or depressed state (Experiment 2). Similarly, recalling a sad life event did not influence subjects' judgments of life satisfaction when they could misattribute the resulting sad feelings to the alleged impact of the experimental room (Experiment 1). In addition, current mood, as assessed at the end of the experiment, was more strongly correlated with judgments of life satisfaction when subjects' attention was *not* directed to a transient source of their feelings than when it was. Conceptual replications of these findings have been reported by Keltner, Locke, and Audrain (1993), Schwarz, Servay, and Kumpf (1985), and Siemer and Reisenzein (1992).

In combination, these findings indicate that individuals may use their current feelings as a basis of judgment unless the diagnostic value of their feelings for the judgment at hand is called into question. This discounting effect (Kelley, 1972) is incompatible with alternative accounts, which hold that mood effects on evaluative judgments are mediated by mood-congruent recall of information from memory (e.g., Bower, 1981; Isen et al., 1978). According to these accounts, people are more likely to recall positive material when in a good mood and negative material when in a bad mood, and this selective recall of mood-congruent "data" results in mood-congruent judgments. Note, however, that the (mis)attribution manipulations used by Schwarz and Clore (1983) only discredited the implications of subjects' current feelings, but not the implications of valenced information about their lives, which may have been recalled from memory. For example, being aware that one's current bad mood may be attributable to lousy weather implies that it may not reflect an overall negative state of one's life. This attribution, however, does not discredit the implications of any recalled failures, for example. Hence, the (mis)attribution effects obtained by Schwarz and Clore (1983) and others indicate that individuals may use their affective state itself as a source of information. They only rely on this source of information, however, to the extent that its informational value is not called into question. Given these findings, it is also not surprising that mood effects on evaluative judgments have been observed in the absence of any evidence for mood effects on the recall of relevant information from memory (e.g., Fiedler, Pampe, & Scherf, 1986), and that the impact of mood on evaluative judgments is a more robust phenomenon than the impact of mood states on the recall of information from memory (see Blaney, 1986; Mayer,

Gaschke, Braverman, & Evans, 1992; Morris, 1989; Clore et al., 1994, for reviews).

As may be expected from a strategy that serves to simplify complex judgmental tasks, reliance on one's affective state as a basis of judgment is more likely when the affective state is more pronounced (e.g., Strack, Schwarz, & Gschneidinger, 1985), when other relevant information is less available (e.g., Schwarz, 1987), the task is more complex (e.g., Schwarz, Strack, Kommer, & Wagner, 1987), and when individuals have fewer attentional resources (e.g., Siemer & Reisenzein, 1992) or less motivation to engage in a more effortful judgmental strategy (see Clore et al., 1994, for a more detailed discussion).

That individuals' perceived affective states may serve as an informational basis for making a wide variety of evaluative judgments suggests that such states may potentially influence the assessment of each and every step of the action sequence. Thus, they may influence, for example, how attractive people find a certain goal, how optimistic they are about the likelihood that they will attain that goal, or how satisfied they are with their performance on a task (see Martin, Ward, Achee, & Wyer, 1993, for a related discussion). If so, the motivational implications of affective states may be considerably more complex than our preceding discussion and the bulk of recent research have suggested. To be sure, there is good reason to assume that different affective states signal different psychological situations and accompanying processing requirements, as suggested above. However, to the extent that individuals bring their moods to bear on a more specific aspect of the situation, we may obtain rather different effects. Below, we explore the likely impact of mood states at different stages of the action sequence and review the limited empirical evidence available. Before doing so, however, we need to review the key steps of the action sequence.

The Steps of the Action Sequence

Various models have been proposed to conceptualize the process by which individuals translate their desires into specific actions. As Gollwitzer (1993, p. 148) observed, most models "describe progress towards goal achievement in terms of discrepancy reducing (i.e., negative) feedback loops" (e.g., Carver & Scheier, 1981; Miller, Galanter, & Pribram, 1960). Reflecting a hierarchical organization of feedback loops, superordinate loops are supposed to set the reference values for subordinate loops. As a result, these models conceptualize successful goal pursuit as "a movement downward from goals that describe an abstract desired end state to goals that specify a distinct behavior. Moreover, at all levels of abstraction the same principle is thought to account for progress towards goal attainment (i.e., the negative feedback loop)" (Gollwitzer, 1993, pp. 148–149).

In contrast, early theorists (e.g., Lewin, 1926; Lewin, Dembo, Festinger, & Sears, 1944) portrayed goal-directed behavior as a horizontal sequence of distinct phases or steps, emphasizing the distinction between "goal setting" (i.e. choosing among various possible goals) and "goal striving" (i.e. moving toward a chosen goal) (for reviews, see Gollwitzer, 1990, 1993, and Chapter 13, this volume). Recent work by Heckhausen and Gollwitzer (Heckhausen, 1989/1991; Heckhausen & Gollwitzer, 1986, 1987; Gollwitzer, 1990, 1993, and Chapter 13, this volume) has re-emphasized the distinction of separate, temporally ordered action phases. In their "Rubicon" model, the action sequence is analyzed from "a temporal perspective that begins with the awakening of a person's wishes prior to goal setting and continues through the evaluative thoughts entertained after goal striving has ended" (Gollwitzer, 1990, p. 55). This analysis yields four distinct phases. A "predecisional phase," in which "people deliberate wishes and desires in an attempt to set priorities" (Gollwitzer, 1993, p. 149), is followed by a "preactional phase," which is "characterized by efforts to promote the initiation of relevant actions via effective planning" (Gollwitzer, 1993, p. 149). During a following "actional phase," individuals focus on achieving the desired outcomes, which they finally evaluate in a "postactional phase" by comparing what has been achieved with what was desired. Each of these phases is assumed to be associated with distinct mental and behavioral activities—deliberating, planning, acting, and evaluating, respectively (Gollwitzer, 1990).

Because these activities are associated with executing different tasks, specific "mind-sets" are postulated to govern each step of the action sequence. Briefly, the deliberative and evaluative mind-sets (related to the first phase and last phase, respectively) are both assumed to be primarily concerned with evaluating the desirability and feasibility of goals. In the predecisional phase the targets of this evaluation are future goals, whereas in the postactional phase its targets are goals already attained. Because of these similarities and their obvious affinity to traditional themes in the psychology of motivation, both action phases and mind-sets were referred to as "motivational" in early versions of the model (e.g., Heckhausen & Gollwitzer, 1987). The remaining two phases are characterized by what have been called "implemental" and "actional" mind-sets, respectively. Both phases are less concerned with evaluation than with the initiation and smooth completion of goal-striving behavior. Therefore, these phases and their accompanying mind-sets were dubbed "volitional" in early renditions of the model (e.g., Heckhausen & Gollwitzer, 1987).

Overall, this model of goal-directed behavior has received ample empirical support (for overviews, see Gollwitzer, 1990, 1993, and Chapter 13, this volume). In the remainder of this chapter, we discuss the potential impact that affective states may have at each phase of the action sequence. We argue that the specific processes by which affect influences the action sequence may be a function of the phase at which it is experienced. A direct impact of mood states on goal-related judgments is most likely to be observed in the two "motivational" phases, because in these phases the individual is preoccupied with making evaluations and proceeds in a relatively open-minded fashion, taking into account a variety of informational input (e.g.,

Gollwitzer & Heckhausen, 1987, cited in Gollwitzer, 1990; Heckhausen & Gollwitzer, 1987). In the two "volitional" phases, on the other hand, this type of mood influence may be less pronounced because individuals tend to be biased toward processing information partial to their goals and toward viewing it in an optimistic fashion (as evidenced, for instance, by dissonance research on postdecisional changes in attractiveness ratings; e.g., Jones & Gerard, 1967; Wicklund & Frey, 1981). In other words, the "conscious" or "strategic" state of optimism linked to the implemental mind-set that governs the postdecisional phases may override or suppress the more "automatic" impact of incidental mood states. Such a priority of controlled as opposed to automatic affective processes is in line with current models in cognitive psychology, which assume that strategic mental processes can correct for automatically suggested ones (e.g., Logan, 1980, 1989; Posner & Snyder, 1975; for an overview, see Bargh, 1984). However, even though strategic effects may dominate at the output level, a certain degree of "facilitation" or "inhibition" may still be observed; that is, the strategic bias of favoring the chosen goal may be amplified by positive moods and attenuated by negative moods.

In addition, incidental mood states may exert a different kind of influence in the postdecisional phases of the action sequence, by affecting the process of recognizing situational opportunities to initiate action. Specifically, the criteria that people use in defining a match between a situation they encounter and the one that was specified in an implementation intention may be more or less stringent as a function of their current mood state. In the following sections, we discuss these possibilities in more detail.

The Predecisional Phase

The predecisional action phase is characterized by the task of evaluating both the desirability and the feasibility of attaining various potential goals. We discuss each of these aspects in turn.

Assessing Goal Desirability

Assessing the attractiveness of some future goal state presents a complex judgmental task that is fraught with uncertainty. When people are trying to determine how much they would enjoy a state that they have not yet experienced, they may have few alternatives but to imagine that they have attained that state and to assess their affective reaction to it. Reliance on such a "How do I feel about it?" heuristic (Schwarz & Clore, 1988), however, is bound to result in more positive evaluations of the imagined state during elated than during depressed moods, as numerous studies on mood effects on evaluative judgments have indicated (reviewed above). Hence, desirable states should seem all the more desirable when individuals are in a good mood, but may seem much less desirable when they are in a bad mood. Conversely, undesirable states may seem all the more repulsive when people are in a bad rather than a good mood. Accordingly, being in an elated mood may increase the power of approach goals, whereas being in a depressed or anxious mood may increase the power of avoidance goals.

Similarly, affective states may not only influence the expected value of goal attainment, but may also affect the evaluation of the process of goal striving. Asking themselves how pleasant or unpleasant the action required for goal achievement may be, people may again consult their apparent affective reactions to the imagined action as a source of relevant information. If so, the effort required for goal achievement may seem less dreadful when they are in a good rather than a bad mood. Findings reported by Hirt, McDonald, and Melton (in press) are consistent with this conjecture. These authors described an experimental task (finding similarities or differences between the characters of TV shows) to subjects in a happy, sad, or neutral mood, and assessed subjects' expectations regarding the enjoyability of the task before they had any actual experience with it. As predicted, happy subjects expected the task to be more fun and more interesting than did subjects in a sad mood, in line with the usually obtained impact of moods on evaluative judgments.

So far, our discussion has assumed that individuals consult their feelings as a source of relevant information in evaluating an unknown future outcome and the effort necessary to obtain it. However, individuals' assessments may be influenced by their mood even if they engage in a more elaborate analysis, based on a wider range of information. Investigating the thought processes that characterize the predecisional phase, Gollwitzer and Heckhausen (1987, cited in Gollwitzer, 1990) observed that subjects who were instructed to deliberate about an unresolved personal problem tended to reflect first about positive consequences of a potential course of action, and only later turned to potential negative outcomes. This process may be influenced by individuals' mood state in several ways. First, individuals in an elated mood are likely to truncate the search process earlier than individuals in a depressed mood. On the one hand, this may reflect the frequently observed differential degree of systematic information processing under elated and depressed moods, as discussed above. On the other hand, individuals may ask themselves, "Is my deliberation of this issue sufficient to allow me to decide what I'm going to do?" As Martin et al. (1993) have demonstrated, the answer to this question is more likely to be positive under a positive rather than a negative mood—an issue to which we return below. In either case, individuals in an elated mood are likely to truncate the search process earlier than individuals in a depressed mood, and hence should base their judgment primarily on the information that is most accessible—which seems to be information bearing on positive consequences of the potential course of action. Moreover, positive material may be more accessible in memory during elated than during depressed moods (Bower, 1981), thus further compounding the likelihood that positive information will dominate under elated moods. As a result, we would expect individuals in an elated mood to arrive at more favorable evaluations, even under conditions where their judgment is based on a wider range of information than the heuristic cue provided by their current affective state itself.

Determining the Likelihood of Goal Attainment: The Aspect of Feasibility

Affective states may also influence the perceived likelihood of goal attainment. In general, the likelihood of goal attainment depends on both personal factors (e.g., ability) and situational factors (e.g., task difficulty, obstacles). With respect to the personal aspect of attainment likelihood, the mood-as-information model predicts that assessments of one's own ability should be more favorable during a positive than during a negative mood. Data bearing on this hypothesis were recently reported by Brown and Mankowski (1993), who studied effects of induced mood and self-esteem on self-appraisals. They found that negative (as compared to positive) mood led to less favorable appraisals of the self on a trait adjective checklist that included ability-related items, such as "smart," "capable," "foolish," and "inadequate." This impact of mood on self-appraisals was particularly pronounced for subjects who were low as opposed to high in self-esteem.

Again, similar effects could be predicted on the basis of models that link mood and memory (Bower, 1981), if we assume that people may base their judgments of feasibility on a wider range of information that comes to mind during deliberation. Indeed, it has been observed that memory-based influences of mood on judgment are most likely if the self is the target of evaluation (Blaney, 1986).

Some suggestive evidence potentially bearing on mood influences on the perception of situational aspects of goal attainment, (e.g., the likelihood of encountering obstacles) comes from research into risk perception. Exploring the impact of affective states on the perceived likelihood of undesirable events, Johnson and Tversky (1983) observed that reading descriptions of negative events, which presumably induced a depressed and slightly anxious mood, increased judgments of risk across a wide set of targets. Not surprisingly, for example, reading about cancer affected judgments of the risk of cancer. More importantly, however, reading about cancer had equally strong effects on judgments of the risk of accidents and divorce. Such thoroughly generalized effects, undiminished over dissimilar content domains, are consistent with the assumption that subjects simplified the difficult task of evaluating unknown risks by consulting the feelings that the stimulus apparently elicited. If they felt depressed and anxious, they concluded that the risk they were asked to evaluate was indeed depressing and threatening, and evaluated it as being more severe, and more likely, than they did during a more positive mood.

In combination, these limited findings suggest that individuals in a depressed mood will be more pessimistic with regard to their own resources, as well as to relevant aspects of the situation, than individuals in a good mood. Hence, being in a good mood should facilitate, and being in a bad mood should impair, the impression that attainment of the goal is feasible.

Setting Performance Standards

A final aspect that needs to be deliberated in concert with goal desirability and feasibility is the height of the performance standard a person considers satisfactory (Gollwitzer, 1990). This aspect may be particularly susceptible to influences of affect, as was recently demonstrated by Cervone, Kopp, Schauman, and Scott (1994). These researchers suggested that in setting a performance standard, individuals may imagine that they reach a certain level of performance and may ask themselves, "How satisfied would I feel about this particular performance?" If so, they should infer less satisfaction if they are in a bad rather than in a good mood, provided that the informational implications of their mood are not called into question. If they infer a low level of satisfaction as a result of being in a bad mood, this inference, in turn, may lead them to adopt higher standards of performance. Hence, individuals in a bad mood should need to meet a higher level of performance to feel satisfied than individuals in a good mood.

Two experiments confirmed this prediction. For example, when asked to indicate "the minimal level of performance with which you would be satisfied; that is, the level of performance that you would have to achieve in order to be truly satisfied with how you had done" (Cervone et al., 1994, p. 501), bad-mood subjects set higher standards for themselves with regard to social skills and academic performance (Experiment 1) as well as a specific lab task (Experiment 2).

Combining these findings with our conjectures concerning judgments of attainment likelihood, we may expect that sad (as compared to happy) individuals set higher performance standards, and at the same time are less likely to judge a given standard as attainable. This is exactly the pattern of results that Cervone et al. (1994) obtained. Although relevant data are not available, we may assume that this process results in a reduced likelihood of forming any goal intentions for people in a sad (as compared to a happy) mood, because among the goals that they could potentially pursue, fewer of these meet the criteria of being both sufficiently attractive and still feasible.

Summary

The considerations above suggest that individuals' mood states may have a pronounced impact on goal adoption. When considering a potential goal state, people are likely to find it more attractive, and the process of obtaining it less unpleasant, when they are in a good rather than a bad mood. And in assessing the feasibility of obtaining the goal, they are likely to arrive at a more favorable assessment of their own resources and the nature of the situation when they feel good rather than bad. Finally, a given standard of performance has been shown to be evaluated as less satisfactory during a bad mood than during a good mood. To the extent that these affective influences reflect the use of feelings as a source of information, however, we should only observe them when the informational value of the feelings has not been called into question. If individuals are aware that their current feelings are attributable to a source that is unrelated to the course of action they are deliberating, they are likely to discount these feelings as a relevant source of information, thus undermining the feelings' impact on evaluative judgments (see Schwarz & Clore, 1988). Note that this latter assumption can be used to distinguish purely judgmental effects of "mood as information" (Schwarz, 1990) from retrieval-based influences of mood as a memory cue (e.g., Bower, 1981; Forgas, 1992), which should be less susceptible to discounting effects.

The Preactional Phase

Once the individual has chosen which goal to pursue and which standard to aspire to, the tasks of implementing this goal and planning the appropriate action become pre-eminent (Gollwitzer, 1990, 1993). The initiation of action is assumed to depend on volitional strength, the perceived favorability of the situation, and the perceived match between the actual situation and the situation that is specified in the person's initiation intention (see Gollwitzer, 1993). The considerations described above suggest that the perceived favorability of the current situation is likely to be affected by individuals' mood states, thus potentially increasing the likelihood of action initiation during elated moods.

Moreover, several studies have demonstrated an impact of mood states on categorization processes (see Isen, 1987, for a review; Hirt et al., in press; Murray, Sujan, Hirt, & Sujan, 1990). For example, Isen and Daubman (1984) found that happy subjects categorized information more broadly than neutral-mood control subjects. Specifically, happy subjects created fewer and more inclusive categories on a category creation task, were more likely to include nonprototypical exemplars in a given category (e.g., "cane" in the category "clothing"), and rated nonprototypical exemplars as being more prototypical. Given these findings, which are compatible with happy people's tendency to use less effortful processing strategies, individuals may be more likely to perceive matches between a given situation and the situation represented as part of their initiation intention when they are in a happy rather than a sad mood.

Such mood-dependent differences in the perception of a situational match or mismatch with an implementation intention may be at the core of an effect that we (Bohner et al., 1992, Experiment 2) observed in an experiment on mood influences in a realistic persuasion setting. In that study, subjects who had been put in a happy or a sad mood were approached by a confederate who asked for a contribution to a charity. The confederate supported her request with either a strong or a weak argument, and presented a list of contributors that suggested high or low consensus. The major result of the study was that sad subjects took the content of the request *and* the situational consensus cue into account in arriving at their action decision, and were likely to donate money only if either a strong argument or high consensus was present. Happy subjects, however, were highly likely to donate, regardless of the specifics of the situation. This behavior may reflect a tendency to form an action decision on the basis of minimal informational input. We suggested that happy subjects may have acted on the basis of a behavioral script (Schank & Abelson, 1977), such as "If someone asks me for a donation to a charity, I donate some money" (with the script including the default assumption that the request is legitimate), whereas sad subjects checked the specific situational information more thoroughly (Bohner, 1990; see Bohner et al., 1992, for an extended discussion). Note that a behavioral script that includes a situational condition for appropriate action may be conceptualized as an implementation intention in the sense of Gollwitzer (1993). Thus, happy subjects in our study may have been more likely to perceive a match between the experimental situation and a previously formed intention.

More recent studies on category formation by Murray et al. (1990; see also Hirt et al., in press), however, suggest that happiness may not always promote action in this way. These researchers tested the interesting hypothesis that happy subjects do not invariably form broad categories, but rather are more *flexible* categorizers. In a task that involved the categorization of television programs, happy subjects formed fewer and more inclusive categories when asked to focus on similarities, but more and more subordinate categories when asked to focus on differences between stimuli. Additional analyses revealed that this greater cognitive flexibility during a happy mood was accompanied by greater intrinsic interest in the categorization task, and that both the similarities and differences produced by happy subjects were more original than those generated by neutral-mood subjects. These findings are in line with the superior performance of happy subjects in creativity tasks (Isen, 1987).

If we apply this happiness–flexibility hypothesis to the perception of opportunities for initiating goal-directed action, we should expect that the direction of mood influences depends on a person's focus of attention. If the person pays more attention to similarities between the actual situation and the one specified in an implementation intention, happy mood should facilitate the perception of a match and thus promote action; if the person pays more attention to differences, however, happy mood should inhibit detection of a match and thus obstruct action. Which of these two possibilities is more likely in natural situations? Given that the postdecisional phases are characterized by a general "optimistic" bias toward processing information in a manner that facilitates rather than impedes action, we may expect a focus on similarities to be the default option. As a result, we would again expect a higher likelihood of action initiation during an elated than during a depressed mood.

The Actional Phase

Successful completion of an initiated course of action is in large part a function of the extent to which the individual commands the relevant skills and is motivated to expend the relevant effort. Of these aspects, the latter is again likely to be influenced by the individual's affective state.

Effort Expenditure

How much effort is expended at the action phase depends on a variety of variables (see Gollwitzer, 1993 and Chapter 13, this volume), of which we only address two. On the one hand, it is likely that individuals expend more effort—work longer on a task, for example—when the action itself is enjoyable rather than unpleasant. On the other hand, effort expenditure is terminated when an individual's performance evaluation indicates that the intended goal is reached. Whereas this latter aspect is typically assigned to the postactional phase in Heckhausen and Gollwitzer's conceptualization, we address it in the context of effort expenditure for the sake of simplicity.

Both the evaluation of one's performance and the assessment of the enjoyability of the action one is engaged in are strongly affected by individuals' mood states, as Martin et al. (1993) recently demonstrated in an ingenious series of experiments. For example, these authors asked subjects to generate a list of birds from memory. Some subjects were instructed to ask themselves how satisfied they were with their performance and to stop when they felt that this was "a good time to stop." Under this performance-oriented decision rule, subjects in a bad mood spent more time listing birds, and listed more birds, than subjects in a good mood. This presumably indicates that bad-mood subjects inferred lower performance satisfaction than good-mood subjects, prompting them to continue in their efforts. Note that his finding is compatible with the observation that sad subjects tend to set higher performance standards for themselves, as discussed above (Cervone et al., 1994). Other subjects, however, were told to stop when they "no longer enjoy[ed] the task." Under this enjoyment-related decision rule, bad-mood subjects spent less time on the task, and listed fewer birds, than good-mood subjects; this presumably indicates that they were more likely to infer that they no longer enjoyed the task. Finally, subjects who were not given an explicit decision rule also spent more time on the task, and listed more birds, when they were in a bad rather than in a good mood, suggesting that they spontaneously adopted a task-oriented decision rule. Hirt et al. (in press) reported a conceptual replication of this interactive impact of mood and decision rule on task performance, using a different task and a different mood induction.

As these findings indicate, the same affective state may result in different performance behavior, depending on the decision rule for which it serves as input: Whereas negative moods result in more effort than positive moods under a performance-oriented rule, the reverse holds true under an enjoyment rule. Depending on the nature of the task and situational circumstances, individuals may spontaneously adopt one or the other rule, resulting in opposite effects of mood on effort expenditure. We may assume, however, that a performance orientation is likely to predominate in most performance settings, hence facilitating effort expenditure during bad mood in most cases, as the research reviewed initially would suggest. To the extent that being in a bad mood signals a problematic situation, we may further assume that the mood state itself may influence which decision rule individuals are likely to adopt spontaneously. In general, a performance-oriented rule may seem more appropriate than an enjoyment-oriented rule in a problematic situation, whereas the reverse holds if an elated mood signals that the environment poses no particular problem. Despite these caveats, the Martin et al. (1993) and Hirt et al. (in press) results, based on decision rules that were explicitly presented by the experimenters, emphasize the extent to which the impact of a given affective state depends on the specific aspect of the action sequence that the state is brought to bear on.

Martin et al.'s (1993) findings also suggest an interesting explanation for the observation that the undermining of intrinsic interest through extrinsic rewards may be attenuated when the person is in a positive mood. Specifically, Pretty and Seligman (1984) suggested that the frequently obtained negative impact of extrinsic rewards on intrinsic task interest is in part mediated through negative affect associated with the task; they provided correlational evidence for this (Experiment 1). Putting subjects into a good mood, however, eliminated the adverse impact of extrinsic rewards on subjects' intrinsic motivation (Experiment 2). Given that the experimental situation in Pretty and Seligman's (1984) study was defined as a play situation, we may assume that subjects endorsed an enjoyment rule. Hence, they stopped playing in response to negative feelings elicited by the task, but continued playing when their positive mood suggested task enjoyment, as has been observed by Martin et al. (1993). These findings suggest that happy individuals' actions may be less dependent on extrinsic rewards, provided that they adopt an enjoyment rule and the informational value of their mood is not called into question. Under these conditions, the apparent enjoyment of the task is likely to motivate further task engagement, regardless of the presence of external rewards. In contrast, being in a sad mood is likely to suggest low task enjoyment, thus prompting disengagement unless extrinsic rewards are sufficient to override the apparent lack of interest.

The Postactional Phase

In the postactional phase, the individual must decide whether the intended outcome has been obtained and whether the goal has been satisfied. As discussed in the context of effort expenditure, these evaluations are likely to be affected by individuals' mood. Consistent with this assumption, Hirt et al. (in press) observed that subjects in an elated mood reported higher satisfaction with their performance on an experimental task, and assumed their performance to be better, than subjects in a depressed mood did. Examining the correlation between estimated and actual performance, these researchers obtained significant correlations (r's ranging from .37 to .39, $p < .01$) under neutral-mood conditions, but not under elated-mood or depressed-mood conditions (r's ranging from −.08 to .15, n.s.). This suggests that happy and sad subjects relied on the information provided by their feelings in estimating their performance, at the expense of more diagnostic performance information.

As discussed in the preceding section, however, the behavioral consequences of mood effects on performance assessments depend on the decision rule used, as Martin et al.'s (1993) and Hirt et al.'s (in press) results have demonstrated. Under a performance-related decision rule, individuals are likely to terminate goal striving when positive feelings suggest that their performance is satisfactory. Obviously, this effect should be more pronounced if the objective criteria of goal attainment are defined less clearly. If an enjoyment-related rule is employed, however, satisfaction with performance is unlikely to be assessed to begin with, and individuals are likely to continue task performance as long as positive feelings suggest that they enjoy it.

CONCLUSIONS

As the present conjectures (and the limited evidence bearing on them) indicate, there is good reason to assume that individuals' affective states may exert an influence at each stage of the action sequence. During the predecisional phase, goals may seem more attractive, and the process of obtaining them less dreadful, when people are in a good rather than a bad mood. Moreover, they may be more optimistic about the likelihood of goal attainment in a good mood, and may arrive at a more favorable assessment of their resources. Indeed, the tendency to consider lower performance standards satisfactory when individuals are in a good rather than a bad mood may render it likely that they will actually meet the standards they set while feeling good. In contrast, higher levels of performance are required to satisfy people when they are in a bad mood (e.g., Cervone et al., 1994; Martin et al., 1993), thus rendering it more likely that they may not live up to them. During the predecisional phase, people may be more likely to see a match between the current situation and the situation specified in their initiation intention when they are in a good mood, reflecting the impact of moods on categorization breadth (e.g., Isen, 1987). Moreover, they may arrive at a more optimistic assessment of the situation's favorability for their intended course of action, thus further increasing the likelihood of action initiation.

Once individuals have embarked on a course of action, their mood state is likely to influence the effort they are willing to expend during the action phase. The specific impact, however, depends on the decision rule employed (e.g., Martin et al., 1993). When people define the situation as a performance situation, feeling good leads them to infer that their performance is satisfactory, resulting in termination of the task. Conversely, feeling bad leads them to infer that their performance does not meet their standards, resulting in continued effort expenditure. If people employ an enjoyment rule, however, feeling good indicates that task performance is enjoyable, resulting in continued performance. Conversely, feeling bad suggests that they no longer enjoy the task, resulting in disengagement. We propose, however, that people's feelings are likely to influence which decision rule they spontaneously adopt if none is explicitly provided. To the extent that negative feelings signal a problematic state of the environment (Schwarz, 1990), individuals may be likely to adopt a performance rather than an enjoyment rule. If so, being in a sad mood should facilitate effort expenditure in most situations, unless the nature of the task or explicit instructions suggest that an enjoyment rule should be adopted. In fact, we conjecture that an enjoyment rule is unlikely to be adopted under negative affect, unless the task seems inconsequential and performance is disemphasized, as was the case under the enjoyment rule conditions of the Martin et al. (1993) and Hirt et al. (in press) studies.

This conjecture is based on the assumption that it would be rather maladaptive to ignore signals that indicate a potentially problematic situation under most other circumstances. Research into the impact of mood states on the adoption of effortful, systematic strategies of information processing is consistent with this assumption. As discussed in the first part of this chapter, most studies in this domain suggest that being in a sad mood facilitates effortful, systematic processing (see Clore et al., 1994, and Schwarz, Bless, Strack, et al., 1991, for reviews). On the other hand, people may be more likely to spontaneously adopt an enjoyment rule when feeling good signals that their current situation poses no problems. If so, they may terminate task performance when the task does not seem enjoyable. In contrast to the information provided by negative feelings, ignoring the information provided by positive feelings is unlikely to be maladaptive. Accordingly, we conjecture that it is easier to override the adoption of an enjoyment rule during a good mood than to override the adoption of a performance rule during a bad mood in potentially consequential situations. Thus, we would expect, for example, that it is easier to induce subjects in a good mood to engage in systematic information processing than to induce subjects in a bad mood to engage in heuristic processing, given that the current situation is characterized as safe or as potentially problematic by their respective mood states. In line with this conjecture, instructing happy subjects to pay attention to argument quality elicited systematic processing in a persuasion experiment, in contrast to the strategy that happy subjects adopted spontaneously (Bless et al., 1990). Thus, happy subjects may be expected to show a considerable degree of flexibility in their choice of processing strategy, whereas sad subjects should show a strong preference for systematic processing strategies (see Hirt et al., in press, for a related discussion).

Finally, when assessing goal attainment during the postactional phase, people are more likely to infer that they have attained their goal when they feel good rather than bad. Indeed, the correlations between estimated and actual performance reported by Hirt et al. (in press) suggest that pronounced mood states may drive assessments, at the expense of more germane information about actual performance. As a result, individuals are more likely to terminate the course of action when positive feelings suggest that they are satisfied with their goal attainment.

In combination, these conjectures suggest that the specific impact of a given mood state depends on the action phase at which individuals consult their feelings in making pertinent decisions. Accordingly, the same mood state may result in very different behavioral effects, depending on the respective stage of the action sequence. Nevertheless, we propose that these different effects can be traced to the same underlying cognitive process. Consistent with the assumption that moods serve information functions (Schwarz & Clore, 1983, 1988), we assume that individuals may ask themselves, "How do I feel about it?" when evaluating a goal, a standard of performance, a course of action, the enjoyability of a task, or their level of performance. In each case, they are likely to arrive at a more positive evaluation when they feel good rather than bad, reflecting that it is difficult to distinguish a pre-existing mood state from an affective reaction to the target that is being evaluated. According to the logic of the feelings-as-information approach, these effects should be eliminated, however, when individuals are aware that their current feelings are attributable to some other source and hence do not reflect their reaction to the target of judgment (Schwarz & Clore, 1983). Accordingly, (mis)attribution experiments, which entail manipulations of subjects' awareness of the source of their moods, are needed to provide stringent tests of the conjectures offered here. As previous research indicated, being aware that one's feelings do not reflect one's reaction to the target is sufficient to eliminate the impact of moods on evaluative judgments (e.g., Schwarz & Clore, 1983), as well as the impact of mood on the choice of different processing strategies (Sinclair, Mark, & Clore, 1994).

Whether future research will support our conjectures is, of course, an empirical question. For the time being, we note that the processes underlying the impact of moods on the course of action taken are likely to be more complex than we assumed in the research reviewed in the first section of this chapter. In this research, we focused on the information that people's moods may provide about the nature of their current psychological situation, and explored how this information affects the choice of information-processing strategies (Schwarz, 1990; Schwarz, Bless, & Bohner, 1991). As Martin and his colleagues demonstrated (see Martin et al., 1993; Hirt et al., in press), however, moods may have different effects, depending on the decision rule for which they serve as relevant information. Extending this theme, the present chapter has identified the key decisions entailed in the action sequence and derived relevant predictions from the mood-as-information approach (Schwarz, 1990; Schwarz & Clore, 1988), which provides a general framework for the conceptualization of mood effects on judgment and behavior.

ACKNOWLEDGMENTS

The research reported was supported by grants Schw. 278/3, Schw. 278/5, and Str. 264/2 from the Deutsche Forschungsgemeinschaft to Norbert Schwarz, Fritz Strack, Gerd Bohner, and Herbert Bless. We thank John Bargh, Daniel Cervone, Peter Gollwitzer, and Ed Hirt for their helpful comments on a previous draft, and Herbert Bless, Tory Higgins, Fritz Strack, and Michaela Wänke for stimulating discussions.

REFERENCES

Arnold, M. B. (1960). *Emotion and personality.* New York: Columbia University Press.

Bargh, J. A. (1984). Automatic and conscious processing of social information. In R. S. Wyer & T. K. Srull (Eds.), *Handbook of social cognition* (pp. 1–43). Hillsdale, NJ: Erlbaum.

Blaney, P. H. (1986). Affect and memory: A review. *Psychological Bulletin, 99,* 229–246.

Bless, H. (1992, September). *Stimmungseinflüsse und die Nutzung kognitiver Repräsentationen in der sozialen Urteilsbildung [Mood effects on the use of cognitive representations].* Paper presented at the convention of the Deutsche Gesellschaft für Psychologie, Trier, Germany.

Bless, H., Bohner, G., Schwarz, N., & Strack, F. (1990). Mood and persuasion: A cognitive response analysis. *Personality and Social Psychology Bulletin, 16,* 331–345.

Bless, H., Mackie, D. M., & Schwarz, N. (1992). Mood effects on encoding and judgmental processes in persuasion. *Journal of Personality and Social Psychology, 63,* 585–595.

Bodenhausen, G. V. (1993). Emotions, arousal, and stereotypic judgments: A heuristic model of affect and stereotyping. In D. M. Mackie & D. L. Hamilton (Eds.), *Affect, cognition, and stereotyping* (pp. 13–37). San Diego, CA: Academic Press.

Bohner, G. (1990). *Einflüsse der Stimmung auf die kognitive Verarbeitung persuasiver Kommunikation und auf nachfolgendes Verhalten [Mood influences on the processing of persuasive communication and on subsequent behavior].* Unpublished doctoral dissertation, University of Heidelberg, Germany.

Bohner, G., Bless, H., Schwarz, N., & Strack, F. (1988). What triggers causal attributions? The impact of valence and subjective probability. *European Journal of Social Psychology, 18,* 335–345.

Bohner, G., Chaiken, S., & Hunyadi, P. (1994). The role of mood and message ambiguity in the interplay of heuristic and systematic processing. *European Journal of Social Psychology, 24,* 207–221.

Bohner, G., Crow, K., Erb, H.-P., & Schwarz, N. (1992). Affect and persuasion: Mood effects on the processing of message content and context cues and on subsequent behavior. *European Journal of Social Psychology, 22,* 511–530.

Bower, G. H. (1981). Mood and memory. *American Psychologist, 36,* 129–148.

Brown, J. D., & Mankowski, T. A. (1993). Self-esteem, mood, and self-evaluation: Changes in mood and the way you see you. *Journal of Personality and Social Psychology, 64,* 421–430.

Carson, T. P., & Adams, H. E. (1980). Activity valence as a function of mood change. *Journal of Abnormal Psychology, 89,* 368–377.

Carver, S., & Scheier, M. F. (1981). *Attention and self-regulation: A control-theory approach to human behavior.* New York: Springer Verlag.

Cervone, D., Kopp, D. A., Schauman, L., & Scott, W. D. (1994). Mood, self-efficacy and performance standards: Lower moods induce higher standards for performance. *Journal of Personality and Social Psychology, 67,* 499–512.

Clark, D. M., & Teasdale, J. D. (1982). Diurnal variation in clinical depression and accessibility of memories of positive and negative experiences. *Journal of Abnormal Psychology, 91,* 87–95.

Clore, G. L., & Byrne, D. (1974). A reinforcement affect model of attraction. In T. L. Huston (Ed.), *Foundations of interpersonal attraction* (pp. 173–170). New York: Academic Press.

Clore, G. L., Schwarz, N., & Conway, M. (1994). Cognitive causes and consequences of emotions. In R. S. Wyer & T. K. Srull (Eds.), *Handbook of social cognition* (2nd ed., pp. 323–417). Hillsdale, NJ: Erlbaum.

Davitz, J. R. (1969). *The language of emotion.* New York: Academic Press.

Eagly, A. H., & Chaiken, S. (1993). *The psychology of attitudes.* Fort Worth, TX: Harcourt Brace Jovanovich.

Easterbrook, J. A. (1959). The effect of emotion on cue utilization and the organization of behavior. *Psychological Review, 66,* 183–201.

Edwards, J. A., & Weary, G. (1993). Depression and the impression formation continuum: Piecemeal processing despite the availability of category information. *Journal of Personality and Social Psychology, 64,* 636–645.

Ekman, P. (1982). *Emotion in the human face.* New York: Cambridge University Press.

Ellis, H. C., & Ashbrook, P. W. (1988). Resource allocation model of the effects of depressed mood states on memory. In K. Fiedler & J. Forgas (Eds.), *Affect, cognition, and social behavior* (pp. 25–43). Toronto: Hogrefe.

Fiedler, K. (1988). Emotional mood, cognitive style, and behavior regulation. In K. Fiedler & J. Forgas (Eds.), *Affect, cognition, and social behavior* (pp. 100–119). Toronto: Hogrefe.

Fiedler, K., Pampe, H., & Scherf, U. (1986). Mood and memory for tightly organized social information. *European Journal of Social Psychology, 16,* 149–164.

Fiske, S. T., & Neuberg, S. L. (1990). A continuum of impression formation, from category-based to individuating processes: Influences of information and motivation on attention and interpretation. In M. P. Zanna (Ed.), *Advances in experimental social psychology* (Vol. 23, pp. 1–74). New York: Academic Press.

Forgas, J. P. (1992). Affect in social judgments and decisions: A multi-process model. In M. P. Zanna (Ed.), *Advances in experimental social psychology* (Vol. 25, pp. 227–275). San Diego: Academic Press.

Frijda, N. H. (1986). *The emotions.* Cambridge, England: Cambridge University Press.

Frijda, N. H. (1987). Emotions, cognitive structure, and action tendency. *Cognition and Emotion, 1,* 235–258.

Frijda, N. H. (1988). The laws of emotion. *American Psychologist, 43,* 349–358.

Gollwitzer, P. M. (1990). Action phases and mind-sets. In E. T. Higgins & R. M. Sorrentino (Eds.), *Handbook of motivation and cognition: Foundations of social behavior* (Vol. 2, pp. 53–92). New York: Guilford Press.

Gollwitzer, P. M. (1993). Goal achievement: The role of intentions. In W. Stroebe & M. Hewstone (Eds.), *European review of social psychology* (Vol. 4, pp. 141–185). Chichester, England: Wiley.

Heckhausen, H. (1991). *Motivation and action* (P. K. Leppmann, Trans.). Berlin: Springer-Verlag. (Original work published 1989)

Heckhausen, H., & Gollwitzer, P. M. (1986). Information processing before and after the formation of an intent. In F. Klix & H. Hagendorf (Eds.), *In memoriam Herrmann Ebbinghaus: Symposium on the structure and functioning of human memory* (pp. 1071–1082). Amsterdam: Elsevier/North-Holland.

Heckhausen, H., & Gollwitzer, P. M. (1987). Thought contents and cognitive functioning in motivational versus volitional states of mind. *Motivation and Emotion, 11,* 101–120.

Higgins, E. T. (1987). Self-discrepancy: A theory relating self and affect. *Psychological Review, 94,* 319–340.

Higgins, E. T. (1989). Knowledge accessibility and activation. In J. S. Uleman & J. A. Bargh (Eds.), *Unintended thought: Limits of awareness, intention, and control* (pp. 75–123). New York: Guilford Press.

Hirt, E. R., McDonald, H. E., & Melton, R. J. (in press). Processing goals and the affect–performance link: Mood as main effect or mood as input? In L. L. Martin & A. Tesser (Eds.), *Affect and social goals.* Hillsdale, NJ: Erlbaum.

Isen, A. M. (1987). Positive affect, cognitive processes, and social behavior. In L. Berkowitz (Ed.), *Advances in experimental social psychology* (Vol. 20, pp. 203–253). San Diego, CA: Academic Press.

Isen, A. M., & Daubman, K. A. (1984). The influence of affect on categorization. *Journal of Personality and Social Psychology, 47,* 1206–1217.

Isen, A. M., Shalker, T. E., Clark, M. S., & Karp, L. (1978). Affect, accessibility of material in memory, and behavior: A cognitive loop? *Journal of Personality and Social Psychology, 36,* 1–12.

Izard, C. E. (1977). *Human emotions.* New York: Plenum.

Jacobsen, E. (1957). Normal and pathological moods: Their nature and function. *Psychoanalytic Study of the Child,* 73–113.

Johnson, E., & Tversky, A. (1983). Affect, generalization, and the perception of risk. *Journal of Personality and Social Psychology, 45,* 20–31.

Jones, E. E., & Gerard, H. B. (1967). *Foundations of social psychology.* New York: Wiley.

Kelley, H. H. (1972). *Causal schemata and the attribution process.* Morristown, NJ: General Learning Press.

Keltner, D., Locke, K. D., & Audrain, P. C. (1993). The influence of attributions on the relevance of negative feelings to satisfaction. *Personality and Social Psychology Bulletin, 19,* 21–30.

Lacey, J. I., & Lacey, B. C. (1970). Some autonomic nervous system relationships. In P. Black (Ed.), *Physiological correlates of emotion* (pp. 205–227). New York: Academic Press.

Lewin, K. (1926). Vorsatz, Wille und Bedürfnis. *Psychologische Forschung, 7,* 330–385.

Lewin, K., Dembo, T., Festinger, L. A., & Sears, P. S. (1944). Level of aspiration. In J. M. Hunt (Ed.), *Personality and the behavior disorders* (pp. 333–378). New York: Ronald Press.

Logan, G. D. (1980). Attention and automaticity in stroop and priming tasks: Theory and data. *Cognitive Psychology, 12,* 523–553.

Logan, G. D. (1989). Automaticity and cognitive control. In J. S. Uleman & J. A. Bargh

(Eds.), *Unintended thought: Limits of awareness, intention, and control* (pp. 52–74). New York: Guilford Press.

Mackie, D., & Worth, L.T. (1989). Processing deficits and the mediation of positive affect in persuasion. *Journal of Personality and Social Psychology, 57,* 27–40.

Martin, L. L., Ward, D. W., Achée, J. W., & Wyer, R. S. (1993). Mood as input: People have to interpret the motivational implications of their moods. *Journal of Personality and Social Psychology, 64,* 317–326.

Mayer, J. D., Gaschke, Y. N., Braverman, D. L., & Evans, T. D. (1992). Mood-congruent judgment is a general effect. *Journal of Personality and Social Psychology, 63,* 119–132.

Miller, G. A., Galanter, E., & Pribram, K. N. (1960). *Plans and the structure of behavior.* New York: Holt, Rinehart & Winston.

Morris, W. N. (1989). *Mood: The frame of mind.* New York: Springer-Verlag.

Murray, N., Sujan, H., Hirt, E. R., & Sujan, M. (1990). The influence of mood on categorization: A cognitive flexibility interpretation. *Journal of Personality and Social Psychology, 59,* 411–425.

Nowlis, V., & Nowlis, H. H. (1956). The description and analysis of mood. *Annals of the New York Academy of Sciences, 65,* 345–355.

Obrist, P. A. (1981). *Cardiovascular psychophysiology.* New York: Plenum.

Ortony, A., Clore, G. L., & Collins A. (1988). *The cognitive structure of emotions.* New York: Cambridge University Press.

Petty, R. E., & Cacioppo, J. T. (1986a). The elaboration likelihood model of persuasion. In L. Berkowitz (Ed.), *Advances in experimental social psychology* (Vol. 19, pp. 124–203). New York: Academic Press.

Petty, R. E., & Cacioppo, J. T. (1986b). *Communication and persuasion.* New York: Springer.

Posner, M. I., & Snyder, C. R. R. (1975). Attention and cognitive control. In R. Solso (Ed.), *Information processing and cognition: The Loyola Symposium* (pp. 55–85). Hillsdale, NJ: Erlbaum.

Pretty, G. H., & Seligman, C. (1984). Affect and the overjustification effect. *Journal of Personality and Social Psychology, 46,* 1241–1253.

Ruehlman, L. S., West, S. G., & Pasahow, R. J. (1985). Depression and evaluative schemata. *Journal of Personality, 53,* 46–92.

Schaller, M., & Cialdini, R. B. (1990). Happiness, sadness, and helping: A motivational integration. In E. T. Higgins & R. Sorrentino (Eds.), *Handbook of motivation and cognition: Foundations of social behavior* (Vol. 2, pp. 265–296). New York: Guilford Press.

Schank, R. & Abelson, R. (1977). *Scripts, plans, goals, and understanding.* Hillsdale, NJ: Erlbaum.

Schwarz, N. (1987). *Stimmung als Information: Untersuchungen zum Einfluß von Stimmungen auf die Bewertung des eigenen Lebens [Mood as information].* Heidelberg: Springer-Verlag.

Schwarz, N. (1990). Feelings as information: Informational and motivational functions of affective states. In E. T. Higgins & R. M. Sorrentino (Eds.), *Handbook of motivation and cognition: Foundations of social behavior* (Vol. 2, pp. 527–561). New York: Guilford Press.

Schwarz, N., & Bless, B. (1991). Happy and mindless, but sad and smart? The impact of affective states on analytic reasoning. In J. Forgas (Ed.), *Emotion and social judgment* (pp. 55–71). Oxford: Pergamon.

Schwarz, N., Bless, H., & Bohner, G. (1991). Mood and persuasion: Affective states influence the processing of persuasive communications. In M. Zanna (Ed.), *Ad-*

vances in experimental social psychology (Vol. 24, pp. 161–199). San Diego, CA: Academic Press.

Schwarz, N., Bless, H., Strack, F., Klumpp, G., Rittenauer-Schatka, H., & Simons, A. (1991). Ease of retrieval as information: Another look at the availability heuristic. *Journal of Personality and Social Psychology, 61,* 195–202.

Schwarz, N., & Clore, G. L. (1983). Mood, misattribution, and judgments of well-being: Informative and directive functions of affective states. *Journal of Personality and Social Psychology, 45,* 513–523.

Schwarz, N., & Clore, G. L. (1988). How do I feel about it? Informative functions of affective states. In K. Fiedler & J. Forgas (Eds.), *Affect, cognition, and social behavior* (pp. 44–62). Toronto: Hogrefe.

Schwarz, N., Servay, W., & Kumpf, M. (1985). Attribution of arousal as a mediator of the effectiveness of fear-arousing communications. *Journal of Applied Social Psychology, 15,* 74–84.

Schwarz, N., Strack, F., Kommer, D., & Wagner, D. (1987). Soccer, rooms and the quality of your life: Mood effects on judgments of satisfaction with life in general and with specific life-domains. *European Journal of Social Psychology, 17,* 69–79.

Siemer, M., & Reisenzein, R. (1992). *Effects of mood on evaluative judgments: Influence of reduced processing capacity and mood salience.* Unpublished manuscript, Free University, Berlin, Germany.

Sinclair, R. C. (1988). Mood, categorization breadth, and performance appraisal: The effects of order of information acquisition and affective state on halo, accuracy, information retrieval, and evaluations. *Organizational Behavior and Human Decision Processes, 42,* 22–46.

Sinclair, R. C., & Mark, M. M. (1992). The influence of mood state on judgment and action: Effects on persuasion, categorization, social justice, person perception, and judgmental accuracy. In L. L. Martin & A. Tesser (Eds.), *The construction of social judgments* (pp. 165–193). Hillsdale, NJ: Erlbaum.

Sinclair, R. C., Mark, M. M., & Clore, G. L. (1994). Mood-related persuasion depends on misattribution. *Social Cognition, 12,* 309–326.

Srull, T. K., & Wyer, R. S., Jr. (1986). The role of chronic and temporary goals in social information processing. In R. M. Sorrentino & E. T. Higgins (Eds.), *Handbook of motivation and cognition: Foundations of social behavior* (Vol. 1, pp. 503–549). New York: Guilford Press.

Strack, F., Schwarz, N., & Gschneidinger, E. (1985). Happiness and reminiscing: The role of time perspective, mood, and mode of thinking. *Journal of Personality and Social Psychology, 49,* 1460–1469.

Tölle, R. (1982). *Psychiatrie* (6th ed.). Heidelberg: Springer-Verlag.

Wicklund, R. A., & Frey, D. (1981). Cognitive consistency: Motivational versus non-motivational perspectives. In J. P. Forgas (Ed.), *Social cognition: Perspectives on everyday understanding* (pp. 141–163). London: Academic Press.

Worth, L. T., & Mackie, D. M. (1987). Cognitive mediation of positive affect in persuasion. *Social Cognition, 5,* 76–94.

Wyer, R. S., & Carlston, D. (1979). *Social cognition, inference, and attribution.* Hillsdale, NJ: Erlbaum.

CHAPTER 7 Depression, Control Motivation, and Person Perception

Gifford Weary
Katherine Gannon

For the past two decades, an enormous amount of theoretical and empirical attention has been directed toward the antecedents, manifestations, and consequences of depression. Much of this work evolved from or tested various aspects of the cognitive theories of depression (e.g., Abramson, Seligman, & Teasdale, 1978; Beck, 1976). As these theories began to incorporate the psychological constructs of causal attributions, self-schemas, and self-focused attentional styles, and particularly as they began to focus on the role of others in the formation or activation of such cognitive processes and structures, depression increasingly became a major focus of inquiry for many social and personality psychologists. This was, of course, a natural development; social and personality psychologists had much to say about how others affect the various cognitive processes postulated to be important to the etiology, maintenance, and exacerbation of depression.

There was, however, at least one additional reason why the phenomenon of depression captured the attention of social and personality researchers and theorists. The study of depression—not as a clinical syndrome, but as an important individual-difference variable—permitted theoretical and empirical consideration of the social-psychological consequences of more intense and chronic affective states, more negative self-representations, and more intense and chronic levels of motivation than can typically be produced or assessed in social psychology laboratory settings and with unselected college student samples. Indeed, research employing depression in this way has proven helpful in elucidating a variety of basic social-cognitive processes (Weary & Edwards, 1994a).

Our own work on the social-cognitive consequences of depression may be considered an example of work employing depression as an individual-difference variable. This work grew out of two important lines of inquiry. One concerned the effects of temporary and relatively mild inductions of control deprivation on social information processing (Pittman, 1993; Pittman & D'Agostino, 1985). The other focused on the cognitive antecedents and correlates of depression (e.g., Warren & McEachren, 1983), among which perceptions and expectations of control loss were prominent.

Like other recent models of motivated social cognition (Chaiken, Liberman, & Eagly, 1989; Fiske & Neuberg, 1990; Nicholls, 1984; Petty & Cacioppo, 1986), ours adopts a pragmatic orientation (Fiske, 1992) in which perceivers' cognitive strategies and subsequent behaviors depend in part upon their goals. This "motivated tactician" (Fiske, 1993) perspective of human social cognition assumes a flexible processor of social information. If simple, relatively quick, and effortless judgments will suffice, then social perceivers will go no further; however, if relevant motives are engaged and if perceivers have the ability, then they can be expected to process relevant, available social information more extensively and complexly.

Our analysis focuses on chronic control concerns that frequently characterize relatively depressed individuals. In particular, our work examines how chronic (and in some cases extreme) differences in the level of control motivation, as exemplified by differences in level of depression, can influence both the content and process of thinking about others, as well as actions toward others.[1]

In this chapter, we intend to accomplish three goals. First, we outline the model (Weary, Marsh, Gleicher, & Edwards, 1993) that has guided most of our and our colleagues' research on the influence of depressives' generalized expectations of uncontrollability on their social perception processes. Second, we provide descriptions of several studies as illustrations of the kind of research that has been conducted to test key aspects of the model; we pay particular attention to studies that have examined the role of the social context in activating depressives' control-motivated social perception processes, and to studies that have examined the relationship between depressives' dispositional control motives and their social behaviors. To our minds, these two research foci represent topics of central importance to the general concerns of this particular volume and significant future research directions. Finally, we discuss briefly the relationship of our work to that on temporary moods and the processing of social information.

THE SOCIAL-COGNITIVE CONSEQUENCES OF DEPRESSION

Background

Although it is not a model of depression, our model does build upon the cognitive theories of depression; for this reason, we would like to present a brief overview of these theories. The major cognitive models—the helplessness–hopelessness model and Beck's model—are quite similar to each other, and for our purposes their differences are not critical. Consequently, for ease of presentation, we use terminology in describing these models that is closer to that of the helplessness–hopelessness model. The most recent formulation of the hopelessness model (Alloy, Kelly, Mineka, & Clements, 1990) is presented in Figure 7.1 in its most general and admittedly abbreviated form.

As can be seen, the model is a cognitive diathesis–stress formulation that identifies the following as distal contributory causes of depression: the presence of negative life events, a depressogenic inferential style, and a generalized tendency to view responses and outcomes as noncontingent. According to the model, the predisposition to explain important negative events in a way that implicates stable (i.e., enduring) and global (i.e., likely to affect many outcomes) factors, and the predisposition to view events as uncontrollable, increase the likelihood that individuals will develop a negative outcome expectancy (a belief that negative-outcomes are likely to occur or that positive outcomes are not likely to happen) and a helplessness expectancy (a belief in the noncontingency of responses and outcomes), respectively. These two expectations are critical elements of a proximal sufficient cause of depression, hopelessness, and they are hypothesized to result in different symptoms of depression. The negative-outcome expectancy is thought to result in sad affect (emotional symptom), and the helplessness expectancy is believed to result in a reduced initiation of voluntary responses (motivational symptom). Finally, low self-esteem is viewed as a likely symptom of depression if the stable and global attribution for the negative event is also internal.

The belief that negative events will occur and that one has no control

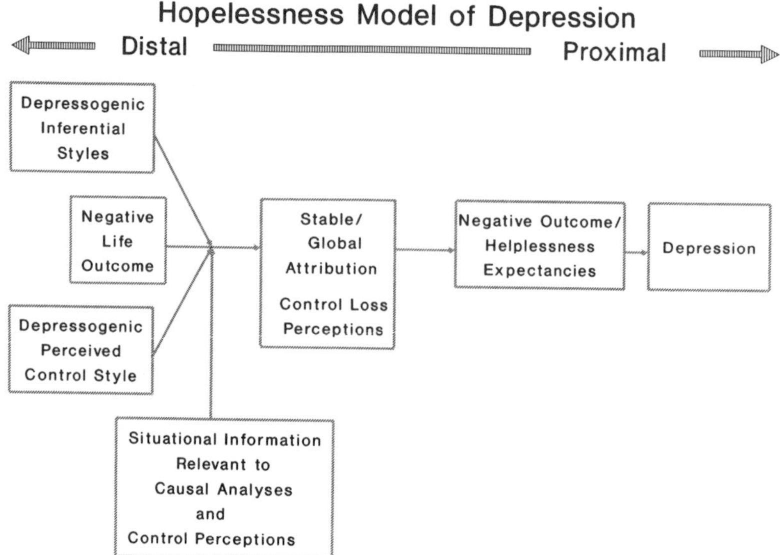

FIGURE 7.1. The hopelessness model of depression. From Alloy et al. (1990). Copyright 1990 by American Psychiatric Press. Adapted by permission.

over their occurrence, then, is seen to play a causal role in the major cognitive theories of depression. What is the empirical evidence for this hypothesized relationship?

We can offer several kinds of empirical evidence as support. First, experimental exposure to high levels of temporary control deprivation has been shown to produce temporarily the motivational and emotional symptoms associated with depression (Burger & Arkin, 1980; Gleicher & Weary, 1991a; Pittman & Pittman, 1980). Second, a number of investigators have demonstrated a concurrent association of depression and measures of less perceived and expected life control (Edwards & Weary, 1993a; Garber, Miller, & Seaman, 1979; Gleicher & Weary, 1991b; Jacobson, Weary, & Edwards, 1995; Marsh & Weary, 1989; Warren & McEachren, 1983; Weisz, Weiss, Wasserman, & Rintoul, 1987), as well as negative-outcome expectancies (Andersen, Spielman, & Bargh, 1992; Hull & Mendolia, 1991; Jacobson et al., 1995; Lewinsohn, Steinmetz, Larson, & Franklin, 1981; Lewinsohn, Hoberman, & Rosenbaum, 1988; Riskind, Rholes, Brannon, & Burdick, 1987). Third, and most important, several studies using longitudinal designs have found that perceptions and expectations of uncontrollability (Brown & Siegel, 1988; Edwards & Weary, 1993a; Lewinsohn et al., 1981, 1988; Pagel, Becker, & Coppel, 1985) and negative-outcome expectancies (Andersen, 1990; Carver & Gaines, 1987; Jacobson et al., 1995; Lewinsohn et al., 1981, 1988) predict the level of subsequent depressive symptomatology even when initial levels of depression are taken into account. Finally, the results of at least one of these studies (Pagel et al., 1985) suggest that the predictive relationship of loss of control is specific to depression; that is, perceived and expected beliefs of uncontrollability were stronger longitudinal predictors of depression than of anxiety or hostility. In sum, although this research cannot conclusively demonstrate the causal role of expectations of uncontrollability in depression and in causal uncertainty, it does provide consistent support for the hypothesized theoretical relationships.

The Model

As we have noted earlier, our model focuses on the social-cognitive consequences of uncontrollability or helplessness expectancies, which the cognitive theories argue are proximal, sufficient causes of depression. Like a number of other dual-process models, this model (see the boldface parts of Figure 7.2) assumes that people are cognitive misers who must be motivated to engage in extensive processing; expectations and perceptions of control loss, as well as resultant causal-uncertainty beliefs and feelings, are viewed as providing such motivation. Before we describe the model in some detail, let us first define a key construct embedded within it: causal uncertainty.

In the context of this model, the notion of "causal uncertainty" contains two components. First, there are causal-uncertainty beliefs, or generalized self-constructs about one's uncertain understanding of or ability to detect

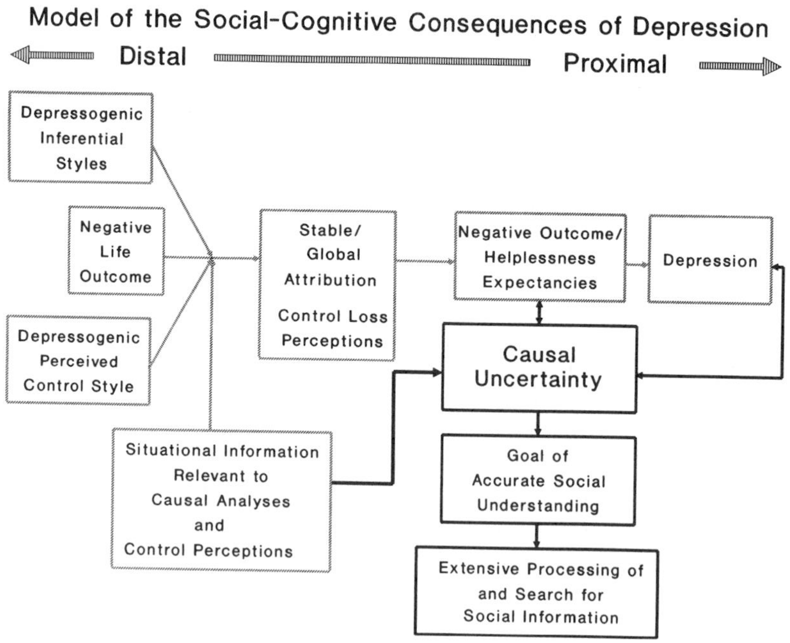

FIGURE 7.2. The model of the social-cognitive consequences of depression. Parts of this figure are adapted from Alloy et al. (1990).

causal relations in the social world (Weary & Edwards, 1994b). This construct is quite similar to Weisz et al.'s (1987) notion of "contingency uncertainty"—uncertainty about the causes of events. Second, there are causal-uncertainty feelings. More specifically, once activated, causal-uncertainty beliefs should give rise to metacognitive feelings of uncertainty (Clore, 1992), which should be experienced as confusion, surprise, or bewilderment.

Weary and Edwards (1996) have proposed that causal-uncertainty beliefs are available for all people, but are more accessible for some people. Specifically, these authors have suggested that individuals who possess chronic expectations that their future responses and outcomes will be noncontingent (e.g., depressed individuals) are more likely to perceive a loss of control and to conclude that they do not fully understand the relevant contingencies. The resulting causal-uncertainty beliefs should be highly accessible because of frequent activation. Although this accessibility notion has not been tested, two recent studies (Edwards & Weary, 1993a; Jacobson et al., 1995) using longitudinal designs have provided support for the hypothesized causal role of expectations of uncontrollability in causal uncertainty.

In the model, we see that an additional factor may contribute to the development and activation of causal uncertainty. Situational information relevant to causal analyses—in particular, information that there are multiple plausible cause or no known reliable causes for a negative outcome—may raise concerns about one's ability to understand contingency relations.

Causal-uncertainty beliefs and feelings, at least at mild and moderate levels, are hypothesized to have two consequences. The first consequence is the exacerbation of perceptions and expectations of uncontrollability: Individuals who believe that they do not understand the operating contingencies should also expect that they will have difficulty producing the desired outcomes (for supportive empirical evidence, see Edwards & Weary, 1993a). The second consequence is the adoption of a goal of "subjective accuracy" (Swann, 1984), or the subjective sense that one understands the social world. More specifically, the activation of causal-uncertainty beliefs and feelings is thought to serve as important input to the perceiver regarding his or her current state of knowledge. This input activates an accuracy goal, or a cognitive representation of the desired state of knowledge, and action plans designed to reduce the discrepancy between the current and desired states are associated with the goal representation. One such plan, and one that Weary and her colleagues have focused on in their research, entails a deliberate, intentional search for and use of social information in an attempt to regain causal understanding and to restore interpretive and predictive control (Rothbaum, Weisz, & Snyder, 1982). Often such an information-processing strategy will require the allocation of conscious attentional resources, and will thus entail a form of more effortful, controlled information processing.

At this point, the careful reader may detect what appears to be a contradiction between the predictions made by our model and those of the cognitive theories of depression. Recall that the cognitive theories predict that helplessness expectancies should result in a reduced motivation to initiate voluntary responses. Indeed, many studies have demonstrated performance deficits associated with depression (for reviews, see Hartlage, Alloy, Vazquez, & Dykman, 1993; Hertel & Rude, 1991; Johnson & Magaro, 1987), and numerous mechanisms have been proposed to account for them (e.g., motivational deficits, reduction in available cognitive capacity, conservative response styles). It is important to note, however, that studies demonstrating such depressive performance deficits have employed tasks that require complex concept-formation, problem-solving, general learning, or hypothesis-testing activities (e.g., anagrams). Importantly, they also have entailed clear performance outcome criteria. Past research has shown that moderately helpless subjects generally perform worse than nonhelpless subjects, primarily when tasks are difficult and when performance is viewed as possibly presenting a threat to further losses of control (Pittman & D'Agostino, 1985; Snyder, Stephan, & Rosenfield, 1978); when performance tasks are relatively simple and do not involve clear outcome criteria, then the performance of helpless subjects is better than that of nonhelpless subjects (Pittman & D'Agostino, 1985).

The performance consequences of helplessness expectancies with which our model and research have been concerned have been more familiar and more routine cognitive activities (e.g., person perception, impression formation processes), for which there have been no clear right or wrong outcomes; in fact, they have probably not even been perceived as performance tasks. Consequently, our model predicts reactance-type effects (enhanced cognitive activity designed to regain secondary forms of control), at least at mild and moderate levels of depression.

For a number of reasons, however, this more extensive processing on the part of mildly and moderately depressed perceivers is not hypothesized in the model to improve judgmental accuracy reliably, and so does not over the longterm lead to reduction in their feelings of uncertainty. Three such reasons are that (1) much of the additional information gathered may be nondiagnostic with respect to correct and incorrect judgments (Kruglanski, 1989); (2) the search for and processing of social information may under certain circumstances itself be biased (Marsh & Weary, 1989); and (3) depressed perceivers' desired levels of confidence may be sufficiently high that their actual confidence, regardless of the sufficiency of the information base, still may not exceed it (see Chaiken et al., 1989 for a discussion of sufficiency thresholds in judgmental confidence).

Finally, we should note that there are at least two important boundary conditions for our hypothesized effects of expectations of uncontrollability and causal-uncertainty beliefs. First, we would not expect to see enhanced processing of and search for social information if perceivers do not believe that such effort expenditure will reasonably render the social world more understandable, predictable, and controllable. Consequently, we would not expect to see enhanced cognitive activity for severely depressed perceivers who harbor extreme expectations of uncontrollability (for supporting evidence, see Marsh & Weary, 1989, 1994). Second, we might not expect to see enhanced sensitivity to social information at extreme levels of causal uncertainty. It seems reasonable to suggest that extreme certainty that one does or does not understand the causes of important outcomes should, on our social perception tasks, result in reduced motivation to process information effortfully.

ILLUSTRATIVE RESEARCH

Empirical Demonstrations of Depressives' Sensitivity to Social Information

As previously mentioned, one important implication of our model is that mildly and moderately depressed individuals, because of their heightened uncertainty about social contingencies, should be particularly sensitive to information that may render the social environment more understandable, predictable, and controllable. Such information may include another's explicit statements about the causal determinants of his or her behaviors, positive and negative social comparison feedback, and negative or unexpected behaviors. Much of our early research on this model, as well as one or two other investigators' research on the social perception processes of depressives, has demonstrated support for the sensitivity of mildly and moderately depressed perceivers to each of these kinds of social information (McCaul, 1983; Weary, Elbin, & Hill, 1987; Weary, Jordan, & Hill, 1985). Let us take one example of this early sensitivity research.

In one of the earliest studies, Weary et al. (1985) examined the reactions of mildly depressed and nondepressed subjects to another's negative, unexpected behavior. In this study, subjects observed (via a videotape) a male student taking a test presumably designed to assess his spatial analysis skills. They also observed the examiner delivering a test score indicating that the student had performed poorly. This feedback was followed by the examiner's asking the student for feedback about the test and about his assessment of the degree to which his ability and effort might have been responsible for his poor performance. Some subjects saw the student indicate a high degree of causal responsibility, while others saw him accept a low degree of responsibility for his test outcome. Following observation of the tape, all subjects were asked to evaluate the student on a number of positively, negatively, and neutrally toned trait adjectives.

Because of a social norm favoring internal attributions for task performance (Jellison & Green, 1981), the investigators expected that all subjects would evaluate the student more negatively when he accepted little responsibility for his poor performance (i.e., when he violated the norm of internality). They also expected that because of chronic, heightened control concerns and resultant feelings of uncertainty, depressed compared to nondepressed perceivers would make more use of or be more sensitive to the available attributional information, and as a consequence would evaluate the actor who violated the norm more negatively. The results were consistent with these predictions.

The results of the Weary et al. (1985) study have since been replicated and extended by Marsh and Weary (1994). In addition, Marsh and Weary have provided important evidence in support of the notion that this sensitivity to available attributional information is attributable to mildly and moderately depressed perceivers' heightened concerns about loss of control.

Empirical Evidence for Assumptions about Cognitive Processing

The research summarized or described above provides initial evidence that moderately depressed individuals are particularly sensitive to information that may reasonably render their worlds more understandable, predictable, and controllable. Through what mechanism, though, do these sensitivity effects occur? Correlational evidence from several of the sensitivity studies suggests that expectations about uncertainty and control loss are implicated in the processes, but the studies do not provide data to address whether the sensitivity effects reflect more systematic and thorough processing of the social information, or merely quick, polarized assessments in response to heuristics (e.g., "Violators of norms are bad"). The former process is more consistent with our reasoning thus far. Let us turn now to studies that provide more direct tests of the processing assumptions implicit in our explanations for depressives' sensitivity to social information.

Three studies have provided evidence relevant to the notion that depression is associated with more effortful processing of social information. First, Gleicher and Weary (1991b) explored possible differences in the amount and kinds of naturally occurring, on-line (Hastie & Park, 1986) inferences generated by depressed and nondepressed perceivers. Because of depressives' chronic expectations of uncontrollability and resultant feelings of uncertainty, Gleicher and Weary predicted that depressed subjects would engage in greater cognitive analyses of the available social information. To test this hypothesis, they asked depressed and nondepressed subjects to watch the videotape employed by Weary et al. (1985). This tape depicted the student performing the spatial analysis aptitude test. After they watched the student deny responsibility for his overall poor performance on the tests (thereby violating the attributional norm of internality; Jellison & Green, 1981), they then were asked to list their thoughts about and impressions of the student and to rate the abstractness of those thoughts and impressions. Analyses revealed that depressed compared to nondepressed perceivers generated a greater number of inferences and a greater number of abstract, dispositional inferences after observing the student's negative, unexpected behavior.

Although the study by Gleicher and Weary (1991b) offers evidence regarding the amount and content of depressed perceivers' thoughts, it does not provide evidence regarding the process or processes by which depressed and nondepressed perceivers arrive at a cognitive representation of another person. A second study attempted to move toward more process-oriented research on the impression formation processes of depressed persons.

This study was based on Fiske and Neuberg's (1990) continuum model of impression formation. This model postulates a processing continuum that runs from category-based to individuating, or "piecemeal," processes. At the category-based end of the continuum, perceivers attempt to place the target other into a social category. This type of processing occurs first and is primary. At the piecemeal end of the continuum, perceivers engage in an attribute-by-attribute analysis of the target other in order to arrive at a final assessment of the person. Piecemeal processing is conceived of as being more effortful than category-based processing, in that it utilizes more information and requires perceivers to construct a judgment algorithmically. Edwards and Weary (1993b) predicted that depressed perceivers, because of their expectations of uncontrollability and consequent feelings of uncertainty, would be more likely than nondepressed perceivers to engage in piecemeal processing when asked to make a judgment about another person.

To test this hypothesis, an idiographic technique developed by Pavelchak (1989) was employed. Specifically, depressed and nondepressed college students were asked to indicate how likable they thought a variety of academic majors and trait attributes were. Two weeks later, they were asked to make likability judgments of several stimulus people who were described by a list of trait attributes. Some subjects were asked to guess each stimulus person's major before rating the person for likability, thereby assigning the person a social category that could be used as the basis of the judgments. The rest of the subjects rated the people for likability and then guessed their majors. The fact that Edwards and Weary already had assessed subjects' liking for the majors and for the traits used to descrive the stimulus people allowed them to determine which type of information had been used by subjects in making their likability judgments.

Analyses of the results indicated that depressed perceivers tended to use piecemeal processing even when they had category information that could have been used to form a judgment. In addition, a path analysis provided support for the notion that depressives' tendency toward piecemeal processing was attributable to their chronic, generalized expectations of control loss. Consistent with our causal arguments, this analysis indicated that a perceived lack of control had a direct effect both on depression and on piecemeal impression formation processes; the path from depression to the index of piecemeal processing was not significant.

One additional study provides evidence that depressed perceivers tend to engage in more effortful processing of available social information. This study, by Yost and Weary (in press), used the attitude attribution paradigm. Studies employing this paradigm have often found that perceivers make dispositional or attitude attributions about a target that are consistent with an essay written by the target, and that they do so even when the essay is written under strong situational constraints. So often does this happen that the effect has been termed the "fundamental attribution error" or "correspondence bias."

Research (Gilbert, Pelham, & Krull, 1988) suggests that this bias or error results from a failure to correct the automatic, dispositional inferences perceivers draw from the target's behavior. That is, perceivers are thought to make an initial categorization of the target's behavior, followed by a characterization of, or drawing of a dispositional inference about, the actor. These two stages are thought to be relatively effortless and automatic. They are followed by an inferential correction stage, wherein perceivers adjust or correct their characterizations to some degree by taking into account important information about situational constraints. According to Gilbert et al. (1988), this correction stage involves more deliberative, effortful cognitive processes.

In their study, Yost and Weary (in press) tested the hypothesis that depressed perceivers, because of their heightened control concerns, would be more motivated to process the available information carefully and extensively, and so would be less likely to make highly correspondent attributions (i.e., would be more likely to correct their initial characterizations) about a target behaving under strong situational constraints than would nondepressed perceivers. When, however, they do not have the requisite cognitive resources to engage in inferential correction, then they should make attributions for the other's behavior that are as correspondent as those of nondepressed perceivers.

Mildly and moderately depressed and nondepressed college students were told that the study concerned impression formation processes, and that they would be asked to read some materials about a male student and then to make some judgments about him. In order to manipulate the cognitive resources available to subjects, half of the depressed and half of the nondepressed subjects were told prior to reading the materials that the study also was concerned with their ability to form impressions under conditions of distraction; they were given a six-digit number to memorize and rehearse during the impression task (cognitive-load condition). The remaining subjects were given no such information (no-load condition). All subjects then read what they believed were opening arguments the student had made during a debate. After reading these arguments, all subjects learned that the debate coach had assigned the student by the flip of a coin to the particular side of the issue he had argued. They then were asked to make attributions about the student's true attitude toward the issue.

The results of this study were entirely consistent with predictions. Mildly and moderately depressed subjects in the no-load condition corrected their initial dispositional characterizations of the other with the situational-constraint information to a greater degree than did nondepressed/no-load subjects. In the cognitive-load condition, however, both depressed and nondepressed subjects made highly correspondent inferences about the debater. Recall that the relatively effortful processing predicted for and exhibited by the depressed/no-load subjects was expected to be attibutable to their chronic experience with and expectations of uncontrollability. The results of path analyses supported these causal arguments: Perceptions of control loss had a direct effect on the correspondence of inferences in the no-load but not in the cognitve-load conditions.

Taken together, then, this group of studies provides converging evidence that mildly and moderately depressed perceivers use a style of information processing that may be characterized as effortful, vigilant, and complex. Moreover, path analyses from two of these studies suggest that this effortful processing is elicited by depressed perceivers' greater control motivation.

It is important to note, however, that in all of our studies, depressed and nondepressed subjects have been asked explicitly to list their thoughts about or to form an impression of another. Although we believe that the research reviewed thus far has demonstrated that such minimal task instructions can activate the chronic control goals of our depressed subjects, our data on this point are correlational. Moreover, there certainly are a host of other situational features—often more subtle, more naturalistic, and more goal-related than task instructions—that also may activate depressives' desires to gain or regain interpretive and predictive control. We now turn to recent work that has begun to examine directly the influence of such situational features on depressives' motivated cognitive strategies.

The Social Context and Activation of Depressives' Dispositional Control Motives: Empirical Evidence

For over two decades, personality theorists and researchers have endorsed the notion that in explaining and predicting human behavior, we must consider the person, the situation, and their interaction (Mischel, 1990). However, until recently there was relatively little progress in understanding what features of situations may be important for what kinds of persons, and what psychological processes may connect persons and situations (Buss, 1991). Perhaps nowhere was this lack of progress more evident than in investigations of the impact of personality variables on person perception. Although researchers have assumed for over five decades that perceivers' personal characteristics influence their social cognitions about others, the empirical evidence for such an influence has been weak and inconsistent. Only recently—as researchers have begun to examine (1) the kinds of personality factors most likely to influence person perception processes (e.g., interpersonal motive and cognitive controls), (2) the important characteristics of the social context (e.g., hedonically relevant features), and (3) the various information-processing stages through which the context is perceived and represented—has research begun to uncover systematic, reliable effects of personality on person perception (Battistich, Assor, Messe, & Aronoff, 1985).

In the research that we describe below, we examined the general thesis that the long-term goals of individuals will determine what aspects of the situational context are important. Like others before us (e.g., Bargh, 1990; Bugental, 1993; Buss, 1991; Dworkin & Goldfinger, 1985; Higgins, 1990; Woike & Aronoff, 1992), we suggest that the psychological meaning or significance of situational input is influenced by an interaction of situational features and perceiver's dispositional goals; when the situation affords an opportunity for goal satisfaction, then goal-directed cognitive strategies will be activated.

In two studies, we (Gannon & Weary, 1993) examined the notion that the social-cognitive differences between depressed and nondepressed perceivers would be greatest when the characteristics of the situation were relevant to depressed perceivers' dispositional motives. More specifically, we examined the effects of performance outcome dependence or independence on depressed and nondepressed perceivers' anticipatory situational involvement (Study 1) and attention to task-relevant or task-irrelevant information about another (Study 2). Past research (for a review, see Depret & Fiske, 1993) has shown that "outcome dependence" (i.e., relying on others for an outcome or correlated outcomes) causes people to feel deprived of control, and leads to more information seeking and greater attention to attribute information in an attempt to regain control or at least to predict the others' behavior. We thought that this would particularly be the case for depressed perceivers, who have chronic and heightened perceptions and expectations of control loss.

Both studies employed a similar procedure. In both, depressed and nondepressed subjects were led to believe that the experiment concerned the effects of working environments on various tasks requiring creativity. In order to create a simulation of naturalistic working environments, they were told that information about another "coworker" would be provided to them, and vice versa. In fact, this information had been pretested to assure that items were perceived by both depressed and nondepressed individuals as either relevant or irrelevant to creativity. In the joint-outcome condition, subjects were told that this information was about the individual with whom they would be working to produce a team output. In the independent-outcome condition, they were told that this information was about another individual in the same session.

At this point the procedures for the two studies differed. In Study 1, subjects were asked to answer, prior to receiving the information about the other person and performing the creativity tasks, several questions about themselves and about what they were thinking. Key items included measures of situational-affordance perception and anticipatory situational involvement.

As expected, both depressed and nondepressed subjects viewed the joint-outcome compared to the independent-outcome condition as relevant to or affording an opportunity for satisfaction of control motives; interestingly, both also viewed the independent-outcome compared to the joint-outcome condition as relevant to self-assessment concerns (i.e., as an opportunity to learn about their level of creativity). Our major prediction, however, was that situational-affordance perception would result in self-reports of greater anticipatory involvement only when the situation activated or corresponded to subjects' dispositional motives. As expected, greater cognitive involvement and interest was reported by depressed compared to nondepressed subjects in the joint-outcome condition; moreover, nondepressed perceivers were more involved in the upcoming situation when there was an opportunity for self-assessment (i.e., in the independent outcome-condition). This latter finding is not terribly surprising; self-assessment via social comparison has long been proposed as a major motive underlying a number of human social behaviors (Festinger, 1954).

Would we find a similar pattern for a behavioral measure of involvement, such as attention to task-relevant information about the target other? In Study 2, after learning that their outcomes were to be either a joint product with or independent from another's performance outcome, subjects simply received items of information about the other individual by hitting a key on a computer. The amount of attention given to each piece of information was recorded.

Analyses of the time spent attending to the target information yielded results consistent with these predictions. As expected, in the joint-outcome condition, depressed compared to nondepressed subjects looked longer at the relevant target information; in the independent-outcome condition, nondepressed compared to depressed subjects looked longer. Although no predictions were made with respect to the irrelevant information, the analyses indicated a main effect of depression: Depressed compared to nondepressed perceivers looked longer at this information.

The results of the research reported above have important implications for the model of depressive person perception presented earlier. This research is the first in our program to examine directly and provide support for the motivational component hypothesized by the model to result in more extensive processing of the available social information. In a situation designed to arouse depressed perceivers' control motivations, compared to one designed not to arouse such motivations, greater anticipatory involvement and attention to information about the target other resulted for depressed subjects. This was the case even for information that was intended to be irrelevant to perceivers' immediate control concerns. With respect to this latter finding, we might speculate that the threshold for what is considered relevant information may decrease as control motivation increases. Future research will need to address this interesting possibility.

Before leaving this research, we need to note one qualification to our findings. We do not want to imply that nondepressed perceivers will never exhibit control-motivated cognitive activities. Nor do we want to suggest, for that matter, that depressed perceivers will never exhibit behaviors directed at self-assessment of their abilities. Both motives surely are important to people generally. Rather, we want to suggest only that our manipulation of control motivation (and self-assessment concerns) was intended to be sufficiently subtle that activation would require a dispositional or chronically accessible goal (Bargh, 1990). Under conditions where the potential for control deprivation is more salient or more extreme, we would expect the congruence between dispositional motives and situational affordances to be less important.

From Motivation and Cognition to Action: Empirical Evidence

The bulk of our research has focused on demonstrations of the depressive sensitivity effect described earlier and on testing the arguments of the model pertaining to cognitive processing. However, two studies have examined overt, behavioral manifestations of depressives' dispositional control motives and consequent cognitive processes. We now present a summary of this work.

In one study, Hildebrand-Saints and Weary (1989) led depressed and nondepressed college students to believe that they were assisting the experimenter in the preparation of a videotape for a subsequent study on interviewing processes. They were assigned the role of interviewer, and they were given an opportunity to select questions that they would then ask a student during the interview; the questions had been preselected to reveal a great deal, a moderate amount, or very little about the interviewee. In addition, half of the subjects were led to believe that they would have to use subsequent to the interview what they had learned about the interviewee, whereas the other half believed that they would have to make no additional use of the information gleaned during the interview.

Hildebrand-Saints and Weary expected that depressed students, because of their greater and more chronic control concerns, would be more motivated than nondepressed students to seek out information in social situations generally. More specifically, they predicted that depressed compared to nondepressed subjects would seek more personal and revealing information from their interaction partners. They also predicted that depressed students would be motivated to engage in this diagnostic information seeking, regardless of the subsequent utility of the information, whereas nondepressed subjects would do so only when the subsequent utility of the information was relatively high (i.e., when their control motivation was activated). The results supported these predictions.

The second study to examine depressives' control-motivated behavioral choices was reported recently by Weary, Marsh, and McCormick (1994). Instead of examining diagnostic information seeking, this study examined depressed and nondepressed students' social comparison choices for a task assessing their causal understanding of several events. Weary et al. argued that depressed and nondepressed individuals' choices of comparison others on such tasks might be determined by different informational motives (Fazio, 1979). More specifically, they argued that depressed compared to nondepressed individuals should be relatively uncertain about their causal understandings for events (Weary et al., 1987), and should therefore be more interested in a comparison other who would satisfy "construction motives" (i.e., motives to obtain objective information about the accuracy of one's judgments), whereas nondepressed individuals should show a preference for comparisons that would satisfy validation concerns.

The results generally supported these predictions. After performing on and receiving feedback about several sample items of a test requiring social understanding, and after receiving information about how three other participants had performed on these same items, depressed and nondepressed students were given an opportunity to select one of these three as a partner in a subsequent, similar test. The results indicated that prior to receiving performance feedback and prior to making their partner choices, depressed subjects expressed more doubt about the adequacy of their causal judgments on the initial test items. Moreover, compared to nondepressed subjects, they indicated a greater preference for the participant who theoretically could provide the most information about the adequacy of their future judgments (a similar participant who had disagreed with their previous judgments). Nondepressed subjects demonstrated a preference for the participant who theoretically could validate or confirm the correctness of their future judgments (a dissimilar other who, despite this dissimilarity, had agreed with the subjects' previous judgments). Analyses of several additional measures provided support for the notion that the informational motives of construction and validation determined depressed and nondepressed subjects' social comparison choices, respectively.

THE ROLE OF NEGATIVE AFFECT

The research summarized and reviewed in this chapter paints a picture of mildly and moderately depressed individuals as active and purposive social perceivers. It suggests that their heightened and chronic control concerns result in the adoption of a particular observational goal (uncertainty reduction via subjective accuracy), and that this goal in turn motivates a relatively effortful and vigilant manner of information processing. Because depression is characterized not only by chronic concerns about control loss, but also by chronic negative affect, it is important to consider briefly the relationship of our work to that concerned with the role of negative moods in the processing of social information. (For a more complete discussion, see Weary et al., 1993.)

Although the influence of affect on information processing has received considerable theoretical and empirical attention during the past 10 years, of most relevance is the work reported by Schwarz and his colleagues (Schwarz, 1990). Schwarz has suggested that moods may function as information about the state of the world. According to this mood-as-information perspective, negative moods suggest to people that there are problems or threats in the environment that require attention, thought, and perhaps remedial action. Positive moods, however, signify to perceivers that the world is fine and that no additional thought or action is required.

This view of positive and negative moods as serving important informational functions has generated a good deal of research, much of it suggesting that general negative mood states increase cognitive activity. These findings, of course, are consistent with the bulk of our work on the influence of depressives' chronic heightened control motivation on their cognitive processes. Indeed, we have conceived of control motivation as a specific motivational state aroused by specific types of negative events and associated with a specific negative affect (causal uncertainty). Moreover, we have proposed that this specific negative affect informs perceivers about the current inadequacy of their state of knowledge, and that it is a cause of depressives' more extensive search for and processing of social information. It is not surprising, therefore, that the results of studies by Schwarz and his colleagues parallel ours. In fact, Weary et al. (1993) have suggested that the effects of control motivation and more diffuse negative moods probably are additive in their instigation of effortful, vigilant information processing under many conditions; however, they also have suggested that the processing consequences of causal-uncertainty feelings may well be more specific to tasks invoking a desire or need for greater causal understanding. Research on this specificity notion, it should be noted, has only just begun (Weary & Edwards, 1996).

CONCLUSION

We have described in this chapter a cognitive model of motivation—in particular, a model that highlights the role of depressed perceivers' chronic control concerns and consequent causal-uncertainty beliefs on their social perception processes. We have also summarized a number of the available research findings. Although there is by now compelling support for a number of key predictions of the model, research focusing on a key construct of the model—causal-uncertainty beliefs and feelings—has had to await the development of an instrument to assess them. Since this is now available (Weary & Edwards, 1994b), we are hopeful that future research will shed light on the role of causal uncertainty in depressives' processing of social information and on the potential distinctiveness of causal-uncertainty feelings and negative affect.

At several points throughout this chapter, we have indicated that we believe future research on this model will attend more to the important role of the social context in activating depressed perceivers' chronic control concerns. We believe that only with such research will we have a complete understanding of the social embeddedness of depressives' control concerns, and that only with such work will we be able to specify when such concerns will guide cognitive acitivity. Indeed, we believe that such work may go a long way toward resolving what one of us has described elsewhere (Weary & Edwards, 1994b) as a looming controversy over the nature and extent of depressives' information processing.

We would like to conclude by noting once again that although the major focus of the model presented herein has been on motivated social-cognitive processes arising from depressives' chronic control concerns, research and theory will need to go beyond this focus and articulate, to a greater extent than it has, the impact of such cognitive activity on overt behavior. Like so many others working within a social-cognitive perspective, we need to be reminded that "thinking is [indeed] for doing, that social understanding operates in the service of social interaction" (Fiske, 1992, p. 877).

There can be little doubt that the cognitive products and processes of our control-motivated social perceivers influence a variety of their social behaviors; to date, we have examined only two of these. Future consideration of the systems that link control-motivated cognition to behavior will do much to elucidate the adequacy of the cognitive and behavioral strategies adopted by our social perceivers to regain a sense of control. A final word of caution, however, seems necessary. We believe it is likely that future investigations of linkages among control motivation, cognition, and overt behavior will also uncover a number of instances where there is no simple or direct relationship between control-motivated social cognition and overt behavior. After all, a host of additional person variables (e.g., number and availability of behavioral action plans) and situational factors (e.g., various environmental presses, target or interactant characteristics) may exert a critical influence on overt behavior. Thus, although it is an exciting and necessary next step, examination of linkages among control motivation, cognition, and action will need to be mindful of the complexity and flexibility of human social beings.

ACKNOWLEDGMENTS

We would like to thank the editors, John Bargh and Peter Gollwitzer, for their thoughtful comments on an earlier draft of this chapter. We also would like to thank John A. Edwards for his generosity and care in providing us with extremely helpful comments on this chapter.

NOTE

1. It should be noted that our model is applicable primarily to individuals who are evidencing only mild or moderate levels of depressive symptomatology. Throughout the remainder of this chapter, our description of individuals as "depressed" should be taken to indicate only these levels.

REFERENCES

Abramson, L. Y., Seligman, M. E. P., & Teasdale, J. (1978). Learned helplessness in humans: Critique and reformulation. *Journal of Abnormal Psychology, 87,* 49–74.

Alloy, L. B., Kelly, K. A., Mineka, S., & Clements, C. M. (1990). Comorbidity of anxiety and depressive disorders: A helplessness–hopelessness perspective. In J. D. Maser & C. R. Cloninger (Eds.), *Comorbidity of mood and anxiety disorders* (pp. 499–544). Washington, DC: American Psychiatric Press.

Andersen, S. M. (1990). The inevitability of future suffering: The role of depressive predictive certainty in depression. *Social Cognition, 8,* 203–228.

Andersen, S. M., Spielman, L. A., & Bargh, J. A. (1992). Future-event schemas and certainty about the future: Automaticity in depressives' future-event predictions. *Journal of Personality and Social Psychology, 63,* 711–723.

Bargh, J. A. (1990). Auto-motives: Preconscious determinants of social interaction. In E. T. Higgins & R. M. Sorrentino (Eds.), *Handbook of motivation and cognition: Foundations of social behavior* (Vol. 2, pp. 93–130). New York: Guilford Press.

Battistich, V., Assor, A., Messe, L. A., & Aronoff, J. (1985). Personality and person perception. In P. Shaver (Ed.), *Self, situations, and social behavior* (pp. 185–208). Beverly Hills, CA: Sage.

Beck, A. T. (1976). *Cognitive therapy and the emotional disorders.* New York: International Universities Press.

Brown, J. D., & Siegel, J. M. (1988). Attributions for negative life events and depression: The róle of perceived control. *Journal of Personality and Social Psychology, 54,* 316–322.

Bugental, D. B. (1993). Communication in abusive relationships: Cognitive constructions of interpersonal power. *American Behavioral Scientist, 36,* 288–308.

Burger, J. M., & Arkin, R. (1980). Desire for control and the use of attributional processes. *Journal of Personality, 56,* 531–546.

Buss, D. M. (1991). Evolutionary personality psychology. *Annual Review of Psychology, 42,* 459–491.

Carver, C. S., & Gaines, J. G. (1987). Optimism, pessimism, and post-partum depression. *Cognitive Therapy and Research, 1,* 449–462.

Chaiken, S., Liberman, A., & Eagly, A. H. (1989). Heuristic and systematic information processing within and beyond the persuasion context. In J. S. Uleman & J. A. Bargh (Eds.), *Unintended thought* (pp. 212–252). New York: Guilford Press.

Clore, G. L. (1992). Cognitive phenomenology: Feelings and the construction of judgment. In L. L. Martin & A. Tesser (Eds.), *The construction of social judgments* (pp. 133–164). Hillsdale, NJ: Erlbaum.

Dworkin, R. H., & Goldfinger, S. H. (1985). Processing bias: Individual differences in the cognition of situations. *Journal of Personality, 53,* 480–502.

Depret, E. F., & Fiske, S. T. (1993). Social cognition and power: Some cognitive consequences of social structure as a source of control deprivation. In G. Weary, F. Gleicher, & K. L. Marsh (Eds.), *Control motivation and social cognition* (pp. 176–202). New York: Springer-Verlag.

Edwards, J., & Weary, G. (1993a). *Relationship between perceived lack of control, causal uncertainty and depression.* Paper presented at the annual meeting of the American Psychological Society, Chicago.

Edwards, J., & Weary, G. (1993b). Depression and the impression formation continuum: Piecemeal processing despite the availability of category information. *Journal of Personality and Social Psychology, 64,* 636–645.

Fazio, R. H. (1979). Motives for social comparison: The construction–validation distinction. *Journal of Personality and Social Psychology, 37,* 1683–1698.

Festinger, L. (1954). A theory of social comparison processes. *Human Relations, 7,* 117–140.

Fiske, S. T. (1992). Thinking is for doing: Portraits of social cognition from daguerrotype to laserphoto. *Journal of Personality and Social Psychology, 63,* 877–889.

Fiske, S. T. (1993). Social cognition and social perception. *Annual Review of Psychology, 44,* 155–194.

Fiske, S. T., & Neuberg, S. L. (1990). A continuum of impression formation from category-based to individuating processes: Influences of information and motivation on attention and interpretation. In M. P. Zanna (Ed.), *Advances in experimental social psychology* (Vol. 23, pp. 1–74). New York: Academic Press.

Gannon, K., & Weary, G. (1993). *Depression and anticipated interaction: The effect of dispositional motives on situational construal.* Paper presented at the annual meeting of the Midwestern Psychological Association, Chicago.

Garber, J., Miller, W. R., & Seaman, S. F. (1979). Learned helplessness, stress, and the depressive disorders. In R. A. Depue (Ed.), *The psychobiology of the depressive disorders: Implications for the effects of stress* (pp. 335–364). New York: Academic Press.

Gilbert, D. T., Pelham, B. W., & Krull, D. S. (1988). Of thoughts unspoken: Social inference and the self-regulation of behavior. *Journal of Personality and Social Psychology, 54,* 733–739.

Gleicher, F., & Weary, G. (1991a). *The effect of noncontingent feedback on expectations of control.* Paper presented at the annual meeting of the Midwestern Psychological Association, Chicago.

Gleicher, F., & Weary, G. (1991b). The effect of depression on the quantity and quality of social inferences. *Journal of Personality and Social Psychology, 61,* 105–114.

Hartlage, S., Alloy, L. B., Vazquez, C., & Dykman, B. (1993). Automatic and effortful processing in depression. *Psychological Bulletin, 113,* 247–278.

Hastie, R., & Park, B. (1986). The relationship between memory and judgment depends on whether the judgment is memory-based or on-line. *Psychological Review, 93,* 258–268.

Hertel, P. T., & Rude, S. S. (1991). Depressive deficits in memory: Focusing attention improves subsequent recall. *Journal of Experimental Psychology: General, 120,* 301–309.

Higgins, E.T. (1990). Personality, social psychology, and person–situation relations: Standards and knowledge activation as a common language. In L. A. Pervin (Ed.), *Handbook of personality: Theory and research* (pp. 301–338). New York: Guilford Press.

Hildebrand-Saints, L., & Weary, G. (1989). Depression and social information gathering. *Personality and Social Psychology Bulletin, 15,* 150–160.

Hull, J. A., & Mendolia, M. (1991). Modeling the relations of attributional style, expectancies, and depression. *Journal of Personality and Social Psychology, 61,* 85–97.

Jacobson, J. A., Weary, G., & Edwards, J. A. (1995). *Causes and concomitants of depression: Causal uncertainty versus negative outcome certainty.* Manuscript submitted for publication.

Jellison, J. M., & Green, J. (1981). A self-presentation approach to the fundamental attribution error: The norm of internality. *Journal of Personality and Social Psychology, 40,* 643–649.

Johnson, M. H., & Magaro, P. A. (1987). Effects of mood and severity on memory processes in depression and mania. *Psychological Bulletin, 101,* 28–40.

Kruglanski, A. W. (1989). *Lay epistemics and human knowledge: Cognitive and motivational bases.* New York: Plenum.

Lewinsohn, P. M., Hoberman, H. M., & Rosenbaum, M. A. (1988). Prospective study of risk factors for unipolar depression. *Journal of Abnormal Psychology, 97,* 251–264.

Lewinsohn, P. M., Steinmetz, J. L., Larson, D. W., & Franklin, J. (1981). Depression-related cognitions: Antecedent or consequence? *Journal of Abnormal Psychology, 90,* 213–219.

Marsh, K. L. & Weary, G. (1989). Depression and attributional complexity. *Personality and Social Psychology Bulletin, 15,* 531–540.

Marsh, K. L., & Weary, G. (1994). Severity of depression and sensitivity to social information. *Journal of Social and Clinical Psychology, 13,* 15–32.

McCaul, K. D. (1983). Observer attributions of depressed students. *Personality and Social Psychology Bulletin, 9,* 74–82.

Mischel, W. (1990). Personality dispositions revisitied and revised: A view after three decades. In L. A. Pervin (Ed.), *Handbook of personality: Theory and research* (pp. 111–134). New York: Guilford Press.

Nicholls, J. G. (1984). Achievement motivation: Conceptions of ability, subjective experience, task choice, and performance. *Psychological Review, 91,* 328–346.

Pagel, M. D., Becker, J., & Coppel, D. B. (1985). Loss of control, self-blame, and depressions: An investigation of spouse caregivers of Alzheimer's disease. *Journal of Abnormal Psychology, 94,* 169–182.

Pavelchak, M. (1989). Piecemeal and category-based evaluation: An idiographic analysis. *Journal of Personality and Social Psychology, 56,* 354–363.

Petty, R. E., & Cacioppo, J. T. (1986). *Communication and persuasion: Central and peripheral routes to attitude change.* New York: Springer-Verlag.

Pittman, T. S. (1993). Control motivation and attitude change. In G. Weary, F. Gleicher, & K. L. Marsh (Eds.), *Control motivation and social cognition* (pp. 157–175). New York: Springer-Verlag.

Pittman, T. S., & D'Agostino, P. R. (1985). Motivation and attribution: The effects of control deprivation on subsequent information processing. In J. H. Harvey & G. Weary (Eds.), *Attribution: Basic and applied issues* (pp. 117–142). San Diego, CA: Academic Press.

Pittman, T. S., & Pittman, N. L. (1980). Deprivation of control and the attribution process. *Journal of Personality and Social Psychology, 39,* 377–389.

Riskind, J. H., Rholes, W. S., Brannon, A. M., & Burdick, C. A. (1987). Attributions and expectations: A confluence of vulnerabilities in mild depression in a college student population. *Journal of Personality and Social Psychology, 53,* 349–354.

Rothbaum, F., Weisz, J. R., & Snyder, S. S. (1982). Changing the world and changing the self: A two-process model of perceived control. *Journal of Personality and Social Psychology, 42,* 5–37.

Schwarz, N. (1990). Feelings as information: Informational and motivational functions of affective states. In E. T. Higgins & R. M. Sorrentino (Eds.), *Handbook of motivation and cognition: Foundations of social behavior* (Vol. 2, pp. 527–561). New York: Guilford Press.

Snyder, M. L., Stephan, W. G., & Rosenfield, D. (1978). Attributional egotism. In J. H. Harvey, W. J. Ickes, & R. F. Kidd (Eds.), *New directions in attributional research* (Vol. 2, pp. 91–120). Hillsdale, NJ: Erlbaum.

Swann, W. B. (1984). Quest for accuracy in person perception: A matter of pragmatics. *Psychological Review, 91,* 457–477.

Warren, L. W., & McEachren, L. (1983). Psychosocial correlates of depressive symptomatology in adult women. *Journal of Abnormal Psychology, 92,* 151–160.

Weary, G., & Edwards, J. A. (1994a). Social cognition and clinical psychology: Anxiety, depression, and the processing of social information. In R. S. Wyer & T. K. Srull (Eds.), *Handbook of social cognition* (2nd ed., pp. 289–338). Hillsdale, NJ: Erlbaum.

Weary, G., & Edwards, J. A. (1994b). Individual differences in causal uncertainty. *Journal of Personality and Social Psychology, 67,* 308–318.

Weary, G., & Edwards, J. A. (in press). Causal uncertainty beliefs and related goal structures. In R. M. Sorrentino & E. T. Higgins (Eds.), *Handbook of motivation and cognition: Vol. 3. The interpersonal context* (pp. 148–181). New York: Guilford Press.

Weary, G., Elbin, S. D., & Hill, M. G. (1987). Attribution and social comparison processes in depression. *Journal of Personality and Social Psychology, 52,* 605–610.

Weary, G., Jordan, J. S., & Hill, M. G. (1985). The attributional norm of internality and depressive sensitivity to social information. *Journal of Personality and Social Psychology, 49,* 1283–1293.

Weary, G., Marsh, K. L., Gleicher, F., & Edwards, J. A. (1993). Depression, control motivation, and the processing of information about others. In G. Weary, F. Gleicher, & K. L. Marsh (Eds.), *Control motivation and social cognition* (pp. 255–290). New York: Springer-Verlag.

Weary, G., Marsh, K. L., & McCormick, L. A. (1994). Depression and social comparison motives. *European Journal of Social Psychology, 24,* 117–129.

Weisz, J. R., Weiss, B., Wasserman, A. A., & Rintoul, B. (1987). Control-related beliefs and depression among clinic-referred children and adolescents. *Journal of Abnormal Psychology, 96,* 58–63.

Woike, B. A., & Aronoff, J. (1992). Antecedents of complex social cognitions. *Journal of Personality and Social Psychology, 63,* 97–104.

Yost, J. H., & Weary, G. (in press). Depression and the correspondent inference bias: Evidence for more effortful processing. *Personality and Social Psychology Bulletin.*

CHAPTER 8

Emotional Influences on Cognitive Processing, with Implications for Theories of Both

Eric Klinger

By "emotions" I refer in part to what most people in the field mean by them and are unable to define satisfactorily: They are far-reaching states of zoological organisms that roughly fit the 8 to 10 or so categories worked out by Tomkins, Izard, and their successors, with both qualitative and arousal dimensions. However, it now appears that this conventional conception describes only the tip of an iceberg. That is, emotions appear to constitute a rather elaborate system intertwined with virtually every other one of an organism's major systems. Each emotional response, in this view, begins nonconsciously and purely centrally as a brain event; it then gradually evolves, subject to a series of decision points, to recruit additional component subsystems until it emerges the way it has been viewed conventionally.

This chapter considers the way emotion is intertwined in particular with one other component subsystem, cognitive processing, and it views both of them in the ultimate context for nearly any zoological organism, motivation. Motivation is the ultimate context because it is the ineluctable consequence of the zoological strategy for survival. There are only two such strategies, both aimed at countering the destructive forces of entropy long enough to permit procreation. One is the "sessile" strategy of sitting in place, waiting for nature to deliver vital substances and conditions. It places a heavy burden on procreation, but in view of the flourishing history of plants, it has to be adjudged successful. The second strategy is the "motile" strategy. In this strategy, organisms achieve a degree of independence from their immediate environment by seeking out the vital substances and conditions they need. It exacts its own biological costs in the complexity of the operations that zoological organisms need to maintain, and it carries with it an imperative: "Seek or perish."

If we may label the target substances and conditions "goals," life for the motile organism is a succession of goal pursuits, and survival depends on their success. This is perhaps the most central distinctive truth of zoology, which means that all zoological evolution must have selected for those properties that facilitate goal pursuits. In this sense, motivation is *the* foundation system for zoological organisms, and all other systems must have evolved in its service.

Space limitations prevent me from fully discussing here the issues of how emotion intertwines with motivation, although some connections will become apparent. However, it is worth pointing out that in the rapidly growing literature on emotion and cognition, only a few other writers have placed the topic in a motivational context (e.g., Brown, 1991; Stein & Levine, 1991). Nevertheless, for motile organisms motivational considerations appear to be functionally primary—the *raison d'être* for everything else.

A PREVIEW OF A MODEL THAT INTEGRATES MOTIVATION, EMOTION, AND COGNITIVE PROCESSING

The pattern of evidence to be described below seems consistent with the following model. When people become committed to pursuing a goal, that event initiates an internal state termed a "current concern," one of whose properties is to potentiate emotional reactivity to cues associated with the goal pursuit. The emotional responses thus emitted begin within about 300 milliseconds (ms) after exposure to the cue—early enough to be considered purely central, nonconscious responses at this stage. Because they appear to be incipient emotional responses but lack many of the properties normally associated with emotion, they are here called "protoemotional" responses.

These go on in parallel with early perceptual and cognitive processing, with which they trade reciprocal influences. The intensity (and possibly other features) of the protoemotional responses affects the probability that the stimulus will continue to be processed cognitively. The results of continued cognitive processing in turn modulate the intensity and character of the emerging emotional response. Should the emotional response pass some as yet unknown kind of threshold (which may well depend on competing responses), it begins to recruit other subsystems, such as autonomic and endocrine responses; nonvolitional motor responses, such as facial and postural expressions; conscious affect; conscious cognitive processing; and ultimately action. By that time, it has emerged as a full-scale emotional response in the classical meaning of the term. While getting there, it will have played a key role in what the individual has processed, retained, noticed, and thought about. What follows is the evidentiary basis for this model.

MOTIVATIONAL INFLUENCES ON COGNITIVE PROCESSING

Motivational factors have been found to be powerful influences on cognitive processing. Investigators have reported a variety of interesting findings: that arousal (which may also be construed as emotional; Revelle & Loftus, 1992) facilitates "detection and encoding for long-term retention" (Revelle & Loftus, 1992, p. 129) but impairs retrievability of information in the short term, perhaps up to 30 minutes; that goal setting affects performance differently at different phases of skill acquisition and for different levels of ability (Kanfer, Chapter 18, this volume; Kanfer & Ackerman, 1989); and that there are distinctly different distributions of cognitive processing and mental content in different phases of goal-striving sequences (Gollwitzer, 1990; Chapter 13, this volume).

Considerable additional evidence is organized around the construct of "current concern" (Klinger, 1971, 1975, 1977, 1987a). This construct refers to the *latent state* of an organism between commitment to striving for a goal and either goal attainment or disengagement from the goal. The construct by itself does not refer to conscious content; although concerns are presumed to exert extensive influence on attention, recall, thought content, and action, the construct is different from (is presumed to underlie) these effects. This view posits a separate concern corresponding to each of a person's current goal pursuits. The goal in question may be as short- or long-term, as narrow or broad, and as trivial or lofty as the person may conceive of it—whether washing the dishes, consolidating a personal relationship, becoming head of state, being popular, or achieving spiritual unity with the universe.

Viewed in this way, current concerns are the results of the motivational factors that are presumed to determine people's choices of goals, such as expectancies and values. Once launched through the process of commitment to a goal (a process that is at this time poorly understood and little investigated), the latent states labeled concerns are presumed to underlie the processes that are once again coming to be called "volitional." Neither commitment nor, of course, the latent state itself is presumed to be conscious, although they generally have their conscious manifestations. Nor are they necessarily verbalizable. Although some kind of cognition must clearly play a role in commitment and goal striving, concerns are not in themselves cognitive; rather, they are dynamic entities, in that they sensitize individuals to cues and potentiate responses (whether emotional, cognitive, or motor).

The initial model for this research program posited that current concerns sensitize people to respond cognitively to cues associated with these concerns, and that under many circumstances a response will include thought content regarding the concern with which the cue is associated. Especially when circumstances militate against taking goal-directed action, the responses potentiated by the concern remain cognitive, including thoughts and images.

Initial investigations of this model employed dichotic listening to two simultaneous 15-minute narratives, one presented to each ear, both of them taken from the same literary work. At intervals, the narratives were modified by inserting words that would presumably be associated with one of the subject's current concerns in one channel; synchronously, the opposite narrative was modified to allude to another individual's concern, designated here as a "nonconcern." These conditions were, of course, balanced with respect to side. Subjects used a toggle switch to signal the channel to which they were currently listening. A few seconds after each of these modified passages (embedding sites), the tape stopped with a signal tone, at which point subjects reported and rated their last thoughts and also reported the last segments of the tape they could recall hearing. This provided information regarding attentional direction, recall, and thought content. Methods for assessing concerns included interviews at first and then questionnaires (Klinger, 1987b), currently including the Motivational Structure Questionnaire (Cox & Klinger, 1988; Klinger & Kroll-Mensing, 1995).

The effects of conditions were quite powerful (Table 8.1, first three rows; Klinger, 1978). Subjects spent significantly more time listening to passages associated with their concerns, recalled those passages much more often, and had thought content that (by ratings of blind judges) was much more often related to them than to the nonconcern-related passages opposite them. Judges found hardly any resemblance of thoughts to passages that subjects had not yet heard, indicating that the cuing effect of concern-related stimuli accounted for the differences. Furthermore, when subjects were exposed to tapes created for other subjects, the embedded passages had no detectable effect, indicating that embedded text as such could not account for the effects.

These results with waking subjects leave unclear to what extent they are attributable to an inexorable, nonconscious mechanism or to a conscious process, such as deliberately focusing on concern-related stimuli. To shed some light on this question, we conducted a sleep experiment (Hoelscher, Klinger, & Barta, 1981). Dreams have more in common with waking thought flow than has generally been recognized, including themes, periodicity, and even dream-like imagery (Klinger, 1971, 1990). It therefore seemed likely that dream content could be influenced by experimentally introduced verbal cues, much as had been shown for waking thought; if that were so, the fact that the effect occurred during sleep would presumably rule out a range of explanations requiring conscious, deliberate self-management. In this investigation, sleeping subjects received spoken words or brief phrases that related to concerns or nonconcerns, as assessed on a previous day. (To minimize recency effects and experimentally induced sensitization, the subjects also read and rated potential nonconcerns—concerns drawn from other subjects—at the previous-day session used for assessing the subjects' concerns. The nonconcerns used to generate nonconcern cues were then drawn from among those potential nonconcerns that subjects actually rated as such.) A few seconds later, they were awakened for a dream report. Subjects much more often reported dreams related to concern-related than to nonconcern-

TABLE 8.1. Cognitive Responsiveness to Concern-Related versus Nonconcern-Related Cues

Dependent variable	Types of cues	
	Concern	Nonconcern
Waking subjects		
Time spent listening (seconds)	74.6	58.9[b]
No. of passages per session recalled	2.78	1.38[c]
Passages per session thought about	3.73	1.95[c]
Sleeping subjects		
Proportion of cues incorporated into REM sleep	.34	.11[a]

Note. Data for waking subjects are from Klinger (1978); data for sleeping subjects are from Hoelscher, Klinger, and Barta (1981). Significance values are for the differences between concern-related and nonconcern-related means.
[a]$p < .05$.
[b]$p < .0005$.
[c]$p < .0001$.

related cues (Table 8.1, last row). Again, a control rating of dreams against cues not yet heard found little resemblance, indicating that the concern-related cues were responsible for the effect. These results confirmed that the effects of concern-related cues on cognitive processing are substantially automatic. That is, they occur in reaction to concern-related cues without the intercession of waking consciousness or of deliberate decision making.

First results from an investigation just completed extend this finding (Brecht, Nikles, Klinger, & Bursell, 1995). The procedure was generally similar to that of the first dream study (Hoelscher et al., 1981), except that on their third and fourth nights in the laboratory, just before they went to bed, subjects were instructed to try to dream about a specified theme. On one of the nights the theme was an important current concern of each subject; on the other night, it was a nonconcern for the subject—a different individual's concern. Subjects were awakened about five times a night for REM dream reports, but after the presleep instructions they received no further instructions or suggestions for dream content and no experimental cues. Subjects incorporated into their dreams significantly more suggested themes when these were concern-related than when they were not. This was true whether the resemblance of dreams to suggestions was rated by subjects themselves or by judges unaware of the experimental conditions. Furthermore, incorporation of suggested concerns was significantly greater following the suggestions than on the baseline night that preceded the suggestions. Clearly, the concern state experimentally induced around the goal of dreaming about certain themes exerted effects in sleep, and to that extent acted automatically, provided that the suggested themes were themselves current concerns.

The automatic character of this process was further buttressed by data from a lexical decision task (Young, 1987). Young's subjects were to decide as quickly as possible whether each occurrence of a letter string on a computer screen was an English word, and to respond by pressing a button (which provided reaction times). The left side of the screen was taken up by a patch containing computer-related verbal "garbage," which subjects were instructed to ignore (and apparently did), but which sometimes contained a word planted to relate to one of a subject's current concerns. When the target string was indeed a word, the reaction time of reporting this was significantly slower if the distractor patch contained a concern-related word. Thus, concern-related stimuli seem to impose an extra load on cognitive processing even when they are peripheral and subjects are consciously ignoring them. This finding adds a further facet to the automaticity of the effect: It is not readily suppressed by disattention, but is instead to some degree irresistible.

This effect was shown in yet another cognitive process, using reaction time with either a modified Stroop or a quasi-Stroop procedure. In the first of these investigations (Riemann & McNally, 1995), student subjects were asked to name the colors of words that varied according to whether they were emotionally neutral or were highly or only slightly related to subjects' positive or negative current concerns. Responses were quickest for neutral words and slowest for words highly related to concerns, regardless of whether the concerns were positive or negative. This relationship was unaffected by whether subjects had gone through a mood induction for neutral, anxious, and happy moods.

In a second such investigation (Johnsen, Laberg, Cox, Vaksdal, & Hugdahl, 1994), alcoholics and nonalcoholics named the colors of computer-displayed neutral words (e.g., "window"), alcohol-related words (e.g., "whiskey"), and, in the standard Stroop manner, mismatched color words (e.g., "red" written in green letters). Reaction times were slower in naming the colors of alcohol-related words than of neutral words for the alcoholics but not for the nonalcoholics. For the alcoholics, the effect was as powerful as was the standard Stroop manipulation. Given that alcohol-related words are also related to the concerns of alcoholics much more intensely than to the concerns of nonalcoholics, these results are consistent with the previous ones.

In the quasi-Stroop investigation (Cox, Blount, & Cools, personal communication, May 1992), alcoholic inpatients were presented with pairs of words, one of them a color word (e.g., "yellow"), and pressed one of two buttons to indicate the identity of the color word. The noncolor word was in either of five conditions: neutral, "color friction" (e.g., "lemon"), alcohol-related (e.g., "drunk"), concern-related (e.g., "daughter"), or presumptively emotionally arousing (e.g., "death"). The color friction condition served as a test of the procedure—as a kind of manipulation check. It was assumed on the basis of previous Stroop research that this quasi-Stroop procedure would produce a slowing of reaction time in the color friction condition, if the design was capable of assessing such an effect; it would therefore assess the validity of the design and provide a standard for other conditions. Reaction time was in fact found to be significantly slower for decisions involving color friction words than for those involving neutral words. The remaining three conditions as a group, which were presumably concern-related for these subjects, also produced significantly slower reactions than neutral words, thereby extending the interference effect to yet another variety of cognitive task.

The interference of incidental concern-related stimuli with cognitive processing appears to be a general phenomenon, at least when the cognitive task is less than fully automatized. It has been shown to occur, in addition to the instances described above, with stimuli constructed to remind anxious subjects of their anxieties; to remind subjects with self-concept problems of the discrepancy between the way they see themselves as being and the way they think they ought to be; and to remind eating- or body-image-disordered subjects of their bodies (Newman et al., 1993). In these experiments, subjects were presented with supraliminal "warning" stimuli followed by target stimuli, strings of either letters or numbers. Their task was to signal as quickly as possible which kind of target string they had just seen. About 75% of the time the target stimuli occurred around the middle of the screen, near the location of the warning stimuli, and about 25% of the time the target stimuli occurred peripherally in a corner of the screen. When the target stimuli occurred peripherally, reaction times were slowed significantly when the warning stimuli (e.g., "mirror" for an eating-disordered subject) were presumably concern-related. There was no effect when the target stimuli were displayed centrally.

Data also link current concerns to electrodermal responses of the kind often identified as orienting responses (Nikula, Klinger, & Larson-Gutman, 1993). When subjects were induced to listen to strings of three-word clusters, those that alluded to one of a subject's current concerns evoked significantly more skin conductance responses than did those chosen to allude to a nonconcern. Furthermore, subjects who were thought-sampled just after a spontaneous skin conductance response were significantly more likely to report just having thought about a current concern than when they were thought-sampled during electrodermally inactive periods. Partialing out self-ratings of emotional arousal at the time of the thought sample did not eliminate this relationship.

EMOTIONAL INFLUENCES ON COGNITIVE PROCESSING

Let us now turn to emotional influences on cognitive processing. The past decade has seen a rapidly developing rapprochement between the research on emotion and that on cognition, which have historically developed in isolation from each other. Although this merger is still nibbling at their edges, it has provoked the publication of a journal (*Cognition and Emotion*) and a number of books devoted to it. At first, much of this interest was in the effects of cognition—especially appraisal and causal attribution—on emotion. But as research has progressed, it has focused increasingly on the impact of emotional states and traits on cognitive processing, with the implication that their influence is reciprocal.

The reciprocity of this relationship between emotion and cognition is gaining increasing neuroanatomical support. Thus, LeDoux (1989, 1992) and Derryberry and Tucker (1992) have emphasized the multiple connections between limbic system areas and the neocortex, both ascending and descending. Especially important here are (1) the proliferation of fibers that lead directly from the thalamus to the amygdala, which presumably represent a flow of information from (as yet only partially analyzed) stimulation obtained very early in cognitive processing to an area heavily implicated in emotional activity; (2) fibers leading from the amygdala to the neocortex, perhaps signaling emotional responses evoked by this preliminary information and timed to influence early stages of cortical processing of stimuli, as well as capable of modulating sensory processes; and (3) fibers leading from the neocortex to the amygdala, which presumably represent cortical feedback from more completely analyzed information to influence emotional response.

Mounting behavioral evidence also supports the connection between affect and cognitive processing, including attention, recall, and thought content. For example, to turn first to memory, retrieval is biased in the direction of mood-congruent content (Bower, 1992). The bias toward mood congruence is not just a matter of valence (positive or negative), but is specific to the type of negative affect: Depressed individuals tend to recall depressive content, and anxious individuals tend to recall anxious content (Ingram, Kendall, Smith, Donnell, & Ronan, 1987). The mood variable used in these studies was assessed rather than induced, so that this evidence is purely correlational; however, selective recall of anxious material by panic disorder patients is enhanced by experimentally induced physical arousal (McNally, Foa, & Donnell, 1989), which suggests a causal influence.

Other relationships between depression and recall have been extensively documented as well (e.g., Alloy, 1988). Of particular interest here is a consistent finding that people in depressed moods recall more negatively toned autobiographical memories, but also that this effect is likelier to be a state than a trait effect (Lewinsohn & Rosenbaum, 1987), because it does not show up after the depression has remitted. Effects of mood may especially affect the *implicit* memories on which naturally occurring, emitted cognitive processing depends (Tobias, Kihlstrom, & Schacter, 1992).

In the case of attention, depressed individuals are more attentive to depressive cues than are nondepressed individuals (Gottlib, McLachlan, & Katz, 1988); moreover, anxious individuals respond more quickly to threat-related than to non-threat-related stimuli (using a probe method) in ways that indicate greater attentiveness to threat cues (Broadbent & Broadbent, 1988; Fox, 1993). It is presumably this differential attentiveness that accounts for panic-disorder patients' selectively slower color naming of threat words in a Stroop-like task (Ehlers, Margraf, Davies, & Roth, 1988). There is developmental evidence that this correlational finding cannot be attributed to anxious individuals' having undergone different experiences that affect cognition independently of the direct emotional effect; rather, the effect seems to be integral to the emotion (Martin, Horder, & Jones, 1993).

At somewhat more global cognitive levels, moods have also been heavily implicated in cognitive organization (Isen, 1991; Kuhl, 1983a, 1983b), such that negative moods are associated with more differentiated, analytic processing and positive moods are associated with more global, synthetic processing. In regard to judgment (Mayer, Gaschke, Braverman, & Evans, 1992), negative moods are associated with more pessimistic, gloomy judgments. Stress states also appear to affect memory (Christianson, 1992), but the effect may be to enhance or to impair memory, depending on numerous factors. Considering the entire pattern of effects of stress, it appears that "emotional events receive some preferential processing" (Christianson, 1992, p. 284).

The relationships sketched above have been reasonably consistent, and they are also consistent with findings arising out of the current-concerns framework. In fact, a number of indications from current-concerns-related data (e.g., the references cited above; see also Klinger, Barta, & Maxeiner, 1980) have suggested that a critical property of current concerns is to dispose individuals to respond emotionally to cues associated with corresponding goal pursuits. The emotional response then induces a number of levels of cognitive processing, ending, at least under some conditions, with conscious thought. That is, the emotional responsivity, which is itself based on goal commitments, mediates the effects on cognition.

This elaborated model gave rise to a number of further investigations. One of these examined the extent to which emotionally arousing distractors placed an automatic load on cognitive processing. Using reaction time methods (Schneider, 1987), subjects pressed buttons to distinguish X's from Y's when they appeared one at a time on the lower half of a computer screen. Distractor stimuli, which subjects were instructed to ignore, often appeared above the letters at the fixation point; many of the distractors were words. After this procedure, subjects rated how much each distractor word aroused them emotionally. More emotionally arousing distractor words were associated with significantly slower reaction times. That this effect really was attributable to something emotional is supported by another feature of the investigation: Subjects who scored high on the Affective Intensity Measure (Larsen & Diener, 1987) were slowed by emotionally arousing distractors significantly more than other subjects were.

Emotional arousal also affects recall. Subjects were asked to perform any of several tasks with word stimuli, such as judging their length, pronounceability, abstractness, or emotional arousal value. After a buffer task, subjects were given a free-recall test for the words, after which they all rated them for their impact on emotional arousal and their relatedness to subjects' individual current concerns. Words rated as either relatively emotionally arousing or concern-related were recalled significantly more often than were other words (Bock & Klinger, 1986). Concern-relatedness and emotional arousal value were strongly intercorrelated. Another, similar investigation (Klinger, Bock, & Bowi, 1990) made possible an assessment of whether either of these variables, concern-relatedness or emotional arousal, mediated the effects of the other. Again, words high on either variable were recalled more often than words low on them, and the two word properties were strongly correlated within subjects, r (1,368) = .54. However, for words that were above average for a subject on one variable but below average on the other, it was possible to examine which combination of highs and lows produced the best recall. For words that had been processed with attention to their meanings, recall was superior when their emotional arousal value was high, regardless of the rating on concern-relatedness. Concern-relatedness, cleaned of emotional arousal variance, had no significant effect on recall. These results suggest that the effect of current concerns on recall is mediated by the emotional responses that the concerns have largely instated.

RELEVANT RESEARCH WITH ALTERNATIVE CONSTRUCTS

Lines of investigation parallel to the one described above have been conducted within other theoretical frameworks centered on the concept of construct and attitude accessibility—the speed and automaticity with which individuals apply categories, especially evaluative categories, to others. This literature has shown that activating accessible constructs or attitudes through one set of stimuli can facilitate cognitive processing of other stimuli under certain circumstances, and can interfere with it under other circumstances. Some of these results support and indeed converge on those described above, which were centered around the constructs of current concern and emotional arousal. That different construct systems can produce rather similar experimental designs and outcomes raises the question as to the relative validity or utility of these competing construct systems.

One branch of the recent research on construct accessibility has its roots in observations that in a Stroop color-naming design, it took subjects longer to name the color of the ink in which a word was printed when the word corresponded to one of a subject's relatively more accessible constructs (Bargh & Pratto, 1986). There was no effort here to control for the extent to which accessible constructs were linked to subjects' current concerns or to the emotional arousal potential of the stimuli. Such an association very likely exists. However, further research (Pratto & John, 1991) showed that this effect was stronger for negatively than for positively valenced words, although the extremity of ratings within the positive and negative word groups had no consistent effects. Negatively valenced words were also recalled more readily in a surprise free-recall test, indicating that the Stroop results are better explained in terms of cognitive interference—priority processing of negatively valenced stimuli—than of perceptual defense. The data are ambiguous with regard to whether they accord better with an explanation based on construct accessibility or one based on current concerns and emotional arousal, but they nevertheless narrow the range of tenable mechanisms by shedding doubt on an explanation based on defense mechanisms.

Another recent line of research arose with methods developed to demonstrate that strongly held attitudes are activated automatically upon exposure to the objects of those attitudes (Fazio, Sanbonmatsu, Powell, & Kardes, 1986). This investigation presented subjects with "attitude objects" (e.g., "cake"), which they had previously rated as "good" or "bad," followed 300 ms after stimulus onset by a positive or negative evaluative adjective (e.g., "awful"), which they were similarly to rate as "good" or "bad." They were also asked to keep rehearsing the word for each attitude object while evaluating the ensuing adjective. When the attitude object was regarded as strongly positive or negative (inferred from response speed in the first rating task), it slowed down response to an ensuing adjective of the opposite valence. The short time interval between them indicated that the effect had to be automatic—that the evaluation evoked by the attitude object could not have been decided deliberately. However, modifications in this procedure (a 2-day lag between evaluation of attitude object and evaluation of adjective, lack of rehearsal of word for the attitude object; Bargh, Chaiken, Govender, & Pratto, 1992) resulted in similar findings for both strongly *and* weakly positive and negative attitude objects. This suggests that the effect is quite general.

Because attitudes are presumed to contain an emotional component, these results could be taken as evidence that emotional reactions to stimuli occur early enough in processing to rule out the intercession of conscious cognition. This conclusion is supported by work described in later sections of this chapter, especially approaches employing evoked potentials.

Not only can the evaluative variables used in the above-described studies (ratings of "good" and "bad," response speed) be readily related to emotional arousal variables, but evidence from Bargh et al.'s (1992) Experiment 3 further buttresses such a connection. In that experiment, in which both strongly (quickly evaluated) and weakly (slowly evaluated) held attitude objects exerted effects on reaction time, the effects were stronger for the stronger than for the weaker attitudes, as would be predicted from the standpoint of emotional arousal. It is therefore ambiguous as to whether these effects are attributable primarily to the accessibility of constructs or to arousal of emotional responses. Moreover, a partial replication of Marcel's (1983) work on subliminal processing showed that subjects can assess the valences of subliminally presented word stimuli with above-chance accuracy, even though at those exposure durations they are unable to identify the word itself (Bargh, Litt, Pratto, & Spielman, 1989; Bock, Klinger, & Schneider, 1992). This finding may shed some doubt on the extent to which the phenomenon depends on the accessibility of constructs (at least of verbally based ones), in contrast to a more primitive process of responding emotionally/evaluatively to certain stimulus patterns following a preliminary semantic analysis.

A third relevant line of investigation asked subjects to form judgments of varying kinds while either trying to keep in mind a string of numbers (cognitive load) or not. In one investigation (Bargh & Tota, 1988), subjects characterized words, including whether a word was self-descriptive or other-descriptive. In another investigation (Andersen, Spielman, & Bargh, 1992), subjects judged whether various future events, both positive and negative, were likely to occur. Cognitive loads tend to slow most subjects' concurrent judgments, but in these studies the interference was less when the subjects both were depressed and made self-referential (but not other-referential) judgments for words associated with depression. Furthermore, cognitive loads produced no interference when depressed individuals predicted future events, which were on average more negative than was true for nondepressed subjects. The investigators interpreted these findings as indicating that depressed individuals have automatized the use of certain constructs for self-perception and of certain schemas for predicting the future.

The conceptual framework in which these results were obtained, and certain of the results themselves, raise the question as to whether the various cognitive effects that have been attributed to current concerns and emotional arousal are indeed thus attributable, or whether they are really the result of confounded correlates of current concerns. Most notably, are the effects really attributable to such cognitive factors as subjects' well-ingrained, especially accessible social-perceptual constructs? Their accessibility might result from a history of frequent use or frequent exposure to them, or it might result from recency effects (the constructs and language most heavily encountered or employed recently). Disentangling these cognitive confounds with concern-relatedness or emotional arousal value is extremely problematic, because an individual's typical current concerns necessarily reflect that individual's characteristic constructs, and the hundreds or thousands of thoughts that the individual is likely to have devoted to an important concern will have been couched in the individual's characteristic vocabulary for that concern, thereby further strengthening the accessibility of the corresponding constructs. Furthermore, if the concern is truly current, the individual's thoughts, conversations, and actions relating to the concern are bound to have occurred on average more recently than would be true for nonconcerns, adding to the accessibility of concern-related constructs.

Factors such as frequency and recency, which affect accessibility, therefore potentially provide an alternative explanation for the purported effects of concerns and emotions. Yet, for the reasons indicated, a direct test of such an alternative is very nearly impossible. A longitudinal study could perhaps control for the frequency with which individuals use or encounter characteristic constructs by comparing the effects of current concerns with those of the same individuals' past concerns, but there would still be a problem of possible recency-related effects. In any event, such research has not yet been done. Nor have investigations of cognitive social constructs or the like controlled systematically for the confounding effects of current concerns and emotional reactivity.

Nevertheless, there are a number of less direct reasons to doubt that the alternative accessibility explanations can replace explanations centered on current concerns and emotional reactivity:

1. The fact that skin conductance responses are associated with current-concern-related content but not past-concern-related content in the thought stream (Nikula et al., 1993) makes it unlikely that at least this effect is mediated by frequency-induced accessibility of constructs—by individuals' characteristic constructs' being responsible for increased skin conductance responses. After all, one would expect past concerns to be about as much related to individuals' construct systems as are current concerns.

2. Young's (1987) data showed that the presence of *disattended* concern-related distractors slows lexical decisions about focal stimuli. It is hard to imagine how construct accessibility could account for such a result without imbuing the construct of "construct accessibility" with motivational properties.

3. Recall of words is associated with both the concern-relatedness of the words and their emotional arousal value (Bock & Klinger, 1986; Klinger et al., 1990), but the association of recall with emotional arousal value remains significant after concern-relatedness is partialed out. This suggests that the emotional arousal value of a stimulus has effects not already contained in the effects of concern-relatedness, and therefore not already contained in whatever social-perceptual constructs they evoke in common.

4. Taylor (1992) reported an effect of anger on recall of stimuli associated with anger-arousing situations, but only if subjects had been experimentally led to expect an opportunity to aggress against the perpetrator. Such a result—involving again a relation of emotion with recall—cannot be explained in terms of enduring cognitive properties of subjects.

5. A number of investigations have found relationships between emotional states and cognitive responsivity in patterns of results that make a cognitive-dispositional explanation improbable. Thus, Lewinsohn and Rosenbaum (1987) found different patterns of recall of parents' behaviors by people who were currently depressed than by those who had at one time been depressed but were now remitted. Mogg, Mathews, and Eysenck (1992) reported that whereas patients diagnosed with generalized anxiety disorder showed a significant attentional sensitivity to threat-related words, this was not the case for former patients who had since recovered. Indeed, the paradigm used by Mogg et al. does not lend itself readily to explanation through accessible constructs: They found faster reaction times to dot-probe stimuli when the dots were located in the previous positions of the threat-related words than when they appeared in the previous position of the neutral words. Furthermore, they found stronger effects when the nature of the threat represented by the previous word (social vs. physical threat) corresponded with the subjects' concerns. It would be hard to argue that the faster these common,

supraliminal words could be understood, the longer the eye would focus on them, but that is what would have had to happen to facilitate reaction time to a dot at that location. It is much easier to argue the contrary view. On the other hand, the result is easily accommodated by current-concerns theory, which would argue that subjects would attend to current- concern-related stimuli more closely than to others. Finally, McNally et al. (1989) showed that panic disorder patients recalled proportionately more anxiety-related words than normal controls did, but that their "false alarms" ("recalls" of words not among the original stimuli) had about the same proportion of anxiety-related words as those produced by normal controls; this suggests that the panic disorder patients were not simply more likely to produce anxiety- related words.

Taken all together, then, these lines of evidence render a cognitive-dispositional explanation (e.g., the accessibility of certain social-perceptual constructs) of results ascribed to current concerns and emotional arousal very unlikely.

Another objection that might be raised to the current-concerns interpretation of the data described above is that current-concerns-related stimuli are also self-referent stimuli. Perhaps, then, reference to oneself is the key mediating factor, given the rich associative network that people develop around their self-concepts. Again, it is hard to disentangle the constructs; current concerns are inherently self-referent. However, there are at least two indications that this explanation is weaker than that offered by the current-concerns framework. McNally et al. (1989), who examined word recall by panic disorder patients and normal control subjects, divided their word stimuli according to how self-referent subjects had rated them as being. They found that "[panic disorder] subjects tended to show a recall bias for self-descriptive anxiety words, whereas [normal control] subjects tended to show a recall bias for self-descriptive nonanxiety words" (p. 39), and that these biases operated only during an exercise arousal condition. In other words, whether or not self-reference plays an independent role in facilitating recall, emotional factors play a separate part. A different kind of recall task (Bock, 1988) led to a similar conclusion. Here subjects had been exposed to pairs of items from a personality inventory; afterwards, the task was to recognize which of two items had been paired with a third item. When correctly and incorrectly recognized pairs were compared, their average self-relevance was virtually identical. It therefore seems unlikely that self-reference can independently account for the effects attributed above to concern-relatedness and emotional arousal value.

IMPLICATIONS FOR THEORIES OF EMOTION AND COGNITION

The patterning of these numerous data has important implications for theories of both emotion and cognition. For cognitive theory, the implication is that emotional responses steer cognitive processing, probably at a number of different stages and levels, including during some of the earliest processing steps (Klinger, 1992). This conclusion is consistent with a continuous-flow model of information processing (e.g., Coles, Gratton, Bashore, Eriksen, & Donchin, 1985), but in a way that provides an evaluative role for essentially emotional responses. Continuous-flow theory posits that as cognitive processing unfolds, its results at every phase become available for further use, such as decision making. Primitive evaluations begin to stimulate reactions even as more refined processing continues. The data described so far suggest that emotional response of some kind plays a role in this primitive processing.

For theory of emotion, the results suggest that essentially emotional responses are continually active without necessarily involving the autonomic, motoric, and humoral responses or the conscious features that are most often identified with emotion. Emotional responses at this early level—designated here as "protoemotional" responses—theoretically recruit the more traditional response components of emotion only if the reciprocal effects of protoemotional evaluation and cognitive processing pass some kind of threshold of urgency, the nature of which is still unclear.

This sequential-component theory of emotion, which posits a very early involvement of essentially emotional responses in cognition, gains support from an investigation of near-liminal perception (Bock, Klinger, & Schneider, 1992). Subjects saw near-liminally and supraliminally exposed images of words and nonword letter strings. They were variously asked to decide whether they had seen a word or nonword, or to rate the emotional valence of the stimulus. Subjects made all their judgments with above-chance average accuracy, even at near-threshold exposures, and they made their judgments in the lexical task faster with longer exposure times; however, the speed of their affective judgments increased little with exposure time. This indicates that the processing on which affective response is based involves rather global stimulus features that are already perceived at very brief exposure times, and that more differentiated stimulus features, which are perceived with longer exposure and which benefit lexical judgments, make little additional contribution to affective response.

Another implication relates to theories in which emotion depends on feedback from motor changes (e.g., Zajonc & Markus, 1984). The rapidity with which protoemotional processes begin to function is probably too great to accommodate interpretations based on motor feedback, except insofar as the motor effects merely modulate emotional responses at later stages of their emergence. On the other hand, it is consistent with evidence that very brief, repeated exposures to unfamiliar stimuli increase subjects' preferences for them (Zajonc, 1980), in that exposures too brief for later recognition nevertheless can modify affective response.

THE USE OF EVOKED POTENTIALS AS AN APPROACH TO PROTOEMOTIONAL PROCESSES: NEUROELECTRIC SUPPORT FOR THE MODEL

The proposed effect of emotion on cognition at the microstructural level of processing, which is nonconscious, lends itself particularly well to investigation by the use of psychophysiological measures, especially averaged evoked potentials (EPs—regularities in electroencephalographic responses to particular classes of stimuli). The time course of certain EP components that are linked to emotion is consistent with the concept of protoemotions.

To be sure, the older EP literature provides little encouragement for such an approach. EPs have commonly been regarded as reflections of cognitive processes (Coles, Gratton, & Fabiani, 1990). The P300 component, for example, has been proposed to indicate "context updating" (perceiving information that requires changing existing models of the environment; e.g., Donchin & Coles, 1988), "context closure" (perceiving the end of a unit of information; Verleger, 1988), responses to high-information priming stimuli (Gratton et al., 1990), subjective probability/uncertainty, stimulus significance, and loss of information (Johnson, 1986), and so on. The arguments have been about what aspects of information processing are the essential conditions for the P300.

However, recent evidence has implicated the P300 component (positive deflections in the neighborhood of 300 ms after stimulus onset), and more generally the late positive complex to emotional variables, in ways that cast doubt on purely cognitive formulations. The P300 has been shown to covary with the emotionality of stimuli, both facial expressions and words (Kestenbaum & Nelson, 1992; Lang, Nelson, & Collins, 1990; Laurian, Bader, Lanares, & Oros, 1991; Naumann, Bartussek, Diedrich, & Laufer, 1992; Naumann, Bartussek, Diedrich, Vogelbacher, & Mehrtens, 1992). Furthermore, the location of maximum effects on P300 amplitude has differed according to experimental procedures. When subjects were instructed to judge the emotional valence or a structural feature of stimuli (higher-level cognitive operations), the emotional processing yielded positivity shifts (as compared with the structural processing) that were primarily frontocentral; however, P300 was also larger for stimuli that subjects later rated as relatively emotionally arousing than for those they rated as relatively neutral, and these effects were mostly parietal (Naumann, Bartussek, Diedrich, Vogelbacher, & Mehrtens, 1992). This may indicate that protoemotional effects show up most clearly at parietal electrode sites.

The divergent interpretations of the P300 raise the question of whether these effects are attributable to cognitive or to emotional differences in the processing of the stimuli. The most common cognitive explanations of the P300 relate, as indicated earlier, to such concepts as context updating, encountering unexpected events, or registering the closure of a communication. But it would be hard to argue that the emotionally toned and neutral stimuli used in the studies by Nelson's and Naumann's groups differed in contextual information, probability, or closure. On the other hand, one could argue that responses to unexpected stimuli, as in the orienting response or in responses upon the completion of a meaningful communication, may regularly have a protoemotional component. Interestingly, just as the emotionality of stimuli is correlated with their retrieval in free recall, so is the size of the P300 component that they elicit (Fabiani, Karis, & Donchin, 1986). It thus seems reasonable to conclude that early cognitive processing and protoemotional processes may well be intertwined, but it is the emotional facet that is reflected in the P300.

There is one more important finding regarding the emotional status of the P300 component. There is increasing evidence that psychopaths suffer from impaired emotional response to at least some classes of emotionally arousing stimuli. Now there is evidence that the difference in EP components (especially 240–300 ms and 650–800 ms—intervals often subsumed under the broad label of P300) between emotionally toned and neutral words is significantly smaller in psychopaths than in others (Williamson, Harpur, & Hare, 1991), once more indicating a relationship between P300-related and emotional (presumably, at about 300 ms, protoemotional) response.

The growing nomological net therefore provides ample reason to suppose that the P300 and potentially other EP components index protoemotional processes. By the same token, it indicates that emotional processes begin to take effect within the first third of a second following stimulus onset.

CONCLUSION

The pattern of evidence seems consistent with the model previewed early in this chapter. When people become committed to pursuing a goal, that event initiates an internal state termed a "current concern," one of whose properties is to potentiate emotional reactivity to cues associated with the goal pursuit. There is now extensive evidence to support the notion that what people notice, recall, and think about is ultimately governed by their concerns, and that this relationship is mediated by the emotional responses evoked by concern-related cues. Because emotional responses are in part innately linked to particular stimuli and are readily conditioned, people also respond to cues that are emotionally arousing without corresponding to a *current* concern. Both behavioral and electrophysiological evidence suggests that the emotional responses thus emitted appear to begin within about 300 ms after exposure to the cue—early enough to be considered purely central, nonconscious, "protoemotional" responses.

To explain the data, protoemotional responses must occur in parallel with early, global perceptual and cognitive analysis and must exert reciprocal influences at several levels of processing. The intensity (and possibly other features) of the protoemotional responses presumably affects the probability that the stimulus will continue to be processed cognitively. The results of continued cognitive processing in turn clearly modulate the intensity and character of the emerging emotional response. Should the emotional response pass some as yet unknown kind of threshold (which may well depend on competing responses), it presumably begins to recruit other, slower subsystems, such as autonomic and endocrine responses; nonvolitional motor responses, such as facial and postural expressions; conscious affect; conscious cognitive processing; and ultimately action. By that time, it has emerged as a full-scale emotional response in the classical meaning of the term. It also presumably affects such cognitive dimensions as speed, coordination, distractibility, and integration.

Most of what needs to be known about these matters remains to be discovered: the precise nature and timing of protoemotional responses; their location, course, and connections through the brain; the precise nature of reciprocal influences with perception and cognition; the criteria that determine whether processing stops at any given point or goes on to biologically and psychologically more costly levels; which emotional subsystems are recruited at which points and according to which criteria; what controls exist that moderate, divert, or inhibit emotional responses at various stages of their unfolding; and the decision rules for admitting emotional responses to consciousness and for giving them priority over competing responses. It is also still unclear at this time just what happens at the point of an individual's commitment to a goal, how the state initiated by this commitment potentiates responses to goal-related cues, under what conditions this potentiation persists, and by what process this potentiation comes to an end (whether following consummation or following disengagement as a result of loss or failure). Many other questions remain. Obviously, there is no shortage of research questions to be answered in this domain.

ACKNOWLEDGMENT

Eric Goetzman and Tanya Hughes assisted in the writing of this chapter.

REFERENCES

Alloy, L. B. (Ed.). (1988). *Cognitive processes in depression.* New York: Guilford Press.

Andersen, S. M., Spielman, L. A., & Bargh, J. A. (1992). Future-event schemas and certainty about the future: Automaticity in depressives' future-event predictions. *Journal of Personality and Social Psychology, 63,* 711–723.

Bargh, J. A., Chaiken, S., Govender, R., & Pratto, F. (1992). The generality of the automatic attitude activation effect. *Journal of Personality and Social Psychology, 62,* 893–912.

Bargh, J. A., Litt, J., Pratto, F., & Spielman, L. A. (1989). On the preconscious evaluation of social stimuli. In A. F. Bennet & K. M. McConkey (Eds.), *Cognition in individual and social contexts* (pp. 357–370). Amsterdam: Elsevier/North-Holland.

Bargh, J. A., & Pratto, F. (1986). Individual construct accessibility and perceptual selection. *Journal of Experimental Social Psychology, 22,* 293–311.

Bargh, J. A., & Tota, M. E. (1988). Context-dependent automatic processing in depression: Accessibility of negative constructs with regard to self but not others. *Journal of Personality and Social Psychology, 54,* 925–939.

Bock, M. (1988). Emotion, self, and memory. In K. Fiedler & J. Forgas (Eds.), *Affect, cognition, and social behavior: New evidence and integrative attempts* (pp. 120–137). Toronto: Hogrefe.

Bock, M., & Klinger, E. (1986). Interaction of emotion and cognition in word recall. *Psychological Research, 48,* 99–106.

Bock, M., Klinger, E., & Schneider, K. (1992, July 21). *Are emotional effects of words mediated by lexical meaning?* Paper presented at the 25th International Congress of Psychology, Brussels.

Bower, G. H. (1992). How might emotions affect learning? In S.-A. Christianson (Ed.), *The handbook of emotion and memory: Research and theory* (pp. 3–32). Hillsdale, NJ: Erlbaum.

Brecht, D. L., Nikles, C. D., II, Klinger, E., & Bursell, A. L. (1995). *The effects of current-concern and nonconcern-related waking suggestions on nocturnal dream content.* Unpublished manuscript.

Broadbent, D., & Broadbent, M. (1988). Anxiety and attentional bias: State and trait. *Cognition and Emotion, 2,* 165–184.

Brown, T. (1991). The biological significance of affectivity. In N. L. Stein, B. Leventhal, & T. Trabasso (Eds.), *Psychological and biological approaches to emotion* (pp. 405–434). Hillsdale, NJ: Erlbaum.

Christianson, S.-Å. (1992). Emotional stress and eyewitness memory: A critical review. *Psychological Bulletin, 112,* 284–309.

Coles, M. G. H., Gratton, G., Bashore, T. R., Eriksen, C. W., & Donchin, E. (1985). A psychophysiological investigation of the continuous flow model of human information processing. *Journal of Experimental Psychology: Human Perception and Performance, 11,* 529–553.

Coles, M. G. H., Gratton, G., & Fabiani, M. (1990). Event-related brain potentials. In J. T. Cacioppo & L. G. Tassinary (Eds.), *Principles of psychophysiology* (pp. 413–455). New York: Cambridge University Press.

Cox, W. M., & Klinger, E. (1988). A motivational model of alcohol use. *Journal of Abnormal Psychology, 97,* 168–180.

Derryberry, D., & Tucker, D. M. (1992). Neural mechanisms of emotion. *Journal of Consulting and Clinical Psychology, 60,* 329–338.

Donchin, E., & Coles, M. G. H. (1988). Is the P300 component a manifestation of context updating? *Behavioral and Brain Sciences, 11,* 357–374.

Ehlers, A. M., Margraf, J., Davies, S., & Roth, W. T. (1988). Selective processing of threat cues in subjects with panic attacks. *Cognition and Emotion, 2,* 201–220.

Fabiani, M., Karis, D., & Donchin, E. (1986). P300 and recall in an incidental memory paradigm. *Psychophysiology, 23,* 298–308.

Fazio, R. H., Sanbonmatsu, D. M., Powell, M. C., & Kardes, F. R. (1986). On the automatic activation of attitudes. *Journal of Personality and Social Psychology, 50,* 229–238.

Fox, E. (1993). Allocation of visual attention and anxiety. *Cognition and Emotion, 7,* 207–216.

Gollwitzer, P. (1990). Action phases and mind-sets. In E. T. Higgins & R. M. Sorrentino (Eds.), *Handbook of motivation and social cognition: Foundations of social behavior* (Vol. 2, pp. 53–92). New York: Guilford Press.

Gottlib, I. H., McLachlan, A. L., & Katz, A. N. (1988). Biases in visual attention in depressed and nondepressed individuals. *Cognition and Emotion, 2,* 185–200.

Gratton, G., Bosco, C. M., Kramer, A. F., Coles, M. G. H., Wickens, C. D., & Donchin, E. (1990). Event-related brain potentials as indices of information extraction and response priming. *Electroencephalography and Clinical Neurophysiology, 75,* 419–432.

Hoelscher, T. J., Klinger, E., & Barta, S. G. (1981). Incorporation of concern- and nonconcern-related verbal stimuli into dream content. *Journal of Abnormal Psychology, 49,* 88–91.

Ingram, R. E., Kendall, P. C., Smith, T. W., Donnell, C., & Ronan, K. (1987). Cognitive specificity in emotional distress. *Journal of Personality and Social Psychology, 53,* 734–742.

Isen, A. M. (1991). The influence of positive and negative affect on cognitive organization: Some implications for development. In N. L. Stein, B. Leventhal, & T. Trabasso (Eds.), *Psychological and biological approaches to emotion* (pp. 75–94). Hillsdale, NJ: Erlbaum.

Johnsen, B. H., Laberg, J. C., Cox, W. M., Vaksdal, A., & Hugdahl, K. (1994). Alcoholics' attentional bias in the processing of alcohol-related words. *Psychology of Addictive Behaviors, 8,* 111–115.

Johnson, R., Jr. (1986). A triarchic model of P300 amplitude. *Psychophysiology, 29,* 367–384.

Kanfer, R., & Ackerman, P. L. (1989). Motivation and cognitive abilities: An integrative/aptitude-treatment interaction approach to skill acquisition [Monograph]. *Journal of Applied Psychology, 74,* 657–690.

Kestenbaum, R., & Nelson, C. A. (1992). Neural and behavioral correlates of emotion recognition in children and adults. *Journal of Experimental Child Psychology, 54,* 1–18.

Klinger, E. (1971). *Structure and functions of fantasy.* New York: Wiley.

Klinger, E. (1975). Consequences of commitment to and disengagement from incentives. *Psychological Review, 82,* 1–25.

Klinger, E. (1977). *Meaning and void: Inner experience and the incentives in people's lives.* Minneapolis: University of Minnesota Press.

Klinger, E. (1978). Modes of normal conscious flow. In K. S. Pope & J. L. Singer (Eds.), *The stream of consciousness: Scientific investigations into the flow of human experience* (pp. 225–258). New York: Plenum.

Klinger, E. (1987a). Current concerns and disengagement from incentives. In F. Halisch & J. Kuhl (Eds.), *Motivation, intention and volition* (pp. 337–347). Berlin: Springer-Verlag.

Klinger, E. (1987b). The interview questionnaire technique: Reliability and validity of a mixed idiographic–nomothetic measure of motivation. In J. N. Butcher & C. D. Spielberger (Eds.), *Advances in personality assessment* (Vol. 6, pp. 31–48). Hillsdale, NJ: Erlbaum.

Klinger, E. (1990). *Daydreaming.* Los Angeles: Tarcher/Putnam.

Klinger, E. (1992). Motivation and imagination. *Psychologische Beiträge, 34,* 127–142.

Klinger, E., Barta, S. G., & Maxeiner, M. E. (1980). Motivational correlates of thought content frequency and commitment. *Journal of Personality and Social Psychology, 39,* 1222–1237.

Klinger, E., Bock M., & Bowi, U. (1990). *Emotional mediation of motivational factors in word recall.* Unpublished manuscript.

Klinger, E., & Kroll-Mensing, D. (1995). Idiothetic assessment: Experience samping and motivational analysis. In J. N. Butcher (Ed.), *Practical considerations in clinical personality assessment* (pp. 267–277). New York: Oxford University Press.

Kuhl, J. (1983b). Emotion, Kognition und Motivation: Auf dem Wege zu einer systemtheoretischen Betrachtung der Emotionsgenese. *Sprache und Kognition, 2,* 1–27.

Kuhl, J. (1983b). Emotion, Kognition und Motivation: II. Die funktionale Bedeutung der Emotionen für das problemlösende Denken und für das konkrete Handeln. *Sprache und Kognition, 4,* 228–253.

Lang, S. F., Nelson, C. A., & Collins, P. F. (1990). Event-related potentials to emotional and neutral stimuli. *Journal of Clinical and Experimental Neuropsychology, 12,* 946–958.

Larsen, R., & Diener, E. (1987). Affect intensity as an individual difference characteristic. *Journal of Research in Personality, 21,* 1–39.

Laurian, S., Bader, M., Lanares, J., & Oros, L. (1991). Topography of event-related potentials elicited by visual emotional stimuli. *International Journal of Psychophysiology, 10,* 231–238.

LeDoux, J. E. (1989). Cognitive–emotional interactions in the brain. *Cognition and Emotion, 3,* 267–289.

LeDoux, J. E. (1992). Emotion as memory: Anatomical systems underlying indelible neural traces. In S.-Å. Christianson (Ed.), *The handbook of emotion and memory: Research and theory* (pp. 269–288). Hillsdale, NJ: Erlbaum.

Lewinsohn, P. M., & Rosenbaum, M. (1987). Recall of parental behavior by acute depressives, remitted depressives, and nondepressives. *Journal of Personality and Social Psychology, 52,* 611–619.

Marcel, A. (1983). Conscious and unconscious perception: An approach to the relations between phenomenal experience and perceptual processes. *Cognitive Psychology, 15,* 238–300.

Martin, M., Horder, P., & Jones, G. V. (1993). Integral bias in naming of phobia-related words. *Cognition and Emotion, 7,* 479–486.

Mayer, J. D., Gaschke, Y. N., Braverman, D. L., & Evans, T. W. (1992). Mood-congruent judgment is a general effect. *Journal of Personality and Social Psychology, 63,* 119–132.

McNally, R. J., Foa, E. B., & Donnell, C. D. (1989). Memory bias for anxiety information in patients with panic disorder. *Cognition and Emotion, 3,* 27–44.

Mogg, K., Mathews, A., & Eysenck, M. (1992). Attentional bias to threat in clinical anxiety states. *Cognition and Emotion, 6,* 149–159.

Naumann, E., Bartussek, D., Diedrich, O., & Laufer, M.E. (1992). Assessing cognitive and affective information processing functions of the brain by means of the late positive complex of the event-related potential. *Journal of Psychophysiology, 6,* 285–298.

Naumann, E., Bartussek, D., Diedrich, O., Vogelbacher, D., & Mehrtens, S. (1992). Emotionality and the late positive complex of the event-related potential. In H.-J. Heinze, T. F. Münte, & G. R. Mengen (Eds.), *New developments in event-related potentials.* Boston: Birkhäuser.

Newman, J. P., Wallace, J. F., Strauman, T. J., Skolaski, R. L., Oreland, K. M., Mattek, P. W., Elder, K. A., & McNeely, J. (1993). Effects of motivationally significant stimuli on the regulation of dominant responses. *Journal of Personality and Social Psychology, 65,* 165–175.

Nikula, R., Klinger, E., & Larson-Gutman, M. K. (1993). Current concerns and electrodermal reactivity: Responses to words and thoughts. *Journal of Personality, 61,* 63–84.

Pratto, F., & John, O. P. (1991). Automatic vigilance: The attention-grabbing power of negative social information. *Journal of Personality and Social Psychology, 61,* 380–391.

Revelle, W., & Loftus, D. A. (1992). Implications of arousal effects for the study of affect and memory. In S.-Å. Christianson (Ed.), *The handbook of emotion and memory: Research and theory* (pp. 113–149). Hillsdale, NJ: Erlbaum.

Riemann, B. C., & McNally, R. J. (1995). Cognitive processing of personally-relevant information. *Cognition and Emotion, 9,* 325–340.

Schneider, W. (1987). *Ablenkung und Handlungskontrolle: Eine 'kognitiv-motivationale perspektive' [Distraction and action control: A "cognitive-motivational perspective"].* Unpublished diploma thesis, University of Bielefeld, Germany.

Stein, N. L., & Levine, L. J. (1991). Making sense out of emotion: The representation and use of goal-structured knowledge. In N. L. Stein, B. Leventhal, & T. Trabasso (Eds.), *Psychological and biological approaches to emotion* (pp. 45–73). Hillsdale, NJ: Erlbaum.

Taylor, L. (1992). Relationship between affect and memory: Motivation-based selective generation. *Journal of Personality and Social Psychology, 62,* 876–882.

Tobias, B. A., Kihlstrom, J. F., & Schacter, D. L. (1992). Emotion and implicit memory. In S.-Å. Christianson (Ed.), *The handbook of emotion and memory: Research and theory* (pp. 67–92). Hillsdale, NJ: Erlbaum.

Verleger, R. (1988). Event-related potentials and cognition: A critique of the context updating hypothesis and an alternative interpretation of P3. *Behavioral and Brain Sciences, 11,* 343–427.

Williamson, S., Harpur, T. J., & Hare, R. D. (1991). Abnormal processing of affective words by psychopaths. *Psychophysiology, 28,* 260–273.

Young, J. (1987). *The role of selective attention in the attitude–behavior relationship.* Unpublished doctoral dissertation, University of Minnesota.

Zajonc, R. B. (1980). Feeling and thinking: Preferences need no inferences. *American Psychologist, 35,* 151–175.

Zajonc, R. B., & Markus, H. (1984). Affect and cognition: The hard interface. In C. E. Izard, J. Kagan, & R. B. Zajonc (Eds.), *Emotions, cognition, and behavior* (pp. 73–102). Cambridge, England: Cambridge University Press.

PART III

Preparing to Act

SECTION A

Mental Construction of the Goal

As pointed out in Part I, people's goal contents may vary according to their needs, their implicit theories about the world, and their styles of framing the goal content. But the same goal may still be mentally represented in various different ways. In his research on delay of gratification, Mischel (Chapter 9) points out that one and the same desired goal object (e.g., cookies) may be represented in a person's mind in different types of cognitions—namely, "cold" versus "hot" cognitions—with drastic consequences for a person's ability to delay gratification. Taylor and Pham (Chapter 10), in their work on mental simulation, differentiate between two forms of thinking about goal attainment. Outcome simulation focuses on being in the goal state; process simulation focuses on getting there. Applied to the goal of getting an A in an exam, for instance, the two different types of thinking about goal attainment affect relevant behaviors (e.g., amount of studying) and quality of performance. Oettingen (Chapter 11) differentiates between fantasies about desired behavioral outcomes and expectations that these outcomes will occur. Whereas positive expectations enhance the likelihood that these outcomes and behaviors will occur, positive fantasies turn out to suppress their occurrence. Finally, Vallacher and Kaufman (Chapter 12) show that any given action goal can be identified at different levels of abstraction. Whereas high-level identifications provide the individual with consistent guidance for purposeful acting, low-level identifications induce erractic, nonintegrated behaviors.

Mischel's research on self-regulation shows that by the age of 6 most children have acquired the ability to strategically vary a goal's mental representation. When children are confronted with a delay-of-gratification problem (e.g., the children face the conflict of either grabbing a smaller, immediate award, such as a single pretzel, or waiting for a larger, delayed award, such as two pretzels), the capacity to wait is determined by the children's strategies of thinking about the delayed reward. Abstract representations of the delayed reward (e.g., imagining pretzels as thin brown logs) increase waiting time, whereas imagining the arousing, sensual aspects of the reward (e.g., the crunchy, salty taste) reduces it. When children are confronted with a temptation problem (e.g., attractive distractions are offered during the performance of a boring task), the capacity to ward off distractions is positively affected by plans that spell out how one intends to deal with the distraction once it occurs (e.g., to ignore it). Both lines of research strongly suggest that once a person has set a goal (e.g., to wait for a bigger reward or to ward off distractions), the capacity to achieve the goal is strongly affected by the mental construction of the goal object or the actions instrumental to goal achievement, respectively. Mischel reminds the reader that these findings demand a rethinking of the classic understanding of willpower. Apparently, willpower is nothing but the skillful control of mental representations of goal contents and goal-directed actions. If this is so, increasing a person's willpower becomes a matter of training individuals in the mental control of cognitions relevant to effective goal achievement. Mischel also proposes the analysis of the development of this type of self-control knowledge, with a focus on long-term implications of preschool delay competence and on high-risk populations, such as children with problems of impulse control.

Taylor and Pham explore whether mental simulation qualifies as a vehicle for linking thought to action. It is suggested that mental simulations enhance the likelihood of actions consistent with the simulation. Mental simulations make the simulated events appear more true or likely; they yield plans; and they invoke emotions and arousal in the service of an action sequence. Three kinds of mental simulations are distinguished. First, mental simulations may be used as goal-focusing techniques (so-called outcome simulations, which envision the intended goal state). Second, process simulations delineate the sequence of events that leads to a desired outcome, thus giving an answer to the question of how a desired outcome can be achieved. Finally, a third kind of simulation combines process and outcome simulations and thus traces the steps for achieving the goal but also pictures goal attainment. In an empirical test of the effectiveness of these various simulations (in the context of preparing for an upcoming exam), process simulations were the winners. Not only did they reduce worries and test anxiety, but they also enhanced test performance (this effect was probably mediated by more intensive and concentrated studying). Outcome simulations, on the other hand, increased self-reported motivation, but this increase in inspiration was not reflected in enhanced studying or better grades. Finally, combined process and outcome simulations were no more effective than the simple process simulations. It appears, then, that mentally rehearsing the process of getting to a desired outcome (e.g., studying for a good grade) is more effective in eliciting the appropriate behaviors than mentally rehearsing the attainment of this outcome (e.g., receiving a good grade). Such process rehearsal may shape concrete plans for acting so as to obtain the desired outcome (e.g., studying), and these plans in turn are enacted with greater likelihood.

Oettingen cuts the pie of thoughts about the future differently. People may entertain spontaneous fantasies about the future that can be experienced as either positive or negative, and they may also hold expectations that certain events will or will not take place. Whereas positive, optimistic expectations favor the execution of behaviors geared toward achieving these events, positive fantasies undermine it. This is demonstrated in various health domains (e.g., losing weight, recovery from a chronic illness), but also in connection with romantic relationships and professional careers (i.e., romantic and professional success). Why does thinking about the future in terms of positive fantasies reduce one's readiness to act on one's thoughts? Positive fantasies about desired outcomes and actions may undermine a person's readiness to act, because indulging in a positive fantasy is consumptive and thus reduces one's urge to implement the fantasy. Moreover, it may conceal the necessity to act and may distract the person from thinking about how to change reality in order to fulfill the fantasy. This is suggested by a series of experimental studies reported by Oettingen. Whenever subjects were requested to contrast their positive fantasies about future outcomes and actions with the present reality, they showed a strong readiness to act—given that outcome expectations were reasonably high. Such positive expectations did not induce actions in subjects, however, when they indulged in positive fantasies only or dwelled solely on the negative reality. Apparently, contrasting fantasy with reality turns positive fantasy into something to be achieved and reality into something to be changed. Positive fantasies, therefore, can affect a person's behavior quite differently, depending on whether the person is confronted with thoughts about a negative reality.

Referring to action identification theory, Vallacher and Kaufman explain that any given action can be identified by the individual either in terms of detailed, mechanistic depictions (low-level identities) or in terms of comprehensive, consequence-defined depictions (high-level identities). Traveling from one city to another can be conceived of, for instance, as going to a conference (high-level) or boarding a train (low-level). Understanding an action in terms of relatively high-level identities leads to focusing on outcomes and consequences of actions. The mental representations of goals based on outcomes and consequences, therefore, qualify as directors of various different actions all serving one and the same purpose. In general, people prefer higher-level identities when thinking about their actions. They move downward only when disruptions and difficulties force them to attend to the intricacies of acting, and even then they are eager to return to higher-level identities. But how do higher-order identifications emerge? Vallacher and Kaufman argue that the first phase of this emergence process is characterized by a turbulent oscillation between diverse higher-order identifications over short periods of time. An experiment employing a new paradigm that traces the moment-to-moment dynamism of a person's flow of thoughts supports this view. When people were induced to understand an action in terms of low-level identities, the subsequent emergence of high-level identifications started off with high volatility (i.e., higher-order identifications were at first unstable, disconnected, and wavering), but it always gave way to a relatively stable higher-order action identification as time passed by.

This observation has important implications. First, if people act out of a state of heightened volatility in which possible higher-level identities are sampled, their actions should be impulsive and erratic, reflecting the unstable succession of different goal representations that vanish as quickly as they appear. The emergence of a stable higher-order identification of future actions seems to be a prerequisite for a goal to provide consistent guidance of a person's actions. Second, the final emergence of higher-order identifications assures that people will not lose sight of their superordinate goals when difficulties force them to move downward to lower-level action identifications. The superordinate goals (being higher-order identifications) have a good chance of being reinstalled by the processes that promote higher-level identifications.

CHAPTER 9 From Good Intentions to Willpower

Walter Mischel

Given that goals are at the core of most approaches to motivation, and that the crucial role of cognitive representation for purposeful behavior has now reached the status of a cliché in psychology, it seems remarkable how little we know about how the cognitive representation of a desired goal influences the individual's ability to continue to pursue it. An adequate theory of goal-directed behavior and motivation needs to explain the specific effects of the mental representation of the goals people seek on their ability to pursue and attain them. Achieving this understanding has been the aim of my research program on self-imposed delay of gratification for the sake of desired but temporally delayed goals. The most basic question has been this: Just how does the mental representation of a blocked goal (or outcome or "reward") influence one's willingness and ability to continue to wait and work for it?

INDIVIDUAL DIFFERENCES IN "WILLPOWER"

Although some individuals seem able to adhere to stringent diets, to give up cigarettes after years of smoking them addictively, or to continue to labor for distant goals even when sorely frustrated, others fail at these efforts although failure may cost them their health and lives. The ancient Greeks considered such failures a character trait, which they called *akrasia* (deficiency of the will), and they philosophized about its possible causes and remedies. Contemporary lay explanations 2,000 years later still use similar concepts of a character trait, offer popular but dubious advice for how to strengthen the will, and leave it equally mysterious. The enduring question for psychology remains how to demystify willpower and understand individual differences among people in their attempts to turn their good intentions into reality in the face of formidable barriers and frustrations.

To answer this question, the research program summarized in this chapter tried to clarify the types of "preliminaries," as William James called them over a century ago (James, 1890, Vol. 2, p. 488), that enable individuals to exercise "willpower" (or "personal agency," its modern name) after they have chosen their goals, believe they can attain them, and proceed to try to do so. We focused on an essential ingredient of volitional self-control: the ability to effectively delay gratification for the sake of better but delayed outcomes that one has chosen to pursue but that prove difficult to attain in the face of immediately available smaller rewards and temptations. In a related vein, we also explored the preliminaries that facilitate delay and resistance to distractions and temptations when children must perform activities that are instrumental to their receiving the desired rewards without succumbing to obstacles along the route (e.g., Mischel & Patterson, 1978). Not only is understanding those "preliminaries" basic for theories of motivation and personality; their absence may underlie many personal and social problems, such as early school failure, conduct disorders, and a wide range of addictive and antisocial behavior patterns (e.g., Bandura, 1986; Bandura & Mischel, 1965; Mischel, 1966, 1968, 1990; Rutter, 1987; Stumphauzer, 1972).

Although the processes that underlie the ability to delay gratification and resist immediate temptation have remained mysterious over many years, the importance of the phenomenon has been recognized in psychology since the beginnings of the field. In Freud's psychodynamic theory of human development, delay of gratification marks the transition from impulse-driven primary process to future-oriented secondary process; Freud assumed it to be at the core of personality development, and indeed a basic foundation for any civilization. Regardless of specific theory, it is widely believed that in all cultures the process of socialization depends on the development of self-imposed delays of gratification in the young child, beginning in such contexts as weaning and toilet training. Effective functioning and indeed survival within a social system require deferring gratification and having the foresight to take account of the future consequences of one's immediate behavior and choices.

Thus self-imposed delay of gratification, concern for the future, and planfulness are essential prerequisites for mature human functioning. However, although the inability to delay may predispose the person to a life of failures, the other extreme—excessive delay of gratification—also has its personal costs and can be disadvantageous. The person who saves money during rampant inflation may be more unwise than the one who lives in the moment and spends it now. Whether one should or should not delay gratification or "exercise the will" in any particular choice is often anything but self-evident. However, unless children develop the competencies to sustain delay when they want and need to do so, the choice itself is lost. With that in mind, the focus of this chapter is not on whether individuals *should* delay gratification, but rather, given that they choose to do so, on the processes that enable them to do so successfully.

STUDYING THE PROCESS OF GOAL-DIRECTED DELAY OF GRATIFICATION

In order to systematically find any of those "preliminaries" of thought and action that might enable people to sustain voluntary delay of gratification, it was necessary to look closely at what people *do* as they actually try to wait to get the delayed outcomes that they have chosen. This required finding a systematic way to observe and study the preliminaries, preferably in young children, as they emerge spontaneously in the normal developmental course. There are many earlier indications of various forms of goal-directed delay behavior in very young children under naturalistic conditions (e.g., waiting to open Christmas presents, refraining from taking cookies from the jar until after dinner). However, we found that the role of cognitive representation in this process with regard to goal-directed self-imposed delay of gratification becomes potentially viable for experimental analysis only after the age of 3 years. At that time, most children become able to clearly comprehend the basic contingency in the delay-of-gratification paradigm, and there are clear individual differences in their ability to continue purposefully to wait for their preferred goals. By age 6, however, most of the children in the middle-class families studied have internalized the essential preliminaries, so that these become less visible for direct observation and experimental analysis. We therefore concentrated on the period from 4 to 5 years as a potential window for studying the processes that enable willpower.

The experimental paradigm we have developed to study the processes that enable delay is as follows: Young children learn to play a game in which the adult experimenter leaves the room, and the children can summon the adult to return by ringing a bell (Mischel, Ebbesen, & Zeiss, 1972; Mischel, Shoda, & Rodriguez, 1989). Then the children are shown two treats (e.g., cookies, marshmallows, or pretzels) that have been chosen through pretests as desirable for children in this age group and that differ in value just enough (e.g., one cookie vs. two) that the children will be faced with a conflict between choosing the smaller, immediate reward and waiting for the larger, delayed reward. They are told that they can receive a treat when the adult returns to the room, and they know that they can summon the adult by ringing the bell. They are also told that if they ring the bell to summon the adult, they will receive the smaller of the two rewards, but that if they can wait until the adult returns to the room on his or her own, they will receive the larger, more desirable reward. The children are not told how long they will have to wait until the adult returns and they can have the larger treat. Once it is clear that each child understands the contingency, the adult leaves the room and does not return until the child rings the bell, or until he or she has waited for a maximum of 20 minutes. The conflict created by this situation is very strong: Children are torn between the temptation to ring the bell and receive the immediately available but smaller reward and the desire to obtain the larger but delayed reward.

KEEPING THE GOAL IN SIGHT: THE EFFECTS OF REWARD PRESENCE

A choice between waiting for two cookies or settling for one now may seem to be artificial and far from the choices adults face in the real world. But this type of problem, when carefully structured in age-appropriate ways, creates a genuine conflict that is as involving to young children as many dilemmas of life are to adults, and provides a route to study the underlying processes in systematic ways. Early trials of the delay situation described above revealed large individual differences in children's willingness and ability to delay (Mischel, 1974; Mischel et al., 1989). The question then became this: What is happening psychologically that makes some children ring soon and others wait for what seems an eternity? This issue became the focus of an extensive research program undertaken with a number of collaborators, including Ebbe Ebbesen, Antonette Zeiss, Bert Moore, Monica Rodriguez, Yuichi Shoda, and Phillip Peake (e.g., Mischel & Ebbesen, 1970; Mischel et al., 1972; Moore, Mischel, & Zeiss, 1976; Rodriguez, Mischel, & Shoda, 1989; Shoda, Mischel, & Peake, 1990).

This was our most basic question: How does attention to the rewards affect the young child's ability to wait for them? Freud provided a rare discussion of how delay of gratification may be learned by children in his analysis of how children bridge the gap from primary to secondary process (Freud 1911/1959). Psychoanalytic theory suggests that when circumstances force an infant to sustain delay before receiving gratification, the infant learns to create and focus on realistic hallucinations (mental representations) of the desired objects (e.g., Freud, 1911/1959; Singer, 1955). The satisfaction infants receive from attending to this mental representation enables them to sustain the delay necessary to receive the real object of desire. Psychoanalytic theory would thus predict that children should be best able to sustain delay when they focus on (or "cathect") the rewards and attend to them during the delay period.

Although cast in quite different language, learning theories have explained the mechanism of sustaining delay even in animals in essentially similar ways. In early behavioral studies with rats running mazes, for example, it was theorized that goal-directed behavior was sustained along the route by anticipatory fractional goal responses—much like partial self-reinforcements (see Mischel, 1974). Contemporary learning theory suggests that people likewise sustain delay by anticipating the reward they will receive if they keep waiting, and that such anticipation can be facilitated by using self-instructions to make the reward more salient (e.g., Bandura, 1986). This view implies that by emphasizing and focusing on desirable features of the delayed outcome, the individuals reinforce themselves during the waiting period, thereby facilitating delay.

Both theoretical approaches, in sum, suggest that any aspects of the situation that enable the individual to focus on the delayed rewards should in turn lead to increased ability to sustain delay. Delay time should be increased by situational factors such as presence of the delayed rewards or instructions to imagine their presence vividly. Early studies on decision making in delay behavior (e.g., Marher, 1956; Mischel, 1966; Mischel & Metzner, 1962; Mischel & Staub, 1965) were likewise consistent with this notion: These studies demonstrated that individuals' *expectation* that they will actually receive the desired delayed reward is an important determinant in their choice to wait for the delayed reward versus taking the immediately available but less desirable reward. It seems likely that the presence of the delayed reward increases the individuals' expectancies about actually receiving it at the end of the waiting period, and thus increases the likelihood of choosing to wait for it. In situations in which the delayed rewards are not physically present, people should be able to improve their ability to sustain delay by generating a vivid psychological representation of the reward.

To test empirically the prediction that attention to rewards will facilitate delay, in early experiments (e.g., Mischel & Ebbesen, 1970) we observed 4-year-old children in variations of the self-imposed delay situation described earlier. We manipulated whether the children were able to see the reward objects while they were waiting to receive them, under the assumption that rewards that can be seen are attended to more easily than those that are present but hidden from view. In one condition, the children were faced with both the smaller, immediately available reward and the larger, delayed reward in full view. In another condition, both the immediate and the delayed rewards were on the table but hidden beneath an opaque tray. There were also two conditions in which one of the rewards (either the immediate reward or the delayed reward) was covered and the other was exposed.

Although the predictions of both psychoanalytic and learning theories, and our own intuitions, led us to expect that the children would wait longest in the conditions in which the larger, delayed reward for which they were waiting was exposed, in fact the results were the opposite. We found that children waited the longest (over 11 minutes on average) when both the delayed and the immediate rewards were obscured from view. By contrast, they tended to wait only a few minutes in conditions in which any of the rewards were in view. There were no significant differences among any of the conditions in which rewards were exposed (immediate reward only, delayed reward only, or both rewards exposed), but delay time in all of these conditions was significantly shorter than when both rewards were obscured from view.

To understand why children had so much more trouble waiting when the rewards were exposed, we decided to look much more closely at what the children were doing while they were waiting. We observed the children directly by means of a one-way mirror throughout the delay period as they sat waiting, focusing on the condition that had proved to be the most difficult for them—namely, when both the immediately available and the delayed rewards faced them.

In one exploratory phase, "Mr. Talk Box" helped us in our observations.

This device consisted of a cheerful clown's face with a tape recorder and a microphone, which announced to the youngsters, "Hi, I'm Mr. Talk Box. I have big ears and I love it when children fill them with all the things they think and feel, no matter what." Then Mr. Talk Box gave accepting and encouraging responses ("Uh-huh," "Ah," etc.) to whatever the children said. Most children seemed quick to confide in Mr. Talk Box and engaged in animated discussions with him as they poured out their hearts and minds and shared their own "preliminaries," as James so aptly called them.

Different children dealt with the delay situation in very different ways, some making it easy for themselves to wait and others using strategies that quickly failed. Some of the most effective strategies that the children used were surprisingly simple. From time to time they reaffirmed their intentions quietly ("I'm waiting for the two cookies"), and occasionally they reiterated the choice contingency aloud ("If I ring the bell I'll get this one, but if I wait I'll get those"). But mostly these 4-year-olds seemed able to wait for long periods by converting the frustrating waiting situation into a more tolerable nonwaiting one, thus making the difficult task easier for themselves. They appeared to achieve this by purposefully creating elaborate self-distractions. Instead of fixing their attention and thoughts on the rewards, as initial theorizing had predicted, they seemed to avoid thinking about them entirely. Some put their hands over their eyes, rested their heads on their arms, and invented other similar techniques for averting their gaze most of the time, occasionally seeming to remind themselves with a quick glance. Some talked quietly to themselves or even sang ("This is such a pretty day, hooray"); others made faces, picked their noses, made up games with their hands and feet, and even tried to doze off while continuing to wait. One of the most successful "delayers" actually managed to nap during the delay time.

THE ROLE OF PURPOSEFUL SELF-DISTRACTION

In sum, these informal observations suggested that in the delay-of-gratification situation, the problem of "willpower" should become easier when attention is diverted from the anticipated rewards to distracting stimuli, thus reducing the frustrative arousal that otherwise occurs and makes further waiting too aversive. In order to test this hypothesis experimentally, and to go beyond the effects of stimulus exposure to explore the impact of the children's reward-relevant cognitions, it was necessary to try to influence the cognitions of the children during the waiting period. We compiled a set of age-appropriate distractions by asking the children themselves what kinds of things made them happy (e.g., "When Mommy pushes me on a swing at a birthday party"). We then used these examples as cues to prime for distraction in the delay situation. One group of children was cued to think about the happy, distracting thoughts while waiting: "If you want to, while you're waiting, you can think about Mommy pushing you on a swing." Another group was cued to think about the treats for which they were waiting: "If you want to, while you're waiting, you can think about the cookies."

We found that delay time was low, regardless of whether the rewards were exposed or covered, when the children were cued to think about the rewards. In contrast, when the rewards were covered they did not seem to need the help of external cues to distract them; they were easily able to supply their own distractors, singing and amusing themselves spontaneously as they waited easily. When we put all these results together, it became clear that attention and thoughts directed toward the rewards substantially reduces, rather than increases, how long young children will wait. And they showed that, in contrast, distractions from the exposed rewards (e.g., prior cues to prime ideation about fun things) help children delay longer (Mischel et al., 1972). Thus, willpower in this situation, when the rewards are exposed and delay is therefore especially frustrative, seems to depend on self-distraction from the aversiveness of the delay situation while maintaining the waiting behavior. This is essentially like being on "automatic pilot": One is waiting without focusing on the aversiveness of having to wait.

FROM DISTRACTION TO ABSTRACTION: THE ROLE OF IMAGES OF THE GOALS

Although the previously discussed studies dealt with attention to the rewards themselves and with cues to attend to them, they made no attempt to study the effects of *images* of the reward objects on children's ability to delay. Yet images of objects were what Freud and the learning theorists hypothesized to be the cognitive mediators of the delay process. Asking children to think about the rewards made it difficult for them to wait, but of course it was not possible to know how the children represented the rewards in their minds. Given that theories of how delay ability develops emphasize the importance of the mental image of the rewards in a child's mind, we wanted to get a better sense of just how the children might represent the rewards mentally in a way that could actually support their delay. With that aim, we showed the children realistic, life-sized pictures of the reward objects, presented with a slide projector, in the hope that this might at least provide a closer analogue to mental representations of images (Mischel & Moore, 1973).

Because the presentation of such images can itself help the delay process by providing distractions, it was essential to control the content of the images to assess their effect on delay time. To test this, we exposed some children to pictures of the anticipated rewards (referred to here as the "relevant" objects), and we exposed a control group to pictures of objects that were comparable in value to the actual rewards, but that were not used in the delay contingency being tested ("control" objects). For example, if a child was waiting for two pretzels eventually rather than one pretzel right away, pretzels were the relevant objects and marshmallows could be the control objects; conversely, if the child was waiting for marshmallows, marshmallows were the relevant objects and pretzels could be the control objects.

To our surprise, we found that although exposure to the actual rewards during the delay made waiting difficult for young children, exposure to images of them had the opposite effect, making it much easier. In addition, children who saw slide-projected images of the relevant rewards for which they were waiting delayed twice as long as those who viewed slides of comparable control objects that were not the rewards for which they were waiting (Mischel & Moore, 1973). Collectively, these results suggest that delay is facilitated by focusing attention on images of the relevant rewards, although it is made difficult by attention to the actual (real) reward objects. Note that this delay-enhancing effect of the relevant reward images cannot be attributed to the possible distraction provided by the presence of images: Focusing attention on images of the anticipated rewards is more effective than focusing attention on images of comparable objects that are not anticipated (i.e., irrelevant rewards).

Because a pictorial image of an object on a screen is at most a crude approximation or analogy for its mental representation, we next wanted to test the effects of mental representations of rewards on delay behavior more directly. With that purpose, we tried to influence the mental representations children generated internally by asking them to pretend that the real rewards were actually pictures, and, conversely, that the pictures were actually real rewards (Moore et al., 1976). Specifically, in one condition, children exposed to real reward objects were told that they could pretend that the rewards were not real, but just pictures. It was suggested that they "put a frame around them in your head, just like a picture." In a second condition, children were exposed to slide representations of the rewards and were asked to pretend that the pictures were real objects and to "make believe they're really there in front of you."

Thinking about the rewards as real made it harder to delay, whereas thinking about them as pictures made it easier, regardless of whether the children were looking at real rewards or slides. Thus the children's cognitive representations of the rewards proved to be more powerful for determining delay time than the actual external rewards or pictures to which they were exposed. Children who were exposed to pictures of the rewards were able to delay almost 18 minutes. Most interestingly, children who waited with the real rewards exposed in front of them, but were cued to imagine them as pictures, also waited almost 18 minutes. In contrast, children who were exposed to pictures but told to pretend that they were real waited less than 6 minutes on average.

EFFECTS OF COGNITIVE FOCUS

To make sense of these results, we hypothesized that two different features of a stimulus lead to opposite effects on self-regulatory behavior. Extrapolating from earlier classic distinctions by Estes (1972) and by Berlyne (1960), we speculated that stimuli can be represented in the mind either in an arousing, motivating, consummatory way or in an abstract, informative, iconic manner. An arousing representation of a rewarding stimulus focuses on its motivating, "hot" features and activates the behaviors associated with experiencing or consuming the reward, such as eating a cookie or climbing a tree. When young children look at the actual goal objects or think about them they may focus spontaneously on these "hot," arousing qualities, thereby increasing their own frustration and arousal, and making it more difficult to continue to wait. Such a "hot" focus thus produces the unwanted effect in the subject of activating the very response he or she is trying to suppress—that is, to ring the bell and end the delay.

In contrast, in an iconic representation, the focus is on the more abstract, informative, "cool," nonconsummatory aspects of the stimulus, which may remind the subject of the contingency, and the reason for delaying the behaviors associated with experiencing the stimulus. Thus the iconic representation (e.g., the slide-presented image of the object) may function to guide and sustain the goal-directed delay behavior, reminding the child of the contingency and of what he or she will get, but without being real and "hot" enough to become arousing and frustrative, and thus activating the behavior the subject is trying to suppress.

The effects of these "hot" and "cool" mental representations were examined next (Mischel & Baker, 1975). To activate a focus on the more abstract qualities of the rewards, we cued some children, if they were waiting for pretzels, for example, to think about the pretzel sticks as long, thin brown logs. If they were waiting for the marshmallows, we suggested that while they were waiting, they could think about the marshmallows as puffy, round clouds, if and when they wanted to.

As predicted, these abstract representations of the rewards made delay much easier for the children. Children waited more than 13 minutes when encouraged to focus on the abstract qualities of the rewards for which they were waiting. In contrast, the children waited less than 5 minutes when asked to focus on abstract qualities of objects that were of comparable value to the anticipated rewards, but were not the rewards themselves. This suggests that the effect of a nonarousing, abstract representation of the actual reward objects cannot be attributed merely to distraction: Focusing on abstract qualities facilitates delay only when the focus is on the actual rewards in the contingency. The effect thus seems more a function of the cognitive abstraction or transformation of the reward to focus on its cool features and associations.

In other conditions, we cued the children to generate a "hot," arousing representation of the rewards. For example, children waiting for marshmallows were cued to focus on the marshmallows' sweet, chewy taste, and children waiting for pretzels were told to think about their crunchy, salty taste. This type of arousing representation of the rewards in the contingency made delay much more difficult for the children.

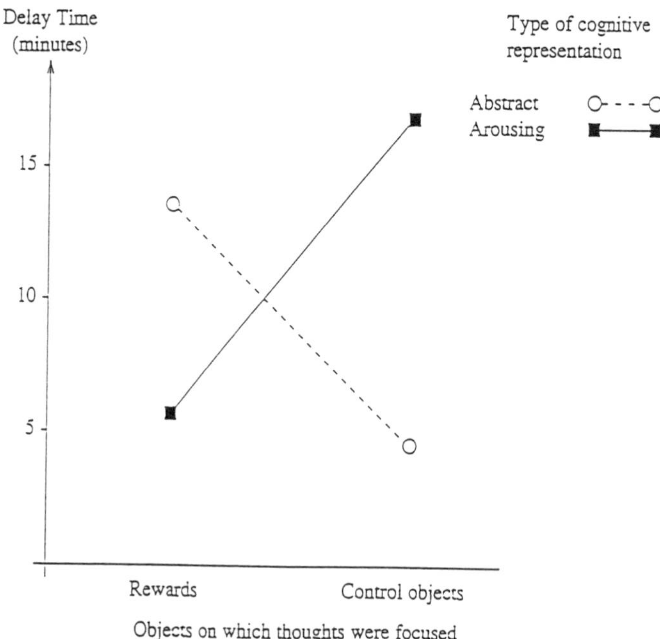

FIGURE 9.1. Delay time as a function of objects on which thoughts were focused and type of representation in thoughts. From Mischel, Shoda, and Rodriguez (1989, p. 244). Copyright 1989 by the American Association for the Advancement of Science. Reprinted by permission.

Figure 9.1 summarizes the results on mental representation with an arousing versus an abstract focus. As the figure shows, whereas an arousing representation of the rewards in the contingency made delay difficult, the same type of "hot" ideation focused on control objects, (e.g, thinking about the sweet, chewy taste of marshmallows while waiting for pretzels) had a delay-enhancing effect, enabling the children to sustain delay almost 17 minutes. This pattern of results suggests that whereas arousing thoughts of the object of desire in the contingency make waiting for it difficult, arousing thoughts about simply unavailable outcomes in the situation (such as the control objects) are the stuff of good fantasies, and make fine distractions for tolerating delay.

Taken collectively, the results led to an important qualification of the previous findings that attention focused on the anticipated rewards will lead to longer delay times. When the real reward objects are exposed to a child, sustaining delay becomes extremely difficult. However, when the child looks at a picture of the rewards, sustaining delay is easier. This paradoxical result can be explained in terms of the *type* of mental representation the child generates when thinking about the rewards.

It is natural for 4-year-old children to think about rewards in terms of their "hot," arousing qualities. In so doing, however, they are actually defeating (without realizing it) their ability to wait for the rewards they really want. Seeing real rewards, or pretending that pictures of them are real, is an arousing activity that only makes children want them more—and want them now. Looking at pictures of the anticipated rewards (without being cued to pretend they are real) enables the children to generate more abstract, less arousing mental representations of them, facilitating delay.

The nature of a child's mental representation of the anticipated rewards can have an even stronger effect than the physical presence of the rewards. Delay is impeded by a focus on the arousing, "hot" aspects of the reward, but is facilitated by focusing on an abstract, "cool" representation of the rewards. Moreover, an abstract cognitive representation of the actual objects provides an excellent bridge for continuing delay that is even better than simple distraction (although not better than arousing thoughts directed at objects that are not in the delay contingency). Learning to generate "cool" representations of anticipated rewards may enable even children who are quickest to ring the bell initially to sustain delay until they can earn the reward they prefer.

INSTRUMENTAL ACTIVITY IN DELAY OF GRATIFICATION AND RESISTANCE TO TEMPTATION: WORKING AND PLANNING

In the research discussed up to this point, the focus was on studying means by which one can facilitate goal-directed delay in a noninstrumental waiting situation, where one has no control over the length of the delay. However, in many self-control situations people do have at least some control over not only the rewards they can receive, but also the length of time they must wait to receive them. In this type of situation people's activity during the delay period is *instrumental* to the delay: Their own behavior can influence the amount of time they will be required to wait. This type of instrumental self-control poses different challenges to people and is facilitated by different means than passively sustained delay. For example, when a focus on the rewards is perceived as instrumental for attaining the delayed outcome, it can substantially enhance rather than impede delay of gratification (Mischel & Underwood, 1974).

In most real-life self-control situations, just thinking about the rewards does not affect the outcome of the delay; more often, it is the case that one must *work* as well as wait to gain desired outcomes. In this vein, we tested preschool children's performance in a resistance-to-distraction paradigm, in which the children's work during the delay period was instrumental to the outcome of their delay. The children were offered an opportunity to play with attractive, desirable toys, contingent upon their completion of a boring, repetitive task such as placing pegs into a pegboard. During the work period the children were systematically interrupted by "Mr. Clown Box," a mechanical clown that talked to the children by means of a tape recording and produced noises and flashing lights to engage their attention. The children were warned not to succumb to the distraction, because they would not be able to complete the task if they did. The dependent variable assessed how well the children resisted the distraction and kept on working (Mischel & Patterson, 1976).

Our basic goal was to identify the cognitive and attentional activities that would facilitate the children's sustained work and continued resistance to Mr. Clown Box's persistent distractions throughout the work period. In a first experiment, plans to resist Mr. Clown Box's temptations were suggested to one group of children, such as saying, "I'm going to keep working so I can play with the fun toys and Mr. Clown Box later." Children who were given plans to resist distraction spent significantly more time working on the task than did children to whom plans were not suggested (Patterson & Mischel, 1975).

A second experiment compared the effectiveness of task-facilitating plans, which directed attention toward performing the task (e.g., "I'm going to look at my work"), and temptation-inhibiting plans, which prohibited focusing attention on the temptation (e.g., "I'm not going to look at Mr. Clown Box"). The results showed that children who were given temptation-inhibiting instructions spent more time working on the task and less time succumbing to distraction than those who were given task-facilitating instructions, which proved to be no more effective than no instructions at all. Interestingly, the number of times the children looked at Mr. Clown Box was roughly the same across all the conditions, but the children who were given temptation-inhibiting instructions returned to work more quickly after looking at the clown (Patterson & Mischel, 1976).

A third experiment manipulated the structure of plans that were suggested to the children (whether they were elaborated and specific or unelaborated and general) and the substance of the plans (whether they were designed to inhibit temptation, facilitate task completion, or focus attention on the rewards). Both structure and substance were found to have significant effects on children's ability to resist temptation (Mischel & Patterson, 1976). Elaborated plans that focused attention on the rewards or that inhibited attention to the distractor led to better self-control than elaborated task-oriented plans. Unelaborated plans of any sort led to self-control that was no better than that in control conditions (irrelevant verbalizations or no plans).

Elaborated plans that focused attention on the rewarding consequences for continuing the task may have been successful in facilitating self-control because of the instrumental nature of the paradigm: The children believed that their success in the situation was contingent upon their completion of the instrumental activity. Ideation about the rewards in this kind of situation may facilitate performance by enhancing resistance to temptation. This contrasts, of course, with the findings by Mischel et al. (1972) discussed previously, which showed that a cognitive focus on the rewards in the contingency impaired children's ability to delay gratification. The important difference between these two paradigms is that whereas children in the Mischel and Patterson (1976) situation believed that their success was contingent upon their performance, children in the Mischel et al. (1972) situation knew that they had no means by which they could decrease the time they had to wait to receive the desired reward. This pattern of results (also supported by the findings of Mischel & Underwood, 1974) suggests that whether a focus on rewards will improve or impair children's efforts to self-regulate depends also upon whether successful performance requires the subjects to perform active, instrumental behaviors or to wait passively: It facilitates the former but can interfere with the latter, depending on just how the rewards are represented cognitively (Mischel et al., 1989).

RECONSTRUING WILLPOWER

Willpower is often construed as a stoic self-denial in the service of a distant goal, a capacity for deliberate endurance, suffering while biting the bullet—a trait some people supposedly have more of than others. But a less heroic approach seemed to characterize those children who waited longest in the self-imposed delay-of-gratification paradigm (Mischel, 1974; Mischel et al., 1989). They managed to wait for 20 minutes in an aversive condition by converting the difficult conflict from one requiring acts of self-denial and grim determination to a more playful, enjoyable time. Their conversations with Mr. Talk Box and with us also suggested that they did seem to keep their goals in mind, but not in the focus of attention, with only occasional reminders of the contingency rules and reaffirmations of their intentions ("I'm waiting for the two cookies"). But most of the time they supported their own effort with various distraction and abstraction strategies, as they invented ways to help themselves to achieve their goal without becoming too upset and discouraged. In addition, our studies of self-control showed that resistance to tempting distractions while working to receive a reward was greatly improved when young children were given plans, especially when these focused on resisting the temptation (Patterson & Mischel, 1975, 1976). Both the structure and substance of those plans predictably influenced the children's self-control (Mischel & Patterson, 1976).

Results like these suggest a quite different view of willpower than has formerly been assumed, as it applies to the ability to delay gratification. Rather than strive to be a stoic, the individual converts the aversive delay situation into a more manageable one by the types of thought and action suggested in this chapter. The child does have to keep the goal in mind, but in the back of the mind, as it were—preventing himself or herself from becoming too aroused while employing strategies that make it easier to continue, and cuing himself or herself abstractly about what he or she is waiting for while avoiding succumbing to temptations and distractions along the route. The use of this type of cognitive transformation of the desired outcomes, and of planful preparation, enables a form of "willpower" that needs to be incorporated into a comprehensive analysis of mental control (see also Ansfield & Wegner, Chapter 21, this volume). The findings suggest that what matter most for purposeful self-regulation and mental control are (1) the cognitive representation of the stimulus and (2) the plans that are readily accessible and activated for effective coping to overcome "stimulus control." Moreover, what matters is not so much *what* is represented as *how* it is represented: Depending on the type of cognitive focus (e.g., "hot" vs. "cool"), and on whether ideation about the stimulus is believed to be instrumental to achieving the desired outcome, the same stimulus can sustain or undo the efforts at self-control (Mischel & Underwood, 1974). Likewise, even in a young child, plans for resistance to temptation and for sustaining effort can be structured to substantially enhance the transition from simply wishing to effectively willing and attaining a desired but delayed outcome.

LONG-TERM IMPLICATIONS OF PRESCHOOL DELAY COMPETENCE

Do these results with 4-year-olds in a playroom with cookies, marshmallows, pretzels, and toys speak to the real dilemmas of life? The experiments described here were done with children from the Stanford University community who were 4 years old during the first assessment of their delay behavior. In a series of follow-up studies (Mischel, Shoda, & Peake, 1988; Shoda et al., 1990), we obtained parental ratings and objective test scores years later for many of the same individuals in adolescence and young adulthood. We expected that the ability to delay gratification requires a set of self-regulatory competencies and strategies that may become relatively stable over time and may be relevant for many important life outcomes (e.g., Mischel et al., 1988; Shoda et al., 1990). In identifying the types of delay conditions in the preschool experiments in which the children's waiting behavior might predict later developmental outcomes we were guided by the results of the earlier experiments.

To identify the delay conditions that would and would not be diagnostic of later outcomes required first understanding the processes that enable delay of gratification and the conditions in which relevant individual differences would be visible. We now know that when preschoolers attempt to delay gratification while facing the exposed rewards, the delay becomes very difficult; when no strategies to facilitate delay are suggested, they therefore must devise their own strategies and put them into effect. We predicted that individual differences in the competencies required to formulate and apply effective delay strategies would be revealed most clearly in the rewards-exposed condition when no strategies were suggested, because then the frustration of delay was maximized, and the least assistance was offered. This condition created a situation in which the individual differences in the ability to cope with this frustration should be activated and visible, so that spontaneously generated (rather than experimenter-supplied) strategies or "preliminaries" would influence the ability to delay. To the extent that this type of competency is stable, we expected that children's ability to sustain delay in this diagnostic condition would predict future outcomes requiring such skills. Ability to delay gratification in the experimental conditions in which strategies were cued was not expected to be diagnostic of future outcomes, because these conditions provided the children with strategies rather than requiring them to generate their own spontaneously. Likewise, delay in the reward-obscured conditions was not expected to be diagnostic of self-regulatory ability, since delay in that condition was not particularly difficult or frustrative for any of the young children we studied.

These predictions were supported clearly in longitudinal studies relating the length of time children were able to delay in the various conditions to indices of their cognitive competence as adolescents. For example, as shown in Table 9.1, seconds of preschool delay time significantly predicted verbal and quantitative scores on the Scholastic Aptitude Test (SAT) administered in adolescence in the diagnostic condition (rewards exposed, no strategies suggested), but not in any of the other conditions (Shoda et al., 1990).[1] Seconds of delay time in the diagnostic condition as preschoolers also correlated significantly with parental ratings of competencies, including ability to use and respond to reason, planfulness, ability to handle stress, ability to delay gratification, self-control in frustrating situations, and ability to concentrate without becoming distracted (Shoda et al., 1990). These correlations remained significant even when variance attributable to SAT scores was statistically controlled for, indicating that the relationship between ability to delay in the preschool diagnostic condition and parental rating of competencies in adolescence cannot be attributed entirely to the type of academic-related competencies measured by the SAT. In contrast, in the conditions identified by the experimental studies as not highly frustrative (e.g., rewards obscured), or in conditions when strategies were supplied, the correlations were nonsignificant.

This pattern of results illustrates that it would be a mistake to apply the standard trait strategy of aggregating diverse measures of delay of gratification to form a broader trait index, because seemingly similar situations actually may engage different processes and have quite different effects. When a child's delay behavior in the multiple delay situations sampled was averaged together (e.g., in conditions when the reward was covered and when it was exposed), the aggregate attenuated the long-term correlations to trivial levels (Shoda et al., 1990).

The fact that delay of gratification in the diagnostic conditions even as early as 4 years of age predicted relevant outcomes more than a decade later in development raises questions about how to understand these long-term links. The significant correlations between preschool delay time and adoles-

TABLE 9.1. Correlations between Preschool Delay Time and Scholastic Aptitude Test (SAT) Scores

	Spontaneous ideation		Suggested ideation	
Measure	Rewards exposed	Rewards obscured	Rewards exposed	Rewards obscured
SAT verbal	.42*	−.12	−.40	−.21
SAT quantitative	.57**	−.31	−.26	−.23
Sample size	35	33	14	12

Note. From Shoda, Mischel, and Peake (1990, p. 984). Copyright 1990 by the American Psychological Association. Reprinted by permission.
*$p < .05$.
**$p < .001$.

cent competencies are exciting, but we can only speculate about the causal links between these early childhood and adolescent abilities. Perhaps the type of home environment that encourages a child to learn to delay gratification at an early age also encourages the child to learn the kinds of activities that contribute to higher SAT scores and parental ratings of competence. In part, children who learn to delay gratification at an early age are at an advantage as they mature and find themselves more often in situations in which it is necessary for them to forgo immediate gratifications in order to pursue long-term goals, such as studying for the SAT.

Individuals who have such self-regulatory competencies (e.g., the attention skills, the necessary metacognitive knowledge) available thus also will be able to use them effectively to manage other academic and social complex tasks requiring extensive delay of gratification (e.g., those needed to achieve high SAT scores and attain good academic grades). But although delay-of-gratification competencies may be necessary preliminaries for such life tasks, the willingness to delay, like all choice behavior from the perspective of cognitive social theory, depends on an individual's expectancies, beliefs, goals, and values, and on the encoding of the particular psychological situation within which the choice occurs (Mischel, 1973, 1990). Thus, the same individuals who are able to delay gratification in the present paradigm may be unwilling to do so when the relative values of the alternatives in the choice are not encoded as adequate to justify the delay, or when their expectancies for attaining the delayed outcomes or goals are insufficient in the particular context (e.g., Mischel, 1973, 1974; Mischel et al., 1989). In fact, the intraindividual discriminativeness, distinctive patterning, and situational specificity of this type of self-regulatory behavior are as impressive as the temporal stability of the competency to delay gratification when and if the individual chooses to do so (e.g., Mischel & Peake, 1982). From the perspective of the social-cognitive theory that guided this work (e.g., Mischel ,1973, 1990), these patterns of preference are expected to form intraindividually stable "if . . . then . . ." relationships in distinctive but predictable combinations—for example, "She waits endlessly if *X*, but not if *Y*" (Mischel & Shoda, 1995; Shoda, Mischel, & Wright, 1994).

METACOGNITIVE DEVELOPMENT OF SELF-CONTROL KNOWLEDGE

In the course of development most children become increasingly aware of the principles of self-regulation needed to sustain self-imposed delay of gratification in the pursuit of a desired but delayed contingent goal. Most interestingly, their growing metacognitive insight into these processes appears to follow an orderly and meaningful progression. To study this type of metacognitive knowledge development, we began by asking children between 3 and 8 years old whether they would prefer to have the rewards exposed or covered if they were required to wait in the self-imposed delay paradigm (H. N. Mischel & Mischel, 1983). Children under age 4 showed no preference for covering or exposing the rewards, and were generally unable to justify their choice, thus essentially guessing. A striking finding was that children between 4 and 4½ years of age showed a strong preference for waiting with the rewards exposed, and thus selected the very strategies that made it most impossible for them to wait. This strong preference for the worst strategy for self-control certainly fits the "negativistic" and stubborn behavior patterns typically attributed to this age group. The clearly self-defeating preference for waiting with the rewards uncovered fortunately waned by the end of the fourth year. Not until the end of the fifth year, however, did children show a clear preference for waiting with the rewards hidden from view, and begin to offer reasons for their choice that showed they understood the frustration-reducing effect of obscuring the desired rewards.

We also studied whether the children would prefer to make use of task-oriented ideation or consummatory ideation (i.e., thinking about how yummy the rewards are). Below age 5, the children showed no preference for task-oriented versus consummatory ideation, but by age 5 they began to show a clear preference for task-oriented ideation. With increasing age, their reasons for making such a choice became more lucid: The older children more often realized that telling themselves how desirable the treats were would only make it harder for them to wait. In a study involving older children (H. N. Mischel & Mischel, 1983), we discovered that by sixth grade, children had also learned the value of choosing abstract ideation (e.g., thinking about marshmallows as clouds) rather than consummatory ideation; knowledge of this rule was not apparent in children at or below the third-grade level. The abstraction rule becomes accessible at about the same stage in development as the one in which Piaget found evidence for the emergence of operational thought—the types of mental operations that would enable the abstraction strategy.

EXTENSIONS TO HIGH-RISK POPULATIONS

In order to elucidate the person variables that contribute to effective delay, we also measured delay behavior of boys with impulse control and adjustment problems, aged approximately 5 to 13 years. Specifically, we studied the interrelationships between several person variables and the ability to sustain delay to receive a larger reward (Rodriguez et al., 1989). The results of this study are shown in a path diagram in Figure 9.2.

Consistent with the earlier studies on younger children, we found that the single most important correlate of delay time in these youngsters was attention deployment (i.e., where the children focused their attention during the delay period). As the earlier experimental results led us to predict, children who attended to the rewards tended to delay for a shorter time than those who focused their attention elsewhere to distract themselves.

As shown in the path diagram, we also found that attention deployment mediated the effects of two person variables, age and verbal intelligence. Verbal intelligence and age, unrelated to each other, were found to be positively related to attention deployment, indicating that older children and more intelligent children were better able to distract themselves from the pull of the rewards, and were thus better able to sustain delay. When the mediating effect of attention deployment was controlled for, verbal intelligence was also found to be directly related to delay time but age was not. Age was related to delay rule knowledge (i.e., understanding that covering

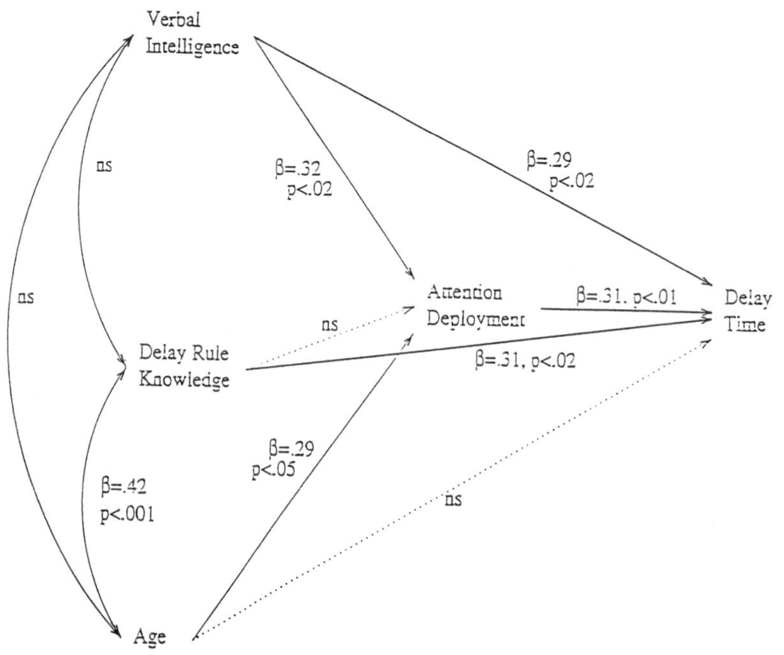

FIGURE 9.2. Path diagram illustrating the relationships among verbal intelligence, delay rule knowledge, age, attention deployment, and delay behavior. From Rodriguez, Mischel, and Shoda (1989, p. 363). Copyright 1989 by the American Psychological Association. Reprinted by permission.

the rewards and thinking about them in an abstract, nonconsummatory way facilitates delay), which also was directly related to delay. Thus, children who understood the rules of the delay situation tended to wait longer, and older children generally had a better understanding of these rules. Although age was not found to be directly related to delay time, it was indirectly related to delay time via its relation to delay rule knowledge and attention deployment.

OVERVIEW AND CONCLUSIONS

To function effectively, individuals must be able voluntarily to postpone immediate gratification and persist in self-directed behavior for the sake of their preferred but delayed goals and outcomes, while resisting the frustration and conflict created by competing temptations and pressures of the moment. To clarify and demystify this type of willpower, the long-term research program reviewed here analyzed the cognitive mediating processes in young children that enable such self-control early in the course of their development. The results identify some of the basic psychological processes that seem to underlie future-oriented self-control, and that can allow the young child to move from wishful intention to effective achievement in the pursuit of temporally distant goals.

Enduring individual differences in this type of competency are visible as early as the preschool years. For example, we found that those 4-year-old children who purposefully delayed gratification longer in certain laboratory situations developed into more cognitively and socially competent adolescents, achieving higher scholastic performance and coping better with frustration and stress later in life. The experimental results that identified specific cognitive and attentional processes underlying the ability to delay gratification also made it possible to specify the particular types of preschool delay situations diagnostic for predicting these aspects of cognitive and social competence later in life.

Correlations of the sort described between seconds of preschool delay in the diagnostic condition and SAT scores allow many different interpretations at many different levels. Nevertheless, it seems reasonable that children will have a distinct advantage beginning early in life if they have available strategies to support their efforts to attain their own chosen goals. Such strategies within their own control may make their efforts less aversive enhance their self-esteem, and allow them a freer hand in building their own futures. But this is a personal hope, not a finding.

To test whether the associations described have serious implications for education, one first would have to show that the types of mental skills and competencies—the "preliminaries" of thought and action considered in this chapter—can be taught in ways that generalize and make a constructive difference. This is what my current colleagues and I are now attempting to study with highly at-risk children in New York City's South Bronx—children who are in danger of becoming early school dropouts unless effective interventions can be found—and in other high-risk populations (e.g., Rodriguez et al., 1989). Although many of these children clearly try hard to wait for the delayed rewards in our delay situation, most surprise and disappoint themselves by how quickly they ring the bell. Whether interventions intended to enhance their ability to exercise their willpower and delay of gratification when they choose to do so will help them to achieve their long-term goals, however, remains to be seen.

ACKNOWLEDGMENTS

Portions of this chapter draw extensively on my earlier publications cited in the references, especially from Mischel (1974) and Mischel, Shoda, and Rodriguez (1989). Preparation of this chapter was supported in part by Grant Nos. MH39349 and MH45994 to me from the National Institute of Mental Health. I am grateful to Kristi Lemm and Alessandra Testa for extensive and constructive editing help with multiple drafts in the preparation of the manuscript, and to my students and colleagues who collaborated in the studies on which this work was based.

NOTE

1. Note that although the negative correlations in the suggested ideation conditions may seem large at first glance, they do not even approach significance with this small sample size.

REFERENCES

Bandura, A. (1986). *Social foundations of thought and action: A social-cognitive theory.* Englewood Cliffs, NJ: Prentice-Hall.

Bandura, A., & Mischel, W. (1965). Modification of self-imposed delay of reward through exposure to live and symbolic models. *Journal of Personality and Social Psychology, 2,* 698–705.

Berlyne, D. (1960). *Conflict, arousal and curiosity.* New York: McGraw-Hill.

Estes, W. K. (1972). Reinforcement in human behavior. *American Scientist, 60,* 723–729.

Freud, S. (1959). Formulations regarding the two principles in mental functioning. In E. Jones (Ed.), *Collected papers of Sigmund Freud* (Vol. 4, pp. 13–21) (J. Riviere, Trans.). New York: Basic Books. (Original work published 1911)

James, W. (1890). *Principles of psychology* (2 vols.). New York: Henry Holt.

Marher, A. R. (1956). The role of expectancy in delayed reinforcement. *Journal of Experimental Psychology, 52,* 101–195.

Mischel, H. N., & Mischel, W. (1983). The development of children's knowledge of self-control strategies. *Child Development, 54,* 603–619.

Mischel, W. (1966). Theory and research on the antecedents of self-imposed delay of reward. In B. A. Maher (Ed.), *Progress in experimental personality research* (Vol. 3, pp. 85–131). New York: Academic Press.

Mischel, W. (1968). *Personality and assessment.* New York: Wiley.

Mischel, W. (1973). Toward a cognitive social learning reconceptualization of personality. *Psychological Review, 80,* 252–283.

Mischel, W. (1974). Processes in delay of gratification. In L. Berkowitz (Ed.), *Advances in experimental social psychology* (Vol. 7, pp. 249–292). New York: Academic Press.

Mischel, W. (1990). Personality dispositions revisited and revised: A view after three decades. In L. Pervin (Ed.), *Handbook of personality psychology: Theory and research* (pp. 111–134). New York: Guilford Press.

Mischel, W., & Baker, N. (1975). Cognitive appraisals and transformations in delay behavior. *Journal of Personality and Social Psychology, 31,* 254–261.

Mischel, W., & Ebbesen, E. B. (1970). Attention in delay of gratification. *Journal of Personality and Social Psychology, 16,* 329–337.

Mischel, W., Ebbesen, E. B., & Zeiss, A. R. (1972). Cognitive and attentional mechanisms in delay of gratification. *Journal of Personality and Social Psychology, 21,* 204–218.

Mischel, W., & Metzner, R. (1962). Preference for delayed reward as a function of age, intelligence, and length of delay interval. *Journal of Abnormal and Social Psychology, 64,* 425–431.

Mischel, W., & Moore, B. (1973). Effects of attention to symbolically-presented rewards on self-control. *Journal of Personality and Social Psychology, 28,* 172–179.

Mischel, W., & Patterson, C. J. (1976). Substantive and structural elements of effective plans for self-control. *Journal of Personality and Social Psychology, 34,* 942–950.

Mischel, W., & Patterson, C. J. (1978). Effective plans for self-control in children. In W. A. Collins (Ed.), *Minnesota Symposia on Child Psychology* (Vol. 11). Hillsdale. NJ: Erlbaum.

Mischel, W., & Peake, P. (1982). In search of consistency: Measure for measure. In M. P. Zanna, E. T. Higgins, & C. P. Herman (Eds.), *The Ontario Symposium: Vol. 2. Consistency in social behavior* (pp. 187–207). Hillsdale, NJ: Erlbaum.

Mischel, W., & Shoda, Y. (1995). A cognitive–affective system theory of personality: Reconceptualizing the invariances in personality and the role of situations. *Psychological Review, 102,* 246–268.

Mischel, W., Shoda, Y., & Peake, P. K. (1988). The nature of adolescent competencies predicted by preschool delay of gratification. *Journal of Personality and Social Psychology, 54,* 687–699.

Mischel, W., Shoda, Y., & Rodriguez, M. L. (1989). Delay of gratification in children. *Science, 244,* 933–938.

Mischel, W., & Staub, E. (1965). Effects of expectancy on working and waiting for larger rewards. *Journal of Personality and Social Psychology, 2,* 625–633.

Mischel, W., & Underwood, B. (1974). Instrumental ideation and delay of gratification. *Child Development, 45,* 1083–1088.

Moore, B., Mischel, W., & Zeiss, A. (1976). Comparative effects of the reward stimulus and its cognitive representation in voluntary delay. *Journal of Personality and Social Psychology, 34,* 419–424.

Patterson, C. J., & Mischel, W. (1975). Plans to resist distraction. *Developmental Psychology, 11,* 369–378.

Patterson, C. J., & Mischel, W. (1976). Effects of temptation-inhibiting and task-facilitating plans on self-control. *Journal of Personality and Social Psychology, 33,* 209–217.

Rodriguez, M. L., Mischel, W., & Shoda, Y. (1989). Cognitive person variables in the delay of gratification of older children at-risk. *Journal of Personality and Social Psychology, 57,* 358–367.

Rutter, M. (1987). Psychological resilience and protective mechanisms. *American Journal of Orthopsychiatry, 57,* 316–331.

Shoda, Y., Mischel, W., & Peake, P. K. (1990). Predicting adolescent cognitive and social competence from preschool delay of gratification: Identifying diagnostic conditions. *Developmental Psychology, 26,* 978–986.

Shoda, Y., Mischel, W., & Wright, J. C. (1994). Intra-individual stability in the organization and patterning of behavior: Incorporating psychological situations into the idiographic analysis of personality. *Journal of Personality and Social Psychology, 67,* 674–687.

Singer, J. L. (1955). Delayed gratification and ego development: Implications for clinical and experimental research. *Journal of Consulting Psychology, 19,* 259–266.

Stumphauzer, J. S. (1972). Increased delay of gratification in young prison inmates through imitation of high-delay peer models. *Journal of Personality and Social Psychology, 21,* 10–17.

CHAPTER 10

Mental Simulation, Motivation, and Action

Shelley E. Taylor
Lien B. Pham

Mental simulation is a fundamental self-regulatory process. As a ubiquitous, mundane cognitive activity, it is used to rehearse future events; to monitor the ongoing present; and to review, cope with, and alter the past. "Mental simulation" refers to the imitative representation of the process of an event or a series of events. It includes both the cognitive construction of hypothetical scenarios and the reconstruction of real ones. These include rehearsals of likely future events, such as what will happen later in the day during a meeting; reconstructions of past events, such as going back over an argument one had with a coworker to figure out what went wrong or to absolve oneself of blame; fantasies, such as imagining oneself in a new city undertaking new employment; and mixtures of real and hypothetical events, such as the reconstruction of a past event (e.g., a rape) with a new ending (e.g., successfully fighting off the attacker).

We maintain that the capacity to simulate events is a distinctive and important feature of cognition for two fundamental reasons. First, mental simulation imitates life as it is experienced. That is, mental simulation occurs at the same level of concreteness and is subject to many of the same causal and temporal constraints as is real behavior; as such, it is conducive to the planning; rehearsal, and reconstruction of behavior. Second, unlike actual behavior, the cognitive system is able to rerun past events, altering their components or changing their endings, and to project multiple versions of imaginary or future events with virtuosity. These features, we argue, make mental simulation a significant coping and self-regulatory resource.

In this chapter, we focus primarily upon mental simulation as a vehicle for linking thought to action. We suggest that when thought is translated into concrete mental simulations, the likelihood of action consistent with the simulation is substantially increased. Moreover, mental simulation appears to achieve these effects to a greater extent than other modes of information representation, such as being instructed to perform tasks related to future events or merely thinking about those future events (e.g., Gregory, Cialdini, & Carpenter, 1982). These effects appear to occur for four reasons, to be discussed further below: Mental simulations make events seem true or likely; they yield plans; they prompt affective responses; and, in so doing, they enhance behavioral confirmation.

SIMULATIONS MAKE EVENTS SEEM TRUE

Research suggesting that mental simulations make events seem real or true is voluminous. A number of experimental studies that have demonstrated these effects have manipulated subjects' simulation of hypothetical events and then asked them to rate the likelihood of those events. Consistently, after imagining that a given event will take place, people are more likely to believe that it will actually occur (e.g., Anderson, 1983; Anderson & Sechler, 1986; Carroll, 1978; Gregory et al., 1982; Hirt & Sherman, 1985; Sherman, Zehner, Johnson, & Hirt, 1983; see Johnson & Sherman, 1990, for a review). For example, Gregory et al. (1982, Study 4) contacted homeowners about their likelihood of subscribing to a cable television service. Some of the homeowners were asked to imagine that they had cable and to envision all the benefits it would bring to them. Other homeowners were given a persuasive communication that described the advantages of subscribing to cable. Results indicated that participants were more likely to intend to purchase cable and more likely actually to do so after performing the simulation exercise than after merely reading about the advantages of cable.

The fact that simulations make events seem true or real may be an important first step in the links between thought and action. First, simulation increases the subjective probability that events will occur, and thus may put people in a state of readiness for action. Second, because simulations actually involve a rehearsal of behavior, they may get people primed for the causal interconnected sequence of events that form the structure of behavior.

SIMULATION AND PLANNING

Mental simulations yield plans. This observation was first made in the classic volume by Miller, Galanter, and Pribram (1960), *Plans and the Structure of Behavior*. It was demonstrated empirically in work by the Hayes-Roths in the 1970s, indicating how simulation-based planning is involved in spontaneous mental activity (Hayes-Roth & Hayes-Roth, 1979).

Imagining *how* events are going to take place provides information about those events. As noted earlier, simulations as representations match the way social reality occurs. Simulations are at the same level of specificity as social interaction, unlike abstract representations, and so they integrate information about social settings, social roles, and specific people. As such, they may be fuller social representations than other cognitive representations people may draw upon for projecting future events. Moreover, a simulation involves a causal sequence of successive interdependent actions, just as real situations do. This causal sequence is essentially a plan. That is, we maintain that the organization of action that occurs in a mental simulation is itself a plan for behavior.

SIMULATION AND EMOTIONAL REGULATION

A major consequence of event simulation appears to be the regulation of emotional states. Imagining a scenario does not produce a dry, cognitive representation; it evokes emotions, often strong and passionate ones. An example of this is the effectiveness with which mood may be manipulated by having people imagine positive or negative events (Larsen & Ketelaar, 1991; Morrow & Nolen-Hoeksema, 1990; Strack, Schwarz, & Gschneidinger, 1985). The degree to which mood is affected by reconstructing positive or negative autobiographical memories (Wright & Mischel, 1982) is also an example of this point.

Imagining events often has an impact on physiological responses, including heart rate, blood pressure, and electrodermal activity. Descriptions of events that include highly specific physiological information, such as "You break into a cold sweat and your heart begins to beat wildly," produce stronger physiological responses than descriptions without such details (Lyman, Bernardin, & Thomas, 1980; see also Strack et al., 1985).

A growing literature on counterfactual reasoning also testifies to the strong impact that the spontaneous or manipulated imagination of nonfactual alternatives to reality can have. Imagining how events may occur or how they could have been otherwise can influence a wide range of emotional states, including sadness, regret, disappointment, comfort, sympathy, and motivation (Campbell & Fairey, 1985; Gleicher et al., 1990; Johnson, 1986; Markman, Gavanski, Sherman, & McMullen, 1993; Miller & McFarland, 1987). When mental simulations are recruited in the rehearsal of future behavior, the arousal and motivation necessary for action may be among the physiological and emotional states evoked.

FROM PROBLEM SOLVING TO ACTION

One of the most important functions of mental simulations may be that they help to bring about behavior (Greenwald, Klinger, Vande Kamp, & Kerr, 1988; Gregory et al., 1982; Sherman, 1980; Sherman & Anderson, 1987). Why exactly do simulations produce links to action? This may derive from the three characteristics of simulations just noted: They enhance the subjective probability of an event's occurrence; they contain an implicit plan; and they invoke specific emotions and can enhance motivation and arousal in service of an action sequence.

Two literatures suggest that the links between thought and action are strengthened by mental simulation. The first is a large popular literature on mental practice, much of it conducted with athletes (Cratty, 1984; Neideffer, 1976; Orlick, Partington, & Salmela, 1983; Singer, 1972). "Mental practice" refers to using mental imagery or simulation to improve performance. In a meta-analysis of 60 studies, mental practice of a motor skill was found to produce performance superior to that in a condition with no practice at all (Feltz & Landers, 1983).

Mental simulation is also systematically incorporated into cognitive-behavior therapy interventions. For example, Marlatt (Marlatt, 1978; Marlatt & Gordon, 1985) has reduced recidivism in alcoholics by incorporating simulation into cognitive coping skills training. Specifically, alcoholics are instructed to imagine situations in which they might be tempted to drink, and then to rehearse how they can avoid giving in to that temptation (see also Brownell, Marlatt, Lichtenstein, & Wilson, 1986).

KINDS OF MENTAL SIMULATIONS

Given that mental simulations can be used to bring about specific action, what form might such mental simulations take? The literature has distinguished among three approaches. The first involves mental simulation as a goal-focusing technique—what we call an "outcome simulation." This approach maintains that if a person envisions the outcome he or she wants to bring about, this may help to bring it about. Thus, for example, a student who imagines himself or herself getting straight A's may be more motivated to achieve the goal of getting straight A's. This view of mental simulation takes an "I can do it" attitude. This approach has been adopted in a wide variety of books on goal setting and time management, such as Alan Lakein's (1973) *How to Get Control of Your Time and Your Life*. This position has also been implicitly incorporated by Markus and Nurius (1986) in their work on "possible selves." They maintain that possible selves function as images of oneself in the future toward which one may strive. The process of envisioning where one wants to be and comparison of it with where one is now may help to yield a plan for closing the gap between one's current and one's anticipated future situation. Markus and her associates (e.g., Markus & Wurf, 1987; Ruvolo & Markus, 1992) propose that mental simulation is one of the vehicles by which both desired and feared future selves may come about.

Mental practice researchers represent the second approach to the use of mental simulation to achieve action—namely, one that emphasizes process. From this viewpoint, it is not the simulation of the outcome, but the simulation of the process—that is, the sequence of events leading up to the outcome—that may enable a person to achieve his or her goal. According to this viewpoint, a student who wishes to achieve straight A's would improve his or her chances by mentally simulating the process of getting straight A's—namely, studying long and hard for exams and working at length on papers—rather than envisioning himself or herself in the desired state. Thus, instead of the "I can do it" approach, the "process simulation" approach asks, "How can I do it?"

A third viewpoint on the links between mental simulation and behavior combines the predictions of the outcome and process viewpoints, arguing that both are necessary conditions for enhancing the links between thought and action. Specifically, one can make the argument (Taylor & Schneider, 1989) that imagining a positive outcome by itself will not bring about a positive outcome unless the outcome is linked to the steps necessary to produce it—namely, the process. By implication, rehearsal of a process may be insufficient to bring out a desired goal state without explicitly envisioning the goal as well. Thus, a combined "process–outcome simulation" might be expected both to enhance motivation and to foster effective action toward a desired goal, by making salient both the goal itself and the steps for achieving it. Shortly, we will describe an experimental study that tested the predictions generated by these three models of the relation between simulation and action.

SIMULATION AND COPING

Thus far, we have discussed mental simulation primarily in the context of effective self-regulation—namely, translating thought into action sequences to achieve goals. But anticipatory self-regulation, particularly in response to forthcoming challenging events, is essentially the same as anticipatory coping. "Self-regulation" refers to the ways in which people control and direct their actions. "Coping" is defined as the process of managing demands that are appraised as taxing or exceeding the resources of a person (Lazarus & Folkman, 1984). These definitions imply that self-regulation is what people do when they are not stressed, and that coping is what takes over when stressful events are anticipated or have occurred. These definitions also imply that self-regulation is an ongoing anticipatory process, and that coping is a reactive, patching-up process. Increasingly, however, psychologists are recognizing that self-regulation is actively involved when people respond to threatening events, and that coping is often anticipatory—that is, directed toward warding off stressful events before they occur (Aspinwall & Taylor, in press). Thus, coping and self-regulation are essentially interchangeable as processes. Coping is both forward-looking and reactive, and self-regulation is often reactive as well as forward-looking. Both processes are called upon to characterize how people manage the ongoing flow of events, anticipate stressful circumstances, ward them off as much as possible, and patch things up when things go wrong. Thus, mental simulation may be thought of as much as a coping technique as a method of self-regulation (Taylor & Schneider, 1989).

Coping researchers distinguish between two types of coping efforts: "problem-solving" efforts and "emotion-focused" coping (Folkman, Schaefer, & Lazarus, 1979; Leventhal & Nerenz, 1982; Pearlin & Schooler, 1978). Problem-solving efforts are attempts to do something active to change stressful or challenging circumstances. Emotion-focused coping involves efforts to regulate the emotional consequences of a stressful event. Often problem-solving efforts and emotional regulation work together. We suggest that the use of mental simulation as a coping technique may be one such instance. For example, when people are using mental simulations to bridge the gap between their thoughts and their actions, they may extract both problem-solving skills and emotional regulation benefits from a mental simulation. Specifically, they may prepare for a forthcoming event by extracting a plan from the simulation. Simultaneously, they may regulate their emotions in anticipation of that action sequence by enhancing their motivation and confidence to perform the actions, and by reducing any anxiety or concern they may have about those actions.

THE EXAM STUDY

We conducted a study to examine how simulation bridges the gap between thought and action. Specifically, we tested the predictions of the three models of simulation and action noted earlier (i.e., the outcome simulation model, the process simulation model, and the outcome–process simulation model) with reference to the fundamental tasks of coping (i.e., emotional regulation and problem solving). We conducted this research in the context of training freshman college students how to cope effectively with the prospect of first-quarter midterm examinations. We recruited 77 undergraduates from introductory psychology courses 5–7 days before their midterm exams. We utilized a 2 × 2 between-participants design, in which participants were trained in either a process simulation, an outcome simulation, both simulations, or a self-monitoring control condition.

Specifically, participants in the process simulation group were instructed to simulate the process of studying for the exam in such a way that it would lead to a positive outcome. They were told to imagine themselves turning off music in their room, sitting down in a quiet place, turning on their light, picking up the book, going through and looking over the material that needed to be studied, and sitting down to read. After participants had been trained in how to do the process simulation exercise, they did it for 5 minutes.

In the outcome simulation condition, participants were asked to simulate a positive exam outcome. They were told to imagine themselves coming up to the building to get their score on the exam, finding the window where the grades were posted, finding their ID number, following the line across, seeing that they had gotten an A, and walking away elated. Students then practiced the simulation for 5 minutes. The outcome simulation and the process simulation were identical in length.

The simulation that combined the outcome and process manipulations was slightly longer than either alone. In this condition, participants were asked first to imagine themselves studying in such a way as to produce a high score, using the same procedures as participants in the process simulation group had done, and then going into the building, seeing the grades posted, and finding that they had gotten an A, as the outcome simulation participants had done.

Participants in the self-monitoring control condition were asked to keep track of how many hours they had studied for the exam on each of the 5–7 days prior to it. We used this control condition because it is commonly adopted as a comparison standard in clinical studies that evaluate coping training. Moreover, self-monitoring alone has often been found to improve performance on a target behavior (e.g., McFall, 1970; Thoresen & Mahoney, 1974), and so the self-monitoring condition provides a conservative control group.

All participants were given a daily calendar sheet and instructed to circle the days and write down the hours they studied for the exam. To assist participants with their planning, they were given a list of chapters that were required for the exam. All participants who had been trained in a simulation technique were told to do the simulation exercise for 5 minutes each remaining day before the exam.

Immediate Consequences of the Simulation Exercise

Immediately after being trained in the simulation exercise (or the self-monitoring control condition), participants were asked to complete several questions regarding their attitudes toward the forthcoming exam and their expectations about their performance on it. There were no differences across the four conditions in participants' anxiety over the exam, how worried they were about it, how much confidence they had in their ability to do well on the exam, the exam score they were striving for, and the exam score they expected to receive. There were, however, systematic differences in self-reports of motivation to study for the exam. Specifically, those students who had been trained in the outcome simulation technique—namely, envisioning themselves doing well on the exam—reported a higher motivation to study for the exam than did the control group and the participants exposed to the process simulation condition.

Longer-Term Effects of the Simulations

All participants were called the night before the exam and again asked about their reactions to the forthcoming exam. By this time, participants who had been trained in the process simulation condition were beginning to experience its effects. Specifically, process simulation participants were the least anxious and worried about the exam, followed by those exposed to the outcome simulation, those who had gotten both simulations, and the control group, in that order.

However, when asked how motivated they were, the participants in the outcome simulation group continued to report that they were more motivated than those in the process simulation group, as had been true immediately after the groups were trained in the simulation exercises. Thus, in terms of the emotional benefits conferred by the simulation exercises on the students as they faced their exams, the outcome simulation appeared to be more inspirational, enhancing self-reported motivation to study; however, the process simulation significantly reduced worry and concern. On other questions, the groups were not different: the exam score participants strove for, their confidence about getting that exam score, and the exam score they expected to receive.

Participants were recontacted the day after the exam and asked to report the contents of their study sheets. The results indicated that the process simulation participants had studied an average of 3 hours longer than participants who had not simulated the process of effective studying for the exam. Process simulation participants had also begun studying for the exam approximately a day and a half earlier than those who did not simulate the process of effective studying. Thus, in terms of problem-solving activities with respect to the forthcoming exam, the process simulation condition clearly fostered effective preparatory action, whereas the outcome simulation condition did not.

Exam Performance and Perceptions of Simulations

We obtained participants' exam grades from their instructors to see whether the simulation exercises had an effect on performance. Having simulated the desired outcome (i.e., getting an A) gave participants a net gain of 2 points on their final exam. However, the process simulation exercise gave participants a net gain of 8 points on the exam. These effects were perfectly additive across the four conditions, with the highest scores achieved in the process–outome simulation condition. In short, then, the process simulation clearly worked in terms of improving the grades that these participants received. However, the outcome simulation had no significant effect and produced only a modest gain in grades.

Participants were asked to evaluate the effectiveness of the simulations. On the question asking them how helpful the exercise had been in their exam preparation, process simulation participants perceived the exercise to have been significantly more helpful than was true for participants in other conditions—an observation that is borne out by the data. In terms of how likely participants would be to use the exercise to study for future exams, both the process simulation participants and the outcome simulation participants indicated that they would be highly likely to use the exercise in the future to study for exams. However, those exposed to the combined condition and the self-monitoring control group indicated that they would not be likely to use those exercises in the future.

KINDS OF MENTAL SIMULATIONS RE-EVALUATED

The results of this investigation are informative regarding the effects of different kinds of mental simulations on emotional regulation and performance, as well as concerning the dynamics concerning how mental simulation builds links between thought and action.

Envisioning a positive outcome in one's future may instill a sense of motivation. It does not necessarily follow that a plan of action is then laid down and diligently pursued. What this implies is that rehearsing one's goals may instill a sense of motivation, but motivation may not be translated into hard work. Rather, what outcome simulation or goal rehearsal may create is "hype" or "free-floating motivation," which makes people feel good and excited without having much effect on their effort and concomitant performance. These results suggest the important point that feelings of being motivated are not necessarily the same as behaving in a motivated manner. There was clear divergence between the perception that one was highly motivated in the outcome condition and the behavioral signs of motivation translated into enhanced effort in the process simulation condition. One might think of this discrepancy as indicating an illusion of motivation, since perceived motivation and actual behavioral indications of it do not show much correspondence, at least in this investigation.

To look at these results from the standpoint of the Markus and Nurius (1986) analysis of possible selves, envisioning a possible self may not inevitably lay down the path to getting there. One might have assumed in the exam study that the path to getting a good grade would have been highly salient—namely, studying more—and that envisioning the outcome of a good grade would have led participants to get on track earlier. But this does not seem to have been the case. The fact that envisioning a positive outcome did not produce much change in a situation in which the process-to-outcome links seem so obvious suggests that psychologists may need to rethink focusing on goals as a technique for motivating people and inducing behavior change. Outcome simulation may not produce a plan of action that enables people to connect their present situation with their desired outcome.

Process simulations, however, may create self-fulfilling prophecies. In the exam study, the participants rehearsed what they would have to do to study, and in fact began studying earlier and more as a result. As such, these findings confirm the thought-to-action links credited to simulations by prior theory. Specifically, the process simulation may have made studying more subjectively likely for the participants, with the result that they did it. Moreover, consistent with research on mental practice effects and on relapse prevention, envisioning how to bring about a course of action may have yielded a plan for so doing.

In an earlier analysis (Taylor & Schneider, 1989), we implied that combining process and outcome elements into a mental simulation might have the effect of maximally enhancing motivation and performance. In the exam study, although the process–outcome condition clearly had the effect of enhancing perceived motivation, and although it clearly "worked" in the sense that these participants scored 10 points higher on their exam, this gain appears to have occurred at the expense of modestly increased worry and anxiety and lower self-confidence. Moreover, these participants reported that they would be less likely to use the technique in the future. Consequently, there does not appear to have been the anticipated synergistic effect of process and outcome elements within a single simulation. It may be that the combined simulation was more effortful and more time-consuming than the outcome or process simulation alone, leading to the unanticipated negative psychological effects it apparently had.

DYNAMICS OF SIMULATION AND ACTION

What is the dynamic process whereby participants' mental simulations of effective behavior lead to effective action—in this case, enhanced studying and exam performance? A first possibility is that the process simulation reduced anxiety and worry, putting participants in a better frame of mind for the exam and yielding a higher performance. Essentially, this line of argument suggests that the emotional regulation benefits of mental simulation as a coping technique bring about successful action. However, covarying out worry and anxiety ratings from the relation between process simulation and performance left the effect unchanged. Thus, it appears that the emotional regulation benefits of the process simulation, though soothing to the participants, did not have a direct effect on their studying or their grades.

A second possibility is that the process simulation produced a plan for effective studying, which was enacted and in turn affected exam performance. For the most part, the results support this mediational process. Although it had no immediate effects on expectations or self-reported motivation, the process simulation did induce participants to begin studying earlier, and on average they studied more. When enhanced study time was covaried out of the relation between process simulation and performance, the relationship was reduced, although still marginally significant. This suggest that, on the whole, enhanced study time produced the better performance on the exam, but that the process simulation may have had beneficial effects in addition to enhanced studying. Because of the content of the simulation, for example, these participants may have reduced the distraction in their environment while they studied, and may have stayed focused on the material better than participants in the other conditions. A related possibility is that because these participants began studying earlier, the material may have been in consciousness longer, and may have been actively or passively rehearsed when the particpants were engaged in activities other than focused studying. In any case, the overall pattern of effects suggests that the thought-to-action links forged by mental simulation may be largely mediated by cognitive factors (such as effective planning), rather than by emotional factors (in this case, reduced worry or concern).

MENTAL SIMULATION AND IMPLEMENTAL INTENTIONS

The similarity of the present analysis to Gollwitzer's work on implementation intentions bears mentioning. In a program of research, Gollwitzer and his associates (see Gollwitzer, Chapter 13, this volume; Gollwitzer, 1993; Gollwitzer, Heckhausen, & Ratajczak, 1990) have found that the simple act of forming an intention to implement an action facilitates the detection of action-related opportunities, intensifies commitment to the action sequence, and leads to a high likelihood of action. Implementation intentions are more effective in this regard than simple goal intentions—that is, the formulation of a goal that one intends at some point to achieve.

The parallels to the present conception should be obvious. Formulating a goal intention is very similar to outcome simulation; it involves individuals' forming a resolution to pursue a desired, specified goal. Implementation intention is very similar to our process simulation, because it involves committing oneself explicitly to when, where, and how to enact a chosen goal.

The results of the two lines of research parallel each other closely as well. In essence, implementation intentions function in a very similar manner to process simulations. That is, both the intention to implement an action sequence and the simulation of the process intended to bring about an action sequence appear to faciliate action better than simply formulating a goal or focusing on that outcome state does. Moreover, and consistent with the results of our exam study, Gollwitzer et al. (1990) have found that increases in outcome value or outcome expectancy do not enhance the effect of action implementation intentions. This finding is similar to our findings that the combined process–outcome simulation achieved trivially greater effects on performance and other outcomes, compared with the process simulation alone. Thus, both lines of work find that thoughts preparatory to action have the effect of bringing about that action, whereas focusing on a goal or adding goal focus to thoughts about action sequences does not enhance the links between thought and action.

The convergence of these two lines of work is encouraging confirmation of their respective analyses, but also demands conceptual analysis of the relation between them. There is nothing in the Gollwitzer paradigms to suggest that participants developing implementation intentions explicitly simulate the process that will be required to achieve effective action. Nor is there any indication in our study that process simulation participants formed implementation intentions; indeed, if anything, there appears to have been a significant absence of implementation intentions, inasmuch as the process simulation, unlike the outcome simulation, had no effect on self-reported motivation to study for the exam.

A possible way to think about the similarities and differences between Gollwitzer's work and our work on mental simulation is in terms of multiple paths to desirable outcomes. Clearly, it is essential both for individual and group survival for individuals to set goals and effectively pursue them. In other words, bridging the gap between thought and action is an essential human task. There is much redundancy in essential human bodily processes (e.g., two eyes, two hands, multiple mechanisms for digesting food), and there may be substantial psychological redundancy in the human being as well, particularly when essential life tasks are implicated. Thus, it should not be surprising to discover that there are at least two psychological routes that may move people in the direction of goal implementation. One of these is characterized by Gollwitzer's implementation intention research. Mental simulation appears to be another such process.

There are important differences in the conceptions of implementation intentions and process simulations, however. Of the two, formulating implementation intentions would seem to be the more deliberative and self-conscious method of getting oneself ready for action—a volitional act that propels an individual to action. Implementation intentions are acts of willing, and an individual engages in them only when he or she runs into difficulties in carrying out goal intentions, or when he or she anticipates obstacles or distractions. In contrast, mental simulation, though amenable to use as a conscious technique of self-motivation, may often be a quite spontaneous, unintentional method of bringing about action. Consider, for example, the context in which mental simulations often spontaneously arise: in the shower, driving to work, going to an appointment, and the like. Un-self-conscious rehearsal of what is going to happen during the day may have the unintended effect of propelling an individual into an action sequence somewhat earlier and more effectively than otherwise might occur. Although this reconciliation between Gollwitzer's research and our own is at present somewhat conjectural, it provides a context for thinking about these clearly related lines of work, their very similar findings, and the different mental processes they posit.

INTERVENTION IMPLICATIONS

The intervention implications of this work are worthy of note. The process simulation appears to be a very simple exercise that can be incorporated into study skills programs or potentially used on its own to help students improve their grades. It is easy to teach and easy to implement, and it appears to reduce worry while simultaneously increasing preparedness and producing beneficial effects on performance. Although previous research has incorporated aspects of mental simulation into multitask interventions with students to reduce anxiety and improve performance, these interventions are typically more time-consuming than the present technique; they involve multiple training sessions and extensive self-monitoring (Dendato & Diener, 1986; Hodges, McCaulay, Ryan, & Strosahl, 1979; Harris & Johnson, 1980; Meichenbaum, 1972; Suinn & Richardson, 1971). Moreover, the multitask nature of the manipulations used in previous intervention studies makes it difficult to identify the active ingredient in those studies that have been successful. Thus, the process simulation bears consideration as a basis for potential interventions with students in the future (cf. Sherman, Skov, Hervitz, & Stock, 1981).

Indeed, any problem area in which bridging the gap between thought and action is the target to be modified could profit from a process rehearsal mechanism analogous to the process simulation adopted here. Process simulations can be incorporated into efforts to change problematic habits or health behaviors (e.g., smoking or overeating) or to induce people to incorporate new health-related activities (e.g., more regular brushing and flossing of teeth). Deficiencies of self-regulation, such as poor planning or procrastination, could conceivably be modified through mental simulation of the processes that would overcome those deficiencies (cf. Meichenbaum & Goodman, 1971).

The modest results of our outcome simulation condition may also have implications for intervening with target populations in the future to enhance effective action. The self-help movement in psychology has relied heavily on people's reports of motivation to change their behavior as an impetus for change, and on the notion that focusing on desired outcomes can be a means to increasing and maintaining that motivation. The present analysis challenges this viewpoint in important respects. It may be that focusing on a goal state produces feelings of being motivated, but provides no staying power that carries people through when the actual steps they must undertake to reach their goals need to be enacted. It may be that the goal itself is distracting because it represents a glorified image of what one would like to be, which makes the "grunt work" of actually achieving the goal pale by comparison (cf. Oettingen, Chapter 11, this volume). Alternatively, it may simply be that a focus on goal states without concomitant attention to the underlying process for achieving them leaves people psychologically up a creek without a paddle, so to speak. The vision is there and the initial feeling of motivation is there, but the means are lacking. Further exploration of the potentially maladaptive effective effects of goal rehearsal is clearly warranted.

CONCLUSIONS

In conclusion, the theoretical and metatheoretical implications of mental simulation should also be noted. Mental simulation may be very functional for anticipatory coping and self-regulation. When intentionally employed in the context of goal seeking, it appears to reliably enhance motivation and action. Mental simulation may help bridge the gap between thought and action by enhancing the subjective likelihood of a set of events, by yielding a plan for bringing about that set of events, and by mustering the emotional concomitants of those events that may provide the fuel for bringing about effective action. Rehearsing the process for getting there may be more effective than goal rehearsal itself, although having a goal in mind is clearly essential for envisioning the process. From the standpoint of effective coping, it appears that mental simulation can have beneficial effects on emotions and can also foster the problem-solving activities that can lead to effective action.

On a metatheoretical level, research on mental simulation underscores the usefulness of a dialogue between researchers who study self-regulation and those who study coping. Coping researchers have carefully elucidated how people deal with intensely stressful circumstances, and self-regulation researchers have begun to articulate the many ways in which people manage information relevant to the tasks of daily life; insights from each of these traditions may help the other to flourish. In this context, the distinction made by coping researchers between problem-solving activities and emotional regulation activities maps on very well to the distinction between motivation and cognitive activities (e.g., planning) as studied by self-regulation researchers. By employing a technique of self-regulation—namely, mental simulation—in the context of coping, we hope to have contributed to this dialogue and to have made some of the links between these two theoretical and empirical traditions clear.

REFERENCES

Anderson, C. A. (1983). Imagination and expectation: The effect of imagining behavioral scripts on personal intentions. *Journal of Personality and Social Psychology, 45,* 293–305.

Anderson, C. A., & Sechler, E. S. (1986). Effects of explanation and counterexplanation on the development and use of social theories. *Journal of Personality and Social Psychology, 50,* 24–34.

Aspinwall, L. G., & Taylor, S. E. (in press). Mediating processes in psychosocial stress: Appraisal, coping, resistance, and vulnerability. In H. B. Kaplan (Ed.), *Perspectives on psychosocial stress.* New York: Academic Press.

Brownell, K. D., Marlatt, G. A., Lichtenstein, E., & Wilson, G. T. (1986). Understanding and preventing relapse. *American Psychologist, 41,* 765–782.

Campbell, J. D., & Fairey, P. J. (1985). Effects of self-esteem, hypothetical explanations, and verbalization of expectances on future performance. *Journal of Personality and Social Psychology, 48,* 1097–1111.

Carroll, J. S. (1978). The effect of imagining an event on expectations for the event: An interpretation in terms of the availability heuristic. *Journal of Experimental Social Psychology, 14,* 88–96.

Cratty, B. J. (1984). *Psychological preparation and athletic excellence.* Ithaca, NY: Mouvement.

Dendato, K. M., & Diener, D. (1986). Effectiveness of cognitive/relaxation therapy and study skills training in reducing self-reported anxiety and improving academic performance of test-anxious students. *Journal of Counseling Psychology, 33,* 131–135.

Feltz, D. L., & Landers, D. M. (1983). The effects of mental practice on motor skill learning and performance: A meta-analysis. *Journal of Sports Psychology, 5,* 25–57.

Folkman, S., Schaefer, C., & Lazarus, R. S. (1979). Cognitive processes as mediators of stress and coping. In V. Hamilton & D. M. Warburton (Eds.), *Human stress and cognition: An information processing approach* (pp. 265–298). Chichester, England: Wiley.

Gleicher, F., Kost, K. A., Baker, S. M., Strathman, A. J., Richman, S. A., & Sherman, S. J. (1990). The role of counterfactual thinking in judgments of affect. *Personality and Social Psychology Bulletin, 16,* 284–295.

Gollwitzer, P. M. (1993). Goal achievement: The role of interventions. In W. Stroebe & M. Hewstone (Eds.), *European review of social psychology* (Vol. 4, pp. 141–185). Chichester, England: Wiley.

Gollwitzer, P. M., Heckhausen, H., & Ratajczak, H. (1990). From weighing to willing: Approaching a change decision through pre- or postdecisional mentation. *Organizational Behavior and Human Decision Processes, 45,* 41–65.

Greenwald, A. G., Klinger, M. R., Vande Kamp, M. E., & Kerr, K. L. (1988). *The self-prophecy effect: Increasing voter turnout by vanity-assisted consciousness raising.* Unpublished manuscript, University of Washington.

Gregory, L. W., Cialdini, R. B., & Carpenter, K. M. (1982). Self-relevant scenarios as mediator of likelihood estimates and compliance: Does imagining make it so? *Journal of Personality and Social Psychology, 43,* 89–99.

Harris, G., & Johnson, S. B. (1980). Comparison of individualized covert modeling, self-control desensitization, and study skills training for alleviation of test anxiety. *Journal of Consulting and Clinical Psychology, 48,* 186–194.

Hayes-Roth, B., & Hayes-Roth, F. (1979). A cognitive model of planning. *Cognitive Science, 3,* 275–310.

Hirt, E. R., & Sherman, S. J. (1985). The role of prior knowledge in explaining hypothetical events. *Journal of Experimental Social Psychology, 21,* 519–543.

Hodges, W. F., McCaulay, M., Ryan, V. L., & Strosahl, K. (1979). Coping imagery, systematic desensitization, and self-concept change. *Cognitive Therapy and Research, 3,* 181–192.

Johnson, J. T. (1986). The knowledge of what might have been: Affective and attributional consequences of near outcomes. *Personality and Social Psychology Bulletin, 12,* 51–62.

Johnson, M. K., & Sherman, S. J. (1990). Constructing and reconstructing the past and the future in the present. In E. T. Higgins & R. M. Sorrentino (Eds.), *Handbook of motivation and social cognition: Foundations of social behavior* (Vol. 2). New York: Guilford Press.

Lakein, A. (1973). *How to get control of your time and your life.* New York: Signet.

Larsen, R. J., & Ketelaar, T. (1991). Personality and susceptibility to positive and negative emotional states. *Journal of Personality and Social Psychology, 61,* 132–140.

Lazarus, R. S., & Folkman, S. (1984). Coping and adaptation. In W. D. Gentry (Ed.), *Handbook of behavioral medicine* (pp. 282–325). New York: Guilford Press.

Leventhal, H., & Nerenz, D. R. (1982). A model for stress research and some implications for the control of stress disorders. In D. Meichenbaum & M. Jaremko (Eds.), *Stress prevention and management: A cognitive behavioral approach* (pp. 5–38). New York: Plenum.

Lyman, B., Bernardin, S., & Thomas, S. (1980). Frequency of imagery in emotional experience. *Perceptual and Motor Skills, 50,* 1159–1162.

Markman, K. D., Gavanski, I., Sherman, S. J., & McMullen, M. N. (1993). The mental simulation of better and worse possible worlds. *Journal of Experimental Social Psychology, 29,* 87–109.

Markus, H., & Nurius, P. (1986). Possible selves. *American Psychologist, 41,* 954–969.

Markus, H., & Wurf, E. (1987). The dynamic self-concept: A social psychological perspective. *Annual Review of Psychology, 38,* 299–337.

Marlatt, G. A. (1978). Craving for alcohol, loss of control, and relapse: A cognitive-behavioral analysis. In P. E. Nathan, G. A. Marlatt, & T. Loberg (Eds.), *Alcoholism: New directions in behavioral research and treatment* (pp. 271–314). New York: Plenum.

Marlatt, G. A., & Gordon, J. R. (Eds.). (1985). *Relapse prevention: Maintenance strategies the treatment of in addictive behaviors.* New York: Guilford Press.

McFall, R. M. (1970). The effects of self-monitoring on normal smoking behavior. *Journal of Consulting and Clinical Psychology, 35,* 135–142.

Meichenbaum, D. H. (1972). Causative modification of test-anxious college students. *Journal of Consulting and Clinical Psychology, 39,* 370–380.

Meichenbaum, D. H., & Goodman, J. (1971). Training impulsive children to talk to themselves: A means of developing self-control. *Journal of Abnormal Psychology, 77,* 115–126.

Miller, D. T., & McFarland, C. (1987). Counterfactual thinking and victim compensation: A test of norm theory. *Personality and Social Psychology Bulletin, 12,* 513–519.

Miller, G. A., Galanter, E., & Pribram, K. H. (1960). *Plans and the structure of behavior.* New York: Holt, Rinehart & Winston.

Morrow, J., & Nolen-Hoeksema, S. (1990). Effects of responses to depression on the remediation of depressive affect. *Journal of Personality and Social Psychology, 58,* 519–527.

Neideffer, R. M. (1976). *The inner athlete: Mind plus muscle for winning.* New York: Cromwell.

Orlick, T., Partington, J. T., & Salmela, J. H. (1983). *Mental training for coaches and athletes.* Ottawa: Coaching Association of Canada.

Pearlin, L. I., & Schooler, C. (1978). The structure of coping. *Journal of Health and Social Behavior, 19,* 2–21.

Ruvolo, A. P., & Markus, H. (1992). Possible selves and performance: The power of self-relevant imagery. *Social Cognition, 10,* 95–124.

Sherman, R. T., & Anderson, C. A. (1987). Decreasing premature termination from psychotherapy. *Journal of Social and Clinical Psychology, 5,* 298–312.

Sherman, S. J. (1980). On the self-erasing nature of errors of prediction. *Journal of Personality and Social Psychology, 39,* 211–221.

Sherman, S. J., Skov, R. B., Hervitz, E. F., & Stock, C. B. (1981). The effects of explaining hypothetical future events: From possibility to actuality and beyond. *Journal of Experimental Social Psychology, 17,* 142–158.

Sherman, S. T., Zehner, K. S., Johnson, J., & Hirt, E. R. (1983). Social explanation: The role of timing, set, and recall on subjective likelihood estimates. *Journal of Personality and Social Psychology, 44,* 1127–1143.

Singer, R. N. (1972). *Coaching, athletes, and psychology.* New York: McGraw-Hill.

Strack, F., Schwarz, N., & Gschneidinger, E. (1985). Happiness and reminiscing: The role of time perspective, affect, and mode of thinking. *Journal of Personality and Social Psychology, 49,* 1460–1469.

Suinn, R. M., & Richardson, F. (1971). Anxiety management training: A nonspecific behavior therapy program for anxiety control. *Behavior Therapy, 2,* 498–510.

Taylor, S. E., & Schneider, S. K. (1989). Coping and the simulation of events. *Social Cognition, 7,* 174–194.

Thoresen, C. E., & Mahoney, M. J. (1974). *Behavioral self-control.* New York: Holt, Rinehart & Winston.

Wright, J., & Mischel, W. (1982). Influence of affect on cognitive social learning person variables. *Journal of Personality and Social Psychology, 43,* 901–914.

CHAPTER 11 Positive Fantasy and Motivation

Gabriele Oettingen

Two different kinds of optimistic thinking about the future, with different impacts on motivation and action, are postulated: optimistic expectations and spontaneously generated positive fantasies. Whereas "optimistic expectations" are beliefs about how likely it is that certain events will happen or not, "spontaneously generated positive fantasies" are daydreams or mental images depicting future events and scenarios. In this chapter, I describe various studies demonstrating that optimistic expectations facilitate successful performance and that spontaneously generated positive fantasies about the future restrain motivation. I then discuss experimental studies investigating the conditions under which spontaneous positive fantasies about the future strengthen the motivation to act. First however, I consider the benefits and perils of optimistic thinking in general.

THE BENEFITS OF OPTIMISTIC THINKING

Empirical research demonstrates that optimistic thinking, even if illusory, has beneficial effects on motivation, cognition, and affect. For example, optimistic thinking is associated with increased persistence in the face of difficulties, better problem solving, heightened creativity, less fear of failure, more effective coping, more prosocial and caring behavior, and higher standards and aspirations. Optimistic thinking is also beneficial to mental and physical health. It is a buffer against depression, alcoholism, and obesity. Moreover, it hinders the emergence of acute and chronic disease and moderates its progress (for reviews, see Bandura, in press; Scheier & Carver, 1992; Peterson & Bossio, 1991; Taylor & Brown, 1988, 1994; Taylor, 1989).

Different theories stress different concepts of optimistic thinking. Taylor and Brown (1988; see also Taylor, 1989) distinguish aggrandizing self-perceptions, illusions of control, and unrealistic optimism about the future. Peterson and Seligman (1984) infer people's optimistic future outlook from their propensity to use stable, global, and internal attributions for explaining positive events to a greater extent than for explaining negative events. Scheier and Carver (1985) ask people directly about their beliefs regarding the quality of their future life. Finally, optimism can be conceptualized as "self-efficacy"—that is, as the self-reported competence to perform a certain action in its relevant context, which is a powerful predictor of successful performance in many life domains (e.g., achievement, mental and physical health) (Bandura, in press; for a trait measure of self-efficacy, see Skinner, Chapman, & Baltes, 1988). All of these concepts of optimistic thinking are common in that they are beliefs about one's self-worth, one's future outlook, or one's range of control.

THE PERILS OF OPTIMISTIC THINKING

Under the influence of humanistic psychologists (e.g., Allport, 1955; Jahoda, 1958; Maslow, 1954; Rogers, 1951), it was widely believed until the beginning of the 1980s that people would benefit from accurately accepting their reality, even if their own personalities had to be looked upon as average, their environment as boring or overwhelming, and their future as grim. Despite the overwhelming empirical evidence for the beneficial effects of optimistic thinking that has accumulated since then, the traditional position stressing the importance of reality acceptance has recently reappeared, and the research that stresses the beneficial effects of illusory optimism has been heavily criticized (e.g., Colvin & Block, 1994). But there are further voices warning against the perils of illusory optimism. For example, Baumeister (1989) argues that overly positive illusions will lead to unsafe behavior and dangerous decision making. He adduces findings that "illusions of unique invulnerability" lead to risky behaviors (Burger & Burns, 1988), and describes examples from history to illustrate the maladaptive consequences of overoptimistic thinking. Research on the "power corrupts" phenomenon (Kipnis, 1972) seems to corroborate Baumeister's position. In persons with high status, overconfidence can lead to a variety of misperceptions of reality, such as devaluing the performance of the less powerful, viewing the less powerful as objects of manipulation, and attributing the agency of others' efforts to their own influence. These misperceptions of reality are conducive to high-risk behaviors on the part of the powerful (e.g., restricting or overworking subordinates). To avoid the dangerous consequences of overconfidence, Baumeister (1989) suggests staying within an "optimal margin of illusion"—a certain *quantity* of illusory optimism that is adaptive for psychological functioning. A moderately positive distortion of the self and the world helps to ensure the benefits of illusory optimism without inducing individuals to act too riskily or on false assumptions.

Gollwitzer and Kinney (1989) present another approach to the advantages and disadvantages of positive illusions. They argue that the benefits of illusory optimism depend on the situation or the task at hand. For example, when people attempt to implement a goal, illusory control helps maintain the determination to pursue the chosen goal (Gollwitzer & Kinney, 1989; Gollwitzer, 1990). When people try to arrive at well-thought-out decisions, however, they need to analyze the positive and negative consequences in an impartial manner; if they choose a path with undue demands, they may suffer for a long time from the adversities of the wrong decision.

In summary, Baumeister (1989) argues that one should look at the quantity of illusory optimism in predicting whether illusory optimism is adaptive or maladaptive. Gollwitzer and Kinney (1989) suggest considering the situation or the task at hand in order to check whether illusory optimism is functional or dysfunctional. But there is still another way to approach this problem. There may be different kinds of optimistic thinking—some associated with perils, others with benefits. It is this issue that I focus on in the present chapter.

DIFFERENT KINDS OF OPTIMISTIC THINKING

Researchers commonly conceptualize optimistic thinking according to control beliefs, self-efficacy beliefs, outcome expectations, or expectations of future life in general. Thoughts about the future, however, do not necessarily have to be beliefs about how likely or unlikely it is that a certain desired event will occur or not, or that a certain behavior will be carried out or not. People also spontaneously imagine their successes and failures, visualize them in their minds' eyes, and play with their memories and mental images of anticipated future events. In their daydreams and wishes, they fancy masterful performances and blissful experiences. But people also picture the falling through of their desires; dreadful news cutting right across their lives; and dreary, everyday, routine work. Such mental images, daydreams, or fantasies may depict incidents with good or bad endings, and thus may possess a positive or negative quality. Fantasies more easily escape the grip of reality than expectations, because fantasies are not constrained by the cognitive mechanisms that make people acknowledge factual information (Klinger, 1971, 1990; Singer, 1966). Accordingly, individuals may indulge in spontaneous positive fantasies, although critical analyses of past performance or thinking about objective likelihoods would lead to low expectations of success.

These considerations suggest that expectations and fantasies are two different ways of thinking about the future. But do they have different effects on motivation and action? High expectations of success signal that a given desired task can be attained, and thus should *increase* motivation (Atkinson, 1957). In contrast, positive fantasies of success constitute an anticipation of having reached it or even an anticipatory consumption of the various positive consequences or experiences, and thus should *reduce* motivation to actually achieve them. In a positive fantasy, a person may "experience" the future event ahead of time and may color the future experience more brightly and joyfully than reality would ever permit. Therefore the need to act is not felt, and the thorny path leading to implementing the fantasy may easily be overlooked. Moreover, positive fantasies may prevent a person from realizing that effortful action precedes most achievements; accordingly, no action plans for how to achieve the imagined fantasies may be formed. This should further reduce the chances of success, as a lack of mentally rehearsed action plans has been linked to decreased performance (Gollwitzer, Heckhausen, & Ratajczak, 1990; Gollwitzer, 1993 and Chapter 13, this volume; Taylor & Schneider, 1989; Taylor & Pham, Chapter 10, this volume; see also Friedman, Scholnick, & Cocking, 1987).

In summary, because positive fantasies imply anticipatory consumption of success, experience of no need to act, and a lack of detailed action plans, they should produce less successful performances than negative fantasies. This should be in contrast to positive expectations, which are known to foster successful performances.

POSITIVE FANTASIES VERSUS POSITIVE EXPECTATIONS

Various studies in different life domains (e.g., health, interpersonal attraction) were conducted to test the hypotheses stated above. In all of these studies, the subjects' expectations and fantasies were assessed for positivity long before (up to 4 years before) we assessed relevant performances (e.g., weight loss, recovery from illness, getting involved with someone). Positive expectations, according to our hypotheses, would predict strong performances. Positive fantasies, on the other hand, would predict weak performances.

Weight Loss

We assessed expectations of success, as well as weight- and food-related fantasies, in 25 obese women who had enrolled in a weight reduction program at the Hospital of the University of Pennsylvania (Oettingen & Wadden, 1991). The women weighed an average of 233 pounds. The weight reduction program, which offered diet prescriptions and weekly behavior therapy, lasted for a full year. In the second year, the patients received weight maintenance therapy.

At pretreatment, each patient had to indicate the number of pounds she wished to lose in the program and her expectations of attaining her weight goal. We used a semiprojective procedure to assess the positivity of patients' fantasies. We wanted subjects to generate spontaneous fantasies *at that very moment* rather than to recall fantasy retrospectively from long-term memory, because such recall is likely to be distorted (see Ericsson & Simon, 1980, 1993). Each patient was asked to imagine herself vividly as the main character in four weight- and food-related scenarios. Two stories were designed to elicit fantasies about the subject's weight loss, whereas the other two stories described encounters with tempting foods. Each story had an open ending, which subjects were asked to complete in writing by describing the stream of thoughts that occurred to them. For example, one scenario read: "You have just completed Penn's weight loss program. A friend of yours has invited you to her annual pool party. You attended this function last year, so you will probably see many familiar faces. As you are on your way to the party, you imagine. . . . " Right after describing their mental images, subjects rated the positivity and negativity of their images, as well as their imagined body shape. From the correlations between these ratings, we learned that positive fantasies meant having images about a slim body. Weight loss was measured three times on a balance beam scale in the clinic: after 3 months, 1 year, and 2 years.

Expectations and fantasies predicted weight loss in opposite directions. After 1 year, patients with high expectations lost about 12 kilograms *more* than patients with low expectations. In contrast, subjects with positive fantasies lost about 11 kilograms *less* than subjects with negative fantasies. After 2 years, the respective differences were 15 and 12 kilograms. These patterns of results stayed unchanged when subjects' weight loss aspirations, as well as their subjective incentives to reach their aspired weight loss, were covaried. The findings thus supported our assumption that optimistic expectations and positive fantasies are different types of optimistic thinking, and that they have differential effects on motivation and action. Apparently, images of getting slim and resisting food temptations hindered weight loss. Subjects seemed to daydream that weight loss had occurred without their having to make any effort. For example, in response to the friend's pool party scenario, one subject with positive fantasies wrote: "I am going swimming in front of everyone!! First I have a drink because I am too excited and have to act like I am not self-conscious. Everyone is going to really check me out. I'll be shining!" Such wishful daydreams did not help subjects to succeed, either in the short or in the long run. On the contrary, positive expectations favored weight loss. This is in line with previous studies demonstrating that people who expect to lose weight are more successful in doing so (Bernier & Avard, 1986; Chambliss & Murray, 1979; Glynn & Ruderman, 1986; Leon, Sternberg, & Rosenthal, 1984; Stotland & Zuroff, 1991).

Recovery from Chronic Illness

Another area where optimistic expectations have beneficial effects is recovery from illness. For example, Scheier et al. (1989), using the Life Orientation Scale (Scheier & Carver, 1985), observed that optimistic patients recovered faster after coronary artery bypass surgery and returned to full-time work somewhat earlier than patients with a pessimistic outlook. Effects of heightened self-efficacy beliefs on physiological functioning have been shown by Bandura, Cioffi, Taylor, and Brouillard (1988), who suggest that even the functioning of the immune system may benefit from optimistic efficacy beliefs. Whatever the path from optimism to recovery may be—physiological or behavioral—it seems that optimistic expectations help to prevent the onset of and the recovery from physical illness (for reviews, see Scheier & Carver, 1992; Taylor, 1989). Data predicting comparatively better health at ages 45 through 60 from an optimistic explanatory style at age 25 further support this claim (Peterson, Seligman, & Vaillant, 1988).

Do positive fantasies retard the recovery from physical illness? In a conceptual replication of the weight loss study, we (Oettingen, Losert, Wood, Nathanson, & Kazak, 1995, Study 1) tested expectations and fantasies in children suffering from chronic asthma and gastrointestinal disease. We recorded children's disease activity at the time of the interview as well as several months later. We operationalized positive expectations using a measure of explanatory style (the children's version of the Attributional Style Questionnaire; Seligman et al., 1984), which assessed to what extent patients perceived hypothetical positive events as more stable, global, and internal than negative events. An optimistic explanatory style conveyed the patients' sense that they would eventually be able to deal with the situation at hand (see Abramson, Seligman, & Teasdale, 1978; Peterson & Seligman, 1984), and thus indicated positive expectations. Positive fantasies concerning patients' future lives were assessed through 12 scenarios, which pertained to the domains of health, interpersonal relations, and achievement (four scenarios each). A typical health scenario read: "Imagine you have been invited to sleep over at a friend's house. But since you have been sick for the past couple of days, your mother calls the doctor to see if you are well enough to go. She hangs up the phone and. . . ." After the children had completed the scenarios in writing, they rated the positivity–negativity of their images. From the doctors' charts, we took a standard measure of disease activity, and also recorded prescribed medicine as an indicator of how well children were doing in fighting their disease. As dependent variables, we used the disease activity and prescription scores several months after the interview, corrected for the respective scores at the time of the interview. The pattern of results was the same as in the weight loss study. Over a period of several months, patients with asthma and gastrointestinal disease who were optimistic in their explanatory style tended to show comparatively better recovery. In contrast, the more positive the patients' fantasies were, the worse their disease activity scores were and the more medicine they had to take over time.

Recovery from Acute Illness

In a study on physical illness, we (Oettingen, Losert, et al., 1995, Study 1) assessed explanatory style and fantasies in children suffering from cancer (i.e., leukemia and lymphoma). The physicians in charge rated patients' probability of survival at two points in time: at the interview and 4 years later.

As the dependent variable, we used probability of survival after 4 years (all patients were still alive), corrected for probability of survival at the time of the interview. The same measures of explanatory style and fantasies that were used in the study of chronically ill children were used here. In the children with cancer, positive fantasies predicted a less favorable recovery rate (p = .10), though explanatory style showed a close to zero correlation to recovery rate. The predictive relation of positive fantasy rested in particular on the four health-related scenarios. Apparently, patients' positive fantasies about their future health did not aid in recovery. Effective recovery from cancer demanded taking action (e.g., complying with the various medical demands and coping with painful procedures), and taking action should have been suppressed by positive fantasies in which future recovery was anticipated to be achieved effortlessly.

To sum up, the studies described to this point supported the hypothesis that positive thinking in terms of expectations is beneficial, whereas positive thinking in terms of fantasies is maladaptive. This pattern of results emerged regardless of whether high-risk health behavior or chronic illness was analyzed. However, all of these data pertained to the health domain only and came from studies with rather small samples. The next question we addressed was how reliable the predictive effects of positive fantasies are when it comes to other domains and larger samples.

Romantic Success

The next study focused on starting a love relationship. Students who had crushes on fellow students of the opposite sex, but who were not yet going out or were not yet involved with them, were tested for their expectations of getting together with their "crushees," as well as for their fantasies about what might happen to them and their crushees in the future. To measure subjects' fantasies, we (Oettingen, Losert, et al., 1995, Study 2) used a procedure similar to that described for the health studies. For example, one item read: "You are at a party. While you are talking to HIM, you see a girl whom you believe HE might like to meet. As she approaches the two of you, you imagine. . . . " After several months, we asked students whether they were successful in getting involved with their crushees. Students who originally had positive expectations were more likely to get together with their crushees than those with more negative expectations. In contrast, students with positive fantasies about themselves and their crushees were less likely to get involved with their crushees than their peers who spontaneously generated less positive fantasies. This pattern of results stayed the same after subjects' perceived incentive to get together with their crushees and subjects' gender were covaried.

Professional Success

Another study (Oettingen, Losert, et al., 1995, Study 3) focused on the topic of "transition into work life." We tested students who were completing their university education and preparing to enter the job market. We assessed subjects' expectations of finding a job and the tone of their spontaneous fantasies related to the future experience of transition into work life. Two years later, subjects were asked to report on the professional opportunities they had been offered and to indicate their current professional status. High expectations of success predicted success, whereas positive fantasies showed an inverse relation to professional achievement. This was true even after subjects' incentive to get a job was statistically controlled for.

Summary

Optimistic expectations fostered the resistance to high-risk health behavior and the combating of chronic disease, as well as interpersonal and professional success, whereas positive fantasies were a clear hindrance. The fact that similar patterns of results emerged in three different life domains (i.e., the health, the interpersonal, and the work domains) supports our hypotheses on the perils of positive fantasy. Moreover, in almost all of our studies, optimistic expectations had beneficial effects. This corresponds to previous findings on optimistic thinking.

OTHER CONCEPTS OF FANTASY

In this section, similarities and differences between our work and three other lines of research involving the concept of fantasy—Thematic Apperception Test (TAT) fantasies, the stream of thought, and current concerns—are discussed.

Thematic Apperception Test Fantasies

Our measure of positive fantasy should not be confused with fantasy generated in response to the TAT, the classic measure of motives (Murray, 1938; McClelland, Atkinson, Clark, & Lowell, 1953). In the TAT approach, fantasies are perceived as reflections of specific personal needs. Accordingly, subjects' fantasies in response to a given picture are content-analyzed to determine to what extent the fantasies contain elements of striving for achievement, affilitation, intimacy, power, and so forth, and to determine whether the fantasies reflect hope (i.e., approach) or fear (i.e., avoidance; see Heckhausen, 1989/1991). Our work is concerned neither with the number of fantasies generated in a given domain (achievement, affiliation, etc.)

nor with whether subjects habitually tend to fantasize about approaching a desired outcome (e.g., having a slim body) versus avoiding an undesired one (e.g., not having an obese body). Rather, we are interested in how positively or negatively subjects fantasize about a certain upcoming event (e.g., their body shape after the weight loss program). As a consequence, the way we measure subjects' positive or negative fantasies is markedly different from the measures used with TAT fantasies. First, we use self-report scales to determine the positivity or negativity of the fantasies. In contrast, the fantasies in response to the TAT are rated according to a prescribed coding scheme applied by trained raters who code various indicators for the respective variables (e.g., "instrumental activity leading to achieving a standard of excellence" as indicative of hope for success in the achievement domain). Second, in our approach fantasies pertain to the self, whereas in the TAT approach they pertain to the people depicted. Third, we have obtained sufficiently high reliability for our fantasy items (Cronbach's alphas of about .70), whereas reliability has always been a problem in the TAT (for a discussion, see McClelland, 1980). Finally, our measure of positive fantasy is different from what are referred to as "incentives" in expectancy–value theories (Heckhausen, 1989/1991). Incentives determine people's beliefs about the expected value (desirability) of a certain future outcome. Our measures of spontaneous positive fantasies do not assess beliefs and thus show only negligible correlations to incentive values. Moreover, expectancy–value theories predict a positive relationship between subjective expected values and success, whereas we have found negative relationships between positive fantasies and success.

The Stream of Thought

Over a century ago, William James (1890/1950) published his revealing ideas about the stream of thought. It took another 60 years for the subject to be examined empirically. Jerome L. Singer, a pioneer in the research on fantasy, and his collaborators showed in experimental and correlational studies that people's inner experience is filled with task-irrelevant thoughts, free-floating images, and fanciful anticipations (see Singer, 1966, 1988, for summaries). Unstructured thoughts and images appear to arise when a person's full attention is not needed to adjust to the present external environment. Memories or environmental stimuli can serve as the starting points for such daydreaming or fantasizing. Therein, past or present experiences are rehearsed, changed, and ingeniously combined to emerge as new creations of the mind, which reshape the past, embellish the present, and fancy the future. Such fantasies can feature extravagant actions, overwhelming successes, and clever strategies, but also shameful failure and painful rejection. Many characteristics of people's fantasy lives, as well as the relationships of these to other personality dimensions, have been identified by self-report instruments measuring daydreaming patterns retrospectively—the Imaginal Processes Inventory (IPI; Singer & Antrobus, 1963, 1972) and the Short Imaginal Processes Inventory (SIPI; Huba, Aneshensel, & Singer, 1981; Huba, Singer, Aneshensel, & Antrobus, 1982) (for a review, see Singer & Bonanno, 1990).

Singer and his collaborators, however, do not focus on the positivity of fantasies. Rather, the SIPI includes a "positive–constructive" daydreaming scale, which combines an accepting attitude toward one's inner experiences with problem-solving, joyful, vivid, and future-oriented daydreaming. The positive–constructive pattern differs from guilty–dysphoric daydreaming, which characterizes people who feel threatened by their fearful and hostile daydreams. Furthermore, fantasy is not distinguished from expectations or self-efficacy beliefs. Rather, both self-efficacy beliefs and fantasies are perceived as important corroborative influences on behavioral change (Singer & Pope, 1978). Finally, rather than prompting the kind of spontaneous fantasies present in our work, the IPI and SIPI ask subjects to retrospectively rate the frequency of certain kinds of daydreams (such as achievement-oriented, sexual, or bizarre).

Current Concerns

The theory of "current concerns," which has its roots in achievement motivation theory (Atkinson, 1957; McClelland et al., 1953), defines such a concern as the state between the act of commitment to a specific goal and the time of achievement of or disengagement from that goal (Klinger, 1975, 1977). Studying the differential effects of optimistic expectations versus spontaneous positive fantasies on behavior is not the objective in Klinger's work. Rather, high expectations of success foster commitment, which as a gate to the state of current concern should then influence the content of fantasies. Other features of current concerns, such as unexpected difficulties in goal achievement, also influence what kind of information the person will process and what the stream of thought will be about (Klinger, Barta, & Maxeiner, 1980). Accordingly, subjects responding to the Concern Dimensions Questionnaire (Klinger et al., 1980) or the Interview Questionnaire (Klinger, 1987) are asked to report about various characteristics of their current concerns, such as value of the goal, subjective probability of success, or intended action regarding the goal. From these self-report answers, subjects' cognitive and physiological reactions as well as the contents of their spontaneous thoughts are predicted.

THE PERILS OF POSITIVE FANTASY: SUPPORTIVE FINDINGS

Thus far in this chapter, I have reported studies explicitly designed to test the predicted negative relation between positive fantasy and performance. But there are various other lines of research that, at least indirectly, add further support to this notion. First, in a prospective study of women with a history of breast carcinoma (Jensen, 1987), comforting daydreaming, as measured by the positive–constructive scale of the SIPI (Huba et al., 1981, 1982), predicted metastatic spread over a period of more than a year. As mentioned earlier, high scores on the positive–constructive scale of the SIPI indicate vivid, enjoyable, problem-solving, and future-oriented daydreaming. Second, wish-fulfilling fantasy has been linked to poor adjustment in patients coping with physical illness and painful medical procedures (Felton & Revenson, 1984), whereas accurate and thus often negative information about the kind of anticipated procedures and about the sensations that patients will experience have beneficial effects on the patients' ability to deal with the hardships (Johnson, Lauver, & Nail, 1989; Suls & Wan, 1989). Similarly, Peterson (1989), summarizing research on how children cope with medical routine, has reported better adjustment in children who seek precise information about upcoming surgical or diagnostic procedures. These results imply that patients who focus on positive images depicting how easy and effortless upcoming medical procedures will be cope less well than patients who generate more negative mental images in response to accurate medical information.

The second line of research comes from the literature on cognitive therapy. By means of various procedures, such as covert modeling, hypnosis, or guided imagery, subjects are led to give up positive fantasies of effortless recovery. Patients are guided to produce mental images about upcoming hardships as a means of preparing them for staying away from high-risk situations and for resisting temptations (for an example, see Brownell, 1989; for a review, see Marlatt & Gordon, 1985; Marlatt, Baer, & Quigley, 1995). Related to this type of research are self-efficacy training programs, in which the overcoming of possible difficulties and pitfalls that hinder successful task performance (e.g., in school, work, or sports) is systematically rehearsed. This should also reduce positive fantasies about the ease of solving such tasks (on changes in self-efficacy, see Bandura, in press; on effects of mental practice, see Corbin, 1972; Feltz & Landers, 1983).

Harmful effects of positive fantasies on performance were reported in an experiment by Goodhart (1986). Subjects with experimentally induced positive images about their own competence did worse on an anagram test than subjects with negative images. However, this was only true when subjects were *not* asked to predict how well they might perform after generating their images—that is, when subjects' positive images were *not* overridden by their expectations. Similar results were obtained by Sherman, Skov, Hervitz, and Stock (1981, Study 1). With respect to an upcoming anagram task, subjects first had to explain hypothetical success or failure, and then either had or did not have to state their expectations of success. Subjects who explained failure did somewhat better than those who explained success when they did *not* have to state their expectations. The reverse was true for subjects who had to state their expectations. Sherman and his collaborators interpreted the findings as follows: Explaining hypothetical failure leads to the consideration of possible failure and consequently to more effort in the upcoming task than does explaining hypothetical success. When explicit expectancies are set, however, subjects' performance tends to confirm their negative expectations generated from explaining undesirable events.

Finally, in working with defensive pessimists, Showers (1992) demonstrated that experimentally induced positive images about performance led to worse performance than negative images did (Study 1). "Defensive pessimists" are generally successful people who strategically reduce their expectations of success (Norem & Cantor, 1986). In Study 2, Showers observed that negative imagery produced more reassuring thoughts than positive imagery. This "plucking up" of courage after having generated negative images should have promoted good performances. Though Showers's findings pertain only to students who have a successful performance history and use a particular performance strategy, they do demonstrate that positive imagery can indeed have harmful effects on performance.

WHY IS POSITIVE FANTASY HARMFUL?

Indulging in positive fantasies should increase the salience of positive outcomes, whereas generating negative fantasies should increase the salience of difficulties and hardships. Subjects with positive fantasies, because they are working out positive events in their minds' eyes, should hardly be motivated to put effort into obtaining success. In contrast, subjects with negative fantasies, because they are perceiving the occurrence of hardship in their minds' eyes, may feel challenged to make efforts to overcome these obstacles (see Sherman et al., 1981). To follow up on this speculation, we asked subjects in our study on finding jobs how many applications they had sent out. Indeed, subjects with positive fantasies reported having sent out fewer job applications than subjects with negative fantasies. At the same time, the subjects with positive daydreams reported having refrained from conflicting commitments (e.g., going on a long vacation) and having already prepared themselves for changes in their private lives that would result from success in finding jobs. It appears, then, that subjects generating positive fantasies about finding a job took success for granted. They presumptuously thought of themselves as having already obtained the desired jobs, and consequently failed to confront the adverse reality that needs to be tackled if success is actually to be achieved.

POSITIVE FANTASY AND NEGATIVE REALITY

At this point, we wondered whether positive fantasy can motivate behavior if it is contrasted with reflections about the negative reality—that is, with reflections on what demands stand in the way of fantasy fulfillment. When positive fantasy and the respective negative reality appear in the mind's eye, positive fantasy should no longer allow indulgence and premature consumption, because it is experienced as something to be achieved in real life. Whereas positive fantasies give action the necessary direction, reflections on reality point to the necessity to act. Moreover, reflections on reality provide clues on how to actually implement one's positive fantasies in real life. Accordingly, focusing on both the positive fantasy and the contradictory negative reality should increase motivation toward implementing the positive fantasy.

If contrasting positive fantasy with negative reality turns positive fantasy into something to be implemented in real life, people who ponder the contrast between fantasy and reality should become tuned to the probabilities of success. The subjective probability of success should now guide motivation and action. Imagine a young man indulging in positive daydreams about getting involved with a young woman. Only after generating both positive fantasies *and* reflections about the actual situation (i.e., being without her) should he perceive his positive fantasies as something to be achieved. Accordingly, he should become attuned to the probability of actually getting involved with the loved one when it comes to the decision of whether to pursue her or not.

In contrast, expectations should leave motivation and action largely untouched when a person prefers to indulge in positive fantasies. Giving free reign to positive images about the future does not suggest a necessity to act nor does it convey any hint on *how* to act. Such positive images are sheer fantasies left to the inner stream of consciousness and thus are not experienced as outcomes to be implemented through laborious efforts. Similarly, expectations should fail to guide motivation and action when a person prefers to brood on the shortcomings of the present reality. Dwelling only on the negative status quo conveys no allusion to *where* to go, that is, in which direction the reality should be changed. There is no guiding future vision that leads a person's efforts to change reality to the better.

These ideas imply that when people are induced to contrast their positive fantasies with reflections on the corresponding negative reality, they should evince high positive correlations between subjective probabilities of fantasy fulfillment and their motivation to achieve their fantasies. In contrast, with people who either generate only positive fantasies or reflect only on their negative reality, no substantial correlations should be observed. Whereas high expectations of success should lead to more motivation when one is contrasting fantasy and reality, as compared to when one is dwelling on fantasy or reality only, low expectations of success should lead to comparatively less motivation.

Interpersonal Concern

In our first experiment on this issue (Oettingen, Böhringer, & Losert, 1995, Study 1), female students were asked to name the interpersonal matter that was presently most important to them (e.g., getting to know somebody) and to state their expectations about whether it would result in a happy ending. Then they were asked to list positive aspects of the happy ending (e.g., love, feeling of being needed) and negative aspects of reality that appeared to stand against the possibility of a happy ending (e.g., being insecure, unattractive). In the fantasy–reality contrast group, subjects had to select two aspects of both the happy ending and the negative reality. To achieve a fantasy–reality contrast, subjects were asked to alternate in their production of spontaneous images between positive aspects of wish fulfillment and negative aspects of reality, beginning with a positive aspect. Thus, both aspects had to be reflected on intermittently. In contrast, in the fantasy-only group, subjects were asked to imagine only positive aspects of the happy ending; in the reality-only group, subjects were asked to reflect only on negative aspects of the actual situation. Dependent variables were measures of activity feelings and immediacy of action. These variables were recorded right after the experiment and during the following weeks.

In the fantasy–reality contrast group, subjects' expectations of success showed a substantial positive correlation with the dependent variables. In both the fantasy-only and the reality-only groups, these correlations were much lower. Furthermore, the latter two groups did not differ in their low correlations. For example, in the fantasy–reality contrast group, subjects with high expectations of success acted sooner than those with low expectations, whereas there was almost no difference in the date of starting action between subjects with high and low expectations in the other two groups. Moreover, subjects with high expectations of success felt more active and started acting earlier in the contrast group as compared to the other two groups, whereas subjects with low expectations felt less active and started acting later in the contrast group than in the other two groups.

Finally, these effects were not attributable to differential effects of the manipulation on subjects' expectations. We found an almost perfect correlation between subjects' expectations measured before and after the experiment. In addition, subjects' expectations measured after the manipulation did not differ among the three groups.

Getting to Know an Attractive Stranger

In the next experiment (Oettingen, Böhringer, & Losert, 1995, Study 2), we used the same salience paradigm as in the preceding study, which had been stimulated by the work of Mischel, Ebbesen, and Zeiss (1972) as well as of Taylor and Fiske (1978). However, instead of asking subjects to name their own interpersonal concerns, we created the same concern for all subjects. The cover story told the female subjects that we were interested in daydreams about getting to know a stranger. Then subjects were shown a picture of an attractive young man whom they did not know, supposedly a young researcher at the Max Planck Institute. Subjects had to indicate their expectations in terms of the probability of successfully getting to know this person, if they had the opportunity. Then they had to go through the same procedures as described in the preceding study. This time, however, the aspects of fantasy fulfillment pertained to how it would be to get to know the person in the picture (e.g., joyful, interesting), whereas the aspects of the status quo pertained to what would stand in the way of getting to know him (e.g., being shy, not having enough time). We also added a fourth group to the design of this study. Subjects in this group were asked to solve arithmetic tasks creating a heavy cognitive load, because we wanted to test whether the high correlations between expectation and motivation observed in the preceding study were indeed attributable to contrasting fantasy–reality images rather than to the sheer listing of the various aspects of fantasy fulfillment and reality. The dependent variable in the present study was the extent to which subjects cared about getting to know the person on the picture. This was assessed immediately after the manipulation and 1 week later.

The results were like those of the preceding experiment: A higher positive correlation between expectation and the dependent variable was obtained for subjects in the fantasy–reality contrast group than for the other groups, which did not differ from each other and which showed correlation coefficients close to zero (including the arithmetic task control group). Furthermore, subjects with high expectations cared more about getting to know the young man in the picture and were more eager to meet him than the respective subjects in the other groups. The opposite was true for subjects with low expectations.

These differences between groups were more pronounced after 1 week than immediately after the experiment. Over time, only subjects with high expectations of success in the fantasy–reality contrast group kept up their motivation to get to know the person in the picture. The remaining subjects cared less about getting to know him and felt less eager to meet him after 1 week had passed.

Combining Work and Family Life

A third experiment used a rationalization paradigm to vary the fantasy–reality contrast. Subjects were female doctoral students who did not have children and who were approaching a critical age for being able to bear children. The study supposedly was concerned with life planning. Subjects were told that we (Oettingen, Böhringer, & Losert, 1995, Study 3) were interested in how individuals of different ages and career paths imagine their futures. More specifically, they were asked to produce positive daydreams or fantasies about their professional and their private lives several years from now, to let these mental images pass in front of their minds' eyes, and then to describe them in writing. Thereafter, subjects rated their confidence that their fantasies and daydreams would come true. Statements then followed that supposedly came from interviews with working mothers. The statements were complaints about the daily hardships of combining work and family life. Two examples were as follows: "Again Nina had to wait all alone in front of the nursery school because I did not get out of the office in time," and "At work I am always so tired and irritated because at night my little son wakes up every other hour."

Subjects in the fantasy–reality contrast group were asked to read through the statements, to let their associations and imaginary thoughts in response to these statements pass freely in front of their minds' eyes, and then to write these images down. Subjects in the fantasy-only group were given the same instructions as the fantasy–reality contrast group. To direct subjects' attention away from the mothers' statements of negative reality, however, we made subjects trivialize the mothers' statements. We added at the beginning of the instructions that in each of the statements, the mother was complaining about the harsh reality of combining professional life and motherhood just as an excuse; in fact, the mother wanted to conceal some other problems she had. Subjects were asked to imagine what each mother's excuse could be about. Finally, subjects in the reality-only group were also given the same instructions as the fantasy–reality contrast group. However, to force subjects' attention away from their positive fantasies, we asked them to depict their thoughts pertaining to the fact that the subjects themselves did not have any children yet. After a couple of weeks, subjects rated their intention to act toward, their thought involvement in, and their caring for the idea to combine work and family life for themselves.

For all three dependent variables, the pattern of results resembled those of the experiments described above: A strong positive correlation with expectation was obtained for the fantasy–reality contrast group, and this was stronger than that found for the two other groups, which did not differ from each other. Furthermore, subjects with high expectations wanted to do more to combine work and family life, their thoughts were more involved in this idea, and they cared more about the idea than the respective subjects in the other groups. However, for subjects with low expectations, the difference between the fantasy–reality contrast group and the other two groups was significant only for subjects' intention to act.

These results pertained only to subjects who fantasized about their future lives in terms of having both a profession *and* a child. Subjects in the fantasy–reality contrast group who fantasized about having a job only (no child) or about having a child only (no profession) showed, like the other group, no correlations between expectations and the dependent variables.

Summary

In each of these studies, optimistic versus pessimistic expectations guided motivation and action more in subjects from the fantasy–reality contrast group than in subjects from the fantasy-only or reality-only group. Furthermore, in the fantasy–reality contrast group, subjects with high expectations were more motivated and subjects with low expectations were by and large less motivated than the respective subjects in the other experimental groups. These effects emerged both when a salience procedure was used and when a rationalization paradigm was employed.

The observed pattern of results was stable over periods of one to several weeks. Whether subjects followed up on their fantasies until they reached a happy ending, we do not know. Our dependent variables focused largely on thought involvement and on activities pertaining to getting things started.

ENGAGEMENT AND DISENGAGEMENT

The observed effects are not attributable to changes in expectations, but to changes in motivation and action *in response* to expectations. Optimistic expectations, then, seem to develop their beneficial effects on motivation and action when positive fantasy points in the direction of acting *and,* at the same time, when reflections on the negative reality show the necessity of acting. The experimental studies also revealed two moderators of the effects of optimistic expectations: Optimistic expectations did not yield their benefits for motivation when subjects indulged in positive fantasies or dwelled on the negative reality. Thus, the observed results should temper the criticism regarding the perils of illusory optimism. Expectations seem to leave motivation and action largely untouched when a person's attention is focused solely on positive fantasies or solely on negative reality. At the same time, however, the results imply that negative thoughts about reality can be beneficial for adjustment. If these reality images are contrasted with positive future fantasies in the mind's eye, expectations gain relevance for action.

To engage a person in a task, then, one would need to create the fantasy–reality contrast plus optimistic expectations; to disengage a person from a concern or a task, one would need to induce the fantasy–reality contrast plus pessimistic expectations. When indulging in positive fantasies or dwelling on negative reality, our subjects behaved unreasonably by not thinking and acting according to the subjective probabilities of success. Subjects with pessimistic expectations were more engaged than their probability judgments suggested, whereas subjects with optimistic expectations were less engaged than their probability judgments suggested. In other words, subjects with low expectations who indulged in positive fantasies, and thus were "pessimistic and hopeful" at the same time, stayed *more* engaged than seemed justified on the basis of their expectations. Interestingly, this was also true for subjects with low expectations who dwelled on the negative reality, and who were thus "pessimistic and worrying" at the same time. Furthermore, subjects with high expectations who indulged in positive fantasies, and thus were "optimistic and hopeful," stayed *less* engaged than seemed justified by their high expectations. They behaved like subjects with high expectations who dwelled on the negative reality, and thus were "optimistic and worrying."

THE FANTASY-REALITY CONTRAST IN DAILY LIFE

Our studies are not relevant to the question of how fantasy–reality contrasts emerge spontaneously. When people are lost in reveries, reality may have to be quite harsh in order to induce them to start reflecting on it. Reality is a nuisance in the sense that it forces people to take sides—that is, either to engage in or to disengage from reaching their fantasies (depending on their expectations). Moreover, engaging and disengaging demand mental, affective, and behavioral efforts. Not surprisingly, then, rationalizations, which allow people to keep daydreaming, are plentiful (Erdelyi, 1990; Kunda, 1990; Taylor, 1983).

And what about people who are lost in dwelling on the negative reality? As they only have to start joyfully daydreaming, shouldn't it be easy for them to create a fantasy–reality contrast? As it turns out, people often have reasons not to fantasize. It may also be that people cannot spontaneously produce positive images about a certain task (e.g., the doctoral students who did not spontaneously envision having both a professional life and a child). Clearly, future studies must examine the processes by which people spontaneously produce fantasies to be contrasted with the grim reality.

Did the successful subjects in our field studies (e.g., the studies of weight loss and romantic success) spontaneously produce a fantasy–reality contrast, whereas the unsuccessful subjects were lost in their positive fantasies? We do not know the exact content of these subjects' mental images. The results of our experiments suggest that indulging in positive fantasies indeed leads to less motivation than can be reasonably inferred from expectations. But this is true only for subjects who have high expectations. For subjects with low expectations, indulging in positive fantasies leads to more motivation than seems reasonable. However, in the long run the latter finding might be poor comfort for the "hopeful and pessimistic" subjects, because pessimistic expectations reflect past failure (e.g., in our weight loss sample; see also Bandura 1977; Mischel, 1973). Over the months and years of harsh confrontation with negative reality, then, these "hopeful and pessimistic" subjects may have started to contrast their positive fantasies with the negative reality. Thus, they may have become attuned to their low expectations, thereby losing much of their initial motivation.

Finally, what happens to the quality of positive fantasies when people contrast them with reflections about the negative reality? As contrasted positive fantasies become something to be achieved, fanciful images should fade, and more realizable features of the happy ending should appear in the stream of thought. Similarly, reflections on the negative reality may change when people contrast them with the respective positive fantasies. Instead of focusing on the stable attributes of the status quo, they now may deal with clues about how to change reality and with preparations for coping with possible hardships. Thus, reflections about the negative reality contrasted with positive fantasies may lead up to what Taylor and Pham (Chapter 10, this volume; see also Taylor & Schneider, 1989) call "process simulations," and what Norem and Cantor (1986) mark out as the strategy of defensive pessimism. These are thoughts of future events and actions that help people to avoid anticipated threat and promote coping with foreseen hardship. Such thoughts and images foster the exploration of alternative routes and hidden opportunities and help control people's actions, all of which should promote the achievement of behavioral change.

HOW POSITIVE FANTASIES TURN INTO GOALS

One might argue that our experimental research shows nothing but the classic notion that deviations from standards are motivating (e.g., Duval & Wicklund, 1972; Higgins, 1987; Locke & Latham, 1990; Markus & Nurius, 1986; Wicklund & Gollwitzer, 1982), particularly when people have high expectations of success (Bandura, 1991; Carver & Scheier, 1981). If this were the case, however, the arithmetic task condition in the study of getting to know an attractive stranger should have generated motivating effects in line with subjects' expectations, because subjects wrote down the discrepant reality at the outset of the experiment. This motivating effect should have been furthered in the positive-fantasy-only group by the subsequent making salient of the standard. The same argument would apply to the negative-reality-only group. If the subjects had already had a set standard or a goal, making the discrepant reality salient should have led to motivating effects guided by subjects' expectations.

The contrasting of mental images about wish fulfillment and the status quo do something to motivation that goes beyond the effects of the sole existence of discrepancies. We know this because the mere availability of the respective positive and negative aspects failed to show the motivational effects of expectations. It may be, then, that when people rehearse the discrepant aspects in their minds' eyes, their positive fantasies are turned into something that definitely needs to be achieved or relinquished, depending on subjects' expectations. In other words, only when expectations are high these fantasies acquire a binding quality and thus become goals: People feel that they have to fulfill these fantasies in real life.

CONCLUSION

To come back to the question of whether realism or illusory optimism is beneficial, it seems that both positions are true. Clearly, optimistic thinking has beneficial effects on health and performance when it is operationalized via expectations. However, a matter-of-fact view of the negative reality is crucial, too. What seems necessary in order to translate both into motivation is fantasy—a positive vision of what the future may hold. Oddly enough, a positive vision also seems necessary to advance pessimistic expectations and reflections on the negative reality into disengagement. Maybe we need to consider not only the question of how much optimistic thinking there is, or in what situation optimistic thinking occurs, but also the question of how various kinds of thinking about the future translate optimistic expectations into motivation and action.

REFERENCES

Abramson, L. Y., Seligman, M. E. P., & Teasdale, J. D. (1978). Learned helplessness in humans: Critique and reformulation. *Journal of Abnormal Psychology, 87,* 49–74.

Allport, G. W. (1955). *Becoming: Basic considerations for a psychology of personality.* New Haven, CT: Yale University Press.

Atkinson, J. W. (1957). Motivational determinants of risk- taking behavior. *Psychological Review, 64,* 359–372.

Bandura, A. (1977). Self-efficacy: Toward a unifying theory of behavioral change. *Psychological Review, 84,* 191–215.

Bandura, A. (1991). Self-regulation of motivation through anticipatory and self-reactive mechanisms. In R. Dienstbier (Ed.), *Nebraska Symposium on Motivation: Vol 38. Perspectives on motivation* (pp. 69–164). Lincoln: University of Nebraska Press.

Bandura, A. (in press). *Self-efficacy: The exercise of control.* New York: W. H. Freeman.

Bandura, A., Cioffi, D., Taylor, C. B., & Brouillard, M. E. (1988). Perceived self-efficacy in coping with cognitive stressors and opioid activation. *Journal of Personality and Social Psychology, 55,* 479–488.

Baumeister, R. F. (1989). The optimal margin of illusion. *Journal of Social and Clinical Psychology, 8,* 176–189.

Bernier, M., & Avard, J. (1986). Self-efficacy, outcome, and attrition in a weight-reduction program. *Cognitive Therapy and Research, 10,* 319–338.

Brownell, K. D. (1989). *The LEARN program for weight control.* Dallas, TX: Brownell & Hager.

Burger, J. M., & Burns, L. (1988). The illusion of unique invulnerability and the use of effective contraception. *Personality and Social Psychology Bulletin, 14,* 264–270.

Carver, C. S., & Scheier, M. F. (1981). *Attention and self-regulation: A control-theory approach to human behavior.* New York: Springer.

Chambliss, C. A., & Murray, E. J. (1979). Efficacy attribution, locus of control, and weight loss. *Cognitive Therapy and Research, 3,* 349–353.

Colvin, C. R., & Block, J. (1994). Do positive illusions foster mental health? An examination of the Taylor and Brown formulation. *Psychological Bulletin, 116,* 3–20.

Corbin, C. B. (1972). Mental practice. In W. P. Morgan (Ed.), *Ergogenic aids and muscular performance* (pp. 93–118). New York: Academic Press.

Duval, S., & Wicklund, R. A. (1972). *A theory of objective self-awareness.* New York: Academic Press.

Erdelyi, M. H. (1990). Repression, reconstruction, and defense: History and the integration of the psychoanalytic and experimental frameworks. In J. L. Singer (Ed.), *Repression and dissociation* (pp. 1–31). Chicago: University of Chicago Press.

Ericsson, K. A., & Simon, H. A. (1980). Verbal reports as data. *Psychological Review, 87,* 215–251.

Ericsson, K. A., & Simon, H. A. (1993). *Protocol analysis: Verbal reports as data.* Cambridge, MA: MIT Press.

Felton, B. J., & Revenson, T. A. (1984). Coping with chronic illness: A study of illness controllability and the influence of coping strategies on psychological adjustment. *Journal of Consulting and Clinical Psychology, 52,* 343–353.

Feltz, D. L., & Landers, D. M. (1983). The effects of mental practice on motor skill learning and performance: A meta-analysis. *Journal of Sport Psychology, 5,* 25–57.

Friedman, S. L., Scholnick, E. K., & Cocking, R. R. (1987). *Blueprints for thinking: The role of planning in cognitive development.* Cambridge, England: Cambridge University Press.

Glynn, S. M., & Ruderman, A. J. (1986). The development and validation of an Eating Self-Efficacy Scale. *Cognitive Therapy and Research, 10,* 403–420.

Gollwitzer, P. M. (1990). Action phases and mind-sets. In E. T. Higgins & R. M. Sorrentino (Eds.), *Handbook of motivation and cognition: Foundations of social behavior* (Vol. 2, pp. 53–92). New York: Guilford Press.

Gollwitzer, P. M. (1993). Goal achievement: The role of intentions. In W. Stroebe & M. Hewstone (Eds.), *European review of social psychology* (Vol. 4, pp. 141–185). Chichester, England: Wiley.

Gollwitzer, P. M., Heckhausen, H., & Ratajczak, H. (1990). From weighing to willing: Approaching a change decision through pre- or postdecisional mentation. *Organizational Behavior and Human Decision Processes, 45,* 41–65.

Gollwitzer, P. M., & Kinney, R. F. (1989). Effects of deliberative and implemental mind-sets on illusion of control. *Journal of Personality and Social Psychology, 56,* 531–542.

Goodhart, D. E. (1986). The effects of positive and negative thinking on performance in an achievement situation. *Journal of Personality and Social Psychology, 51,* 117–124.

Heckhausen, H. (1991). *Motivation and action* (P. K. Leppmann, Trans.). Berlin: Springer-Verlag. (Original work published 1989)

Higgins, E. T. (1987). Self-discrepancy: A theory relating self and affect. *Psychological Review, 94,* 319–340.

Huba, G. J., Aneshensel, C. S., & Singer, J. L. (1981). Development of scales for three second-order factors of inner experience. *Multivariate Behavioral Research, 16,* 181–206.

Huba, G. J., Singer, J. L., Aneshensel, C. S., & Antrobus, J. S. (1982). *The Short Imaginal Processes Inventory.* Port Huron, MI: Research Psychologists Press.

Jahoda, M. (1958). *Current concepts of positive mental health.* New York: Basic Books.

James, W. (1950). *The principles of psychology* (2 vols.). New York: Dover. (Original work published 1890)

Jensen, M. R. (1987). Psychobiological factors predicting the course of breast cancer. *Journal of Personality, 55,* 317–342.

Johnson, J. E., Lauver, D. R., & Nail, L. M. (1989). Process of coping with radiation therapy. *Journal of Consulting and Clinical Psychology, 57,* 358–364.

Kipnis, D. (1972). Does power corrupt? *Journal of Personality and Social Psychology, 24,* 33–41.

Klinger, E. (1971). *Structure and functions of fantasy.* New York: Wiley.

Klinger, E. (1975). Consequences of commitment to and disengagement from incentives. *Psychological Review, 82,* 1–25.
Klinger, E. (1977). *Meaning and void: Inner experience and the incentives in people's lives.* Minneapolis: University of Minnesota Press.
Klinger, E. (1987). The interview questionnaire technique: Reliability and validity of a mixed idiographic–nomothetic measure of motivation. In J. N. Butcher & C. D. Spielberger (Eds.), *Advances in personality assessment* (Vol. 6, pp. 31–47). Hillsdale, NJ: Erlbaum.
Klinger, E. (1990). *Daydreaming: Using waking fantasy and imagery for self-knowledge and creativity.* Los Angeles: Tarcher.
Klinger, E., Barta, S. G., & Maxeiner, M. E. (1980). Motivational correlates of thought content frequency and commitment. *Journal of Personality and Social Psychology, 39,* 1222–1237.
Kunda, Z. (1990). The case for motivated reasoning. *Psychological Bulletin, 108,* 480–498.
Leon, G. R., Sternberg, B., & Rosenthal, B. S. (1984). Prognostic indicators of success or relapse in weight reduction. *International Journal of Eating Disorders, 3,* 15–24.
Locke, E. A., & Latham, G. P. (1990). *A theory of goal setting and task performance.* Englewood Cliffs, NJ: Prentice-Hall.
Markus, H., & Nurius, P. (1986). Possible selves. *American Psychologist, 41,* 954–969.
Marlatt, G. A., Baer, J. S., & Quigley, L. A. (1995). Self-efficacy and addictive behavior. In A. Bandura (Ed.), *Self-efficacy in changing societies.* New York: Cambridge.
Marlatt, G. A., & Gordon, J. R. (Eds.). (1985). *Relapse prevention: Maintenance strategies in the treatment of addictive behaviors.* New York: Guilford Press.
Maslow, A. H. (1954). *Motivation and personality.* New York: Harper & Row.
McClelland, D. C. (1980). Motive dispositions: The merits of operant and respondent measures. In L. Wheeler (Ed.), *Review of personality and social psychology* (Vol. 1, pp. 10–41). Beverly Hills, CA: Sage.
McClelland, D. C., Atkinson, J. W., Clark, R. A., & Lowell, E. L. (1953). *The achievement motive.* New York: Appleton-Century-Crofts.
Mischel, W. (1973). Toward a cognitive social learning reconceptualization of personality. *Psychological Review, 80,* 252–283.
Mischel, W., Ebbesen, E. B., & Zeiss, A. R. (1972). Cognitive and attentional mechanisms in delay of gratification. *Journal of Personality and Social Psychology, 21,* 204–218.
Murray, H. A. (1938). *Explorations in personality.* New York: Oxford University Press.
Norem, J. K., & Cantor, N. (1986). Anticipatory and post hoc cushioning strategies: Optimism and defensive pessimism in "risky" situations. *Cognitive Therapy and Research, 10,* 347–362.
Oettingen, G., Böhringer, B., & Losert, A. (1995). *The emergence of motivation: The interplay of fantasies about the future and reflections on the presence.* Unpublished manuscript, Max Planck Institute for Human Development and Education at Berlin, Germany.
Oettingen, G., Losert, A., Wood, B., Kazak, A. E., & Nathanson, M. (1995). *Expectancy, fantasy, and success in three life domains: The impact of positive thinking is not always positive.* Unpublished manuscript, Max Planck Institute for Human Development and Education at Berlin, Germany.
Oettingen, G., & Wadden, T. A. (1991). Expectation, fantasy, and weight loss: Is the impact of positive thinking always positive? *Cognitive Therapy and Research, 15,* 167–175.
Peterson, C., & Bossio, L. M. (1991). *Health and optimism.* New York: Free Press.

Peterson, C., & Seligman, M. E. P. (1984). Causal explanations as a risk factor for depression: Theory and evidence. *Psychological Review, 91,* 347–374.

Peterson, C., Seligman, M. E. P., & Vaillant, G. E. (1988). Pessimistic explanatory style is a risk factor for physical illness: A thirty-five-year longitudinal study. *Journal of Personality and Social Psychology, 55,* 23–27.

Peterson, L. (1989). Coping by children undergoing stressful medical procedures: Some conceptual, methodological, and therapeutic issues. *Journal of Consulting and Clinical Psychology, 57,* 380–387.

Rogers, C. R. (1951). *Client-centered therapy: Its current practice, implications, and theory.* Boston: Houghton Mifflin.

Scheier, M. F., & Carver, C. S. (1985). Optimism, coping, and health: Assessment and implications of generalized outcome expectancies. *Health Psychology, 4,* 219–247.

Scheier, M. F., & Carver, C. S. (1992). Effects of optimism on psychological and physical well-being: Theoretical overview and empirical update. *Cognitive Therapy and Research, 16,* 201–228.

Scheier, M. F., Matthews, K. A., Owens, J. F., Magovern, G. J., Sr., Lefebvre, R. C., Abbott, R. A., & Carver, C. S. (1989). Dispositional optimism and recovery from coronary artery bypass surgery: The beneficial effects on physical and psychological well-being. *Journal of Personality and Social Psychology, 57,* 1024–1040.

Seligman, M. E. P., Peterson, C., Kaslow, N. J., Tanenbaum, R. L., Alloy, L. B., & Abramson, L. Y. (1984). Attributional style and depressive symptoms among children. *Journal of Abnormal Psychology, 93,* 235–238.

Sherman, S. J., Skov, R. B., Hervitz, E. F., & Stock, C. B. (1981). The effects of explaining hypothetical future events: From possibility to probability to actuality and beyond. *Journal of Experimental Social Psychology, 17,* 142–158.

Showers, C. (1992). The motivational and emotional consequences of considering positive or negative possibilities for an upcoming event. *Journal of Personality and Social Psychology, 63,* 474–484.

Singer, J. L. (1966). *Daydreaming.* New York: Random House.

Singer, J. L. (1988). Sampling ongoing consciousness and emotional experience: Implications for health. In M. J. Horowitz (Ed.), *Psychodynamics and cognition* (pp. 297–346). Chicago: University of Chicago Press.

Singer, J. L., & Antrobus, J. S. (1963). A factor-analytic study of daydreaming and conceptually-related cognitive and personality variables. *Perceptual and Motor Skills, 17,* 187–209 (Monograph Suppl. 3-V17).

Singer, J. L., & Antrobus, J. S. (1972). Daydreaming, imaginal processes, and personality: A normative study. In P. Sheehan (Ed.), *The function and nature of imagery* (pp. 175–202). New York: Academic Press.

Singer, J. L., & Bonanno, G. A. (1990). Personality and private experience: Individual variations in consciousness and in attention to subjective phenomena. In L. A. Pervin (Ed.), *Handbook of personality: Theory and research* (pp. 419–444). New York: Guilford Press.

Singer, J. L., & Pope, K. S. (1978). The use of imagery and fantasy techniques in psychotherapy. In J. L. Singer & K. S. Pope (Eds.), *The power of human imagination: New methods in psychotherapy* (pp. 3–34). New York: Plenum Press.

Skinner, E. A., Chapman, M., & Baltes, P. B. (1988). Control, means–ends, and agency beliefs: A new conceptualization and its measurement during childhood. *Journal of Personality and Social Psychology, 54,* 117–133.

Stotland, S., & Zuroff, D. C. (1991). Relations between multiple measures of dieting self-efficacy and weight change in a behavioral weight control program. *Behavior Therapy, 22,* 47–59.

Suls, J., & Wan, C. K. (1989). Effects of sensory and procedural information on coping with stressful medical procedures and pain: A meta-analysis. *Journal of Consulting and Clinical Psychology, 57,* 372–379.

Taylor, S. E. (1983). Adjustment to threatening events: A theory of cognitive adaptation. *American Psychologist, 11,* 1161–1173.

Taylor, S. E. (1989). *Positive illusions: Creative self-deception and the healthy mind.* New York: Basic Books.

Taylor, S. E., & Brown, J. D. (1988). Illusion and well-being: A social psychological perspective on mental health. *Psychological Bulletin, 103,* 193–210.

Taylor, S. E., & Brown, J. D. (1994). Positive illusions and well-being revisited: Separating fact from fiction. *Psychological Bulletin, 116,* 21–27.

Taylor, S. E., & Fiske, S. T. (1978). Salience, attention, and attribution: Top of the head phenomena. *Advances in Experimental Social Psychology, 11,* 249–288.

Taylor, S. E., & Schneider, S. K. (1989). Coping and the simulation of events. *Social Cognition, 7,* 174–194.

Wicklund, R. A., & Gollwitzer, P. M. (1982). *Symbolic self-completion.* Hillsdale, NJ: Erlbaum.

CHAPTER 12

Dynamics of Action Identification

Volatility and Structure in the Mental Representation of Behavior

Robin R. Vallacher
James Kaufman

Introspection tells us that the mind is a busy place. Holding onto a single thought or image, and in effect freezing the stream of consciousness, is an impossible task (the dubious claims of Zen masters aside). No matter how familiar, simple, or mundane the topic, one's thoughts seem to arise spontaneously, briefly present themselves on the Cartesian theater screen (Dennett, 1991), and then vanish back into the subconscious realm, only to be replaced immediately by other seizing but ephemeral thoughts. Particularly when thinking about one's own behavior—past acts, current conduct, or impending courses of action—the turnover in mental content can have an unpredictable, almost chaotic feel to it, as disparate memories, images, and concerns stumble over one another in seemingly whimsical fashion. The flow of thought, moreover, does not stop for lack of new information, but instead seems to have a rhythm all its own, coursing through one's consciousness unabated even when cut off from external prompts and instigations (cf. Wegner, 1994).

Psychology, however, tells us that the mind is a place of equilibrium. One may experience fairly steady turnover in thought, but, far from being a turbulent flow, this succession is orderly and highly constrained. In contrast to James's (1890/1950) stream of consciousness, the image here is one of architecture, with the various elements fitting together to form a reasonably coherent and stable structure. And whereas introspection suggests heightened volatility when the object of thought is one's own behavior, psychological wisdom suggests that thoughts become particularly coherent and stable when considering personal conduct. The assumption of cognitive equilibrium in personal action understanding finds explicit expression in schema theories (e.g., Markus, 1980; Taylor & Crocker, 1981), as well as in the various permutations of dissonance theory (e.g., Aronson, 1992; Festinger, 1957; Schlenker, 1992), and is implicit in a host of theories trading on such notions as balance, consistency, congruity, and verification (e.g., Heider, 1958; Rokeach, 1968; Swann, 1990). With the emphasis on inertia and equilibrium in action understanding, the undeniable volatility in thought is given relatively short shrift; it is often simply dismissed as noise obscuring a stable signal.

We suggest that the personal sense of turbulence in thought is a valid insight into the nature of action understanding. But we also suggest that such volatility is not inconsistent with psychology's assumptions concerning mental equilibrium and stability. Indeed, volatility and structure are complementary aspects of mind; working in tandem, they enable cognitive and behavioral accommodation to new events and contingencies, and thereby serve to regulate one's interactions with the world. Our aim in this chapter is to explore the interplay between dynamism and structure that provides the basis for effective and meaningful action. We begin by providing some theoretical background for the mental representation and control of action.

BASICS OF ACTION UNDERSTANDING AND CONTROL

Two people performing what appears to be the same act may have vastly different notions of what they are doing. One person may be thinking of his or her behavior as "taking a train from Copenhagen to Munich," for instance, while someone else may think of the same behavior as "getting to a conference." It is also the case that the same person performing the same act can have different representations of the act at different times. What starts out as "getting to a conference," for instance, may become "taking a train," "traveling for 10 hours," "becoming sleep-deprived," or "having an adventure" at various times before, during, and after the act. These observations signal two basic points about the personal understanding of action. First, there are a number of possible ways of identifying a given action. Second, there must be some process at work that determines which identification is embraced by the performer as the act's prepotent identity in a given circumstance or at a given time. Both these points are addressed in action identification theory (Vallacher & Wegner, 1985, 1987; Wegner & Vallacher, 1986).

Levels of Action Representation

On the first point, it is helpful to note that the various identities for an act can be arranged in a cognitive hierarchy ranging from detailed, mechanistic depictions of the action ("low-level identities") to comprehensive, consequence-defined depictions ("high-level identities"). Thus, taking a train to Munich could be identified in molecular terms as "sitting in a seat," "looking out the window," "dealing with the toilet facilities," and "communicating with cabin mates"; in somewhat higher-level terms as "traveling" or "getting to a conference"; and in yet higher-level terms as "adding to one's life experiences" or "straining international relations."

A partial resolution of the second point centers on the factors shown to influence the level at which an action is identified (e.g., Vallacher & Wegner, 1987). Foremost among these are those associated with the personal difficulty of the action. If the act is unfamiliar, time-consuming, or effortful, for example, it is likely to be identified in relatively low-level terms. If the action is familiar and can be executed with relatively little effort, on the other hand, it is likely to be identified in terms of its higher-level goals, effects, and implications. Even an action that is well learned and relatively easy, however, can come to be identified in low-level terms if the performance of the action is disrupted in some way (e.g., Wegner, Vallacher, Macomber, Wood, & Arps, 1984). So, although there is commonly a host of potential ways of identifying a given action, the particular identity that assumes prepotence is constrained by the personal ease with which the action can be performed at a particular time.

The concept of identification level is useful in thinking about the mental control of action. Undertaking an action with a relatively high-level identity for the act in mind is tantamount to having a goal or plan for the action, and thus is consistent with theories that emphasize goal-directedness and purposefulness in human action (e.g., Carver & Scheier, 1981; Emmons, Chapter 14, this volume; Gollwitzer, Chapter 13, this volume). The fact that actions can also be undertaken with relatively low-level identities in mind, however, serves as a reminder that broad goals must often be broken down into more basic subgoals in order to be implemented successfully. In such instances, action can become reactive to immediate situational cues and contingencies, including those that hold potential for subverting the broader concern one originally had in mind (cf. Vallacher, 1993). When this occurs, action can appear to be unplanned, reactive, or even impulsive, rather than simply the strategic implementation of a broad goal or plan.

Of course, any action can be represented in terms of larger goals and plans as long as one does not have to perform it. But in the conduct of action itself, a sustained high-level orientation is typically limited to acts that can be performed relatively effortlessly and automatically, with lower-level control (concern with details and immediate situational constraints) assuming prepotence for actions that are difficult or novel or that have been disrupted in some way. Although lower-level control may help to achieve one's higher-level objectives, it is also possible for the original plan to become derailed instead, with action taking off in a new direction that is at odds with what one had in mind at the outset.

The relation between action difficulty and identification level also specifies the likely quality of attempts at action control. When an action is personally easy or familiar, performance tends to be facilitated by a high-level (goal) orientation; when an action is personally difficult or unfamiliar, performance tends to be undermined by prepotent high-level identification and facilitated by maintaining a lower-level orientation (e.g., Vallacher, Wegner, & Somoza, 1989; Vallacher, Wegner, McMahan, Cotter, & Larsen, 1992). Thus, blanket statements about the relative merits of focusing on a goal versus attending to detail provide unsatisfactory generalizations about optimal performance. The optimal mode of action control instead is dictated by the amount of attention necessary to execute the action effectively.

The Emergence Process

Despite the utility of low-level identification in many instances, it does not seem to be a personally satisfactory way of thinking about one's behavior (see Vallacher & Wegner, 1985, 1987; Wegner & Vallacher, 1986). People seem to prefer instead to think about their action in more comprehensive, meaning-laden terms, even when such higher-level identities provide insufficient guides to action performance. In talking with someone, for example, one normally thinks about one's action as "exchanging information," "impressing someone," "having a good time," and so forth, rather than as "uttering words" or "moving one's lips" (Vallacher et al., 1992). In effect, people maintain their actions with respect to lower-level identities only when they have to because of difficulty or disruption. When a more comprehensive identity for an action is available, that identity provides an avenue of emergence from the low-level state.

There is little mystery regarding the basic features of action emergence. A number of investigations have shown that when people are induced to think about what they are doing in relatively low-level terms, they become acutely sensitive to the context surrounding the act and embrace whatever cues to higher-level identification the context provides (see Vallacher, 1993). Subjects who were asked to think about the details of their participation in a recent social interaction, for example, became very accepting of feedback suggesting that they had demonstrated either cooperative or competitive personality tendencies in their behavior (Wegner, Vallacher, Kiersted, & Dizadji, 1986). The subjects apparently were eager to appreciate the higher-level meaning of their specific acts and so became especially vulnerable to whatever high-level cues were provided, even if these had questionable connection to the lower-level details.

Explanations for the preference of high- over low-level identities have largely appealed to analogous phenomena in other areas of psychology. Thus, the idea that people are always sensitive to the larger meanings and implications of what they are doing is reflected, implicitly if not explicitly, in such diverse domains as learning theory (a basic act becomes redefined in terms of its consequences), the mastery of skilled action (discrete acts become automated and integrated into a larger action unit), Gestalt psychology (parts become unified to produce a whole), and existentialism (themes common to distinct actions become the basis for broader awareness of what one has done and who one is). What these phenomena have in common is a tendency to move from the particular to the general, to combine basic features into a larger pattern. This tendency has intuitive appeal in its favor, but begs for a somewhat more fundamental explanation. In the following section, we attempt to develop such a rationale for the emergence process—one that reflects a proposed interplay between volatility and structure in action understanding.

THE DYNAMICS OF ACTION UNDERSTANDING

Viewed only in terms of endpoints, the emergence process seems somewhat magical. One moment a person is thinking about uttering words; the next moment he or she is thinking about impressing a conversation partner or winning an argument. The motive for such a leap in understanding is easy to appreciate, but what enables it to occur? How does a person go from a mechanistic depiction of his or her behavior to a single comprehensive identity for the act? We suggest that the seemingly sudden and effortless emergence of high-level identification for an act obscures relatively volatile mental activity occurring on a very short time scale in a state of low-level identification. This volatility sets the stage for the emergence of higher-level understanding of the action in question.

Instability and Low-Level Understanding

The tendency to identify one's action in low-level terms only when necessary, and to move to a state of higher-level identification when possible, suggests that low-level identification is an unstable state (Vallacher, 1989, 1993). Apart from being transient, however, what are the critical features of low-level identification that qualify it as an unstable state? What role do these features play in shaping the particular state of high-level identification that emerges to form a more stable action representation? In addressing these questions, we provide a way of thinking about the functional interplay between turbulence and structure in action understanding.

"Instability" with respect to natural phenomena means that the system in question fluctuates between qualitatively different states on a relatively rapid and irregular time scale. To say that the weather is unstable, for example, is to note that rain, cloudiness, and sunshine alternate over short intervals of time, and do so in an erratic manner. In analogous fashion, an unstable ceiling fan or a perturbed pendulum rotates in accordance with a number of different orbits, some of which repeat but do so on an irregular basis. Instability has a similar meaning in social systems (Vallacher & Nowak, in press). Instability in public opinion, for example, means that there are dramatic swings over short intervals of time in the prevailing sentiment regarding some event or issue (e.g., Nowak, Lewenstein, & Frejlak, 1995). An unstable society is one in which there is rapid and dramatic turnover in leaders, policies, and even forms of government (e.g., Nowak, Lewenstein, & Szamrej, in press). The instability of dyadic relations can be characterized in much the same way. In an unstable love relationship, for example, the partners may fluctuate between various extremes (passion vs. coldness, jealousy vs. trust, love vs. hate) in a heartbeat, and may do so in a seemingly random temporal pattern (e.g., Vallacher, 1995).

Such instances of instability represent more than noise or breakdown in a system. To the contrary, far from being unavoidable at best or dysfunctional at worst, instability plays a critical role in the functioning of many different kinds of systems. Simply put, the fluctuation among different states and patterns characterizing an unstable system provides the raw material for subsequent self-organization in the system (see, e.g., Davies, 1988; Haken, 1984; Kelso, 1995; Prigogine & Stengers, 1984; Thompson & Stewart, 1987). Self-organization occurs when one of the internally generated states or patterns is locked in by the environment and comes to provide order and stability for the system.

This scenario has recently been documented in research on the neurobiological basis of learning (e.g., Bressler & Freeman, 1991; Skarda & Freeman, 1987). Skarda and Freeman (1987), for example, provided evidence that odor recognition and discrimination (at least in rabbits) is dependent on low-dimensional chaos in the electroencephalographic activity in the olfactory bulb. They suggest that chaos provides the system with a deterministic "I don't know" state, within which new activity patterns can be generated when a novel odor is encountered. Depending on the timing of cue and reinforcement conditions associated with a particular odor, one of the neural activity patterns present in the background chaotic state becomes linked to the odor. Subsequent encounters with that odor thus reinstantiate the selected neural activity pattern.

There is some controversy as to whether deterministic chaos is essential to the emergence of order in biological (and other) systems (see, e.g., commentaries in Skarda & Freeman, 1987). There appears to be little doubt, however, that the generation of new behavior in a system is linked to "critical fluctuations" signaling instability in the system. Thus, the development of interlimb coordination to produce movement (Kelso & DeGuzman, 1991; Turvey, 1990), the synchronization of individual behavior to produce dyadic behavior (Newtson, 1994), the formation of perceptual Gestalten (Hock, Kelso, & Schoner, 1993), and the sudden changes associated with new stages in children's cognitive and motoric development (Thelen, 1992; van Geert, 1991) all represent cases in which the degrees of freedom in a system are suddenly reduced to produce a single pattern that provides coherence and stability for the system. Presumably, such self-organization in biological and psychological systems could not occur without the proliferation of possible organizing patterns. In effect, instability provides the menu from which a particular item is chosen to enslave the lower-level elements in the system.

It is a straightforward matter to cast the transition from low- to high-level action understanding in these terms. One need only assume that low-level identification is an unstable state punctuated by frequent and irregular bursts of possible high-level identities. The sample of high-level states generated in this manner provides the menu from which a particular form of integrative understanding is subsequently selected. The selection criteria are provided by informational cues in the action context (e.g., social feedback, social comparison, criteria of success vs. failure), stored memories relevant to the action (e.g., previous consequences associated with the action), and whatever biases are salient at the time for the person (e.g., self-esteem maintenance, mastery, self-presentation of modesty). With the availability of such criteria, the instability inherent in the low-level identification state eventually gives way to a stable and comprehensive understanding of what one is about to do, is doing, or has done.

Consider, for example, the train ride from Copenhagen. At some point after completion of the trip, the traveler will no doubt settle on a stable, comprehensive view of the act. Prior to achieving such stability, however, he or she may experience a number of different higher-level integrations of the act, each occupying center stage for a brief period of time. Particularly if cues to a single high-level identity are lacking (e.g., the traveler has no prior experience of this kind and has yet to receive feedback from other people), the traveler may entertain a host of evaluatively inconsistent high-level depictions of the act (e.g., yet another demonstration of poor planning vs. a valuable learning experience). More generally, in the process of developing a comprehensive understanding of what one has done, several different and even conflicting provisional integrations may come to mind in relatively rapid succession. This volatile mental activity provides a sample of higher-level identities, one of which is ultimately selected by the environment to provide a stable view of the act. It is in this sense that the state of low-level identification reflects the mental turbulence alluded to at the outset.

Assessment of Dynamism

It is difficult to document empirically the scenario we have described. Assessment of people's act identities, like the assessment of other forms of social thinking, relies on self-report methodology. Beyond the well-documented issues concerning the validity of self-report (social desirability, limits to introspective access, etc.), this assessment strategy cannot hope to capture the fine-grained dynamics purported to be at work in action understanding. The turnover in thought that people experience during periods of instability likely operates on very short time scales, perhaps those involving milliseconds. Even if the validity of self-reports were beyond reproach, it is simply impossible to obtain self-reports of action identification (or of any other cognitive process) with anything approaching that degree of temporal resolution.

A possible solution to this problem is provided by a paradigm recently developed to capture the moment-to-moment fluctuations in judgment of social stimuli (Vallacher & Nowak, 1994b). This approach centers on a computer mouse used to control a cursor on a computer screen. Two symbols are presented on the screen: a small circle positioned in the middle of the screen, and an arrow showing the position of the cursor. The circle is said to represent a particular target of judgment, and the arrow is said to represent the subject. Subjects read a description of the target person, or of an event involving themselves and the target person, and then are asked to think about and evaluate the target person. As they do so, they adjust the arrow in relation to the target circle by moving the mouse so as to express their moment-to-moment feelings about the target over a 2-minute period.

Instructions for the task trade on the idea that evaluation is an implicit approach–avoidance response (cf. Hovland, Janis, & Kelley, 1953). The experimenter informs subjects that if they feel positive about the target, they should move the arrow toward the circle by moving the mouse. By the same token, if subjects feel negative about the target, they should move the arrow away from the target. Subjects' placement of the cursor in relation to the target circle, in other words, represents their global evaluation at each point in time; the closer the cursor is placed to the circle, the more positive the evaluation. If their feelings about the target change, meanwhile, they are instructed to move the arrow toward or away from the target to express these changes. Subjects are free to adjust their position relative to the target as often and as much as is necessary to reflect their feelings about the target as they continue to think about him or her. Movement of the cursor, then, signals instability in global evaluation; the more movement in a given period of time, the greater the instability in judgment.

A 20-second practice session is typically provided, during which subjects move the mouse and observe the corresponding movement on the screen. The screen then clears, a description of the target person appears, and subjects begin the 2-minute mouse procedure. The location of the arrow is assessed 10 times per second for a total of 1,200 potential data points. The program preserves the Cartesian coordinates of each data point, although for purposes of our research thus far, only the absolute distance from the target has been considered. This distance provides a measure of subjects' moment-to-moment feelings about the target. Changes in this distance, in turn, reveal the volatility in subjects' feelings. Special emphasis is given to the speed and acceleration of mouse movements, as these measures provide intuitive and direct assessments of the turnover in subjects' feelings. The greater the speed, the more rapid the turnover; the greater the acceleration, the more unstable the rate of turnover.

Preliminary research suggests that this paradigm provides a window into the dynamic nature of social thinking (Vallacher & Nowak, 1994b; Vallacher, Nowak, & Kaufman, 1994). One study particularly relevant to present concerns looked at the respective dynamism associated with judgments of targets likely to generate univalent versus ambivalent feelings in subjects (Vallacher et al., 1994). Subjects were asked to think about one of three acquaintances: someone they liked (univalent positive), someone they disliked (univalent negative), or someone about whom they felt ambivalent. As they thought about the target, they used the mouse to express their moment-to-moment feelings about him or her.

For each target, we expected to find evidence of initial instability in evaluation as subjects experienced a succession of different thoughts about him or her. The degree of instability was reflected in the speed and acceleration of mouse movements, with rapid and irregular changes in evaluation signaling greater instability. For the univalent (liked and disliked) targets, this instability was expected to be short-lived as subjects settled on a relatively stable judgment of the person. For the mixed-valence target, however, the instability in judgment was not expected to dissipate, but rather to remain relatively high throughout the 2-minute period as subjects continued to experience diverse feelings about the target.

These predictions were confirmed in analyses that examined the distance, speed, and acceleration measures during the first 40 seconds and again during the final 40 seconds of the mouse task. Each target was associated with a unique pattern of dynamism. Initial judgments of the univalent positive target tended to oscillate at a moderate and stable frequency (moderate speed, low acceleration), and on average were relatively positive (close to the target circle). By the final period, however, this oscillation had dampened considerably, with the evaluation stabilizing on a more extreme positive position (closer to the target circle). A similar form of oscillation at the outset was observed for the univalent negative target, although the judgment on average was far more negative (distant from the target circle). This oscillation also tended to dampen over time, with judgment stabilizing on a more negative value (farther from the target circle). For the univalent targets, then, there was evidence of initial dynamism giving way to a relatively stable and polarized judgment.

A fundamentally different pattern was observed for the mixed-valence target. The oscillation in judgment at the outset was faster and less stable (higher speed and acceleration), indicating that subjects were experiencing a rapid and irregular succession of different feelings about the target. Nor did this oscillation pattern change over time; the speed and acceleration of movement at the end of the mouse period was the same as that at the beginning. Finally, unlike the results obtained for the univalent targets, average evaluation (distance from the target circle) did not change over time, but remained approximately halfway between the respective evaluations of the two univalent targets. It is worth noting here that polarization in judgment has been observed in research on thought-induced attitude change, but only for social stimuli associated with well-developed schemas and conflict-free representations (e.g., Tesser & Leone, 1977; Liberman & Chaiken, 1991). The effects we observed concerning change in average evaluation and dynamism for univalent versus mixed-valence targets in this study are consistent with such findings.

The results of the Vallacher et al. (1994) study suggest that the mouse paradigm is a viable means of assessing the moment-to-moment dynamism of social thinking (see Vallacher & Nowak, 1994b, for a summary of research to date employing this approach). In a more specific sense, the study provides encouraging support for the idea that instability in evaluation is associated with fluctuation between different global states. Although instability of this kind can be an unpleasant experience, particularly if extended for long periods of time, it may be a necessary precondition for cognitive growth. Moment-to-moment variation in feelings about a social stimulus (e.g., a new acquaintance, a political figure, an unusual event) represents a condition in which the cognitive system is not ready to settle down on a stable equilibrium, but rather samples different evaluative states. If the various states can be integrated, or if one of the states becomes locked in by some environmental influence (e.g., social feedback, new information), movement between different evaluative states sets the stage for the evolution of a representation that provides coherent and stable understanding.

Dynamism and Identification Level

The state of low-level identification, as we have described it, would seem to have much in common dynamically with ambivalence. In both cases, there is instability in thought as the mind samples different comprehensive ways of thinking about the focal target (i.e., the person or action). Like the ambivalent judge, then, we would expect a person in a low-level state to show rapid and irregular changes in evaluation as different considerations of the action succeed one another in the stream of consciousness.

Low-level identification differs from ambivalence in a crucial respect, however. "Ambivalence" refers to a state in which higher-level meanings are not easily integrated (e.g., Scott, Osgood, & Peterson, 1979). An acquaintance about whom a person feels ambivalent, for instance, is judged to have both good and bad qualities, neither of which set is sufficiently salient or significant to reduce the salience of the other. So although the judge is sampling different higher-level images of the person, there is no guarantee that one of them will come to supplant the others and establish judgmental coherence. In contrast, low-level identification lends itself to the emergence of a single prepotent high-level identity. The sampling of higher-level identities that occurs in this state is not an indication of conflict, then, but rather a necessary stage in the evolution of thought concerning a course of action. Presumably, once a signal in the environment locks in a particular high-level identity, the person's thoughts will stabilize. In this sense, the temporal trajectory of someone in a state of low-level identification should more closely resemble that of someone judging a univalent target than that of someone judging a mixed valence target.

We recently tested this reasoning regarding dynamism and low-level identification (Vallacher, Kaufman, Canaday, & Bagby, 1993). Subjects were asked to think about a recent interaction with someone of the same sex and to provide five one-sentence descriptions of their behavior in this interaction. Half the subjects were instructed to generate low-level descriptions (e.g., particular words and gestures), and half were instructed to generate higher-level descriptions (e.g., opinions and attitudes conveyed). In both cases, they used the keyboard to enter the descriptions into the computer. The descriptions were displayed on the monitor for the next minute, during which time subjects were instructed to look at and think about each description.[1]

All subjects then used the mouse procedure to indicate their moment-to-moment feelings about themselves having performed the action they had just described. For this purpose, the instructions used in the Vallacher et al. (1994) study were modified so that the target circle represented themselves rather than an acquaintance. Thus, positive feelings about themselves were expressed by moving the cursor closer to the circle, whereas negative feelings were expressed by moving the cursor farther from the circle. As in the earlier study, the primary dependent measures were average distance from the target and the speed and acceleration of mouse movements, computed both during the first 40 seconds and the final 40 seconds of the 2-minute mouse task.

We had no reason to expect differences between the high- and low-level conditions with respect to the central tendency in subjects' feelings about themselves, and none were observed. When the data were collapsed over time, the cursor was positioned relatively close to the target circle for subjects in both conditions, suggesting moderately positive feelings on average. Differences between the high- and low-level conditions were expected with respect to the dynamism measures, however. Subjects in the low-level condition were expected to show rapid and irregular fluctuations in their moment-to-moment feelings at the outset, similar to the pattern observed for ambivalence in the earlier study. Over time, however, these subjects were expected to show signs of emergence to a relatively stable identity for their action. Hence, fluctuation in feelings about themselves were expected to give way to a relatively stable position vis-à-vis the target circle. In contrast, we expected subjects in the high-level condition to demonstrate less volatility in their moment-to-moment feelings about the self, as they presumably had a relatively stable way of thinking about their action by the time they began the mouse procedure. Their degree of volatility, moreover, was expected to be fairly constant from the initial to the final 40-second mouse period.

The results were consistent with these expectations. Subjects in the low-level condition demonstrated greater speed and acceleration during the initial portion of the judgment period than did subjects in the high level condition. Presumably, low-level subjects were moving between different higher-level considerations of the act, each associated with a somewhat different valence. By the end of the 2-minute period, however, the speed and acceleration of mouse movements for these subjects had significantly diminished—although acceleration was still somewhat higher than that observed in the final period for high-level subjects. From the sample of higher-level states, the low-level subjects had begun to lock in on one that provided comprehensive understanding of the act, but this process of emergence apparently was not entirely complete. For their part, subjects in the high-level condition displayed a relatively low degree of speed and acceleration that did not reliably change from the initial to the final 40-second period. High-level subjects presumably went into the mouse task with a fairly comprehensive way of thinking about their behavior, and thus did not entertain alternative identities associated with differing valences.

To provide a feel for the dynamism associated with low- versus high-level action identification, Figures 12.1 and 12.2 show the time series of a representative low-level and a representative high-level subject, respectively. The *x*-axis in these figures represents time (0 to 1,200 seconds), and the *y*-axis represents absolute distance from the target. Inspection of Figure 12.1 reveals the rapid and irregular oscillation characterizing the mouse movements of the low-level subject during the early portion of the judgment period, and the decrease in this dynamism by the end of the period. Figure 12.2, meanwhile, shows the less rapid and more regular oscillations associated with the mouse movements of the high-level subject—a pattern that persisted throughout the judgment period.

Subjects in this study also responded to self-report questions concern-

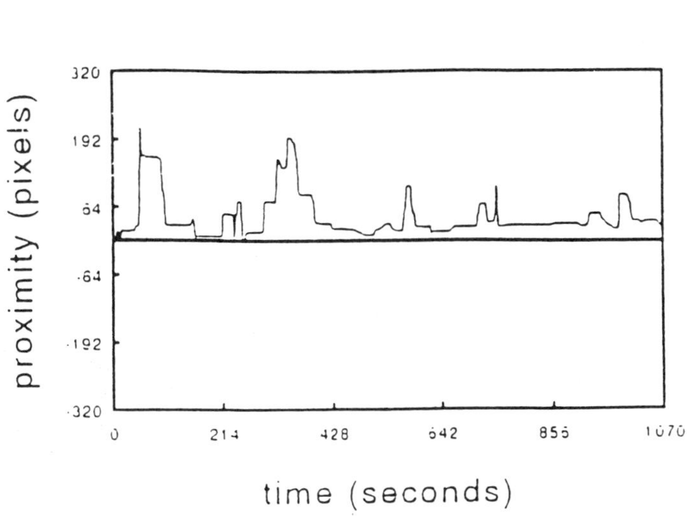

FIGURE 12.1. Distance from target (self) by time for a subject in the low-level condition. Data from Vallacher et al. (1993).

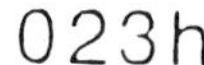

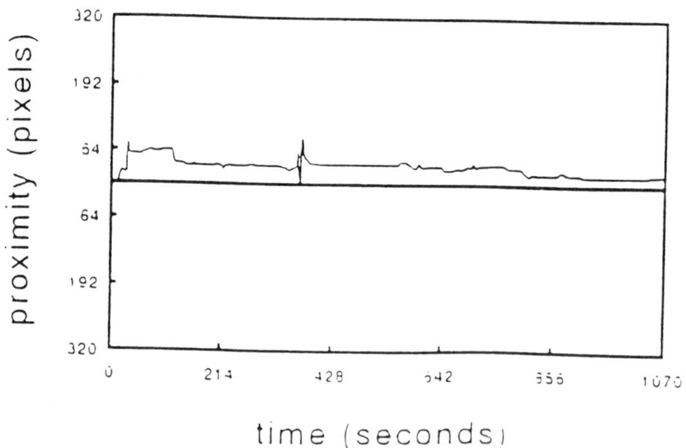

FIGURE 12.2. Distance from target (self) by time for a subject in the high-level condition. Data from Vallacher et al. (1993).

ing the act and themselves. They did so either before or after completing the mouse task. One set of questions assessed whether subjects felt the act they described reflected on themselves; another set assessed the certainty and stability of subjects' evaluation of the act and of themselves for having performed the act. We expected that subjects in the high-level condition would see the act as more indicative of what they were like than would subjects in the low-level condition. We also expected the high-level subjects to indicate greater certainty and stability in their judgment of the act and their performance of it. These predictions are consistent with research on the self-relevance of behavior (e.g., Vallacher & Wegner, 1989).

The predicted differences were observed—but only among subjects who responded to the self-report items before performing the mouse task. For these subjects, the manipulation of identification level was fresh when they were asked to report on their behavior. Low-level subjects, then, were still in a pre-emergence state and so, unlike the high-level subjects, did not have a clear and stable sense of the action's higher-level meanings, including its self-relevant implications (cf. Wegner et al., 1986). Among subjects who completed the mouse task first, however, the impact of the identification level manipulation was notably diminished by the time the self-report questions were encountered. Presumably, subjects in the low-level condition demonstrated at least partial emergence to a stable higher-level understanding by the end of the mouse task. This interpretation, of course, is consistent with what we observed for the dynamism measures.

Caveats on Generalizability

We should note that this study employed a manipulation intended to induce "pure" (nonoverlapping) levels of action identification. Thus, subjects were induced to think about a recent behavior either in exclusively high-level terms or in exclusively low-level terms. This approach is reasonable if one's concern is highlighting the differences (in this case, with respect to dynamics) between these states, but it is potentially misleading in two respects. First, cognitive representations of behavior in everyday life are rarely this pure. People probably undertake and reflect on a majority of their actions under identities that reflect a mix of different levels, with sensitivity both to the implications and to the details of what they are doing or have done. In thinking about a recent interaction, for instance, a person might be sensitive both to the consequences of his or her behavior (e.g., "establishing a relationship") and to the specific behaviors he or she enacted (e.g., "talking rapidly," "maintaining eye contact"), and perhaps to identities intermediate in level (e.g., "discussing campus politics") as well. To say that someone is at a high or a low level, then, is to emphasize the identities most salient for him or her, or to note the relative proportions of identities at different levels (Vallacher & Wegner, 1985).

Our manipulation of identification level could be considered misleading in a more subtle and potentially more significant way. There are two general scenarios under which people identify their actions in relatively low-level terms. People may undertake an action or reflect on its occurrence, first of all, without the benefit of higher-level goals, plans, or considerations. Sometimes people do things on impulse, for example, or are induced without warning to reflect on the details of a past action. This is the basis for the low-level manipulation we employed in the Vallacher et al. (1993) study. Under these conditions, people are especially vulnerable to contextual cues to integrative higher-level identities for the act (e.g., Wegner et al., 1986). Lacking clear avenues of emergence from the low-level state, people in such instances sample possible high-level meanings, each of which may convey different implications for self-evaluation, until they embrace one over the others. This, of course, is the process documented in the Vallacher et al. (1993) study.

There is a second, rather different scenario for low-level identification, however. Quite simply, people tend to adopt lower-level identities out of necessity when their higher-level goals and plans are disrupted or prove too complex to achieve without focusing on means of implementation. In such instances, the high-level orientation may remain in the mental background, ready to reassume prepotence once the lower-level means are implemented. Presumably, with this basis for low-level identification, one would be less inclined to sample alternative higher-level identities as potential avenues of emergence, and thus would be correspondingly less likely to demonstrate the degree of volatility we observed among low-level subjects. A person may have a clear goal for his or her interaction with someone, for example, and then think about his or her behavior in terms of the specific acts necessary to accomplish the goal. Assuming that the person does not lose sight of the larger plan generating the specific acts, he or she is unlikely to demonstrate notable moment-to-moment changes in self-evaluation when prompted later to think about the lower-level features of his or her behavior in the interaction.

Even here, however, there is potential for the kind of volatility demonstrated in the Vallacher et al. (1993) study. Research on action identification has shown that firmly anchored high-level identities can be dislodged by factors that disrupt the conduct of the intended action (e.g., Vallacher et al., 1989, 1992; Wegner et al., 1984). When this occurs, the person becomes as sensitive to new higher-level identities as someone who undertook the act without a higher-level goal or understanding. Presumably, then, if the context fails to provide a salient single identity for the act, the person will sample different possible higher-level meanings in much the same way as did subjects in our study. It remains for future research, of course, to test this possibility, and more generally to delineate the conditions under which goals and plans are effectively erased and subsequently replaced when people are induced to identify their actions in low-level terms.

BACK TO BASICS

Contemporary treatments of human action invariably assign a pivotal role to mental representations in the control of overt behavior (see Atkinson & Birch, 1970; Beckmann & Gollwitzer, 1987; Carver & Scheier, 1981; Frese & Sabini, 1986; Gauld & Shotter, 1977; Ginsburg, Brenner, & von Cranach, 1986; Heckhausen & Gollwitzer, 1987; Norman & Shallice, 1986; Vallacher & Wegner, 1985; von Cranach & Harre, 1982; Wegner & Vallacher, 1987). Particular emphasis is commonly placed on cognitive structures that provide a frame of reference for the generation and understanding of intentional acts. Such a theoretical emphasis has much to recommend it—provided that the dynamics by which structures are created and expressed are given equal billing. Although we have yet to collect data linking the dynamics of action identification to the expression of overt behavior, the rationale outlined above has fairly straightforward implications for such linkage. In this section, we provide a broad outline of these implications, and thereby suggest how the dynamics of mind are tied to the dynamics of action.

States of Mental Dynamics

Not all mental states are equally conducive to the expression of goal-directed behavior. This point is acknowledged, implicitly if not explicitly, in many treatments of human action (e.g., Atkinson & Birch, 1970; Jones & Gerard,

1967; Klinger, 1986; Reither & Staudel, 1986), although the mapping between mental states and action is rarely couched in concrete empirical and operational terms. A noteworthy exception, and one that fits well with our perspective on mental dynamics, is the research program of Gollwitzer and his colleagues (e.g., Beckmann & Gollwitzer, 1987; Heckhausen & Gollwitzer, 1987; Gollwitzer, Chapter 13, this volume). Building on the distinction between "predecisional" and "pre-actional" stages of thought (e.g., Festinger, 1964; Frey, 1986; Jones & Gerard, 1967), this work has identified qualitatively different mind-sets associated with these stages.

In the predecisional stage, the actor is said to have a deliberative state of mind, in which he or she considers possible action goals that are salient and impartially processes information relevant to each of these goals. Thus, the actor entertains, often in fairly rapid succession, the positive and negative implications associated with different courses of action or with different goals for the same action. In deciding how to approach an upcoming interaction, for example, the person may think about the pros and cons associated with such diverse interaction goals as showing sensitivity, offering criticism, and demonstrating wit.

The person's mind-set changes dramatically after he or she has chosen a course of action and decided on a goal for the action. In this pre-actional stage, the person is said to become oriented toward implementing the chosen goal. The vacillation among good and bad features of the action possibilities associated with the predecisional phase thus gives way to an unquestioned commitment to the goal and a focus on its performance-relevant features. It is important to note that, in contrast to dissonance theory, this selectivity in information processing and thought is not in the service of justifying the chosen goal by emphasizing only its positive features. Rather, the goal is accepted as a given, with subsequent thought devoted to how best to achieve the goal. Once the person has decided to show sensitivity in an interaction, for instance, his or her thoughts no longer center on the likely benefits (or possible drawbacks) of having this goal, but rather are given over to the best way of achieving the goal.

The distinction between deliberative and implementational mind-sets corresponds nicely to the distinct patterns of mental dynamics demonstrated in the Vallacher et al. (1993) study. Thus, considering possible actions and goals constitutes a particular manifestation of sampling alternative higher-level identities, whereas maintaining an unequivocal commitment to a single goal represents a manifestation of stable high-level identification. In the former state, the mind is likely to demonstrate evaluative volatility as the person considers the positive and negative implications of various goals (high-level identities), whereas in the latter state the person's mental state is likely to demonstrate little evaluative variability over time because he or she has locked in on a particular high-level orientation. Of course, the sampling of high-level states purportedly demonstrated by subjects in our research was retrospective rather than predecisional. However, given the potential for erasure of high-level identities through low-level inductions (cf. Vallacher, 1993), the volatility we demonstrated for low-level subjects is consistent in principle with the deliberative mind-set observed for subjects in Gollwitzer's research who have yet to commit to a single goal.[2]

Dynamics and the Expression of Action

The action stages perspective suggests, almost by definition, that action is more likely to take place when the person's mind-set is implementational (the pre-actional stage) as opposed to deliberative (the predecisional stage). In terms of action identification dynamics, we would expect the expression of overt behavior to be unlikely when the person is demonstrating heightened volatility reflecting the sampling of different higher-level identities for the action in question. Once the person locks onto a high-level identity that provides integration for the lower-level identities, however, the likelihood of overt behavior should increase dramatically.[3]

It would be unforgivably naive, however, to suggest that people always inhibit behavior during periods of heightened mental dynamism. People clearly act on occasion without the benefit of an unequivocal behavior orientation (Jones & Gerard, 1967), and sometimes with little if any regard for the consequences of their behavior. Indeed, psychologists and laypeople alike commonly sort behavior into two distinct types—one corresponding to goal-directed action, the other to unplanned and impulsive behavior. Strictly speaking, of course, even impulsive behavior is in the service of goals, in the sense that the person undertakes the act with some (low-level) identity for the act in mind (Vallacher & Wegner, 1985). Impulsive behavior, though, tends to be inconsistent and erratic; this suggests that the underlying mental state generating the behavior is similarly inconsistent and erratic, displaying substantial variation on a relatively short time scale. Goal-directed action, in contrast, tends to be relatively stable over long periods of time, reflecting an integrated mental state that dampens moment-to-moment volatility in thought process.

The focus on dynamics, in sum, provides a new perspective on the link among cognition, motivation, and action. In particular, it suggests that the mental states generating action can be characterized in terms of their relative dynamism, and that such differences in dynamism are associated with differences in motivational propensities and action tendencies. Some states are characterized by heightened volatility, with oscillation between evaluatively diverse representations occurring over short intervals of time. This happens when the person has only low-level identities for what he or she has done, is doing, or contemplates doing, and samples possible higher-level identities for the act in question. Because the concern here is with achieving an unambiguous action orientation, the expression of action itself tends to be inhibited. If action does occur, it tends to be impulsive and erratic, reflecting the unstable succession of different representations (goals, concerns, etc.) that can vanish as quickly as they arise.

Things are quite different for mental states characterized by relatively little dynamism. The person in such a state presumably has a more or less stable cognitive structure for his or her behavior. In reflecting on past action, the person is sensitive to an evaluatively consistent set of consequences or self-evaluative implications; in thinking about ongoing or future action, the person is committed to a single goal or anticipated outcome. Because of the integration, stability, and consistency of action understanding in this state, there is less equivocation in the expression of action. Assuming that integration takes the form of a desired goal, the person's motivation in this state centers on implementation, with mental deliberation devoted to how best to achieve one's aims. Because behavior in this state is goal-directed and reflects a stable cognitive structure, it captures what many commentators feel to be the essence of human action.

SUMMING UP: DYNAMICS AND PSYCHOLOGICAL PROCESS

It makes little sense to talk of process without giving explicit consideration to the dimension of time. Yet such consideration is rarely incorporated into research ostensibly concerned with cognitive and behavioral dynamics in social psychology. Everyone acknowledges, of course, that psychological processes occur in real time, but surprisingly little is known about the actual time scales on which these processes unfold and evolve. In the canonical research paradigm, one or more independent variables are assessed at Time 1, and the effects of these manipulations on the dependent variables are assessed at some Time 2. The timing of manipulation and assessment in this approach is typically a matter of convenience and thus may not correspond with the true time scale of the phenomenon under investigation. Even if theoretically meaningful effects are observed, moreover, this approach does not illuminate the intermediate steps in the process that may be occurring on a shorter time scale. So although the traditional approach may be well suited for capturing macro-level changes in phenomena, it is almost certain to miss important elements of the process on a shorter time scale (cf. Vallacher & Nowak, 1994a).

This point can be framed more constructively, in the form of a suggestion for empirical work. In analyzing any phenomenon—be it social judgment, social interaction, intimate relationships, or action identification—it is important to adjust one's temporal resolution as necessary to gain deep insight into the dynamics at work. At the least, investigation of a hypothesized process should not be confined to its overall form (what might be called its macro dynamics), but rather should also attempt to identify any embedded time scales (its micro dynamics). Such work is likely to find that different phenomena are each associated with unique time scales. The course of a social interaction, for example, has an ebb and flow that may be revealed only by analyzing the transaction over small units of time, perhaps minutes or even seconds (cf. Newtson, 1994), whereas the temporal evolution of a romantic relationship may show meaningful punctuation points on a much longer time frame, involving days, weeks, or even months (cf. Baron, Amazeen, & Beek, 1994).

It is also reasonable to suggest that more than one time scale may be operative for a given phenomenon. A social interaction, for example, may be understood in terms of some fairly macro time frame, such as the beginning, middle, and end of the encounter, but also in terms of its shorter-term aspects, such as turn taking in speaking or the moment-to-moment coordination of gestures and facial expressions. Similarly, although a relationship tends to evolve over fairly large units of time, there are nonetheless important fluctuations occurring with finer temporal resolution (e.g., a particular power struggle or an attempt at conflict resolution). It is only by understanding a social-psychological phenomenon with respect to all of its relevant time scales that a true appreciation of the dynamics underlying the phenomenon can be attained (Nowak, Lewenstein, & Vallacher, 1994).

The process of action understanding provides a case in point. Research on action identification theory has succeeded in documenting the general form of the emergence process as it occurs on a broad time scale (see Vallacher, 1993). Without assessing the moment-to-moment dynamics of subjects in a state of low-level identification, however, we would have overlooked the mental turbulence associated with this state—a turbulence that takes the form of sampling high-level states that makes emergence on a longer time scale possible. The paradigm we have developed to provide access to the phenomenology of low-level identification has also revealed a change in time scale once emergence has occurred. It appears that with the emergence of a higher-level depiction of what one has done, the mind effectively slows down, displaying a rate of turnover in mental content that is in line with what models emphasizing the structure and stability of social judgment would suggest.

The importance of exploring the micro dynamics as well as the macro dynamics of action identification—indeed, of any social-psychological process—should come as no surprise. In daily life, after all, we attempt to understand personally relevant and interesting events with varying degrees of temporal resolution, focusing both on rapidly changing components and on the various longer-term effects and consequences. There is no reason why this approach to understanding, which serves us well in our role as lay epistemologists, should not be employed in our role as investigators to understand the process of understanding itself.

ACKNOWLEDGMENTS

We thank John Bargh, Charles Carver, Peter Gollwitzer, and Dan Wegner for their helpful comments on an earlier draft of this chapter.

NOTES

1. Our preliminary research on this topic suggested that this period of time (i.e., approximately 1 minute) is typically necessary for subjects in the low-level condition to begin considering possible higher-level integrations of the basic descriptions they have provided. Prior to that, low-level subjects tend to be too caught up in the details of their behavior to sample possible higher-level identities of the act in question.

2. Gollwitzer and his colleagues identify two other mind-sets, corresponding to the actual conduct of action and the completion of the action (e.g., Beckmann & Gollwitzer, 1987). In terms of the present analysis, we would expect the "actional" mind-set to be associated with relatively low-level identification (assuming the act requires at least some attention to detail) and the "postactional" mind-set to be associated with remergence to relatively high-level identification. In both cases, evaluative volatility should be nominal, although this has yet to be demonstrated in our research program.

3. To demonstrate this mapping of mental dynamics onto behavior, of course, it would be necessary to have subjects think about an action they have an opportunity to perform subsequently, rather than asking them to reflect on a past action, as in the Vallacher et al. (1993) study.

REFERENCES

Atkinson, J. W., & Birch, D. (1970). *The dynamics of action.* New York: Wiley.

Aronson, E. (1992). Return of the oppressed: Dissonance theory makes a comeback. *Psychological Inquiry, 3,* 303–311.

Baron, R. M., Amazeen, P. G., & Beek, P. J. (1994). Local and global dynamics of social relations. In R. R. Vallacher & A. Nowak (Eds.), *Dynamical systems in social psychology* (pp. 111–138). San Diego, CA: Academic Press.

Beckmann, J., & Gollwitzer, P. M. (1987). Deliberative versus implemental states of mind: The issue of impartiality in predecisional and postdecisional information processing. *Social Cognition, 5,* 259–279.

Bressler, S. L., & Freeman, W. J. (1991). Mechanisms of chaotic dynamics in the olfactory system as shown by simultaneous recordings from bulb and cortex. In D. Duke & W. Pritchard (Eds.), *Measuring chaos in the human brain* (pp. 6–16). Singapore: World Scientific.

Carver, C. S., & Scheier, M. F. (1981). *Attention and self-regulation: A control-theory approach to human behavior.* New York: Springer-Verlag.

Davies, P. (1988). *The cosmic blueprint: New discoveries in nature's creative ability to order the universe.* New York: Simon & Schuster.

Dennett, D. C. (1991). *Consciousness explained.* Boston: Little, Brown.

Festinger, L. (1957). *A theory of cognitive dissonance.* Stanford, CA: Stanford University Press.

Festinger, L. (Ed.). (1964). *Conflict, decision, and dissonance.* Stanford, CA: Stanford University Press.

Frese, M., & Sabini, J. (Eds.). (1986). *Goal-directed behavior: The concept of action in psychology.* Hillsdale, NJ: Erlbaum.

Frey, D. (1986). Recent research on selective exposure to information. In L. Berkowitz (Ed.), *Advances in experimental social psychology* (Vol. 19, pp. 41–80). New York: Academic Press.

Gauld, A., & Shotter, J. (1977). *Human action and its psychological investigation.* London: Routledge & Kegan Paul.

Ginsburg, G. P., Brenner, M. J., & von Cranach, M. (Eds.). (1986). *Discovery strategies in the analysis of action.* New York: Academic Press.

Haken, H. (1984). *The science of structure: Synergetics.* New York: Van Nostrand Reinhold.

Heckhausen, H., & Gollwitzer, P. M. (1987). Thought contents and cognitive functioning in motivational versus volitional states of mind. *Motivation and Emotion, 11,* 101–120.

Heider, F. (1958). *The psychology of interpersonal relations.* New York: Wiley.

Hock, H. S., Kelso, J. A. S., & Schoner, G. (1993). Bistability and hysteresis in the organization of apparent motion patterns. *Journal of Experimental Psychology: Human Perception and Performance, 19,* 63–80.

Hovland, C., Janis, I., & Kelley, H. H. (1953). *Communication and persuasion.* New Haven, CT: Yale University Press.

James, W. (1950). *The principles of psychology* (2 vols.). New York: Dover. (Original work published 1890)

Jones, E. E., & Gerard, H. B. (1967). *Foundations of social psychology.* New York: Wiley.

Kelso, J. A. S. (1995). *Dynamic patterns: The self-organization of brain and behavior.* Cambridge, MA: MIT Press.

Kelso, J. A. S., & DeGuzman, G. C. (1991). An intermittency mechanism for coherent and flexible brain and behavioral function. In J. Requin & G. E. Stalmach (Eds.), *Tutorials in motor neuroscience* (pp. 305–310). Dordrecht, The Netherlands: Kluwer.

Klinger, E. (1986). Missing links in action theory. In M. Frese & J. Sabini (Eds.), *Goal-directed behavior: The concept of action in psychology* (pp. 311–319). Hillsdale, NJ: Erlbaum.

Liberman, A., & Chaiken, S. (1991). Value conflict and thought-induced attitude change. *Journal of Experimental Social Psychology, 27,* 203–216.

Markus, H. (1980). The self in thought and memory. In D. M. Wegner & R. R. Vallacher (Eds.), *The self in social psychology* (pp. 102–130). New York: Oxford University Press.

Norman, D. A., & Shallice, T. (1986). Attention to action: Willed and automatic control of behavior. In R. J. Davidson, G. E. Schwartz, & D. Shapiro (Eds.), *Consciousness and self-regulation* (Vol. 4, pp. 1–18). New York: Plenum.

Nowak, A., Lewenstein, M., & Frejlak, P. (1995). Dynamics of public opinion and social change. In R. Hegselman & U. Miller (Eds.), *Chaos and order in nature and theory.* Vienna: Helbin.

Nowak, A., Lewenstein, M., & Szamrej, J. (in press). Bubbles: A model for social transitions. *Scientific American.*

Nowak, A., Lewenstein, M., & Vallacher, R. R. (1994). Toward a dynamical social psychology. In R. R. Vallacher & A. Nowak (Eds.), *Dynamical systems in social psychology* (pp. 279–293). San Diego, CA: Academic Press.

Newtson, D. (1994). The perception and coupling of behavior waves. In R. R. Vallacher & A. Nowak (Eds.), *Dynamical systems in social psychology* (pp. 139–167). San Diego, CA: Academic Press.

Prigogine, I., & Stengers, I. (1984). *Order out of chaos.* New York: Bantam.

Reither, F., & Staudel, T. (1986). Thinking and action. In M. Frese & J. Sabini (Eds.), *Goal-directed behavior: The concept of action in psychology* (pp. 110–122). Hillsdale, NJ: Erlbaum.

Rokeach, M. (1968). *Beliefs, attitudes, and values.* San Francisco: Jossey-Bass.

Schlenker, B. R. (1992). Of shape shifters and theories. *Psychological Inquiry, 3,* 342–344.

Scott, W. A., Osgood, D. W., & Peterson, C. (1979). *Cognitive structure: Theory and measurement of individual differences.* Washington, DC: V. H. Winston.

Skarda, C. A., & Freeman, W. J. (1987). How brains make chaos in order to make sense of the world. *Behavioral and Brain Sciences, 10,* 161–195.

Swann, W. B., Jr. (1990). To be adored or to be known? The interplay of self-enhancement and self-verification. In E. T. Higgins & R. M. Sorrentino (Eds.), *Handbook of motivation and cognition: Foundations of social behavior* (Vol. 2, pp. 408–448). New York: Guilford Press.

Taylor, S. E., & Crocker, J. (1981). Schematic bases of social information processing. In E. T. Higgins, C. P. Herman, & M. P. Zanna (Eds.), *Social cognition: The Ontario Symposium* (Vol. 1, pp. 89–134). Hillsdale, NJ: Erlbaum.

Tesser, A., & Leone, C. (1977). Cognitive schemas and thought as determinants of attitude change. *Journal of Experimental Social Psychology, 13,* 340–356.

Thelen, E. (1992). Development as a dynamic system. *Current Directions in Psychological Science, 1,* 189–193.

Thompson, J. M. P., & Stewart, H. B. (1987). *Nonlinear dynamics and chaos.* New York: Wiley.

Turvey, M. T. (1990). Coordination. *American Psychologist, 45,* 938–953.

Vallacher, R. R. (1989). Action identification as theory and metatheory. In D. W. Schumann (Ed.), *Proceedings of the Society for Consumer Psychology* (pp. 63–68). Washington, DC: American Psychological Association.

Vallacher, R. R. (1993). Mental calibration: Forging a working relationship between mind and action. In D. M. Wegner & J. W. Pennebaker (Eds.), *Handbook of mental control* (pp. 443–472). Englewood Cliffs, NJ: Prentice-Hall.

Vallacher, R. R. (1995, June). Mental dynamics in close relationships. In *Dynamics and temporal systems in personal relationships.* Symposium, International Network on Personal Relationships, Williamsburg, VA.

Vallacher, R. R., Kaufman, J., Canaday, J., & Bagby, S. (1993). [Intrinsic dynamics of action identification]. Unpublished raw data.

Vallacher, R. R., & Nowak, A. (1994a). The chaos in social psychology. In R. R. Vallacher & A. Nowak (Eds), *Dynamical systems in social psychology* (pp. 1–16). San Diego, CA: Academic Press.

Vallacher, R. R., & Nowak, A. (1994b). The stream of social judgment. In R. R. Vallacher & A. Nowak (Eds.), *Dynamical systems in social psychology* (pp. 251–277). San Diego, CA: Academic Press.

Vallacher, R. R., & Nowak, A. (in press). The emergence of dynamical social psychology. *Psychological Inquiry.*

Vallacher, R. R., Nowak, A., & Kaufman, J. (1994). Intrinsic dynamics of social judgment. *Journal of Personality and Social Psychology, 67,* 20–34.

Vallacher, R. R., & Wegner, D. M. (1985). *A theory of action identification.* Hillsdale, NJ: Erlbaum.

Vallacher, R. R., & Wegner, D. M. (1987). What do people think they're doing? Action identification and human behavior. *Psychological Review, 94,* 3–15.

Vallacher, R. R., & Wegner, D. M. (1989). Levels of personal agency: Individual variation in action identification. *Journal of Personality and Social Psychology, 57,* 660–671.

Vallacher, R. R., Wegner, D. M., & Somoza, M. P. (1989). That's easy for you to say: Action identification and speech fluency. *Journal of Personality and Social Psychology, 56,* 199–208.

Vallacher, R. R., Wegner, D. M., McMahan, S. C., Cotter, J., & Larsen, K. A. (1992). On winning friends and influencing people: Action identification and self-presentation success. *Social Cognition, 10,* 335–355.

van Geert, P. (1991). A dynamic systems model of cognitive and language growth. *Psychological Review, 98,* 3–53.

von Cranach, M., & Harre, R. (Eds.). (1982). *The analysis of action.* Cambridge, England: Cambridge University Press.

Wegner, D. M. (1994). Ironic processes of mental control. *Psychological Review, 101,* 34–52.

Wegner, D. M., & Vallacher, R. R. (1986). Action identification. In R. M. Sorrentino & E. T. Higgins (Eds.), *Handbook of motivation and cognition: Foundations of social behavior* (Vol. 1, pp. 550–582). New York: Guilford Press.

Wegner, D. M., & Vallacher, R. R. (1987). The trouble with action. *Social Cognition, 5,* 179–190.

Wegner, D. M., Vallacher, R. R., Kiersted, G., & Dizadji, D. (1986). Action identification in the emergence of social behavior. *Social Cognition, 4,* 18–38.

Wegner, D. M., Vallacher, R. R., Macomber, G., Wood, R., & Arps, K. (1984). The emergence of action. *Journal of Personality and Social Psychology, 46,* 269–279.

SECTION B

Planning and Coordinating Action

Preparing to act on one's goals does not only concern the mental construction of goal contents. It also extends to thinking and reflecting about the implementation of these goals. This has been alluded to in some of the chapters in Section A of Part III, and it is discussed extensively in the chapters in Section B. As long as the implementation of goals does not take habitual routes, conflicts may arise: Should we act here or there, now or later, this way or another? And how should we deal with obstacles and disruptions? Gollwitzer (Chapter 13) discusses how planning, in the sense of committing oneself to specific implementational routes, effectively alleviates such conflicts. But effective planning needs to consider the implementation of goals in concert, because making progress with one goal (or set of goals) may hinder the successful implementation of others. Emmons (Chapter 14) points out that this is particularly true for enduring and recurring goals, which he calls "personal strivings." Only if the various strivings of a person are integrated into a meaningful whole may the individual derive satisfaction from his or her goal pursuits. The question of how multiple goal pursuits are negotiated most effectively is analyzed by Cantor and Blanton (Chapter 15). These authors focus on the many goals originating from a person's various life tasks. Typical strategies of negotiating multiple goal pursuits are distinguished, and their benefits and costs are discussed in comparison.

Gollwitzer raises the question of whether planning promotes goal achievement by alleviating volitional problems. These problems are linked to getting started effectively with one's goal pursuit (e.g., warding off distractions) and bringing a goal pursuit already begun to successful completion (e.g., overcoming obstacles, such as unexpected difficulties or disruptions). The results of a series of experiments suggest that initiating goal-directed actions is facilitated because planning creates a perceptual readiness for and guides a person's attention toward relevant opportunities and means. In addition, planning heightens the individual's readiness to respond effectively once these opportunities and means are encountered, and it suppresses distractive doubts about the goal's feasibility and desirability. Planning also facilitates the completion of an initiated goal pursuit, as it helps to mobilize effort in the face of difficulties, wards off distractions by focusing the individual's attention on the ongoing goal pursuit, and furthers the undelayed resumption of a goal pursuit when disruption occurs. Gollwitzer explains the effects of planning by employing two different concepts (i.e., implemental mind-sets and implementation intentions), which are derived from a model of action phases. This model breaks down the course of goal achievement into a number of consecutive tasks, one of which is planning the implementation of the goal. Implemental mind-sets are understood as a set of general cognitive orientations activated by planning when, where, and how the goal should be implemented. Implementation intentions, on the other hand, are considered to be acts of willing that link anticipated opportunities to act with specific goal-directed actions. As the experimental work reported by Gollwitzer suggests, the cognitive orientations associated with implemental mind-sets and the various cognitive processes induced by the links created in implementation intentions effectively alleviate the numerous volitional problems of goal achievement.

Emmons focuses on goals that specify what a person is typically trying to do. Examples are "trying to overcome shyness with strangers," "avoiding being dependent on others," and "making others feel good about themselves." These goals, which cannot be achieved by a single course of action, are enduring and recurring. Again, Emmons calls these goals "personal strivings"; he proposes that they are, like other personality attributes, relatively stable over time and consistently expressed in a variety of situations. The central question of Emmons's analysis is how personal strivings affect a person's subjective well-being. Emmons argues that it is not the actual fulfillment of these goals that is critical, but the kind of strivings people hold, how they frame them, and, most importantly, how they handle the conflicts between them. Inability to resolve chronic conflicts between or among personal strivings (i.e., a goal the person wishes to accomplish interferes with at least one other goal) is associated with poor well-being, as is ambivalence about the pursuit of a given goal (approach–avoidance conflict). One type of approach–avoidance conflict is found to be particularly closely related to psychological distress: the ambivalence over emotional expression. Emmons suggests that the negative relation between conflict and subjective well-being may be mediated by the conflicted individual's failure to solicit and utilize social support. In addition, he argues that creative integrations of personal projects may reverse the negative effects of conflict. The observation that generativity strivings are associated with higher levels of subjective well-being is cited in support of this proposition, because generativity may be understood as the creative blending of intimacy strivings and power strivings. Through the creative integration of agentic (power) and communal (intimacy) strivings, the generative individual is able to achieve a reconciliation between power and intimacy. Emmons also points out that certain personality traits (e.g., neuroticism) and implicit beliefs regarding the incompatibility of goals may account for both the generation of conflict and the individual's potential for resolution. But even for individuals whose goals are not in conflict, Emmons observes low subjective well-being in individuals who let their goals stand unrelated next to each other. This leads Emmons to argue that the experience of subjective well-being needs more than the possession of and progression toward important life goals. Rather, people need to integrate separate goal strivings into a coherent Gestalt or philosophy of life.

Cantor and Blanton discuss action goals originating from a person's life tasks. Life tasks, such as doing well academically, exert specific influences on behavior as they are interpreted differently over the life course and across situational contexts. The accomplishment of life tasks is often obstructed by difficulties, frustrations, anxieties, and self-doubts, and the individual's style of appraising these hindrances leads to typical patterns of action goals aimed at overcoming these obstacles. For instance, college students who worry about their abilities when they experience failures (i.e., outcome-focused individuals) may, in a strategic effort to meet their academic life task, turn for reassurance to others whom they regard as confidants and encouragers. In contrast, college students who worry about losing their composure and thus failing to perform well in an upcoming test or exam (i.e., defensive pessimists) may instead try to meet their academic life task by mentally playing through worst-case scenarios prior to taking the test. Apparently, people tune the goal pursuits in the service of life tasks to their idiographic appraisals of experienced obstacles, thus trying to find the most suitable solutions for them personally. But this is just one aspect of coordinating actions in the realm of life tasks. Another aspect concerns constructively dealing with the fact that people commonly try to meet more than just one life task. One problem of negotiating multiple life tasks is rooted in resource limitations: There is not enough time or energy to meet the demands of different life tasks (e.g., the academic and job tasks vs. the friendship and intimacy tasks). This strain may be reduced by the strategy of setting priorities (i.e., dropping pursuits or taking turns) or consolidating pursuits (e.g., bringing academics to one's social life, or one's friends to academics). Another problem of negotiating life tasks is rooted in spillover. In consolidated life tasks, promoting one task is often achieved at the expense of the other. But life task pursuits can be paired together in ways that create positive rather than negative spillover, as, for instance, when social pursuits are used as a means of improving mood for academic work. Cantor and Blanton point out that the individual's style of appraising obstacles to a given life task often predetermines or limits the options of negotiating among life tasks. In addition, Cantor and Blanton emphasize the differences between the effortful pursuit of life tasks and strivings triggered by natural incentives grounded in a person's motives (e.g., need for power, intimacy, achievement).

CHAPTER 13 The Volitional Benefits of Planning

Peter M. Gollwitzer

Assume that you have decided to accomplish a personal wish or desire that has been on your mind for quite some time. Should you go ahead and plan the execution of behaviors that will eventually lead to your desire? Or would planning only be a waste of time, as you already feel highly committed to act and ready to go? Would passively waiting for a good opportunity to get started not be sufficient? As planning might not add anything to the commitment implied by your decision, the time and effort devoted to planning might be unnecessary. The present chapter focuses on this issue: Does planning promote the willful implementation of a person's goals and thus provide volitional benefits?

My colleagues and I believe that planning helps to alleviate crucial volitional problems of goal achievement, such as being too easily distracted from a goal pursuit or giving up in the face of difficulties when increased effort and persistence are needed instead. The conceptual analysis of this question relies on ideas that have evolved around the model of action phases (Heckhausen & Gollwitzer, 1987). In particular, we use two different but related concepts to understand the processes by which planning unfolds its beneficial effects on goal achievement: "implemental mind-sets" (Gollwitzer, 1990) and "implementation intentions" (Gollwitzer, 1993).

THE STRUCTURE AND FUNCTIONS OF PLANS

Planning is a mental strategy that prepares the individual for future action. For instance, a person who faces the task of retrieving a book from the library can mentally prepare this activity by planning. Planning commonly precedes the execution of a course of action and thus anticipates future relevant situational contexts (e.g., the physical and organizational features of the library), as well as the course of action to be executed. The end result of this mental activity is a plan stored in memory. Such plans may differ on a variety of structural features, however. Plans may be either complete (i.e., they specify each individual link of a course of action) or incomplete (i.e., some steps remain unspecified). These steps are filled by later planning or interspersed on-line into an individual's actual acting. Plans may vary in terms of their complexity (i.e., they may entail one, a few, or many different steps of action) or specificity (i.e., the anticipated situational contexts and the various actions to be executed are specified in detail or left rather vague). Moreover, some plans entail a number of choice points and can thus be modified flexibly in response to situational demands once the individual has started to act, whereas others entail one single, select course of action and thus cannot be easily modified when failure is encountered during the enactment of the plan. Also, plans may be linked to one another and organized in some temporal or hierarchical order; finally, plans may entail either well-practiced, reliable solutions or newly developed insights (for reviews, see Berger, 1988; Friedman, Scholnick, & Cocking, 1987).

As different as plans are, they all serve the same primary function: to facilitate the performance of the task or goal at hand. The person who plans prior to retrieving a book from the library does so in order to locate the book more effectively. The person confronted with the Tower of Hanoi problem plans before starting on the task in order to avoid unnecessary moves. The present examples highlight the cognitive aspects of task performance and show that planning can help people to deal successfully with the *intellectual* demands of the tasks to be accomplished. The analysis of this function of planning has been of major interest to cognitive psychologists (e.g., Hayes-Roth & Hayes-Roth, 1979; Mannes & Kintsch, 1991; Kreitler & Kreitler, 1987; Bruce & Newman, 1978) and researchers interested in artifical intelligence (Wilensky, 1983). Of central interest are questions of how plans are constructed (e.g., top-down or event-driven), what kinds of plans are constructed for different types of tasks (e.g., retrieving a book from the library vs. solving the Tower of Hanoi problem), and whether or not plans that are effectively constructed help to overcome the intellectual problems of achieving the task at hand.

Performing a task successfully, however, also requires overcoming volitional problems. Typical volitional problems include getting started with a task despite distractions, persisting at a task in spite of difficulties, and successfully resuming a task after a disruption. In the present chapter, it is demonstrated that planning also serves the function of alleviating these volitional problems of successful task performance. The volitional function of planning is explicated within the framework of a motivational–volitional theory of goal achievement, the model of action phases (Heckhausen & Gollwitzer, 1987; Gollwitzer, 1990).

THE MODEL OF ACTION PHASES

This model is based on the conceptual distinction between the motivational issue of goal setting and the volitional (willful) issue of goal striving (Lewin,

Dembo, Festinger, & Sears, 1944). It is assumed that the principles guiding goal selection and those guiding goal achievement are qualitatively different (Kuhl, 1984). The model provides a temporal perspective that starts with the awakening of a people's wishes prior to goal setting and continues to the evaluative thoughts people have once goal striving has led to some kind of outcome. The sequence of events within this comprehensive time frame is spelled out in four successive, discrete tasks that need to be accomplished in order to promote wish fulfillment (see Figure 13.1).

The first of these tasks, to be accomplished in the "predecisional" phase, consists of deliberating wishes and setting preferences. People cannot act on all of their wishes at once; some wishes may contradict each other, others are too difficult to implement, and life is simply too short to follow all of their wishes. They have to decide which of their many wishes they prefer to pursue. Preferences are established by employing the evaluative criteria of feasibility and desirability. A wish's feasibility is determined by reflecting on the chances that it can be realized (e.g., "Do I possess the necessary skills and talents, time, access to means, and opportunities?"). Desirability relates to the expected value of wish fulfillment (i.e., the likelihood of the positive and negative consequences of having achieved the desired wish, such as an anticipated positive or negative self-evaluation, evaluation through others, progress toward some important life goal, excitement of acting on the wish, and external costs or rewards). The perceived feasibility and desirability of a given wish are not fixed givens, but depend on whether the wish is scrutinized in the context of other complementary or contradicting wishes.

The model suggests that progress toward fulfilling a wish will not occur simply through judging a wish high in desirability and feasibility. Rather, progress demands a decision to act on a given wish. The model speaks of a transition from wishes and desires to binding goals, the latter being accompanied by a feeling of determination or obligation to fulfill the implied wish. Forming a goal commitment, however, is just a prerequisite for mak-

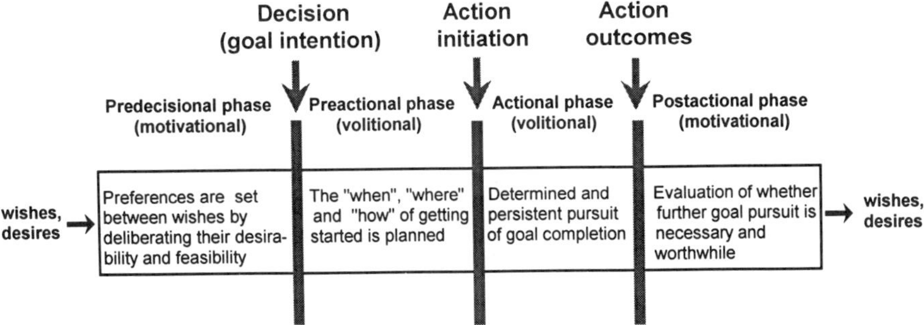

FIGURE 13.1. The model of action phases dissects the course of wish fulfillment into two motivational and two volitional phases. The boxes between the transition points (decision, action initiation, and action outcomes) describe the distinct tasks associated with each of the four phases (predecisional, preactional, actional, and postactional).

ing progress toward wish fulfillment. Once a decision has been made, the next task to be solved is promoting the initiation and successful execution of goal-directed actions. This may be quite simple when the necessary goal-directed actions are well practiced or routine. However, things may get rather tricky when people are still undecided about where and how to act. In such cases, the execution of goal-directed actions needs to be prepared. The model of action phases speaks of this period prior to the initiation of goal-directed action as the "preactional" phase. To advance further on the way from wishes to action, individuals reflect and decide on *when, where, how,* and *how long* to act, thus creating plans for action.

With the initiation of goal-directed behaviors, individuals enter the "actional" phase. The task associated with the actional phase is bringing goal-directed behaviors to a successful conclusion. For this purpose, it is necessary to respond readily to situational opportunities and demands. People should jump at all opportunities that allow progress toward their goals, and when difficulties and hindrances are encountered, they should readily increase their efforts. This responsiveness to situational opportunities and demands promotes goal achievement.

The final action phase is called "postactional." Here the task is to evaluate goal achievement. This is done by comparing what has been achieved to what was desired. Often reality does not live up to people's wishes and desires even when they are determined to act on them. They may have to admit that they simply did not perform as well as they had hoped or that the environment was not as supportive as they had expected, and that therefore they fell short of attaining their goals. But even if they do fully attain their goals, they may learn that their successes are not as sweet as they had hoped. In the postactional phase, people look back at the original deliberation of their respective wishes and desires. This triggers renewed deliberation and re-evaluation of their feasibility and desirability. As a consequence, individuals may reduce their standards of performance with respect to the goal at hand, but they may also start to consider other, competing wishes and desires that now appear comparatively more feasible and desirable. Apparently, the postactional phase directs individuals toward the past as well as the future; most importantly, it brings them back to where they started—their wishes and desires.

The central theme in the postactional phase (i.e., a primary concern for goal selection) is therefore the same as in the predecisional phase. Accordingly, the model describes both of these phases as motivational (i.e., goal-selection-oriented), whereas the preactional and actional phases in between are considered to be volitional in nature. In the latter two phases, the primary concern is to implement a chosen goal successfully (i.e., an orientation toward goal achievement).

In summary, the model of action phases attempts to delineate distinct tasks within the course of wish fulfillment. In temporal order, these tasks are as follows: setting preferences between or among wishes, making plans for goal-directed actions, effectively executing goal-directed actions, and evaluating performances and outcomes. The model's primary objective is to identify the typical problems people encounter when attempting to translate their wishes and desires into reality. But the model has also stimulated two theoretical concepts that explain people's functioning at various stages of wish fulfillment. These are the concepts of "mind-set" and "implementation intention." Both are particularly useful for understanding the beneficial effects of planning on the implementation of goals.

The Concept of Mind-Set

The concept of "mind-set" was suggested by the Würzburg school of thought (Külpe, 1904; Watt, 1905). It was an attempt to explain the experimental observation that instructing subjects to solve a specific task creates a related cognitive set that furthers the solution of the task at hand, but hampers solving other, unrelated tasks. Apparently, when a person becomes involved with a given task, relevant cognitive procedures are activated and hence become more easily accessible. When this idea is applied to the model of action phases, it follows that different mind-sets (i.e., general cognitive orientations with distinct features) should emerge when a person addresses the different tasks associated with the various action phases. These mind-sets should be endowed with cognitive features that facilitate the respective tasks.

Elsewhere, I (Gollwitzer, 1990) have employed this idea to demonstrate that the task addressed in the predecisional phase (setting preferences between or among wishes) is indeed different from the task addressed in the preactional phase (planning the execution of goal-directed actions). In various studies, it was demonstrated that subjects who had been asked to deliberate a personal wish developed a different cognitive orientation (i.e., a "deliberative" mind-set) than subjects who had been induced to plan the execution of a personal goal (i.e., an "implemental" mind-set). Comparing the features of the deliberative versus the implemental mind-set, my colleagues and I observed the following: open-mindedness versus closed-mindedness with respect to processing available information (Heckhausen & Gollwitzer, 1987); cognitive tuning toward feasibility- and desirability-related issues versus cognitive tuning toward implementation-related issues (Gollwitzer, Heckhausen, & Steller, 1990); impartial analysis of desirability-related information versus partial analysis of this information (Beckmann & Gollwitzer, 1987); and accurate analysis of feasibility-related information versus a self-serving, optimistic analysis (Gollwitzer & Kinney, 1989). These findings support the assertion of the model of action phases that the predecisional and the preactional phases are qualitatively distinct.

These data, however, can also be utilized to find an answer to the question of the present chapter: Does planning have volitional benefits? We only have to delineate the crucial problems of implementation and then scrutinize the accumulated implemental mind-set findings in terms of whether the discovered cognitive features potentially alleviate these problems. If the answer is positive, we can be assured that planning furthers the implementation of goal-directed actions, at least via the induction of implemental mind-sets.

The Concept of Implementation Intention

There should be more to planning than just creating the cognitive orientation of the implemental mind-set. People may strongly commit themselves to their specific plans, and this commitment may also trigger cognitive processes that help them perform goal-directed actions. These implementation-related commitments are not of primary concern to the model of action phases, as the model focuses on goal commitments (i.e., goal intentions). It postulates that progress toward goal attainment first of all requires a decision that transforms the deliberated wish or desire into a binding goal, which ends conflict among competing wishes and desires. Such a decision takes the format of "I intend to achieve *X*!" and therefore is best conceived of as a goal intention. The *X* specifies a desired end-state, which may be the execution of a concrete behavior or the attainment of a desired outcome. Accordingly, the consequence of having formed a goal intention is a feeling of commitment to achieve this end-state.

However, as long as the implementation of a chosen goal does not follow habitualized routes, an individual will have to make further decisions. This time the choice is between or among competing ways of realizing the goal. Such decisions take the format of "I intend to do *X* when situation *Y* is encountered!", and I have referred to them as "implementation intentions" (Gollwitzer, 1993). In an implementation intention, an anticipated future situation (opportunity) is linked to a certain goal-directed behavior. Holding implementation intentions commits the individual to perform certain goal-directed behaviors when the critical situation is actually encountered.

We discovered the concept of implementation intention in a study on the transition from weighing to willing (Gollwitzer, Heckhausen, & Ratajczak, 1990). In this study, subjects first had to name an unresolved personal problem of the following format: "Should I try to attain some desirable *X* or not?" We hoped that this would elicit unfulfilled wishes and desires. Indeed, subjects named problems such as "Should I move in with my boyfriend?", "Should I switch my major?", and "Should I go on a skiing vacation?" Then we asked subjects to indicate how far they felt from making a commitment to act on their wishes (i.e., forming a goal intention). All subjects were far from making a goal commitment. Finally, we had subjects think in various ways about the events associated with goal implementation. One group of subjects had to imagine the positive consequences that they expected to come true once their wish had been implemented. Another group had to simulate various possible ways of implementing their wishes. In a final group, subjects had to decide on one specific route of implementation.

When we assessed again how far subjects felt from making a goal commitment, we discovered that only subjects in the final group had advanced significantly. Apparently, committing themselves to a certain way of implementing a wish strengthened these subjects' readiness to transform the wish into a binding goal. Mediational analyses revealed that this effect was not due to changes in the feasibility or desirability of the wishes and desires named; rather, it was attributable to how strongly subjects felt committed to when, where, and how they intended to implement their wishes and desires.

Subsequently, we (see Gollwitzer, 1993) explored whether implementation intentions could also promote the achievement of chosen projects (i.e., goal intentions). For this purpose, we asked college students prior to Christmas break to name projects they intended to achieve during vacation. Subjects indicated such projects as writing a seminar paper or settling a family conflict. When we asked subjects whether they had formed intentions on when and where to get started (i.e., implementation intentions), about two-thirds responded positively. After the Christmas vacation, we contacted the subjects and checked on project completion. Of the subjects who had formed implementation intentions, two out of three had carried out their projects. Subjects without implementation intentions mostly failed to complete their projects (only one-fourth were successful).

The findings of this latter study were corroborated in an analogous experiment. In this experiment all subjects were asked, again prior to Christmas break, to complete the same type of project. More specifically, subjects were requested to write a report on how they spent Christmas Eve. This report was to be written no later than 48 hours after the event and then sent to the experimenters, who were presumably conducting a demographic study on how people spend their Christmas holidays. Half of the subjects were randomly chosen and then instructed to form implementation intentions. They were handed a questionnaire that requested them to specify when and where during the 48 hours they intended to write the report. The other half of the subjects were not requested to pick a specific time and place for implementing this project. When we received subjects' reports after Christmas, we analyzed them in terms of the dates when they were written. It turned out that three-quarters of the implementation intention subjects wrote the report in the requested time period, whereas only one-third of the control subjects managed to do so. It would be tempting to explain this finding in terms of obedience to the authority of the experimenters; being aware of this problem, we granted subjects absolute anonymity.

Impressed by the powerful effects of implementation intentions, we raised the question of how these effects come about. Our theory proposes (Gollwitzer, 1993) that implementation intentions are formed to alleviate the volitional problems of goal achievement. As soon as people anticipate such problems, they should form implementation intentions to protect themselves from falling prey to these problems. Because implementation intentions spell out plans that link situational cues to goal-directed behaviors, we postulated that implementation intentions pass on the control of goal-directed behavior to environmental cues. On a more micro level of analysis, we hypothesized that the mental representation of the specified situational cues becomes highly activated, thus making these cues easily accessible. In addition, we hypothesized that linking situational cues to goal-directed behaviors will facilitate the initiation of these behaviors in the presence of these cues. This implies that once these cues are encountered, goal-directed behavior is initiated relatively swiftly and effortlessly; moreover, action initiation is triggered without conscious intent.

THE VOLITIONAL PROBLEMS OF GOAL ACHIEVEMENT

Problems of volition can be classified into two categories. The first set of problems involves getting started. For a number of reasons, people continue to miss good opportunities to act, and thus delay goal achievement. The second set of problems involves bringing started goal pursuits to successful completion. People often give up in the face of difficulties, fail to ward off distractions, and have trouble resuming the pursuit of their goals once disruptions have occurred. How can implementation intentions and implemental mind-sets alleviate such problems?

Getting Started: Positive Effects of Implementation Intentions

As postulated above (see also Gollwitzer, 1993), implementation intentions are expected to lead to heightened accessibility of the specified situational cues (i.e., good opportunities). This implies that implementation intentions are particularly helpful when opportunities to act are hard to detect, and when people find it difficult to attend to these opportunities. Finally, as the situation–behavior links are expected to facilitate action initiation, the benefits of implementation intentions should prevail in situations that require fast and efficient responding. In the following subsections, experimental studies are presented that demonstrate these beneficial effects of implementation intentions.

Perceptual Readiness

Good opportunities to act on a goal are lost when people do not recognize them. This may happen even when they are actively looking for a good opportunity to get started. Think of a situation, for example, where two people who are communicating with each other are searching for a good opportunity to influence the other (e.g., ask for a favor, make a compliment and ingratiate the other, retaliate, or aggress)—often with little success. Planning that links certain situational cues to specific behaviors serving these interaction goals should facilitate goal pursuit, given that such linkages lead to a heightened cognitive accessibility of these cues.

Steller (1992) analyzed the perceptual readiness for situational cues specified in implementation intentions. She followed the postulate of the "New Look" research on perception (Bruner, 1957), which states that heightened accessibility of a concept induces a perceptual readiness that allows for the swift and easy recognition of relevant stimuli. Because implementation intentions are thought to furnish intended opportunities with heightened accessibility, increased perceptual readiness was expected for these opportunities—much as a person's expectations, need states, interests, and values produce an increase in perceptual readiness for relevant objects (e.g., Bruner, 1951; Bruner & Goodman, 1947; Bruner & Postman, 1948).

More specifically, Steller employed the so-called embedded figures test (Gottschaldt, 1926; Witkin, 1950). This test consists of complex geometrical figures (b-figures) that contain a smaller partial figure (a-figure). The a-figure is hidden within the b-figures according to Gestalt principles and is thus difficult to detect. Gottschaldt (1926) reported that even excessive familiarizing (over 300 trials) with the a-figure did not alleviate the difficulty of detecting it within the b-figures. Still, following the idea that implementation intentions would lead to heightened accessibility and thus better detection of the a-figure, Steller predicted that subjects who formed relevant implementation intentions would show enhanced detection performance. More specifically, subjects were requested to form implementation intentions on how to turn the a-figure into a new traffic sign. Subjects put down in writing how they intended to draw their traffic sign (i.e., they had to make a choice of color, etc.). The control subjects were requested to form the goal intention to draw a traffic sign, but were discouraged from forming implementation intentions on how they wanted to do that. To account for the possibility that implementation subjects' thinking about how to draw the sign without committing themselves to one specific behavioral route would produce heightened accessibility in and of itself, a second group of implementation intention subjects was asked to enhance their commitment to their plans of drawing the sign. That is, they were requested to mobilize maximal willpower for each detail of the plan by saying to themselves, "I will do it in exactly this way!" It was hoped that this procedure would induce highly mandated plans and would thus lead to the best detection performance of the three groups of subjects.

Before subjects were allowed to paint a paper model of their traffic sign, they were first asked to work on a visual search task consisting of b-figures that either contained the a-figure (the traffic sign) or not. Detection performance for the a-figure was highest in the intensified implementation intention condition and lowest in the goal intention condition, with the regular implementation intention condition in between. Assuming that the shape of the a-figure qualified as the situational cue for the intended actions specified in subjects' implementation intentions, this pattern of data suggests that the strength of commitment to plans spelled out in implementation intentions is positively related to the accessibility of the specified situational cues.

Disruption of Focused Attention

When people are highly absorbed in some ongoing activity, wrapped up in demanding ruminations, gripped by an intense emotional experience, or simply tired, chances are high that they do not seize an available good opportunity to act, simply because it fails to attract attention. The reason for this is that their attention is focused on other things that have nothing to do with the question of how to achieve the intended goal. Can implementation intentions disrupt focused attention?

The so-called dichotic listening task, in which words are presented to both ears simultaneously, can be used to study the disruption of focused attention. Subjects are instructed to repeat (i.e., shadow) the words presented to one ear (i.e., the attended channel) and to ignore the words presented to the other ear (i.e., the nonattended channel). Focusing attention on the shadowed ear becomes difficult when the words presented to the nonattended ear attract attention to themselves. This is the case for words that relate to temporarily or chronically active categories or schemas (e.g., Bargh, 1982; Johnston, 1978; Nielsen & Sarason, 1981; for a review, see Johnston & Dark, 1986). Whether an item presented on the nonattended channel has the potential to attract attention, and thus to disrupt focused attention, can be assessed in two different ways: first, by checking whether shadowing becomes faulty and shadowing speed decreases while shadowing mistakes increase (see Dawson & Schell, 1982); second, by assessing whether subjects' performance on a subsidiary secondary task (e.g., quickly turning off a probing light that goes on at irregular intervals) deteriorates. It is assumed that the more attentional effort is required by the shadowing task, the less capacity remains to respond to a subsidiary probe stimulus (see Kahneman, 1973; Logan, 1979).

Assuming that opportunities specified in an implementation intention acquire heightened accessibility, I (with Marit Mertin and Birgit Steller) presented words related to such opportunities to the nonattended channel in a dichotic listening task. These words were obtained in the following manner. First, subjects had to name a project (i.e., a goal intention) that they wanted to complete in the near future. Then they were asked to divide the implementation of this project into five major steps and commit themselves (in writing) to when, where, and how they intended to implement each of these steps. From these implementation intentions, we abstracted the critical words (i.e., the specified opportunities) for the dichotic listening task, which demanded the shadowing of several word blocks. On the nonattended channel, half of the simultaneously presented word blocks contained critical words; the other half contained neutral words.

The critical words turned out to be highly disruptive to focused attention. Not only did they reduce the subjects' speed in turning off the probing light, but they also worsened their shadowing performance (in terms of slowing down reading speed and increasing shadowing errors). When we applied a recognition test for the words presented on the nonattended channel, we observed a better recognition performance for critical than for noncritical words, which indicated shifts of attention to the nonattended channel. Thus it appeared that even when efforts to direct attention to the shadowing task were stepped up (as indicated by the reduced speed in turning off the probing light), the critical words still managed to attract attention (as indicated by a weak shadowing performance and a high recognition performance).

One has to keep in mind that in this research the critical opportunities were presented to subjects in terms of a verbal description only. When a person actually enters a situational context that entails these opportunities in reality, their potential to attract attention should be even stronger. This implies that opportunities specified in implementation intentions will not easily escape people's attention even when they are focusing on other things (e.g., worries, strong emotions, the conscious pursuit of other goals) besides the respective goal pursuit.

Behavioral Readiness

The potential to disrupt focused attention will certainly make it less likely that good opportunities remain unnoticed. But this will not protect people from letting slip those opportunities that present themselves only for a short moment. What is needed here is a swift initiation of the planned goal-directed behaviors. Implementation intentions not only specify when and where people plan to get started on goal achievement; they also lay down how this should be done, and thus also specify the intended goal-directed behavior. More importantly, they create a link between the situational context and the goal-directed behavior, and people feel committed to initiate this behavior once the situational cues are encountered. Does forming such linkages facilitate the initiation of the goal-directed behaviors, given the presence of the specified opportunity? If so, this would guarantee that people could effectively respond to good opportunities even if these present themselves for only a short moment.

Brandstätter (1992, Study 1) explored this question in an experiment in which subjects were requested to take a convincing counterposition on racist remarks made by a confederate presented on videotape. All subjects readily agreed to do so. Subjects were then made familiar with these remarks in a first viewing of the video. A second run was carried out so that subjects could mark those points on the tape that they considered to be suitable (i.e., good opportunities) for a counterargument. To induce implementation intentions, one group of subjects was requested to form intentions that linked the marked situational cues to specific counterarguments. Control subjects did not form such implementation intentions, but were encouraged to think of good counterarguments to be delivered later in writing. In a third viewing of the video, the subjects were finally allowed to stop the videotape at any point and deliver their counterarguments on audiotape.

Without subjects' being aware of it, a computer recorded the marks they had made on the videotape and also the times at which they started to speak. Implementation intention subjects managed to place their counterarguments within a narrowly defined critical time period surrounding the points previously marked more frequently than control subjects. One has to keep in mind that all subjects intended to achieve the goal of taking a convincing counterposition to a racist view. Still, good opportunities elicited goal-directed behaviors (i.e., presentations of counterarguments) with greater speed when subjects had linked critical situations (good opportunities) to behaviors (counterarguments) by forming implementation intentions. The mental act of forming such linkages obviously managed to increase the speed of action initiation.

It should be highly beneficial if this "speed-up" effect remains active even when people are busy with other things. This should allow people to seize short-lived opportunities even when there is a high cognitive load from being involved with other demanding tasks. Following the logic of the dual-task paradigm (e.g., Kahneman & Treisman, 1984; Posner, 1978; Shiffrin & Schneider, 1977), Brandstätter (1992, Study 2) explored whether the "speed-up" effect originating from an implementation intention is effortless in the sense that it does not put much cognitive load on limited processing resources, and thus persists even when the cognitive demands of the primary task in a pair of tasks are high. In this study, subjects were asked to work simultaneously on two tasks, which were both presented on a computer monitor in two adjacent windows. The primary task consisted of working on meaningless syllables and was presented to each subject at low and high difficulty levels. The secondary task was to press a button as quickly as possible when numbers rather than letters were shown.

Half of the subjects were instructed to respond as quickly as possible to a specific number; the other half (the control group) were asked to familiarize themselves with this critical number by repeatedly writing it on a sheet of paper. Both groups of subjects were asked to do this for the purpose of speeding up their responses to this number. Implementation intention subjects showed a marked acceleration to the critical number, and this "speed-up" effect was not affected by the level of difficulty of the primary task. For control subjects, no acceleration in responding to the critical number was observed. Reaction times to critical and noncritical numbers did not differ, and they corresponded to the reaction times for noncritical numbers in the implementation intention condition.

Why do implementation intentions lead to fast and effortless initiation of goal-directed behaviors? It seems possible that the commitment (or willpower) people attach to the situation–behavior contingencies that they proclaim in their implementation intentions creates very strong links, which normally can only be attained through frequent and consistent situation–response pairings. As this latter procedure leads to the automatic, direct environmental control of behavior (Bargh, 1992, 1994), one could argue that implementation intentions also achieve this effect. In other words, implementation intentions may be conscious mental acts that set up contingencies, which will then lead to the automatic, environmental control of behavior.

One feature of automatic control of behavior is high efficiency (i.e., the behavior is excuted fast and effortlessly), and Brandstätter's (1992) studies clearly suggest that implementation intentions lead to this type of action initiation. One further feature of automatic control of behavior, however, is that it is triggered without any conscious intent once the critical situational context is encountered. Could it be that implementation intentions also manage to bring about this latter feature of automatic action control? Malzacher (1992) explored whether the opportunity specified in an implementation intention prompts supportive cognitive processes without conscious intent. The processes considered were the automatic activation of knowledge that is instrumental to the effective initiation of the intended action and the automatic inhibition of knowledge that potentially disturbs the initiation of actions. Malzacher employed a retaliation paradigm modeled after that of Zillman and Cantor (1976). The intended action consisted of responding to an insult in the form of a complaint spoken directly to the transgressor. Accordingly, facilitative knowledge entailed attributes to be ascribed to an unfriendly person, whereas inhibitory knowledge entailed attributes one would ascribe to a friendly person.

Subjects who were insulted by a first experimenter were then induced to form the following implementation intention: "As soon as I see this person again, I'll tell her what an unfriendly person she is!" In an allegedly independent second study run by another experimenter, subjects had to read a series of successively presented adjectives as quickly as possible from a screen. The adjectives were either positive or negative words, all suitable for describing people. Shortly (about 100 milliseconds) before each adjective, either a neutral face or the face of the unfriendly experimenter was subliminally presented (presentation time was less than 10 milliseconds on average, and the faces were pattern-masked). Negative adjectives presented directly after the face of the unfriendly experimenter tended to be read faster than those presented directly after the neutral face, and positive adjectives were read much more slowly after the unfriendly experimenter's face than after the neutral face. This pattern of data was not observed in a first control group of subjects, who were not insulted, or in a second control group of subjects, who formed goal intentions to retaliate as a response to the experienced insult but did not furnish these with implementation intentions. Apparently, the situational cue specified in an implementation intention directly elicits, without conscious intent, cognitive processes (in this case, the activation of relevant knowledge and the inhibition of irrelevant knowledge) that facilitate the initiation of the intended action. The mere formation of a goal intention is not sufficient to produce this effect.

In summary, it has been observed that the situational cues specified in implementation intentions lead to fast and effortless responding (Brandstätter, 1992, Studies 1 and 2). Even prior to the individual's becoming aware of these cues, they manage to trigger cognitive processes that support the initiation of the intended actions (Malzacher, 1992). The findings on heightened behavioral readiness as a consequence of implementation intentions suggest that people can switch from the effortful, conscious control of goal-directed action to automatic environmental control—simply by forming implementation intentions. A recent dissertation by Lengfelder (1994) supports this conclusion. Lengfelder discovered that frontal lobe patients can also benefit from implementation intentions. More specifically, the "speed-up" effect reported above (Brandstätter, 1992, Study 2) was also observed with frontal lobe patients. Because these patients are known to be deficient in the conscious control of action, this finding adds to the proposition that implementation intentions induce direct, automatic action control.

The automatic action control associated with implementation intentions has an interesting implication that pertains to the control of unwanted habitual responses. When certain behaviors, goals, and cognitive concepts are repeatedly and consistently instigated in the same situational context, they fall under the direct control of the respective situational cues (Bargh & Gollwitzer, 1994). If people want to inhibit these behaviors, goals, and cognitive concepts, they may turn to implementation intentions. If these intentions link the critical situational cues to antagonistic behaviors, goals, and concepts, they can start a race between the (unwanted) habitual response and the intended alternative (antagonistic) response. This race should be won by the intended antagonistic response when the link created by the implementation intention is stronger then the link established through repeated and consistent pairing of the critical situational cues and the (now unwanted) original response. We are currently exploring this line of thought by studying the inhibiting effects of implementation intentions on the suppression of habitual behaviors and the so-called automatic activation of stereotypes (e.g., gender or professional stereotypes).

Getting Started: Positive Effects of Implemental Mind-Sets

The effects of implementation intentions are very specific. They only relate to the particular situations and behaviors implied. These situations will be more easily recognized and more readily attended to, and the behaviors will be executed more efficiently. But forming implementation intentions also has some general effects. As pointed out above, intensive involvement with the planning of the implementation of one's goals creates a so-called implemental mind-set. The features of the implemental mind-set also help people to get started on their goals, because these features alleviate one very crucial problem of getting started. Often people fail to act on a given goal even though the present situational context would allow it, only because they experience doubts about either the feasibility or the desirability of the goal. Numerous mind-set experiments suggest that various aspects of the cognitive orientation of the implemental mind-set suppress such doubts.

Positive Illusions

We (Gollwitzer & Kinney, 1989) put one group of our university student subjects into an implemental mind-set by asking them to plan the implementation of a decision they had already made (e.g., to move from home). More specifically, subjects had to divide this project into five steps, and to list when, where, and how they intended to initiate goal-directed actions for each of these steps. The second group of subjects was put into a deliberative mind-set. These subjects were asked to contemplate the pros and cons of making a major change in their lives (e.g., to move from home). Subsequent to the mind-set manipulations, subjects participated in an ostensibly unrelated task that required them to estimate their degree of personal control. The final group of subjects, the control group, immediately started to work on this task.

The task was modeled after Alloy and Abramson's (1979) contingency learning paradigm and requested subjects to turn on a target light by either pressing or not pressing a button. Although light onset was noncontingent to subjects' behavior (i.e., pressing or not pressing the button), implemental mind-set subjects inferred that they had successfully exerted personal control over the light task when light onset was frequent, whereas subjects in the deliberative mind-set condition did not succumb to this illusion of control. Implemental mind-set subjects' illusion of control tended to be even stronger than that of control subjects.

We (Taylor & Gollwitzer, 1995) recently extended this research by encompassing other indications of positive illusions. The same type of mind-set manipulation was used as in the Gollwitzer and Kinney (1989) study. Subsequently, subjects had to fill out various questionnaires. On one questionnaire, subjects rated themselves in comparison to the average college student of their age and gender on a series of 21 qualities and skills (e.g., cheerfulness, academic ability). Another questionnaire assessed how likely it was that they or the average college student of their age would encounter various controllable risks (e.g., divorce) or uncontrollable risks (e.g., losing a partner to an early death). Implemental mind-set subjects described their own personal qualities and skills more positively than they did those of the average college student, and they did this to a larger degree than both deliberative mind-set and control subjects did. The same pattern of data emerged for perceived invulnerability to both controllable and uncontrollable risks. Finally, implemental mind-set subjects reported themselves to be in a better mood than both deliberative mind-set and control subjects. The differences in mood did not account, however, for the differences in self-perception and perceived invulnerability to risks.

All of these findings suggest that implemental mind-set subjects are very certain about the feasibility of their goals. They believe themselves to be very capable, rather invulnerable to controllable as well as uncontrollable risks, and in control over (uncontrollable) action outcomes. This rampant optimism associated with the implemental mind-set should relieve a planning person's mind from any doubts about being able to reach a desired goal, and thus should favor the efficient initiation of goal-directed actions. As has been shown over and over again, optimism about the feasibility of goals leads to more successful goal achievement than pessimism (for reviews, see Carver & Scheier, 1989; Bandura, 1991; Taylor & Brown, 1988; Seligman, 1990).

Unequivocal Behavioral Orientation

When it comes to acting on a chosen goal, people need to concern themselves with issues of how to achieve the goal. This implies that the question of whether the goal is indeed attractive should be settled for good. Deliberating the desirability of the chosen goal anew would only hamper the efficient initiation of goal-directed actions as doubts about the goal's desirability are raised. Does the implemental mind-set direct a person's thoughts away from the deliberative issue of estimating the expected value of the goal to the implementational issues of when, where, and how to act on the goal?

We (Gollwitzer, Heckhausen, & Steller, 1990) reported two experiments in which deliberative and implemental mind-set subjects' readiness to process expected-value-related information as compared to implementation-related information was studied. In the first study, subjects were presented with the beginnings of three different fairy tales and were asked to continue these tales with three sentences each. Implementational themes were more frequently observed in the sentences of implemental mind-set subjects than in those of deliberative mind-set subjects, with those of control subjects in between. The opposite was found for deliberative themes. In the second study, subjects' recall performance for information on the expected value as compared to information on the implementation of goals was assessed. Implemental and deliberative mind-set subjects showed better recall for the congruent information than for the incongruent, with the control subjects again in between.

These data strongly suggest that implemental mind-sets favor the processing of information relevant to executing a person's goals, and hamper the processing of expected-value-related (i.e., deliberative) information. Planning apparently orients people toward issues of implementation as processing of implementation-related information becomes easier, whereas the opposite is true for expected-value-related information. But there is a second principle serving this end. As researchers on cognitive dissonance have observed, postdecisional (pre-actional) subjects' perception of the attractiveness of the chosen alternative increases, whereas the attractiveness of the nonchosen alternative decreases (Brehm, 1956). Some dissonance researchers have interpreted this finding as an attempt to arrive at an "unequivocal behavioral orientation" that precludes further deliberation of the choice alternatives (Jones & Gerard, 1967; Wicklund & Frey, 1981). Recent findings (Taylor & Gollwitzer, 1995, Study 3) support this view. When subjects who had started to plan the execution of a choice (e.g., to switch their major) were asked to deliberate its expected value, they did not think about pros and cons to an equal degree, but strongly favored pros over cons. In addition, they thought more about implementation-related issues than about the expected value of their choices. Apparently planning protects people from returning to the deliberation of a chosen goal by focusing them on both the pros of their choice and the implied implementational issues.

Completion of Goal Pursuit: Positive Effects of Implemental Mind-Sets and Implementation Intentions

Volitional problems are not only associated with getting started. When the first steps toward goal achievement are implemented successfully, further volitional obstacles may be encountered. First, people may have to step up their efforts when unexpected increases in task difficulty threaten successful task performance. Second, they may have to ward off distractions. Because most situations allow for more than one goal pursuit, people need to prevent the primary goal pursuit from getting derailed. Third, if they fail at these two problems, a further volitional problem presents itself: The interrupted goal pursuit needs to be resumed. Can planning possibly alleviate these volitional problems?

Effort Mobilization

Energization theory (see Wright, Chapter 19, this volume) holds that as perceived task difficulty increases, so does a person's effort (i.e., actual motivation)—at least up to a point. This cutoff point is reached when the person no longer sees further effort mobilization as worthwhile. In other words, this cutoff point describes a person's potential motivation and is reached rather early with unattractive tasks, but much later with attractive tasks. When this line of thought is combined with the observation that implemental mind-set subjects feel very positive about the expected value of their goals and are very optimistic about actually attaining them, it follows that people in an implemental mind-set should reach the cutoff point comparatively later. As a consequence, people in an implemental mind-set should show high persistence in the face of difficulties.

But effort mobilization may also be achieved via implementation intentions. If a person anticipates the critical difficulty and links it to a behavioral response that implies heightened effort, the initiation of this behavior should be facilitated once the difficulty is encountered. In other words, an implementation intention that links an anticipated difficulty with a behavioral response associated with high effort should lead to effort mobilization in the presence of this difficulty (see the study by Schaal, 1993, described later).

Warding Off Distractions

Kuhl (for reviews, see Kuhl & Beckmann, 1985, 1994) has applied his theory of action control to the issue of warding off distractions. The theory distinguishes a number of different mental strategies (e.g., attention control, emotion control), which are assumed to effectively shield a person's ongoing goal pursuit from distractions stemming from potential alternative pursuits. Action-oriented people are found to use these strategies more effectively than state-oriented people, as the latter tend to become wrapped up in ruminative thoughts about past failures and desired successes or in the deliberation of a decision.

Can planning also strengthen a person's shielding of an ongoing goal pursuit? We conducted a number of mind-set studies to explore this issue (see Gollwitzer, 1991, Ch. 4). In the first study, deliberative and implemental mind-set subjects were asked to memorize a coherent story consisting of several sentences that were each presented centrally on an individual slide. At the upper left and lower right corner of each slide, we placed single two-syllable nouns. Recognition performance for these peripherally presented nouns was worse for implemental than for deliberative mind-set subjects, indicating that planning leads to more closed-mindedness in the sense of concentrating on the task at hand (i.e., memorizing the centrally presented sentences).

Follow-up studies (see Gollwitzer, 1991, Ch. 7) employed a modified Müller–Lyer illusion. The classic figure was redrawn so that a narrow field of attention (i.e., only exploring the center of the figure) produced different illusions than a broader field of attention (i.e., also exploring the periphery of the figure). Each subject was placed into a deliberative as well as an implemental mind-set, and after each mind-set manipulation a series of modified Müller–Lyer figures was presented on slides. The implemental mind-set produced more illusions associated with a narrow field of attention than the deliberative mind-set did.

The results of these studies suggest that planning creates a certain closed-mindedness, which is based on a narrowed field of attention. This effect of planning, transported via the implemental mind-set, should facilitate warding off all kinds of distractions (even unanticipated distractions); the goal that is currently pursued commonly takes center stage, whereas distractions originate from the periphery. But planning can also aim directly at particular anticipated distractions. Implementation intentions that specify a feared distraction as the situational cue to which a protective response is linked should provide an effective strategy for escaping these distractions.

Patterson and Mischel (1976) thought of this possibility some time ago when they equipped children with plans to help them escape the temptations of "Mr. Clown Box." The children were trying to put as many pegs into a pegboard as possible in order to get permission to play with some attractive toys. However, a box dressed up as a clown was challenging the children's devotion to the pegboard task. Mr. Clown Box spoke to the children (e.g., asked them to disrupt their task and press his nose) and displayed various distractive stimuli (e.g., attractive toys in an illuminated window). The experimenter told children to form specific plans to escape the clown's distractions. Two different types of plans were formed: temptation-inhibiting plans ("When Mr. Clown Box says to look at him and play with him, then I just won't look at him, and say, 'I'm not going to look at Mr. Clown Box!' ") and task-facilitating plans ("When Mr. Clown Box says to look at him and play with him, then I just look at my pegboard and say, 'I'm going to look at my work.' "). As it turned out, the temptation-inhibiting plan facilitated children's pegboard performance (in terms of amount of pegboard work completed), compared to that of control children who were not equipped with plans. Furthermore, children with a temptation-inhibiting plan performed better than children with a task-facilitating plan, who were no more effective than children with no plans at all.

Apparently, people have to be cautious with respect to the specification of the behavioral side of their implementation intentions when it comes to warding off distractions. This was also observed in a recent experiment by Schaal (1993). University students were placed in front of a computer terminal and asked to solve as many of the arithmetic problems presented as possible. These problems were simple, but demanded much attention. For 15 minutes a series of problems was presented in a self-paced procedure (i.e., when one problem was answered, the next was offered). On top of the terminal a TV screen was mounted, showing very attractive, award-winning commercials in random intervals. Subjects were requested to form implementation intentions to protect themselves from these distractions. The implementation intentions were either disruption-inhibiting ("As soon as a commercial comes on, I will ignore it!") or task-facilitating ("As soon as a commercial comes on, I will concentrate on my work!"). The control subjects solely set the goal not to let themselves be distracted from working on the arithmetic problems (i.e., they formed a goal intention).

Subjects with distraction-inhibiting implementation intentions worked harder than control subjects (i.e., they answered more arithmetic problems), and subjects with task-facilitating implementation intentions were in between. As in the Patterson and Mischel (1976) study, the way in which the behavioral aspect of the plan was phrased mattered. Future research will have to find out why the distraction-inhibiting phrase ("When . . . , I will ignore the distraction!") is superior to the task-facilitating phrase ("When . . . , I will attend to my task!"), as well as when the task-facilitating phrase achieves an effect and when it does not.

Resumption of Disrupted Goal Pursuits

Following Lewin's (1926) tension system theory of intention, Ovsiankina (1928) and others (Mahler, 1933; Lissner, 1933) observed in their experiments that the resumption rate of an interrupted task was close to perfect, with the exception of cases where substitute completion occurred (i.e., a similar alternative task was performed instead). Ovsiankina and others inferred from these studies that people are rather effective in resuming interrupted tasks. However, if one considers delay instead of rate of resumption, a less positive picture presents itself. People often take a lifetime to return to a disrupted goal pursuit. Focusing on the delay of resumption thus suggests that people are rather ineffective in resuming interrupted goal pursuits.

My colleagues and I believe that *un*delayed resumption implies warding off distractions stemming from other unfinished business. Accordingly, we hypothesized that an implemental mind-set should facilitate quick resumption of a disrupted task in the presence of other unfinished tasks. To test this line of thought, Pösel (1994) ran an experiment in which university students were requested (by a first experimenter) to name various personal projects that still demanded action. These projects had to be such that a first implementational step could be effectively initiated by writing a letter. Once subjects had named their projects, two equally important projects were selected, and subjects were asked to start writing a letter for each project by putting the addresses of the recipients on two separate sheets of papers. At this point subjects were interrupted and led to a different room, where a second experimenter placed them into either a deliberative or an implemental mind-set; control subjects were requested to solve simple arithmetic problems.

When subjects returned to the first experimenter, she led them to a table with either both incomplete letters sitting on it (i.e., the conflict condition) or only one of them (i.e., the no-conflict condition). Then she timed both when subjects grabbed a letter and when they actually started writing. There was no difference among groups in terms of grabbing a letter, although subjects in all three groups took longer in the conflict condition than in the no-conflict condition. However, an interesting interaction effect was observed with respect to when subjects actually started to write (i.e., put the pencil on the sheet of paper). Conflict between letters slowed down deliberative mind-set subjects as well as control subjects, but not implemental mind-set subjects. The latter started writing as fast in the conflict condition as they did in the no-conflict condition. In other words, implemental mind-set subjects in the conflict condition resumed work on the incomplete letter at hand as if there were no second incomplete letter sitting on the table. This pattern of data suggests that an implemental mind-set does not create a general urge to complete unfinished business. Rather, it helps subjects to shield the resumption of an interrupted task from competing unfinished business. This finding parallels the observations reported in the subsection on warding off distractions, suggesting that implemental mind-set subjects are characterized by a narrowed field of attention.

It seems plausible to assume, however, that the implemental mind-set aids efficient resumption of a disrupted project not only via the attentional mechanism discovered in the Pösel (1994) experiment. When individuals have doubts either about the feasibility or the desirability of resumption, the implemental mind-set's positive illusions and unequivocal behavioral orientation, respectively, should destroy these doubts and thus facilitate resumption. Finally, effective resumption should also be favored by implementation intentions that link critical situations to behaviors that qualify as effective resumptions.

CONCLUSION AND PROSPECTS FOR FUTURE RESEARCH

At the beginning of the present chapter, the following question has been raised: Given that a person feels highly committed to a goal, is planning how to achieve this goal just a waste of time? Analysis of this question strongly suggests that people can derive additional volitional benefits from planning. First, initiating goal-directed behaviors is facilitated, because planning creates a perceptual readiness for and guides people's attention toward relevant opportunities and means. In addition, it sets up a special behavioral readiness to respond effectively once these opportunities and means are encountered. Finally, the illusionary optimism and the unequivocal behavoiral orientation associated with planning suppress dysfunctional doubts about the goal's feasibility and desirability. Second, bringing initiated goal pursuits to successful completion is facilitated, because planning helps to mobilize effort in the face of difficulties and to ward off distractions. Moreover, if disruptions to goal-directed actions occur, planning furthers undelayed resumption.

The experiments discussed in the present chapter have demonstrated that many of the beneficial effects of planning are based on the cognitive features of the *implemental mind-set.* But what makes an implemental mind-set particularly powerful? Mind-sets are general cognitive orientations that originate when people become involved with solving a given task. Powerful mind-sets are rather stable over time and generalize across situations. The task that leads to the implemental mind-set is planning the execution of behaviors that lead to efficient goal achievement. Accordingly, we may assume that the more involved a person becomes with this task, the more pronounced the implemental mind-set is.

In our mind-set studies, my colleagues and I requested subjects to think of the five most important implementational steps of their goal, and then to commit themselves to plans specifying, when, where, and how they intended to execute these steps (i.e., the subjects were asked to form implementation intentions). Can other forms of planning also lead to an implemental mind-set? The task of planning can also be approached with a more hesitant, reflective attitude, as is entailed in mental simulations that explore possible routes to achieving one's goal (see Taylor & Pham's conceptualization of process simulation, Chapter 10, this volume; Taylor & Schneider, 1989). Such mental simulations should not be accompanied with the strong sense of commitment typically attached to the plans specified in implementation intentions. However, mental simulations can be applied repeatedly (see Taylor & Pham, Chapter 10, this volume), which should bring out one particular route to implementation. When this very same route is reiterated in numerous mental simulations, strong links between certain situational cues and goal-directed behaviors should emerge. Accordingly, the mental strategy of repeated simulation of the same implementational route should also result in firm plans. In other words, there may be two different types of planning—one based on the repeated simulation of a specific course of implementation, and the other based on the willful acts of forming implementation intentions—both of which possess the potential to induce strong implemental mind-sets.

The amount of involvement with the task of planning should, however, be affected not only by the planning strategies employed. The features of the planning task at hand should also matter. Some goals simply do not need much planning. When the implementation of the goal is determined from the outside (i.e., when other people determine how it is done), or when there exists one well-practiced implementational routine (e.g., when a person is driving to work), no thorough planning should be needed, and therefore no strong implemental mind-set should emerge. But even with goals that demand intensive planning, we should expect differences in the amount of planning activity. More important goals should induce a stronger motivation to plan thoroughly. Furthermore, some people may generally be more prone to planning than others (e.g., Kuhl's action-oriented individuals).

The experiments discussed in the present chapter have also demonstrated that many of the beneficial effects of planning are based on the various cognitive processes originating from *implementation intentions.* What makes for particularly powerful implemetation intentions? Because implementation intentions link situational cues to behvavioral responses, the strength of an implementation intention should depend on the quality of the link between these situational cues and the intended goal-directed behaviors. Strong links should lead to more powerful effects of implementation intentions. As these links are established by an act of will ("I intend to do *X* when I encounter the situation *Y*!") and induce a commitment to act in the specified way, more intensive willing ("I really intend to . . . ") should lead to stronger commitments and thus to more effective implementation intentions.

In a recent study (Seehausen, Bayer, & Gollwitzer, 1994), we systematically varied people's readiness to commit themselves to the plans spelled out in their implementation intentions. Prior to the experiment, subjects were told (based on their performance on a ficticious personality test) that when it came to achieving goals they would either benefit from firmly committing themselves to fixed plans or suffer unnecessary rigidity from doing so. In a subsequent experiment, subjects first chose a goal (task) and were then asked to form several relevant implementation intentions. Either immediately after a short distraction task or 48 hours later, subjects were asked to recall the situational cues they had specified in their implementation intentions. This was done to assess a classic effect of implementation intentions—the heightened accessibility of the specified situational cues (see the section on perceptual readiness, above). Subjects who believed that committing themselves strongly to their plans would facilitate goal achievement recalled more of these situational cues than subjects who thought that strong commitments would be a hindrance. This pattern of results was the same regardless of whether the recall test was applied immediately or after a 48-hour delay. Data from the study by Steller (1992; reported above) parallel these findings. Subjects who intensified their implementation intentions by "really" wanting to draw the new traffic sign as planned showed the strongest effects (i.e., the highest perceptual readiness for the traffic sign).

Apparently, the strength of the links specified in implementation intentions is dependent on the amount of willing or commitment a person manages to mobilize. This triggers the question of whether the commitment to the superordinate goal intention, in the service of which implementation intentions are formed, also feeds into the strength of a person's implementation intentions. Does a person's readiness to form and hold strong links require a vital goal commitment? Findings of the Seehausen et al. (1994) study support this view. When subjects were told that the goal would no longer have to be implemented, as other subjects had already taken on this task, the recall effect of having committed themselves strongly to implementational plans (i.e., having formed strong implementation intentions) was weakened immediately after the distraction task and completely wiped out 48 hours later.

In summary, the issue of the strength of implementation intentions seems first and foremost an issue of commitment. Feeling strongly about achieving the superordinate goal appears to be the prerequisite for powerful implementation intentions. On the basis of such strong goal commitments, forming and holding highly mandated links between situational cues and goal-directed behaviors produce strong implementation intention effects. As a consequence, the types of variables known to induce strong goal commitments (e.g., high desirability), as well as the variables that induce the formation of highly mandated plans (e.g., fears of missing an anticipated good opportunity to act), qualify as determinants of the strength of implementation intentions.

REFERENCES

Alloy, L. B., & Abramson, L. Y. (1979). Judgments of contingency in depressed and nondepressed students: Sadder but wiser? *Journal of Experimental Psychology: General, 108,* 441–485.

Bandura, A. (1991). Self-regulation of motivation through anticipatory and self-reactive mechanisms. In R. Dienstbier (Ed.), *Nebraska Symposium on Motivation* (Vol. 38, pp. 69–164). Lincoln: University of Nebraska Press.

Bargh, J. A. (1982). Attention and automaticity in the processing of self-relevant information. *Journal of Personality and Social Psychology, 43,* 425–436.

Bargh, J. A. (1992). Being unaware of the stimulus versus unaware of its interpretation: Does subliminality *per se* matter to social psychology? In R. Bornstein & T. Pittman (Eds.), *Perception without awareness* (pp. 236–255). New York: Guilford Press.

Bargh, J. A. (1994). The four horsemen of automaticity: Awareness, intention, efficiency, and control in social cognition. In R. S. Wyer, Jr., & T. K. Srull (Eds.), *Handbook of social cognition* (2nd ed.). Hillsdale, NJ: Erlbaum.

Bargh, J. A., & Gollwitzer, P. M. (1994). Environmental control of goal-directed action: Automatic and strategic contingencies between situations and behavior. In W. D. Spaulding (Ed.), *Nebraska Symposium on Motivation: Vol. 41. Integrative views of motivation, cognition, and emotion* (pp. 71–124). Lincoln: University of Nebraska Press.

Beckmann, J., & Gollwitzer, P. M. (1987). Deliberative versus implemental states of mind: The issue of impartiality in pre- and postdecisional information processing. *Social Cognition, 5,* 259–279.

Berger, C. R. (1988). Planning, affect, and social action generation. In L. Donohew, H. Sypher, & E. T. Higgins (Eds.), *Communication, social cognition, and affect* (pp. 93–116). Hillsdale, NJ: Erlbaum.

Brehm, J. W. (1956). Postdecision changes in the desirability of alternatives. *Journal of Abnormal and Social Psychology, 52,* 384–389.

Brandstätter, V. (1992). *Der Einfluß von Vorsätzen auf die Handlungsinitiierung. Ein Beitrag zur willenspsychologischen Frage der Realisierung von Absichten.* Frankfurt: Peter Lang.

Bruce, B., & Newman, D. (1978). Interacting plans. *Cognitive Science, 2,* 195–233.

Bruner, J. S. (1951). Personality dynamics and the process of perceiving. In R. R. Blake & G. V. Ramsey (Eds.), *Perception: An approach to personality* (pp. 121–147). New York: Ronald Press.

Bruner, J. S. (1957). On perceptual readiness. *Psychological Review, 64,* 123–152.

Bruner, J. S., & Goodman, C. C. (1947). Value and need as organizing factors in perception. *Journal of Abnormal and Social Psychology, 42,* 33–44.

Bruner, J. S., & Postman, L. (1948). Symbolic value as an organizing factor in perception. *Journal of Social Psychology, 27,* 203–208.

Carver, C. S., & Scheier, M. F. (1989). Expectancies and coping: From test anxiety to pessimism. In R. Schwarzer, H. M. van der Ploeg, & C. D. Spielberger (Eds.), *Advances in test anxiety research* (Vol. 6, pp. 3–11). Amsterdam: Swets & Zeitlinger.

Dawson, M. E., & Schell, A. M. (1982). Electrodermal responses to attended and nonattended significant stimuli during dichotic listening. *Journal of Experimental Psychology: Human Perception and Performance, 8,* 315–324.

Friedman, S. L., Scholnick, E. K., & Cocking, R. R. (Eds.). (1987). *Blueprints for thinking: The role of planning in cognitive development.* Cambridge, England: Cambridge University Press.

Gollwitzer, P. M. (1990). Action phases and mind-sets. In E. T. Higgins & R. M. Sorrentino (Eds.), *Handbook of motivation and cognition: Foundations of social behavior* (Vol. 2, pp. 53–92). New York: Guilford Press.

Gollwitzer, P. M. (1991). *Abwägen und Planen: Bewußtseinslagen in verschiedenen Handlungsphasen.* Göttingen: Hogrefe.

Gollwitzer, P. M. (1993). Goal achievement: The role of intentions. In W. Stroebe & M. Hewstone (Eds.), *European review of social psychology* (Vol. 4, pp. 141–185). Chichester, England: Wiley.

Gollwitzer, P. M., Heckhausen, H., & Ratajczak, H. (1990). From weighing to willing: Approaching a change decision through pre- or postdecisional mentation. *Organizational Behavior and Human Decision Processes, 45,* 41–65.

Gollwitzer, P. M., Heckhausen, H., & Steller, B. (1990). Deliberative vs. implemental mind-sets: Cognitive tuning toward congruous thoughts and information. *Journal of Personality and Social Psychology, 59,* 1119–1127.

Gollwitzer, P. M., & Kinney, R. F. (1989). Effects of deliberative and implemental mind-sets on the illusion of control. *Journal of Personality and Social Psychology, 56,* 531–542.

Gottschaldt, K. (1926). Über den Einfluß der Erfahrung auf die Wahrnehmung von Figuren: I. Über den Einfluß gehäufter Einprägung von Figuren auf ihre Sichtbarkeit in umfassenden Konfigurationen. *Psychologische Forschung, 8,* 261–317.

Hayes-Roth, B., & Hayes-Roth, F. (1979). A cognitive model of planning. *Cognitive Science, 3,* 275–310.

Heckhausen, H., & Gollwitzer, P. M. (1987). Thought contents and cognitive functioning in motivational versus volitional states of mind. *Motivation and Emotion, 11,* 101–120.

Johnston, W. A. (1978). The intrusiveness of familiar nontarget information. *Memory and Cognition, 6,* 38–42.

Johnston, W. A., & Dark, V. J. (1986). Selective attention. *Annual Review of Psychology, 37,* 43–75.

Jones, E. E., & Gerard, H. B. (1967). *Foundations of social psychology.* New York: Wiley.

Kahneman, D. (1973). *Attention and effort.* Englewood Cliffs, NJ: Prentice-Hall.

Kahnemann, D., & Treisman, A. M. (1984). Changing views of attention and automaticity. In R. Parasuraman, R. Davies, & J. Beatty (Eds.), *Varieties of attention* (pp. 29–61). New York: Academic Press.

Kreitler, S., & Kreitler, H. (1987). Conceptions and processes of planning. In S. L. Friedman, E. K. Scholnick, & R. R. Cocking (Eds.), *Blueprints for thinking: The role of planning in cognitive development* (pp. 205–272). Cambridge, England: Cambridge University Press.

Kuhl, J. (1984). Volitional aspects of achievement motivation and learned helplessness: Toward a comprehensive theory of action control. In B. A. Maher & W. B. Maher (Eds.), *Progress in experimental personality research* (pp. 99–171). New York: Academic Press.

Kuhl, J., & Beckmann, J. (Eds.). (1985). *Action control: From cognition to behavior.* Berlin: Springer-Verlag.

Kuhl, J., & Beckmann, J. (Eds.). (1994). *Volition and personality.* Toronto: Hogrefe.

Külpe, O. (1904). Versuch über Abstraktion. In F. Schumann (Ed.), *Bericht über den 1. Kongre ß für experimentelle Psychologie* (pp. 56–71). Leipzig: Barth.

Lengfelder, A. (1994). *Die Bedeutung des Frontalhirns beim Abwägen und Planen.* Unpublished doctoral dissertation, Ludwig-Maximilians-Universität, München.

Lewin, K. (1926). Vorsatz, Wille und Bedürfnis. *Psychologische Forschung, 7,* 330–385.

Lewin, K., Dembo, T., Festinger, L.A., & Sears, P.S. (1944). Level of aspiration. In J. M. Hunt (Ed.), *Personality and the behavior disorders* (pp. 333–378). New York: Ronald Press.

Lissner, K. (1933). Die Entspannung von Bedürfnissen durch Ersatzhandlungen. *Psychologische Forschung, 18,* 218–250.

Logan, G. D. (1979). On the use of a concurrent memory load to measure attention and automaticity. *Journal of Experimental Psychology: Human Perception and Performance, 5,* 189–207.

Mahler, W. (1933). Ersatzhandlungen verschiedenen Realitätsgrades. *Psychologische Forschung, 18,* 27–89.

Malzacher, J. T. (1992). *Erleichtern Vorsätze die Handungsinitiierung? Zur Aktivierung der Vornahmehandlung.* Unpublished doctoral dissertation, Ludwig-Maximilians-Universität, München.

Mannes, S. M., & Kintsch, W. (1991). Routine computing tasks: Planning as understanding. *Cognitive Science, 15,* 305–342.

Nielsen, S. L., & Sarason, I. G. (1981). Emotion, personality, and selective attention. *Journal of Personality and Social Psychology, 41,* 945–960.

Ovsiankina, M. (1928). Die Wiederaufnahme unterbrochener Handlungen. *Psychologische Forschung, 11,* 302–379.

Patterson, C. J., & Mischel, W. (1976). Effects of temptation-inhibiting and task-facilitating plans on self-control. *Journal of Personality and Social Psychology, 33,* 209–217.

Pösel, I. (1994). *Wiederaufnahme unterbrochener Handlungen: Effekte der Bewußtseinslagen des Abwägens und Planens.* Unpublished master's thesis, Universität Regensburg.

Posner, M. I. (1978). *Chronometric explorations of mind.* Hillsdale, NJ: Erlbaum.

Schaal, B. (1993). *Impulskontrolle: Wie Vorsätze beherrschtes Handeln erleichtern.* Unpublished master's thesis, Ludwigs-Maximilians-Universität, München.

Seehausen, R., Bayer, U., & Gollwitzer, P. M. (1994, September). *Experimentelle Arbeiten zur vorsätzlichen Handlungsregulation.* Paper presented at the biannual meeting of the German Psychological Association, Hamburg.

Seligman, M. E. P. (1990). *Learned optimism.* New York: Knopf.

Shiffrin, R. M., & Schneider, W. (1977). Controlled and automatic human information processing: II. Perceptual learning, automatic attending, and a general theory. *Psychological Review, 84,* 127–190.

Steller, B. (1992). *Vorsätze und die Wahrnehmung günstiger Gelegenheiten.* München: Tuduv Verlagsgesellschaft.

Taylor, S. E., & Brown, J. D. (1988). Illusion and well-being: A social psychological perspective on mental health. *Psychological Bulletin, 103,* 193–210.

Taylor, S. E., & Gollwitzer, P. M. (1995). The effects of mind-sets on positive illusions. *Journal of Personality and Social Psychology, 69,* 213–226.

Taylor, S. E., & Schneider, S. K. (1989). Coping and the simulation of events. *Social Cognition, 7,* 176–196.

Watt, H. J. (1905). Experimentelle Beiträge zu einer Theorie des Denkens. *Archiv für die gesamte Psychologie, 4,* 289–436.

Wicklund, R. A., & Frey, D. (1981). Cognitive consistency: Motivational versus non-motivational perspectives. In J. P. Forgas (Ed.), *Social cognition: Perspectives on everyday understanding* (pp. 141–163). London: Academic Press.

Wilensky, R. (1983). *Planning and understanding.* Reading, MA: Addison-Wesley.

Witkin, H. A. (1950). Individual differences in ease of perception of embedded figures. *Journal of Personality, 19,* 1–15.

Zillmann, D., & Cantor, J. R. (1976). Effect of timing of information about mitigating circumstances on emotional responses to provocation and retaliatory behavior. *Journal of Experimental Social Psychology, 12,* 38–55.

CHAPTER 14 Striving and Feeling

Personal Goals and Subjective Well-Being

Robert A. Emmons

It is clear from this volume that goal structures are indispensable theoretical constructs for understanding action patterns. Impressive research programs (e.g. see Locke & Kristof, Chapter 16, this volume) have linked goals to a variety of cognitive and behavioral outcomes. It is also clear, however, that goal-directed action cannot be understood apart from affect. As Pervin (1983), Klinger (1977), and Kruglanski (Chapter 26, this volume) have argued, affect is central to goals. At a minimum, affect is related to goals in the following ways: It plays a role in determining one's commitment to goals; it energizes goal-directed behavior; and it serves as feedback informing a person of the status of their goals. Theories of emotion and theories of subjective well-being (SWB) are increasingly adopting the position that affective states are a function of the status and nature of one's goal strivings. Whether affect is examined in terms of discrete short-term states (emotions) or as long-term individual-difference characteristics (SWB), there is widespread agreement that goals and related constructs such as concerns and commitments play an essential role in determining the quality and intensity of affective experience (Frijda, 1986; Klinger, 1977; Lazarus, 1991; Oatley, 1992; Ortony, Clore, & Collins, 1988).

Within the domain of SWB, characteristics of personal goal systems are being explored as precursors of life satisfaction and of long-term positive and negative affective states (Brunstein, 1993; Emmons, 1986; Little, 1989; Omodei & Wearing, 1990; Yetim, 1993). Similarly, goal theories of emotion postulate that discrete emotional states are the results of goal-relevant appraisals (Lazarus, 1991; Oatley, 1992). My interest has been in exploring individual differences in emotional well-being, or long-term positive and negative affective states, as a function of both the structural and functional properties of one's goal system. In this chapter, I do not focus on work that has been primarily concerned with short-term mood states or discrete emotions. Rather, my primary purpose is to review the empirical evidence that has linked goals with long-term affective outcomes.

PERSONAL GOALS

The Importance of Goals

Why are goals important for SWB? Human beings are, by nature, goal-oriented organisms. Goals are desired states that people seek to obtain, maintain, or avoid. People's lives are structured around the pursuit of incentives—incentives that reflect fundamental human needs. Ryan (1992, Ryan, Sheldon, Kasser, & Deci, Chapter 1, this volume) contends that goals instantiate the needs for autonomy, competence, and relatedness, and that an individual's sense of well-being depends upon the ability of the individual to make progress toward these goals. Goal theories (e.g., Pervin, 1983) assume the following: (1) Behavior is organized around the pursuit of goals, with goals being defined as objectives that a person strives to attain or avoid; (2) goals influence ongoing thought and emotional reactions in addition to behavior; (3) goals exist within a system of hierarchically organized superordinate and subordinate goals, where functioning in one aspect of the system has ramifications for other parts of the system; and (4) goals are accessible to conscious awareness, though there is no requirement that a goal be represented in consciousness while a person is in active pursuit of it.

A prominent recent trend in the field of personality has been the adoption of idiographic goal units of human motivation. Many of the cognitive–motivational units of personality being studied today are what have been termed "middle-level" units of analysis (Buss & Cantor, 1989) for personality psychology. They are termed "middle-level" in that they are typically at a middle level of abstraction in a structural hierarchy, can be concretized with reference to specific activities and situations, and can be generalized with reference to higher-order themes and meanings in life. These consciously articulated cognitive–motivational units include the constructs of possible selves, personal strivings, personal projects, current concerns, life tasks, self-defining goals, and various schemas and scripts (e.g., as core organizing themes, core conditional patterns, and core conflictual relationship themes) (see Emmons & King, 1992, for a review). These are all ways of representing affectively charged goals and themes that are central to the person's life while emerging from and determining the nature of the person's transactions with his or her social worlds. As such, they are ideal units for studying both intrapsychic and interpersonal conflict. Goals, with links to affect, cognition, and behavior, are central to understanding motivated behavior. The hierarchical structure of goals, with links to both higher and lower levels; the flexibility, discriminativeness, and yet coherence that the goal concept implies; and its amenability to measurement and individual differences make it a highly desirable unit of analysis for researchers interested in examining motivational models of SWB, and more generally in examining the relation between motivational and emotional processes. However, as I argue, the ultimate fulfillment of these goals may not be what is critical for SWB. Thus, goals may be viewed as necessary yet insufficient for high levels of SWB. Goals provide meaning and purpose in life (Baumeister, 1991; Klinger, 1977). In the absence of personally significant goals, the individual must look for other sources of meaning. This is a theme to which I return in a later section of the chapter.

Personal Strivings as Goal Units

Over the past several years, I have been developing a model of personality and SWB in which goals play a central role in determining the degree to which a person is satisfied with his or her life, and the degree to which that person experiences positive and negative emotional states. In our laboratory, my colleagues and I have been examining the relation between goals and SWB by using the "personal strivings" construct. In this approach, goals are conceptualized as personal strivings, defined as "what a person is typically or characteristically trying to do" (Emmons, 1989, p. 92). Personal strivings consist of recurring objectives that characterize a person's intentional behavior. For example, a person may be trying to "find that special someone," "overcome shyness around strangers," or "be a good Christian example." Other examples of personal strivings are shown in Table 14.1. According to the personal-striving perspective, personality is organized into idiographically coherent patterns of goal strivings. More discriminating than global motives, yet more stable than specific plans or behaviors, personal strivings occupy a desirable position in the hierarchy of personality functioning. A personal striving is a unifying construct—it unites what may be phenotypically different goals or actions around a common quality or theme. The personal-striving approach is guided by the control theory of behavioral self-regulation (Carver & Scheier, 1981, 1982, 1990; Powers, 1973). According to control theory, various levels of reference values that regulate action exist in a hierarchy ranging from the narrowest, most specific actions to the broadest, most abstract principles. Behavior is a process of discrepancy reduction in which individuals act to minimize the discrepancy between their present condition and a desired standard or goal. Personal strivings can be thought of as one of these reference values that are used to guide action. A personal striving describes enduring and recurring personality characteristics: Strivings are durable concerns that are relatively stable over time and consistently expressed in a variety of situations.

The personal-striving construct was initially proposed in order to offer both an additional unit of personality (to complement trait-based levels of analysis) and a construct that could account for individual differences in SWB. Personal goals have been assessed normatively as well as idiographic-

TABLE 14.1. Examples of Personal Strivings

Be physically attractive
Present myself as intelligent
Avoid conflicts with people
Be empathetic to others
Remain open-minded no matter what the circumstances
Show compassion towards others
Be assertive
Exercise three times a week
Avoid people who provoke bad habits in me
Not be the center of attention
Help my friends and family
Not procrastinate
Not lose my temper
Find time for myself alone
Do something spontaneously, once a week

ally in previous research. Goals tend to be generated idiographically and then are rated on common dimensions that permit comparisons across individuals. The content of goal systems, and the structural and functional properties of goals, have been examined with respect to well-being. Research on personal goal strivings and well-being can be divided into three areas: goal content and SWB, goal orientation and SWB, and goal parameters and SWB.

GOAL CONTENT AND SUBJECTIVE WELL-BEING

Main Effects

One way to examine the relation between personal goals and SWB is in terms of goal content. Is the content of what people are trying to do related to their level of SWB? In terms of personal goals, this requires moving from an idiographic to a nomothetic level of analysis—a move that is made possible when strivings are coded into broader, thematic categories. We have developed a coding system for classifying personal strivings into 12 content categories. These include the "Big Three" (McAdams, 1994) motive dispositions (achievement, affiliation/intimacy, and power), as well as other higher-order themes, such as independence, self-presentation, and generativity. Unlike many thematic measures of motivation (Smith, 1992), however, this results in the clustering together of strivings on the basis of surface similarities rather than underlying motivational content.

In a number of different samples, we have found that the strongest predictor of positive well-being is the proportion of intimacy strivings in a person's striving system (Colby, Emmons, & Rabin, 1994), whereas the proportions of achievement and power strivings tend to be related to higher levels of negative well-being (Emmons, 1991). Intimacy strivings reflect a concern for establishing deep and mutually gratifying relationships, whereas affiliation reflects more of a desire to be popular and to avoid loneliness (McAdams, 1994). Generativity strivings, defined as those strivings that involve creating, giving of oneself to others, and having an influence on future generations, were related to higher levels of life satisfaction and to measures of positive affectivity, but were unrelated to negative affect (Stemmerich & Emmons, 1993). That intimacy strivings are related to higher levels of well-being should come as no surprise. The ability to engage in close intimate relationships is the hallmark of psychosocial maturity and a key component to psychological growth, according to a variety of theorists. The link between achievement strivings, and lower well-being, on the other hand, is somewhat more surprising. Perhaps these individuals are "linkers," to use McIntosh and Martin's (1992) term, in that they believe that the attainment of an achievement goal is necessary for happiness, and that happiness is not possible in the absence of such an outcome. Putting one's affective fate in the hands of external contingencies is a sure formula for failure. Persons with many agentic strivings may experience less positive well-being for another reason—namely, that they are overinvested in individual striving to the exclusion of developing interdependent strivings. Indeed, in her analysis of implicit and explicit measures of motivation, King (1991) argued that in some individuals achievement strivings represent an explicit rejection of affiliative concerns, in that individuals preoccupied with achievement turn away from opportunities to develop relational ties. Cantor et al. (1991) have also shown that preoccupation with achievement life tasks to the exclusion of intimacy-based tasks is associated with greater stress levels.

Kasser and Ryan (1993) demonstrated that the extrinsically oriented goals of achieving financial success and social recognition were negatively related to several measures of well-being, including vitality and self-actualization. Alternatively, subjects who possessed the intrinsic goals of personal growth and community contribution reported higher levels of well-being. Despite these scattered studies, however, relatively little research in the literature on personal goals has examined the relationship between the *content* of personal goals and well-being indicators.

One additional study should be mentioned here. Beginning with different assumptions than Kasser and Ryan, Diener and Fujita (1995) proposed that personal strivings mediate the relation between resources and well-being. They hypothesized that resources such as money, good looks, health, or intelligence should be related to well-being only to the extent to which these resources enable an individual's personal strivings. Subjects rated the relevance of each of 21 resources for the attainment of each of their 15 strivings. The degree to which the subjects possessed various resources was based on judgments by knowledgeable informants rather than through self-reports. Significant correlations were found between goal relevance of resources on the one hand and negative affect and life satisfaction on the other; higher correlations were also observed between goal-relevant resources and well-being than between less relevant resources and well-being. The possession of resources per se, independent of goal strivings, was unrelated to SWB. Thus, the greater the congruence between a person's goals and his or her resources, the higher the SWB that person tends to experience. It is interesting to note that, consistent with the study by Kasser and Ryan (1993) cited earlier, the "intrinsic" resources of self-confidence, social skills, and self-discipline received the highest relevance ratings, whereas the "extrinsic" resources of material possessions, physical attractiveness, and money were rated as mostly irrelevant to the attainment of one's goals. Both studies seriously question whether the "American dream" of fame, fortune, and image is a desirable state of affairs to strive toward.

Rarely have studies on goal content and SWB included non-college-based samples. One exception is the work of Rapkin and Fischer (1992). In an elderly community sample, these authors found that elders leading satisfying lives were most concerned with the maintenance of social goals, whereas the disengagement from social roles and relationships was associated with higher levels of depression.

Interactional Models

In addition to examining the main effects of goal type on SWB, a few studies have tested interactional models, in which SWB is predicted to be dependent on the interaction between goals and stressful life events that impinge upon these goals. Much of this work has been implicitly or explicitly rooted in a transactional framework of stress and coping (Lazarus, 1993). In such an approach, chronic goal concerns are seen as mediators determining the relevance of objective life events for SWB. Elsewhere (Emmons, 1991), I proposed that life events are appraised with respect to the significance they hold for a person's personal strivings, and that people attach significance to events that have implications for their strivings. This general hypothesis was supported in a study of daily life events and mood (Emmons, 1991). The degree to which individuals experienced positive and negative moods on a day-to-day basis was contingent upon positive and negative life events in domains relevant to their goals. For example, the moods of affiliative and intimacy-oriented individuals were most affected by interpersonal events, and those of achievement-oriented individuals were most susceptible to academic and task-related events. Similarly, Lavallee and Campbell (1994) found that self-relevant negative events (i.e., those that impinge upon personal goals) are more threatening to the self-concept and are associated with more self-focused attention and more rumination. Thus, although there may be some main effects of goal type on SWB, interactional models may hold more promise for explaining daily variations in SWB (Affleck, Tennen, Urrows, & Higgins, 1994; Marco & Suls, 1993).

In an attempt to expand the interactional model, we are currently examining the link between traumatic life experiences and personal strivings. Our goal-based model of trauma (Emmons, 1994) assumes that traumatic life experiences cause individuals to reorganize their personal strivings, and that strivings also play a major role in facilitating adaptation to trauma. We are examining changes in striving content and appraisals as a function of traumatic experiences, with an eye toward identifying the nature of goal system change that promotes personal growth and recovery.

GOAL ORIENTATION AND SUBJECTIVE WELL-BEING

The second way in which personal goals are related to SWB is through goal orientation. "Goal orientation" refers to individual differences in the manner in which goals are represented consciously by the individual and described linguistically when the individual is communicating his or her goals to others. Thus, orientation refers to individual differences in the mental representations of goals. Goal orientations have been identified with respect to both goal setting and goal striving. In this section of the chapter, I describe three orientations, each of which has relevance for SWB. These three are level of goal specification, approach versus avoidance goals, and the degree of relative autonomy of one's goals.

Level of Goal Specification

The first orientation describes differences in what I have called "level of goal specification." According to Little (1989), some of us dedicate our lives to "magnificent obsessions," whereas others are content to muddle through life working on "trivial pursuits." This distinction represents two extremes along a dimension that can be characterized as level of abstraction of one's goal strivings. In examining strivings that subjects have spontaneously generated in past studies, my colleagues and I have found that people frame their goals at various levels of generality. Some individuals describe their goals in primarily broad, abstract, and expansive ways. These individuals are referred to here as "high-level strivers." Others tend to frame their goals in concrete, specific, and more superficial terms. These individuals are referred to as "low-level strivers." High- and low-level strivers may describe what are functionally equivalent goals in very different ways. Some individuals may be trying to "ward off the ravages of time," whereas others may simply be trying to "stay out of the sun." Although these are ostensibly similar goals, the goals are framed at different levels of abstraction. "Keep my books straightened on my shelves" and "write 10 pages a day for my new book" are low-level goals, whereas "be an organized person" and "try to make a contribution to future generations" are examples of higher level strivings. Table 14.2 shows goals characteristic of high- and low-level strivers.

TABLE 14.2. Examples of High- and Low-Level Strivings

High level

1. Seek out new ways of bettering my spiritual growth, attitudes, behavior
2. Be postitive and optimistic in the way I approach daily goals
3. Spend time with and care for animals
4. Knowledge education in area of interest
5. Reassure kids and grandkids of my feelings and concerns
6. Come to terms with suppressed feelings and emotions
7. Daydream about my future—how I would like it to be
8. Increase quality of life for others less fortunate
9. Continually talk to self regarding anger and resentments
10. Alleviate obsessive behaviors
11. Maintain personal appearance
12. Bring happiness to those around me—tell them how important they are
13. Be actively involved in outdoor activities
14. Remove self-centered thoughts
15. Face my character flaws and evaluate their origins

Low level

1. Stay in shape (exercise, eat healthy)
2. Keep up in my classes
3. Get along with my brother
4. Keep my room clean
5. Read the newspaper and keep up on current events
6. Not watch too much TV
7. Pay attention in class
8. Get enough sleep
9. Have balance in my life between school and socializing
10. Have a good life
11. Travel as much as possible
12. Persuade others to my line of thinking

This distinction between high- and low-level goals is reminiscent of Vallacher and Wegner's (1985) levels of action identification theory, in which actions can be identified at various levels of analysis, ranging from the molecular to the molar (see Emmons, 1989, for a detailed comparison of the personal-strivings approach and action identification theory). There is considerable support for the notion of levels of abstraction within many different areas of psychology, including personality, clinical, social, and cognitive psychology. Cutting across these areas, levels of abstraction can be viewed within control theory (Carver & Scheier, 1982, 1990; Martin & Tesser, 1989; Powers, 1973). Control theory formulations posit a hierarchy of levels of control, with various levels of standards or goals arranged from the most concrete and narrow to the broadest and most abstract organizing principles. The lowest levels indicate how the action is to be carried out, while the higher levels provide information on the purposes or implications of the action. Goals or standards can be characterized at different levels within this hierarchy. People may be said to differ in terms of the level at which they tend to characterize their goals within the hierarchy.

However, within the control theory literature, the interest has not been in individual differences in tendencies to phrase goals at different levels of abstraction. In a variety of different samples (reported in Emmons, 1992), high-level striving tended to be associated with psychological distress, particularly anxiety and depression. Low-level striving, on the other hand, has been linked to greater levels of psychological well-being, but also to more physical illness. I have referred to this pattern as the "illness versus depression" tradeoff. What it really reflects, though, is the tradeoff described earlier by Little (1989) between having manageable versus meaningful goals. Higher-level goals are rated as more difficult to accomplish and lower in clarity of means to accomplish them; these factors may account for their link to negative affectivity. High-level goals are also associated with higher ratings on purpose in life measures, suggesting that a meaningful life need not be based solely on short-term, pleasant emotional states. Notice the spiritual nature of many of the high-level strivings in Table 14.2. Religiosity is often linked to well-being by providing meaning or purpose in life. Low-level goals, particularly those indicating an absence of emotional self-awareness, may be linked to physical illness through mechanisms of repression/defensiveness. Presented with the psychologically charged task of confronting one's innermost aspirations, repressors are likely to find the task threatening, to engage in avoidant processing, and to produce less revealing and more superficial goals. If low-level striving is indicative of a repressive personality, then low-level strivers should also appraise their strivings more positively than high-level strivers, as repressors tend to deny negative characteristics in themselves.

In order to test this hypothesis, Gomersall (1993) explored the relation between personal-striving system variables (including level of goal specification) and repression/defensiveness. Repressors, as measured by the combination of scores on the Marlowe–Crowne Social Desirability Scale and the Taylor Manifest Anxiety Scale, had fewer strivings with emotional content and fewer negative, avoidant strivings (see below) than did nonrepressors. Repressors also rated themselves as being more satisfied with the degree of progress made toward their strivings, rated their strivings as less difficult, and reported higher levels of instrumentality among their strivings. Examples of strivings reported by repressors include "think positives about myself," "not be quick to anger because it is not a good feeling," "not show negative emotions so much," "please people," and "seek other people's approval." The theme of emotional avoidance is prevalent throughout these strivings, as is the need for social approval. The fact that repressors have insight into their mood regulation strategies suggests that avoidance is not an entirely unconscious process. It is also interesting that it is the emotionality component of the construct of levels that is responsible for the links with repressive coping. There is a substantial literature on avoidant coping styles, autonomic arousal, and physical health (Krohne, 1993; Pennebaker & Traue, 1993), which implicates repressiveness as a risk factor for various physical illnesses.

Approach and Avoidance Goals

A second goal orientation that we have studied is the degree to which individuals are striving toward positive, appetitive goals as opposed to striving to avoid negative, aversive goals. For instance, a person may be trying to "spend time with others" versus "avoid being lonely," or trying to "avoid letting anything upset me" versus "stay calm even under trying circumstances." The motivation literature has demonstrated that these differing orientations lead to very different behavioral patterns and consequences, even when similar goal content is involved. Similarly, we have found that individuals who are concerned with avoiding negative outcomes have higher levels of psychological distress, compared to persons with primarily approach orientations. The purpose of our research (Emmons & Kaiser, 1994) was to investigate the relation between approach and avoidance strivings and indicators of psychological and physical well-being. We predicted that individuals whose striving lists contained a large number of avoidant strivings would experience more psychological distress, particularly anxiety, than individuals with predominantly appetitive striving systems. This prediction was based on Gray's (1987) theory of the behavioral activation and inhibition systems, and their hypothesized effect on emotional experience.

Two hundred and sixty-one undergraduates in several studies on mood and goals at the University of Illinois and the University of California at Davis, and 100 community couples in Davis, California, served as subjects. After completing the Striving Assessment Packet (Emmons, 1989), subjects completed either a daily mood report for periods ranging from 3 to 6 weeks or a global measure of positive and negative affect. Subjects completed physical symptom reports in a similar manner, by indicating whether or not they had experienced any physical symptoms (eight categories) on the daily form. Subjects in all samples completed a number of well-being questionnaires.

The open-ended lists of strivings were coded for approach–avoidance according to the guidelines in the Personal Striving Coding Manual (Emmons, 1989). Examples of two subjects with a high proportion of avoidance strivings are shown in Table 14.3. Interrater reliability was 100% for this coding task. The proportion of avoidance strivings ranged from 9% to 15% in the various samples.

What does it mean to be oriented toward avoiding outcomes? What are the consequences of possessing a high number of avoidance strivings? Zero-order product–moment correlations between avoidance strivings and the measures of psychological well-being are shown in Table 14.4. The correlations between avoidance strivings and physical well-being are shown in Table 14.5. Subjects with a high proportion of avoidance strivings tended to report

TABLE 14.3. Subjects with a Large Percentage of Avoidant Strivings

S#10754

1. Be an honest person.
2. Do unto others as I would like to be done to me.
3. Curb my habit of telling my personal thoughts and opinions to people I just meet.
4. Share everything with my family.
5. Not get angry at myself for being out of shape.
6. Always be prompt.
7. Want the best of life for myself and my family.
8. Not have so many expectations of my son.
9. Be a friend to my friends.
10. Avoid feeling guilt.
11. Curb my desire to spend money.
12. Avoid comparing myself to my sister.
13. Avoid the overwhelming feeling of wondering if my father approves of my decisions.
14. Want better for my son.

S#0381

1. Be understanding of others accepting them as they are.
2. Avoid offending others by maintaining my distance.
3. Always live in the past or future, but not for today.
4. Look at matters realistically rather than accept things for what they appear to be.
5. Appear knowledgeable of any and all subjects to others.
6. Avoid taking sides in an issue even though I may feel very strongly about one side.
7. Put myself down by appearing "bumbling" as if age were causing me to slip.
8. Avoid eye contact—more with strangers than with people I know.
9. Be all things to all people, i.e., react rather than proact.
10. Give others what I think they want from me.
11. Tone down any enthusiasm I may spontaneously generate about anything I may be doing.
12. Avoid arguments or even spirited discussions.
13. Be the great mediator when thinking no one else can do the job.
14. Keep things light, rather than engage in a searching, serious discussion of issues.

lower well-being across most measures and most samples. The strongest pattern of correlations was found in the community sample of adults. In that sample, adults who strove to avoid negative goals reported lower positive moods, less life satisfaction, and more anxiety compared to appetitively motivated individuals. They were also higher on all five measures of physical symptomatology, as seen in Table 14.5.

Thus, negative strivings appear to constitute a risk factor for psychological and physical distress. Individuals who are concerned with avoiding negative outcomes have higher levels of negative well-being, compared to persons with primarily approach orientations. There are at least two reasons for this pattern. Norbert Schwarz's (1990) account of the cognitive asymmetry of approach and avoidance situations is one possibility. According to Schwarz, in order to obtain a certain positive outcome, there need be only

TABLE 14.4. Correlations between Proportion of Avoidance Strivings and Psychological Well-Being

Measure	Sample 1 (n = 40)	Sample 2 (n = 105)	Sample 3 (n = 116)	Sample 4 (n = 200)
Positive affect	−.16	−.23[a]	−.18	−.47[b]
Negative affect	.27	.12	.01	.10
Life satisfaction	.00	−.09	−.19	−.56[b]
Depression	.34[a]	.19	.12	.13
Anxiety	.17	.29[b]	.25[b]	.28[b]
Differntial Personality Scale; Well-being	−.30[a]	−.21[a]	−.24[a]	−.57[b]
Observer positive affect			−.30[a]	−.25[a]
Observer negative affect			.07	.02

Note. Samples 1–3 consisted of college students; Sample 4 consisted of 100 married community couples.
[a]$p < .05$.
[b]$p < .01$.

a single accessible route to that goal. However, in order to avoid or prevent an undesired outcome from happening, all possible routes to that goals must be identified and blocked. Thus, avoidance goals require a very different form of analytical reasoning than approach goals. In addition to this cognitive explanation, these preferences could also reflect different brain processes, such as the behavioral inhibition and activation systems (Gray, 1987). Perhaps individuals preoccupied by avoidant goals have more reactive inhibition systems, and are thus preoccupied with avoiding aversive outcomes. In support of this conjecture, we (Emmons & McAdams, 1991) found that inhibition scores from a Thematic Apperception Test-like picture story exercise were significantly correlated with proportion of negative strivings. On the other hand, individuals whose striving system contained predominantly approach goals were more sensitive to rewards. Recently, Carver and White (1994) developed a questionnaire measure of Gray's behavioral activation and inhibition systems. We are currently exploring how scores on this measure are related to approach and avoidance strivings.

TABLE 14.5. Correlations between Proportion of Avoidance Strivings and Physical Well-Being

Measure	Sample 1 (n = 40)	Sample 2 (n = 105)	Sample 3 (n = 116)	Sample 4 (n = 200)
Somatization	−.14	.18	.01	.31[b]
PILL[a]		.23[b]	.08	.30[b]
Missed work			.15	.21[b]
Physician visits			.07	.24[b]
Spouse-rated symptoms				.25[b]

[a]PILL, Pennebaker Inventory of Limbic Languidness.
[b]$p < .05$.

Degree of Relative Autonomy

A third and final goal orientation that has been linked to well-being is derived from Deci and Ryan's (1991) self-determination theory. Deci and Ryan have proposed that motivated behaviors vary in the degree to which they are self-determined, or autonomous, versus controlled. Ryan et al. (Chapter 1, this volume) contend that "The amount or level of motivation does not necessarily differ when people are autonomous versus controlled, but the type or orientation of motivation does, and this results in a different quality of functioning" (p. 9). Ryan and Connell (1989) have developed a continuum of reasons for acting, ranging from extrinsic, controlling reasons to intrinsic, self-determined reasons. Acting for more autonomous reasons has been associated with more favorable outcomes in terms of academic motivation and religiosity (see Deci & Ryan, 1991, for a review). Applying this continuum to personal strivings, Sheldon and Kasser (1993) asked subjects to rate the degree to which they strove for each of their goals, either because the goal was personally interesting, important, and valued, or because they felt compelled to for either interpersonal or intrapsychic reasons. Having more autonomous reasons for one's strivings was positively associated with several measures of psychological well-being, including life satisfaction, vitality, and self-actualizing tendencies.

GOAL PARAMETERS

The final domain of goal processes that are related to well-being, and that account for the majority of research on goals and SWB, is the domain of goal parameters. "Goal parameters" is the general term I use to refer to those goal appraisal dimensions identified by some theorists (e.g., Klinger, 1977) as dimensions that link goals to affect, cognition, and action. These nomothetic dimensions permit comparisons across persons even though they possess idiographic sets of personal goals.These include goal conflict/ambivalence, expectancies for success, goal commitment, goal differentiation, past attainment, and clarity of means for achieving goals. These dimensions incorporate both the structural and functional attributes (Karoly, 1991) of goal systems. Of the structural attributes, conflict/ambivalence and differentiation stand out as especially powerful predictors of SWB.

Goal Conflict and Ambivalence

Intrapsychic goal conflict is an inevitable by-product of motivational life. Peopel desire many things, but often their other desires keep them from obtaining all that they want. Conflict may be as trivial as the decision of whether to have Chinese or Italian food for dinner, or it may be as monumental as the decision of whether or not to run for president of the United States.

Individuals whose goals are in conflict spend more time ruminating about their goals and less time working toward achieving them (Emmons & King, 1988). This inhibitory behavior only serves to perpetuate the conflicts, since such persons fail to act toward resolving the conflicts and ares also unable to make progress toward achieving any goal. Personal goals serve as an ideal vehicle for examining intrapsychic conflict, since both major and minor life decisions revolve around fundamental values, goals, desires, and other personally motivating factors.

Arising from within various theoretical perspectives, from psychodynamic to cognitive-behavioral, many terms have been offered to describe oppositional tendencies within the mind. These include "discrepancies," "disregulations," "disconnections," "contradictions," "incongruities," "incompatibilities," "imbalances," and "discontinuities." Regardless of terminological differences, these perspectives are all dealing with internal incompatibilities or the terms we have used, "conflict" and "ambivalence" (the latter being a subset of the former). The term "goal conflict" is used here to refer to two processes. First, an individual may be ambivalent about achieving a particular goal. Meehl (1964, p. 10) defined intense ambivalence as "the existence of simultaneous or rapidly interchangeable positive and negative feelings toward the same object or activity, with the added proviso that both the positive and negative feelings be strong." Clearly, this definition conjures up a conflict situation. Ambivalence can also be thought of as an approach–avoidance conflict—wanting but at the same time not wanting the same goal object. For example, a person may be ambivalent about the goal "express my true feelings" because of the potential negative consequences that such free expression might entail. In addition, an individual may be ambivalent about the goal "finish my dissertation as soon as possible" not because the end is viewed as potentially negative, but because the process of achieving the goal may seem unusually daunting. The second use of the term "conflict" refers to the situation in which a goal that a person wishes to accomplish interferes with the attainment of at least one other goal that the individual simultaneously wishes to accomplish. For example, the goal of trying to spend time with one's family may interfere with the goal of doing well in one's career.

The debilitating effects of conflict on self-regulatory processes have been discussed in some detail by various authors (Bargh & Gollwitzer, 1994; Emmons, King, & Sheldon, 1993; Gollwitzer, 1993; Karoly, 1993). We (Emmons, King, & Sheldon, 1993) and Gollwitzer (1993) describe how individuals may resolve conflicts between competing intentions in the service of attaining valued personal goals. The inability to resolve chronic conflicts is associated with poorer well-being. In our lab, we have found that conflict between and within personal strivings is related to measures of negative affectivity and physical symptomatology, both concurrently and prospectively. Conflict (between goals) and ambivalence (approach–avoidance conflict) were associated with a variety of physical symptoms, as well as an increase in health center visits, at a 1-year follow-up (Emmons & King, 1988). Interpersonal goal conflict is also related to lower psychological well-being and to physical illness (King & Emmons, 1991).

Conflict over Expressing Emotion

One type of conflict, ambivalence over emotional expression, seems to be an especailly pernicious form of conflict that is especially strongly related to psychological distress. A content analysis of the types of strivings that individuals rated high in ambivalence in earlier research (Emmons & King, 1988) revealed a theme of conflict over expressing emotion. Given our culture's emphasis on the containment of emotional expression, coupled with a natural tendency to seek expression, it is not surprising that individuals become ambivalent over emotional expression. Goals pertaining to emotional expression provide a pointed demonstration of the translation of cultural ambivalence into individual lives. For example, rated high in ambivalence were strivings such as "keep my anger under control," "express myself honestly," "control my temper," "always appear cool," "not let my emotions take over," "always wear a smile on my face," "be honest and open about my feelings," and "let my anger out before it all builds up inside me." These goals illustrate the belief that emotion should be honestly expressed, but also the belief that expression implies vulnerability. We (King & Emmons, 1990) suggested that inhibition of emotional expression may be understood as a result of an individual's competing desires to express and not to express emotions. Thus, inexpressiveness that may be pathogenic is distinguished from "comfortable" inexpressiveness by the conflict dynamic that exists beneath the overt expressiveness style. The Ambivalence over Expressing Emotion Questionnaire (AEQ; King & Emmons, 1990) is a 28-item self-report measure designed to assess wanting to express and failing to, as well as expressing and later regretting having done so.

Although it has been found to relate negatively to emotional expressiveness, conflict over emotional expression, measured via the AEQ, has been distinguished from simple inexpressiveness in studies demonstrating that ambivalence over emotional expression is related to depression, anxiety, guilt, other measures of distress, and symptom reports, when self-reported expressiveness is controlled for (King & Emmons, 1990). Thus, whether the ambivalent individual is expressive or not, he or she may experience the distress associated with the underlying conflict dynamic. Importantly, these relations between distress/symptoms and ambivalence over expression persist even when overall negative affectivity is controlled for, supporting the utility of the ambivalence construct.

Recently, Katz and Campbell (1994) demonstrated that emotionally ambivalent individuals showed less of a connection between daily stressful events and negative affect. These authors attributed the lower level of covariation between event stress and mood to the emotional perseveration or rumination (King, Emmons, & Woodley, 1992) that characterizes ambivalent individuals. The inability of ambivalent individuals to complete the emotion sequence (Greenberg, 1993) results in prolonged emotional experiences and a slower resolution of the emotional experience. Future research might profit by distinguishing among different forms of ambivalence. For example, the rumination characteristic of regretted expression ("I wish I hadn't gotten angry at her") may have different consequences than the behavioral inhibition associated with failing to express these angry feelings in the first place may have.

We (Emmons & Colby, 1995) have presented a model in which emotional conflict, including ambivalence over expressing emotion and fear of intimacy (Descutner & Thelen, 1991), are linked with distress via interpersonal pathways. This model attempts to link intrapsychic conflict with its interpersonal consequences. Specifically, a reduction in social support stemming from conflicted individuals' failure to solicit and utilize available aid has been shown to mediate the relationship between conflict and well-being.

The pervasive relationship between conflict and lower well-being may account for the finding, mentioned earlier, that generativity strivings are related to higher levels of well-being. According to McAdams and de St. Aubin (1992), generativity involves the creative blending, or coalescing, of intimacy and power motivation. Generativity is both the creating and giving up of a product, and surrendering control. These two processes represent an agentic as well as an intimate act. To quote McAdams (1989):

> Generativity challenges us to be both powerful and intimate, expansive and surrendering at the same time. In motivational terms, generativity draws on our desire to be strong and our desire to be close to others, mandating that we integrate and reconcile power and intimacy motivation. (p. 163)

Through the creative integration of agentic and communal needs, the generative individual is able to override the potential for conflict between these two motivational themes, thus achieving a reconciliation of the often competing needs for power and intimacy. Perhaps those individuals who are able to harmoniously integrate their power and intimacy strivings during adolescence and early adulthood will be those most likely to develop into generative adults. In a similar vein, Guisinger and Blatt (1994) argue that generativity emerges out of an integration or consolidation of the individuality and relatedness developmental lines. The study by Diener and Fujita (1994), described earlier, similarly supports the general supposition that integration between components of the self (in that case, personal strivings and resources) is a necessary prerequisite for SWB.

Future Research on Goal Conflict

Future research on the relation between conflict and SWB may profit by taking a developmental perspective on goal conflict. To understand more completely how goals are related to well-being, it will be necessary to track the attainment or nonattainment of goals over time, as well as shifts in their importance within goal hierarchies as the individual negotiates various life transitions in which various conflicts may be activated. The study of stability and change in adult personality should include goal concepts such as conflict in its models and measures. Conflict within and among personally relevant strivings, tasks, projects, and selves should be employed in understanding stability and change across the lifespan. Helson (1987) demonstrated the role that creativity can play in resolving developmental conflicts related to separation and autonomy in adult women's lives. The reconciliation of the conflicting needs of independence and relatedness that arises during various life transitions depends in part on a person's level of creative motivation. In the absence of high levels of creativity, these developmental conflicts are likely to remain unresolved. As another example of a developmental perspective on conflict, Deci and Ryan (1991) outlined howparental behaviors such as making affection contingent on performance can lead toconflict in children between the needs for autonomy and relatedness. Research on developmental processes in personality that focuses only on what traits or selves the individual currently possesses is missing an important piece of the picture—that of dealing with future orientation and the striving, and conflicts that emerge within these.

Efforts to resolve conflict must be cognizant of the role that stable personality factors play in its generation. The implication of this is that attempts to eliminate isolated conflicts may not be successful in the long run, without change in those elements of personality that are generating the conflict. In our current work, we are exploring two hypothesized sources of goal conflict: personality traits and implicit beliefs regarding the (in)compatibility of goals between various life domains (Emmons, Murphy, & King, 1993). For instance, to what degree do people believe that it is possible to successfully balance work and relationships? (See Cantor & Blanton, Chapter 15, this volume, for a discussion of balance between life domains.) Personality traits may be related to conflict in several ways. Self-defeating characteristics such as neuroticism and ruminative thinking may lead a person to frame their goals in competing and mutually exclusive ways. Other traits, such as constructive thinking and positive coping skills may facilitate conflict resolution. Taken together, these two lines promise to provide considerable insight into both the generation of conflict and its potential for resolution. Personality may moderate the effects of conflict on physical and psychological well-being. Personality characteristics, such as hardiness (Maddi, 1990), constructive thinking (Epstein & Meier, 1989), or creativity (Sheldon, in press) might buffer individuals against the negative effects of conflict while other characteristics, such as the tendency to ruminate over conflict (Nolen-Hoeksema, 1992) may exacerbate the effects of conflict. Establishing a link between conflict and personality also highlights the difficulty individuals may have in resolving conflict in their own lives. Karen Horney stated that a crucial step for a client to overcome conflict was to be shown the "incapacitating effects of his (or her) drives and conflicts" (1945, p. 233). Our results suggest that recognizing conflict may be only the first step, however, because conflict prone individuals may be less likely to see a variety of options, to come up with constructive solutions, or to hold much hope for their ability to resolve the conflict. The negative effects of intrapsychic conflict on psychological and physical well-being become all the more understandable within the context of a larger personality style, which includes a disposition toward negative emotions, low self-esteem, and few resources to overcome this debilitating condition.

Additional Goal Parameters

Other goal parameters that have been linked to well-being include effort, which is related to higher levels of positive affect, and goal importance, which is associated with higher levels of life satisfaction (Emmons, 1986). Karoly (1991) includes these among various "functional" attributes of goal systems in that these characteristics lead to functional relations with various outcomes measures, including psychological and physical health.

The majority of relations between goal attributes and well-being outcomes have been correlational, leaving unanswered the question of what leads to what: Does conflict lead to lower well-being or do chronic dysphoric states lead a person to appraise their goals more negatively, including seeing more conflict between those goals? Myriam Mongrain and I recently attempted to answer this question in a mood induction study (Mongrain & Emmons, 1993). Pleasant and unpleasant moods were induced through a combination of music and autobiographical recall. No changes from baseline in goal appraisals were observed in the depressed condition. In the elated condition, subjects rated their goals less ambivalently and higher on clarity of means compared to baseline. Thus, it appears that the alleviation of negative affect results in more favorable evaluations of one's goals, a finding consistent with the literature on affect and judgment (cf. Schwarz, 1990).

Another attempt to disentangle the causal direction between goal appraisals and SWB was undertaken by Brunstein (1993). In a longitudinal study, he examined the interactive effects of goal commitment, attainability, and progress on SWB. Measures of SWB were taken at 4 points in time over a period of 14 weeks. Commitment was found to mediate the relationship between attainability and SWB. Specifically, students who possessed a high level of commitment and attained their goals showed positive changes in well-being over time. On the other hand, students with high levels of commitment and with fewer opportunities for goal attainment showed a decrement in SWB over time. Commitment per se was unrelated to SWB. The results support the position that perceived progress in attainment acts to cause changes in SWB rather than vice-versa.

Goal Differentiation

A final goal parameter that has ramifications for well-being is the differentiation or distinctiveness that exists within one's goal system. "Goal differentiation" refers to the degree of interrelation that exists among individual goals in the system. A high degree of differentiation exists in systems in which goals are not highly related to one another, and are thus relatively independent. Highly differentiated persons possess a variety of strivings in a variety of domains. A low degree of differentiation, on the other hand, is characteristic of systems in which the goals are highly related to one another or are interdependent. Differentiation is one component of structural complexity, along with integration (Werner & Kaplan, 1956).

We (Emmons & King, 1989) assessed the degree of differentiation both within and between strivings by having subjects assess the degree of (dis)similarity between all possible pairs of strivings. Subjects also indicated the number of distinct strategies they possessed for achieving each striving ("plan differentiation"). Using both an experience-sampling and a daily diary methodology, we found that striving differentiation was positively related to affective reactivity. Individuals who possessed highly differentiated goal systems tended to experience more extreme affective states, and in general were characterized by lower levels of psychological well-being. In another study, we (Sheldon & Emmons, 1993) found that differentiated persons tended to appraise their strivings more negatively on a number of striving dimensions. More specifically, they reported less successful attainment, reported lower expectancies for future attainment, and rated their strivings as more difficult than did less differentiated subjects. Donahue, Robins, Roberts, and John (1993) recently demonstrated that differentiation in the self-concept is negatively related to a variety of adjustment indicators, including emotional distress and interpersonal and occupational difficulties. Their work is further evidence that the "fragmentation of the self," whether conceptualized in terms of goal conflicts or discrepancies in trait attributes (see also Higgins, Chapter 5, this volume), is associated with internal as well as external costs.

PERSONALITY INTEGRATION AND SUBJECTIVE WELL-BEING

At the beginning of this chapter, a question has been posed: Why are goals important for well-being? Simply, it is because that is how people are designed. Goal-directedness is a human enterprise. Yet something more than the possession of and progression toward important life goals is needed in order for individuals to experience well-being, and in order to distinguish them from nonhuman goal-directed organisms. People are more than just collections of personal goals. What seems to be missing is an overall organizing principle that brings together and integrates separate goal strivings into a coherent structure. A goal-based account of SWB or affect is incomplete if it does not deal with the issue of unity, coherence, and integration between goals and other aspects of personality. This is the job of identity or the self—creating an overall life purpose. This organizing principle—be it identity, the self, or a similar structure—is that which links individual goals together and to future states and desired outcomes. It enables people to see beyond the immediate present and to interpret the present with respect to the future. It enables them to connect their current goal pursuits with images of who they hope to become. Conflict and differentiation are such prepotent predictors of well-being precisely because they reflect incoherence and lack of harmony in the system. However, linking differentiated goals with future positive selves (Sheldon & Emmons, 1993) appears to circumvent the deleterious effects of differentiation on well-being. Individuals with more links between their goals and future selves—the ability to see their current intentional actions as relating to images of who they wish to become— may reclaim a sense of successful striving. Similarly, when personal projects are linked to future self-representations, rated progress toward them is higher (Yetim, 1993). It is clear that people should strive for outcomes that are consistent with the types of persons they envision becoming. Personality integration has long been viewed as an important precondition for optimal psychological health. In their classic work, Kluckhohn and Murray (1953) stated that

> the chief overall function of personality, then, is to, create a design for living which permits the periodic and harmonious appeasement of most of its needs as well as the gradual progression towards distal goals. At the highest level of integration, a design of this sort is equivalent to a philosophy of life. (p. 32)

The work of Sheldon and Kasser (1994; see also Ryan et al., Chapter 1, this volume) is especially noteworthy in that they have attempted to operationalize personality integration and relate it to psychological adjustment. According to Sheldon and Kasser, integration consists of two components: "coherence" and "congruence." Coherence represents the degree to which proximal goals contribute toward or are instrumental for longer-term, more distal goals, and the degree to which lower-level, subordinate goals are instrumental for higher-level, superordinate strivings (vertical coherence). Horizontal coherence occurs when success at particular goals contributes to success at other goals at the same level in the system (essentially the opposite of conflicting goals). Congruence in the system occurs when goals are genuinely chosen by the person and fulfill the basic needs of autonomy and relatedness (Deci & Ryan, 1991). Sheldon and Kasser (1994) found that congruence and coherence were related to questionnaire measures of health and well-being, and to daily measures of mood, vitality, and engagement in meaningful as opposed to distracting activities.

CONCLUSION

It is evident from a review of the literature that the *content* of what a person is trying to do, the motivations underlying the strivings, and the framework within which the goals are organized are all essential elements of a goal-based theory of SWB. It is equally evident that SWB involves more than the presence of positive feelings and the absence of negative feelings. It involves the search for meaningfulness in one's life. Meaning comes from involvement in personally fulfilling goals, the integration of these goals into a coherent self-system, and the integration of these goals into a broader social system. It is meaning or purpose that gives life unity and coherence, despite its paradoxes and seeming inconsistencies. Goal attainment per se will not lead to subjectively satisfying long-term states unless these goals are intrinsically meaningful and integrated within an overall structure of the individual in his or her social context. Although meaningfulness may not guarantee high levels of affective well-being, a lack of meaning surely guarantees an absence of well-being.

ACKNOWLEDGMENTS

Research reported in this chapter was supported in part by a grant to me from the National Institute of Mental Health (No. MH47263-01). I would like to thank Patricia M. Colby, Myriam M. Mongrain, and the editors of this volume for their helpful comments on an earlier draft.

REFERENCES

Affleck, G., Tennen, H., Urrows, S., & Higgins, P. (1994). Person and contextual features of daily stress reactivity: Individual differences in relations of undesirable life events with mood disturbance and chronic pain intensity. *Journal of Personality and Social Psychology, 66,* 329–340.

Bargh, J.A., & Gollwitzer, P.M. (1994). Environmental control of goal-directed action: Automatic and strategic contingencies between situations and behavior. In W. D. Spaulding (Ed.), *Nebraska Symposium on Motivation: Vol. 41. Integrative views of motivation, cognition, and emotion* (pp. 71–124). Lincoln: University of Nebraska Press.

Baumeister, R. F. (1991). *Meanings of life.* New York: Guilford Press.

Brunstein, J. C. (1993). Personal goals and subjective well-being: A longitudinal study. *Journal of Personality and Social Psychology, 65,* 1061–1070.

Buss, D. M., & Cantor, N. (Eds.). (1989). *Personality psychology: Recent trends and emerging directions.* New York: Springer-Verlag.

Cantor, N., Norem, J., Langston, C., Zirkel, S., Fleeson, W., & Cook-Flannagan, C. (1991). Life tasks and daily experience. *Journal of Personality, 59,* 425–452.

Carver, C. S., & Scheier, M. F. (1981). *Attention and self-regulation: A control theory approach to human behavior.* New York: Springer-Verlag.

Carver, C. S., & Scheier, M. F. (1982). Control theory: A useful conceptual framework for personality–social, clinical, and health psychology. *Psychological Bulletin, 92,* 111–135.

Carver, C. S., & Scheier, M.F. (1990). On the origins of positive and negative affect: A control-process view. *Psychological Review, 97,* 19–35.

Carver, C. S., & White, T. L. (1994). Behavioral inhibition, behavioral activation, and affective responses to impending reward and punishment: The BIS/BAS scales. *Journal of Personality and Social Psychology, 67,* 319–333.

Colby, P. M., Emmons, R. A., & Rabin, N. (1994, August). *Intimacy strivings and well-being: The role of social support.* Poster presented at the 102nd Annual Convention of the American Psychological Association, Los Angeles.

Deci, E. L., & Ryan, R. M. (1991). A motivational approach to the self: Integration in personality. In R. Dienstbier (Ed.), *Nebraska Symposium on Motivation: Vol. 38. Perspectives on motivation* (pp. 237–288). Lincoln: University of Nebraska Press.

Descutner, C. J., & Thelen, M. H. (1991). Development and validation of a fear of intimacy scale. *Psychological Assessment: A Journal of Consulting and Clinical Psychology, 3,* 218–225.

Diener, E., & Fujita, F. (1994). *Resources, personal strivings, and subjective well-being: A nomothetic and idiographic approach. Journal of Personality and Social Psychology, 68,* 926–935.

Donahue, E. M., Robins, R. W., Roberts, B. W., & John, O. P. (1993). The divided self: Concurrent and longitudinal effects of psychological adjustment and social roles on self-concept differentiation. *Journal of Personality and Social Psychology, 64,* 834–846.

Emmons, R. A. (1986). Personal strivings: An approach to personality and subjective well-being. *Journal of Personality and Social Psychology, 51,* 1058–1068.

Emmons, R. A. (1989). The personal striving approach to personality. In L. A. Pervin (Ed.), *Goal concepts in personality and social psychology* (pp. 87–126). Hillsdale, NJ: Erlbaum.

Emmons, R. A. (1991). Personal strivings, daily life events, and psychological and physical well-being. *Journal of Personality, 59,* 453–472.

Emmons, R. A. (1992). Abstract versus concrete goals: Personal striving level, physical illness, and psychological well-being. *Journal of Personality and Social Psychology, 62,* 292–300.

Emmons, R. A. (1994, August). *Traumatic life events and personal goals: When losses lead to gains.* Poster presented at the 102nd Annual Convention of the American Psychological Association, Los Angeles.

Emmons, R. A., & Colby, P. M. (1995). Emotional conflict and well-being: Relation to perceived availability, daily utilization, and observer reports of social support. *Journal of Personality and Social Psychology, 68,* 947–959.

Emmons, R. A., & Kaiser, H. (1994, August). *Approach and avoidance strivings and subjective well-being.* Poster presented at the 102nd Annual Convention of the American Psychological Association, Los Angeles.

Emmons, R. A., & King, L. A. (1988). Conflict among personal strivings: Immediate and long-term implications for psychological and physical well-being. *Journal of Personality and Social Psychology, 54,* 1040–1048.

Emmons, R. A., & King, L. A. (1989). Personal striving differentiation and affective reactivity. *Journal of Personality and Social Psychology, 56,* 478–484.

Emmons, R. A., & King, L. A. (1992). Thematic analysis, experience sampling, and personal goals. In C. P. Smith (Ed.), *Motivation and personality: Handbook of thematic content analysis* (pp. 73–86). New York: Cambridge University Press.

Emmons, R. A., King, L. A., & Sheldon, K. (1993). Goal conflict and the self-regulation of action. In D. M. Wegner & J. W. Pennebaker (Eds.), *Handbook of mental control* (pp. 528–551). Englewood Cliffs, NJ: Prentice-Hall.

Emmons, R. A., & McAdams, D. P. (1991). Personal strivings and motive dispositions: Exploring the links. *Personality and Social Psychology Bulletin, 17,* 648–654.

Emmons, R. A., Murphy, M. D., & King, L. A. (1993, August). *Personality styles related to intrapsychic goal conflict and ambivalence.* Poster presented at the 101st Annual Convention of the American Psychological Association, Toronto.

Epstein, S., & Meier, P. (1989). Constructive thinking: A broad coping variable with specific components. *Journal of Personality and Social Psychology, 57,* 332–350.

Frijda, N. (1986). *The emotions.* New York: Cambridge University Press.

Gollwitzer, P. M. (1993). Goal achievement: The role of intentions. In W. Stroebe & M. Hewstone (Eds.), *European review of social psychology* (Vol. 4., pp. 141–185). Chicester, England: Wiley.

Gomersall, T. E. (1993). *Personal strivings and repression: Identifying the repressive coping style within the personal strivings framework.* Unpublished master's thesis, Humboldt State University.

Gray, J. A. (1987). *The psychology of fear and stress.* New York: Cambridge University Press.

Greenberg, L. S. (1993). Emotion and change processes in psychotherapy. In M. Lewis & J. M. Haviland (Eds.), *Handbook of emotions* (pp. 499–508). New York: Guilford Press.

Guisinger, S., & Blatt, S. J. (1994). Individuality and relatedness: Evolution of a fundamental dialectic. *American Psychologist, 49,* 104–111.

Helson, R. (1987). Which of those young women with creative potential became productive? In R. Hogan & W. H. Jones (Eds.), *Perspectives in personality* (Vol. 2, pp. 51–92). Greenwich, CT: JAI Press.

Karoly, P. (1991). Goal systems and health outcomes across the life span: A proposal. In H. E. Schroeder (Ed.), *New directions in health psychology assessment* (pp. 65–91). New York: Hemisphere.

Karoly, P. (1993). Mechanisms of self-regulation: A systems view. *Annual Review of Psychology, 44,* 23–52.

Kasser, T., & Ryan, R. M. (1993). A dark side of the American dream: Correlates of financial success as a central life aspiration. *Journal of Personality and Social Psychology, 65,* 410–422.

Katz, I. L., & Campbell, J. D. (1994). Ambivalence over emotional expression and well-being: Nomothetic and idiographic tests of the stress-buffering hypothesis. *Journal of Personality and Social Psychology, 67,* 513–524.

King, L. A. (1991). *Investigations in the relations, predictive validity, and implications of explicit and implicit motives.* Unpublished doctoral dissertation, University of California at Davis.

King, L. A., & Emmons, R. A. (1990). Ambivalence over expressing emotion: Physical and psychological correlates. *Journal of Personality and Social Psychology, 58,* 864–877.

King, L. A., & Emmons, R. A. (1991). Psychological, physical, and interpersonal correlates of emotional expressiveness, conflict, and control. *European Journal of Personality, 5,* 131–150.

King, L. A., Emmons, R. A., & Woodley, S. (1992). The structure of inhibition. *Journal of Research in Personality, 26,* 85–102.

Klinger, E. (1977). *Meaning and void: Inner experience and the incentives in people's lives.* Minneapolis: University of Minnesota Press.

Kluckhohn, C. & Murray, H. A. (1953). Outline of a conception of personality. In H. A. Murray & C. Kluckhohn (Eds.), *Personality in nature, society, and culture* (2nd ed., pp. 3–32). New York: Knopf.

Krohne, H. W. (Ed.). (1993). *Attention and avoidance.* Seattle, WA: Hogrefe & Huber.

Lavallee, L. F., & Campbell, J. D. (1994). *The impact of personal goals on self-regulation processes elicited by negative events.* Unpublished manuscript, University of British Columbia.

Lazarus, R. A. (1991). *Emotion and adaptation.* New York: Oxford University Press.

Lazarus, R. S. (1993). Coping theory and research: Past, present, and future. *Psychosomatic Medicine, 55,* 234–247.

Little, B. R. (1989). Personal projects analysis: Trivial pursuits, magnificent obsessions, and the search for coherence. In D. M. Buss & N. Cantor (Eds.), *Personality psychology: Recent trends and emerging directions* (pp. 15–31). New York: Springer-Verlag.

Maddi, S. R. (1990). Issues and interventions in stress mastery. In H. S. Friedman (Ed.), *Personality and disease* (pp. 121–154). New York: Wiley.

Marco, C., & Suls, J. (1993). Daily stress and the trajectory of mood: Spillover, response assimilation, contrast, and chronic negative affectivity. *Journal of Personality and Social Psychology, 64,* 1053–1063.

Martin, L. L., & Tesser, A. (1989). Toward a motivational and structural theory of ruminative thought. In J. Uleman & J. A. Bargh (Eds.), *Unintended thought* (pp. 306–326). New York: Guilford Press.

McAdams, D. P. (1989). *Intimacy: The need to be close.* New York: Doubleday.

McAdams, D. P. (1994). *The person: An introduction to personality psychology* (2nd ed.). Fort Worth, TX: Harcourt, Brace.

McAdams, D. P., & de St. Aubin, E. (1992). A theory of generativity and its assessment through self-report, behavioral acts, and narrative themes in autobiography. *Journal of Personality and Social Psychology, 62,* 1003–1015.

McIntosh, W. D., & Martin, L. L. (1992). The cybernetics of happiness: The relation of goal attainment, rumination, and affect. In M.S. Clark (Ed.), *Emotion and social behavior* (pp. 222–246). Newbury Park, CA: Sage.

Meehl, P. E. (1964). *Manual for use with checklist of schizotypic signs.* Minneapolis: University of Minnesota Medical School, Psychiatric Research Unit.

Mongrain, M., & Emmons, R. A. (1993). *The influence of induced mood on dependency, self-criticism, ambivalence, and goal appraisals.* Unpublished manuscript, University of California at Davis.

Nolen-Hoeksema, S. (1993). Sex differences in the control of depression. In D. M. Wegner & J. W. Pennebaker (Eds.), *Handbook of mental control* (pp. 306–324). Englewood Cliffs, NJ: Prentice-Hall.

Oatley, K. (1992). *Best laid schemes: The psychology of emotions.* New York: Cambridge University Press.

Omodei, M. M., & Wearing, A. J. (1990). Need satisfaction and involvement in personal projects: Toward an integrative model of subjective well-being. *Journal of Personality and Social Psychology, 59,* 762–769.

Ortony, A., Clore, G. L., & Collins, A. (1988). *The cognitive structure of emotions.* New York: Cambridge University Press.

Pennebaker, J. W., & Traue, H. C. (Eds.) (1993). *Emotion, inhibition, and health.* Seattle, WA: Hogrefe & Huber.

Pervin, L. A. (1983). The stasis and flow of behavior: Toward a theory of goals. In M. M. Page (Ed.), *Nebraska Symposium on Motivation* (Vol. 30, pp. 1–53). Lincoln: University of Nebraska Press.

Powers, W. T. (1973). *Behavior: The control of perception.* Chicago: Aldine.

Rapkin, B. D., & Fischer, K. (1992). Framing the construct of life satisfaction in terms of older adults' personal goals. *Psychology and Aging, 7,* 138–149.

Ryan, R. M. (1992). The nature of the self in actionary and relatedness. In G. Goethals (Ed.), *Multidisciplinary perspectives in the self* (pp. 208–238). New York: Springer-Verlag.

Ryan, R. M, & Connell, J. P. (1989). Perceived locus of causality and internalization: Examining reasons for acting in two domains. *Journal of Personality and Social Psychology, 57,* 749–761.

Schwarz, N. (1990). Feelings as information: Informational and motivational functions of affective states. In E. T. Higgins & R. Sorrentino (Eds.), *Handbook of motivatio and cognition: Foundations of social behavior* (Vol. 2, pp. 527–561). New York: Guilford Press.

Sheldon, K. M. (in press). Creativity and goal conflict. *Creativity Research Journal.*

Sheldon, K. M., & Emmons, R. A. (1995). Comparing differentiation and integration within personal goal systems. *Personality and Individual Differences, 18,* 39–46.

Sheldon, K. M., & Kasser, T. (1994). Coherence and congruence: Two aspects of personality integration. *Journal of Personality and Social Psychology, 68,* 531–543.

Smith, C. P. (Ed.). (1992). *Motivation and personality: Handbook of thematic content analysis.* New York: Cambridge University Press.

Stemmerich, E. D., & Emmons, R. A. (1993, August). *Generativity and power and intimacy strivings: Implications for subjective well-being.* Poster presented at the 101st Annual Convention of the American Psychological Association, Toronto, Ontario.

Vallacher, R. R., & Wegner, D. M. (1985). *A theory of action identification.* Hillsdale, NJ: Erlbaum.

Werner, H., & Kaplan, B. (1956). The developmental approach to cognition: Its relevance to the psychological interpretation of anthropological and ethnolinguistic data. *American Anthropologist, 58,* 866–880.

Yetim, U. (1993). Life satisfaction: A study based on the organization of personal projects. *Social Indicators Research, 29,* 277–289.

CHAPTER 15

Effortful Pursuit of Personal Goals in Daily Life

Nancy Cantor
Hart Blanton

When we reflect on motivation and action, it is striking how much people seem to live their daily lives in one of two extreme states—either appetitively drawn to activities that involve natural incentives for affective fulfillment (McClelland, 1985; Weinberger & McClelland, 1990), or, in contrast, disengaging from frustrated goal pursuit (Kuhl, 1985; Klinger, 1975). As different as these two states can be in hedonic tone, they share an important feature: Phenomenologically, they are experienced as "spontaneously happening." Outcomes are independent of self-regulation, personal commitment, or judgement and choice. Motives can be pursued or tasks disrupted without recognition (Fleeson, 1992). As a result, the psychological and behavioral consequences of particular motivations are hard to avoid, prevent, interrupt, or overcome.

While recognizing the prevalence of these effortless motivational states, we have come to focus our thinking and empirical work on a separate type of motivated behavior—one that implicates the self and requires self-reflection, commitment, and effort (Cantor & Fleeson, 1994). We have focused on individuals' attempts to mobilize energy for the tasks in their current lives that are at once important to them and yet not straightforward for them to undertake and/or to accomplish in their daily lives (Cantor & Harlow, 1994). Individuals often knowingly pursue such goals because they regard them as important, and they persist despite natural tendencies to withdraw effort in the face of setbacks (Cantor, 1990; Dweck & Leggett, 1988; Bandura, 1986). Progress often comes at some cost and requires effortful negotiation of obstacles, coordination of competing goals, and management of self-doubt and anxiety (Blanton, 1994; Harlow & Cantor, 1994a). This is the sort of arousal or "energization" that Wright and Brehm (1989) describe as associated with the pursuit of outcomes that are perceived by individuals as difficult, possible, and worthwhile.

We believe that a significant piece of motivation involves this effortful goal pursuit. This is because many goals that are important simply cannot be attained without considerable self-regulation and effort. Consider, for example, Mischel's work on willpower and delay of gratification (e.g., Mischel, Chapter 9, this volume). He consistently shows that people, be they 4-year-olds waiting for pretzels or adults attempting to improve their health habits, find it necessary to exert considerable cognitive-behavioral effort to resist the motivational pressure to disengage or the temptation to settle for less. We find analogous examples in our own work, which focuses on the achievement of self-relevant tasks in daily life. We often find individuals committed to tasks that they find intimidating and challenging, and our work has focused on explicating the strategies they use for overcoming these obstacles and persisting when they might otherwise disengage (Cantor & Harlow, 1994).

SPONTANEOUS MOTIVATION

McClelland and colleagues (McClelland, Koestner, & Weinberger, 1989; Weinberger & McClelland, 1990; Koestner, Weinberger, & McClelland, 1991) highlight effortless pursuit by drawing a contrast between two systems of motivation. The "traditional" implicit system is one that spontaneously reacts with "direct experience of affect" to "natural incentives" in unconstrained situations. They contrast this with a self-regulated ("cognitive") system attuned to specific task demands and self-obstacles, and "equipped to make plans or set specific goals that can take contextual circumstances into account" (Weinberger & McClelland, 1990, p. 589).

In the traditional system, motivation and action are triggered by environmental cues. These cues signal the possibility of experiencing specific natural incentives (e.g., being in meaningful relationships, having an impact on others), which are biologically based motivations, grounded in each individual's needs for procreation and survival (e.g., need for intimacy, need for power, etc.). Natural incentives are inherently pleasing and associated with specific pleasant affective experiences. Thus, cues that signal the possibility of experiencing natural incentives cause an emotional charge or "energization." This anticipatory state causes people to seek the "kick" or "natural high" that accompanies natural incentives. Behavior is thus influenced by incentive cues, regardless of the situational context (McClelland et al., 1989). People approach *all* situations with the same readiness to be influenced by incentive cues.

Individuals differ in their predisposition to seek particular incentives, because of their differential sensitivity to these incentive cues (Weinberger & McClelland, 1990). Thus, within a particular context, the likelihood that an individual will pursue a specific natural incentive depends partly on cues available in the situation and partly on the individual's emotional readiness to respond with energization to the cues present. To the extent that a specific situation provides cues for competing incentives, the motive that "wins out" over the others will simply be the one that evokes the strongest anticipatory energization (Weinberger & McClelland, 1990). There is no regulatory system that prioritizes or "orchestrates" pursuit of multiple motivations. People pursue the motive that offers the best opportunity of creating pleasant affect. To the extent that the cues create equal but opposing behavioral tendencies, the individual, in theory, should become immobilized (Norem, 1989).

Traditional motives are "effortless" because they orient generalized approach tendencies, which require no self-reflection or self-regulation. To be affected by a cue, individuals need not reflect on the meaning of the cue, know that the cue typically makes them act in certain ways, infer that their behavior is patterned to experience the incentive, or consider themselves the types of persons who react to cues in particular ways (McClelland et al., 1989; Fleeson, 1992). It is for this reason that McClelland and colleagues refer to these motivations as "implicit" (Weinberger & McClelland, 1990). For an implicit motivation to affect behavior, it is only necessary that persons feel energized to seek the natural incentive. At no level must they know why, how, or even *that* a desire was evoked.

EFFORTFUL MOTIVATION

Following Weinberger and McClelland (1990), our work has focused on a second motivational system (Cantor & Kihlstrom, 1987), which is "cognitive" in nature, in that it is based on individuals' self-articulated goals and aspirations. It centers on individuals' desires to take part in the "life tasks" of their age-graded culture (Erikson, 1950; Havighurst, 1953; Higgins & Parsons, 1983). This is motivation that comes through the self-system, in that it is directed by cognitive representations of the self—who individuals want to be and what they would like to accomplish (e.g., Cantor, Markus, Niedenthal, & Nurius, 1986; Markus & Nurius, 1986; Higgins, 1987). We do not suggest that the pursuit of life tasks subsumes all "cognitive" motivations (cf. Pervin, 1989; Read & Miller, 1989; Little, 1989). However, we do feel that it provides a solid framework for studying the "effortful" slice of motivation, in that it is grounded in the tasks, norms, and rituals of culture (Zirkel & Cantor, 1990). Making progress, achieving success, and even simply participating in these tasks can be quite difficult, requiring effortful problem solving and strategic action. Thus, we contrast the "spontaneous pursuit" of natural incentives with the more effortful "strategic pursuit" of life tasks (Cantor, 1994). Examples include the college student who faces the age-typical concern of developing both independence from family and a sense of personal identity (Zirkel & Cantor, 1990), or the mature adult who seeks a sense of personal generativity and opportunities to educate younger generations (Erikson, 1980; Hooker, Kaus, & Morfei, 1993).

Like natural incentives, life tasks create goal-directed behavior. However, because they are representations of the self in specific, often culturally regulated contexts, they influence behavior with similar specificity (Cantor et al., 1986). Life tasks exert *situationally, developmentally,* and *personally* specific influences on behavior. For instance, students' representations of themselves in pursuit of academics are situationally specific, in that these will influence their responses to events in their academic life task but not necessarily their reactions to situations relevant to their social, family, or intimacy life tasks (Cantor, Norem, Niedenthal, Langston, & Brower, 1987). A life task is developmentally specific because how and when it is pursued is largely determined by age-graded cultural expectations. High school students and college students have different representations of themselves in academics, in large part because of the differing cultural expectations of what this pursuit should mean at these different stages in the life course (Havighurst, 1972; Zirkel, 1992). Finally, pursuit is personally specific because each individual's representation of the self in pursuit of the task is the product of his or her unique life experiences. In our work, we often find that even with well-defined tasks such as "doing well at school" and "making friends," students differ enormously in how they pursue these tasks, and this difference can be accounted for through analysis of each student's "self-at-task" representations (Cantor & Fleeson, 1994).

Specificity of this sort contrasts with implicit motives, which exert pan-situational, -developmental, and -personal influences on action. For instance, someone high in need for power will approach academic situations, as well as social, family, and intimacy situations, with a sensitivity to cues suggesting opportunities to have an impact on others (McClelland et al., 1989). This motive involves a readiness that is activated quite early in life and that continues to exert influences on the individual throughout the lifespan (Weinberger & McClelland, 1990). Moreover, regardless of personal history, need for power should translate specifically into a readiness to "have an impact on others" (McClelland, 1985; cf. Veroff, 1983).

By drawing a contrast between these two motivational systems, we do not mean to suggest that they operate completely independently of each other. A natural incentive can push individuals to "take on" tasks that are conducive to its expression (Fleeson, 1992; Emmons & McAdams, 1991). Moreover, *how* individuals pursue each task may be influenced in part by the relative strength of their implicit motivations (Fleeson, 1992). However, to say that one system influences the other does not mean that one accounts for the other. Individuals' representations of themselves in pursuit of life tasks exert highly structured influences on behavior. Although the choices of tasks and strategies an individual pursues may be partly influenced by natural incentives, they are not reducible to the more generalized tendency to seek affective fulfillment (Fleeson, 1992). In fact, a central point of this chapter is that life tasks often direct behavior in ways that are not conducive to immediate hedonic fulfillment. The academic defensive pessimist, for instance, is driven to pursue academic success, even though doing so engenders a great deal of stress and anxiety before academic challenges, and strategic effort is required to persist at the task (Cantor et al., 1987). Although it might be reasonable to characterize such an individual as high in need for achievement and avoidance motivation, such as fear of failure (Atkinson & Litwin, 1960), this implicit-motive profile tells us little or nothing about the particulars of the tasks and contexts that evoke a conflict for defensive pessimists, or about their strategy that serves to enable continued task pursuit in those same contexts (Norem, 1989). The development of life tasks and the choice of strategies may be influenced by implicit motives as well as by cultural norms and personal experiences. However, once established, life tasks direct action in ways that cannot be fully attributed to the influence of natural incentives, and strategies facilitate persistence even when immediate hedonic fulfillment is seen to be unlikely.

Unlike natural incentives, which are cued by anticipated fulfillment, life tasks are pursued even when the possibility of success is uncertain and task pursuit is frustrating. Life tasks orient individuals toward the pursuit of specific goals, but often provide few clues about how best to proceed. For instance, consider students who have just made the transition from college to the workplace. They now approach their social lives with a new set of challenges arising from the cultural pressure to develop intimate relationships (Havighurst, 1972). Even though they have faced social dating for years with relatively little anxiety, their "romantic pursuits" have taken on a new meaning in light of the current life task concern for "mature intimacy" (Zirkel, 1992). To proceed, the individuals must find new ways of pursuing this task that can help them make progress in the face of considerable anxiety. Being cued to pursue a particular task often begs more questions than it answers. As this example shows, making progress can require considerable effort in the form of strategic problem solving and action.

Life Task Strategies: Effortful Interventions

Life tasks are potent sources of effortful pursuit because progress must be made in the face of personal experiences of anxiety, frustration, and self-doubt (Fleeson, 1992). The exact nature of these difficulties is reflected in a person's life task appraisal. We use the term "appraisal" to characterize individuals' cognitive representations of themselves pursuing a task (Little, 1989). This develops over time as a result of both social feedback and personal experience with the task. Consider, for instance, students with an excellent record of academic performance who know that they have done very well but still harbor fears of not being able to "perform" during a task so as to meet their own high standards. Phillips and her colleagues (e.g., Phillips & Zimmerman, 1990), for example, have studied a group of talented high school students who nonetheless possess an "illusion of incompetence." This self-at-academics appraisal may have developed as a result of early self-evaluations of academic success as being highly dependent on exerting substantial personal effort to prepare for each task (Weiner, 1986)—an attributional pattern that could have been inadvertently reinforced by parents (Parsons, Adler, & Kaczala, 1982; Phillips, 1987) and teachers (Parsons, Kaczala, & Meece, 1982; Heyman, Dweck, & Cain, 1992). As young adults, pursuing a life task of "doing well in academics," such students are at risk for experiencing considerable self-doubts about taking on new challenges that might demand more than they can muster. These self-doubts and the accompanying anxiety could easily lead to disengagement and frustrated pursuit, without some effort to protect the self and motivate task commitment.

As debilitating as this appraisal pattern may potentially be, it will not always adversely affect academic pursuit. In our work, we have examined individuals' strategic responses in the face of personal obstacles—that is, specific events or situations that evoke the motivational or emotional barriers associated with the individuals' appraisal patterns (Cantor & Harlow, 1994). For instance, we might expect persons with doubts about being able to rise sufficiently high to perform up to par in each new academic hurdle to react with anxiety before pressured academic tasks. Tests and exams that would be "part of the territory" for most students are, for these students, ripe with opportunities to "choke." It is in response to these obstacles that they must develop behavioral strategies that will overcome their anticipatory anxiety. In a sense, they must create their own clinical "intervention"—one that will address their anxiety and override any tendency just to avoid such academic hurdles altogether. One such strategy has already been mentioned: namely, defensive pessimism (Norem & Cantor, 1986a, 1986b; Norem, 1989). Defensive pessimists overcome their anticipatory anxiety about "choking" during critical academic tasks by playing through possible outcomes in advance and thereby "freeing" themselves to take on challenges with full effort (Norem & Illingworth, 1993). Their strategic intervention overcomes the obstacle set in place by their academic appraisal. As a result, they are able to persist and succeed, even during those times when they most fear not being able to "rise to the task" and meet their personal standards of excellence.

Effortful Pursuit as Patterned Behavior

It is by showing that the appraisal pattern predicts behavior, *in a way that is patterned to overcome the particulars of an individual's obstacle,* that we find evidence of strategic effort. This is done by establishing temporal, situational, and interpersonal specificity of behavior (the "when, where, and with whom" of strategic behavior; Cantor & Fleeson, 1991; see also Gollwitzer, 1993). Behavior is "strategic" when it addresses a distinct motivational or emotional obstacle, and is specifically observed in pursuits that evoke that obstacle. Our strategy analyses, in both interpersonal and achievement task domains, follow a particular form (Cantor & Harlow, 1994). First, we identify individuals who are committed to a life task and yet report particular appraisal patterns that suggest the presence of motivational or emotional obstacles. Next, we study their daily life pursuits, using event-sampling techniques to identify patterning in their responses to events that suggests strategic effort to overcome the life task obstacle.

To illustrate, Harlow and Cantor (1994a; 1994b) have recently studied the daily life academic pursuits of a group of women in a campus sorority whom they labeled as "outcome-focused" in the academic task domain. These women fit a pattern of outcome focus because their academic appraisals were distinct from those of their peers in the excessive concern with achieving good outcomes and avoiding bad outcomes on academic tasks, and in the belief that this would be difficult to accomplish (see Dweck & Leggett, 1988, on performance goals; Deci & Ryan, 1985, on ego involvement). This appraisal pattern put them at risk for experiencing potentially debilitating anxiety in response to specific academic situations—namely, performance setbacks, which for these women called their abilities into question. In contrast, for example, to defensive pessimists, who are typically self-focused and concerned about doing the task itself rather than about protecting themselves in the face of performance outcomes (Norem & Cantor, 1986a), these outcome-focused women needed ability-relevant feedback and bolstering from others in the face of academic setbacks and performance disappointments (cf. Butler, 1992). In fact, their response was contextually patterned in a way that would seem ideally suited to address precisely this motivational self-obstacle. In ostensibly social situations, they sought reassurances after negative academic outcomes with individuals (typically not themselves outcome-focused) whom these women regarded as confidants and "encouragers." Their strategic response to setbacks was temporally, situationally, and interpersonally patterned in this way so as to redirect behavior away from their self-doubts and toward the fulfillment of a personally meaningful pursuit—in this case, academics.

It is partly through such behavioral specificity that strategic pursuit can be contrasted with the spontaneous pursuit of natural incentives (Weinberger & McClelland, 1990). However, we appreciate that strategic pursuit may be influenced by implicit motivations. For instance, both the reassurance seeking of outcome-focused individuals and the worst-case reflections of defensive pessimists are strategies for dealing with academic stress, but they differ in that one is necessarily affiliative and the other is not. Therefore, it may be that people high in need for affiliation will be more likely to adopt a strategy of reassurance seeking, which involves seeking contact with others, than one of defensive pessimism, which depends upon self-focused task preparation. Moreover, differences of this sort may be reflected in each group's unique appraisal of academics, in that reassurance seekers' appraisal tends to emphasize others' views and the need for gaining external approval (Harlow & Cantor, 1994a, 1994b).

However, viewing the strategic effort of Harlow and Cantor's outcome-focused subjects through the lens of need for affiliation provides only a very sketchy overview, because the subjects "affiliated" at very specific times and then for a purpose in a particular task context—namely, to gain personal reassurances about academic setbacks. To say that they were intrinsically drawn to social contact explains very little of their strategy, either in terms of the specific conditions that evoked reassurance seeking for them or in terms of the particular people with whom they sought social contact. For example, they could just as well have sought social contact indirectly by studying with others who might have provided instrumental, informational help by modeling successful academic pursuits (cf. Butler, 1993; Cantor, 1994; Harlow & Cantor, 1995). Instead, these outcome-focused women sought reassurance in social settings from close confidants, precisely because they were so distressed by an academic setback that they specifically needed emotional support before continuing any academic pursuits (Harlow & Cantor, 1994b; for work on strategies with a similar outcome focus, see also Butler, 1992; Dweck & Leggett, 1988; and Higgins, Chapter 5, this volume).

Behavioral specificity of this sort suggests a personally tuned strategic intervention. Were their responses not limited to academics—for instance, if these women had sought reassurance after any negative event, even those about which they were not outcome-focused—their behavior would not have been strategic. It is by showing that a behavior solves a particular problem ("appraisal"), which in this case was confined to academic tasks, that we see evidence of coordinated effort. Strategically intervening to find "solutions" that override anxiety and self-doubt in the face of personal obstacles takes effort. However, because people respond in ways that address these difficulties, it is clear that they are exerting the effort necessary to make progress on (or at least to continue participating in) these important life tasks.

NEGOTIATING MULTIPLE PURSUITS

Both the implicit-motive model and the life task model of motivation assume that people possess more than one motivation. In the traditional system, this number is limited because of the finite number of biological needs (Weinberger & McClelland, 1990), whereas individuals are able to take on or create any number of life tasks (Cantor, 1990). Nonetheless, the presence of multiple motives in each system highlights the importance of considering the dynamic interplay among multiple pursuits. In the implicit-motive system, there is no structure designed to regulate or coordinate multiple motives. People pursue the natural incentive that offers the greatest opportunity of evoking positive affect, which is partly a function of motive strength and partly of the particular cues that are currently available (Weinberger & McClelland, 1990).

Although people cannot structure their various natural incentives, it is possible to think of ways in which different motives do affect one another. For instance, a person who is high in many needs may be more prone to immobilization, because of the heightened likelihood that competing cues will be of equal strength (Norem, 1989). Moreover, work by Zeldow, Daugherty, and McAdams (1988) suggests that such difficulties may be particularly acute with the juxtapositioning of specific implicit-motive pairs. They found, for instance, that medical students were at particular risk for experiencing symptoms of neuroticism and depression when they were high in both intimacy and power motives. Similarly, Atkinson and colleagues (e.g., Atkinson & Litwin, 1960) have predicted that a combination of need for achievement and high fear of failure interacts uniquely to predict behavioral immobilization. It seems likely, then, that multiple implicit motives affect one another. However, because they are spontaneous reactions elicited by environmental cues, people cannot "prioritize" or "coordinate" their multiple motivations in a meaningful way.

In the following subsections, we explore ways in which people can and do negotiate multiple life tasks. In our work with college students, we often find that issues of task negotiation revolve around ways of managing both achievement-related (i.e., academic and job task) pursuits and social-related (i.e., friendship and intimacy task) pursuits (e.g., Cantor, Acker, & Cook-Flannagan, 1992; Harlow & Cantor, 1994a; Blanton, 1994). Conflicts of this sort are common throughout the life course, though the forms they take vary considerably across age-graded contexts. Zirkel's (1992) longitudinal analysis of the changing meaning of independence as a life task, from late adolescence to young adulthood, provides one example of the persistence in a new form of these familiar conflicts. She found that whereas her subjects as college students were absorbed with differentiating from the intimacy of family in favor of the independence of academics, as young adults they were determined to find romantic intimacy, albeit in a context of demanding career pressures. Similarly, much work in role theory has focused on the stress associated with balancing career and family concerns (e.g., Kandel, Davies, & Raveis, 1985; Verbrugge, 1983).

By focusing on this aspect of college life, we are acknowledging that it is a particularly central conflict at this age. Nonetheless, we assume that this conflict (and the need for task negotiation) is quite likely to reappear in new forms and life settings in subsequent life periods (Hooker et al., 1993; Havighurst, 1972). Moreover, it is also certainly true that task negotiation is not by any means limited to these "classic" conflicts between work and play, intimacy and identity, at any point in the life course. College students have conflicts between maintaining good health habits on the one hand, and obtaining social acceptance and fitting in with the group on the other hand. Midlife adults worry about finding the energy to be generative both with aging parents and with developing children (Bumpass, 1994). Task negotiation is a ubiquitous aspect of life task pursuit, even though the content of and contexts for multiple pursuits may change substantially.

We believe that the need to coordinate strategies for making progress on multiple life tasks adds a further constraint on motivated behavior. Because life tasks require long-term commitment, are culturally prescribed and personally meaningful, and often evoke feelings of anxiety and threat, multiple pursuits may easily lead to role strain. Moreover, difficulties in one task may "spill over" and become obstacles in the pursuit of others. However, as in the case of isolated pursuits, people may well develop personal strategic interventions to address the demands of competing life tasks. To date, our research has indirectly addressed this next level of strategic effort by examining the ways in which strategies, fine-tuned to address particular task obstacles, turn out to have a highly specific impact on individuals' coordination of multiple task demands. Examination of these strategies, therefore, indirectly addresses two types of additional obstacles uniquely associated with contemporaneous pursuit of multiple life tasks: the obstacles of role strain that occur because of generalized resource limitations, and those of "spillover" that occur because of specific life task interrelations.

Resource Limitations and Role Strain

To the extent that multiple pursuits mean multiple demands, strategic pursuit of one task should lead to personal fatigue as well as debilitation in other task domains. This would be consistent with theories of role accumulation suggesting that multiple roles lead inevitably to role strain (Goode, 1960; Merton, 1957; Sarbin & Allen, 1968), and with models of stress that emphasize the importance of "resource depletion" (Hobfoll, 1989). For example, the burdens of multiple pursuits are commonly experienced by students who are highly involved in both social and academic life task pursuits (Cantor et al., 1992). Fortunately, however, these same students do develop strategies for overcoming the obstacles inherent in these multiple demands.

In its simplest form, this takes the shape of *prioritizing* pursuits. One can avoid debilitation or resource demands by strategically withdrawing from tasks that exacerbate efforts in more pressing domains. Evidence of such "narrowing of interest" was found by Cantor et al. (1992) in a study of the pursuit of intimacy by individuals experiencing considerable conflict about this highly self-relevant task. In their sample, students who expressed conflict about the intimacy life task while currently pursuing a serious relationship resolved their difficulties in part by withdrawing effort from other important life task activities—in particular, academic ones. By systematically disengaging from competing life tasks, they were able to continue working on a task that was particularly demanding for them. As might be expected, however, this strategy was not without its costs. Subjects sacrificed involvement in academics for the sake of making progress on the intimacy life task. In so doing, they may have eliminated some role strain, but only by restricting their other life-task activities. However, it is important to remember that this study focused on life task negotiation in one delimited life period. It is quite possible that strategic withdrawal of this sort is used only as a temporary "solution" to current resource demands. Cantor and Malley (1991), for example, analyzed data from a longitudinal study of adult women (Stewart, 1989), and observed a pattern of *alternating* emphasis on personal identity tasks and interpersonal relationship tasks over time.

Evidence of change across the lifespan suggests that prioritizing need not be a permanent solution to resource demands. Nonetheless, even in the moment, there may be other ways of negotiating task demands that do not require such a narrowing of interests. One possible alternative to dropping or alternating tasks is to find ways of *consolidating* the pursuit of multiple tasks. By adopting strategies that address obstacles in one life task, but that involve contemporaneous pursuit of other important tasks, individuals can reduce the strain inherent in life task accumulation, and thereby reduce the need to sacrifice or shortchange less pressing pursuits. An example of such a strategy can be found in the strategic reassurance seeking of outcome-focused women (Harlow & Cantor, 1994a). As noted earlier, these students addressed obstacles in their academic lives by altering their style of social pursuit. By consolidating the pursuit of social and academic life tasks, these women were able to make progress on academics even while maintaining high levels of social pursuit. Had they kept these two tasks independent of each other, the demand of making progress in both social and academic pursuits might have led to role strain. As will be discussed later, although their reassurance seeking minimized the strain of maintaining two independent pursuits, it nonetheless created difficulties of its own.

A similar consolidation of social and academic pursuits was found with a group of students who, rather than focusing on gaining reassurance after academic setbacks, focused intently on self-improvement following such challenges (Cantor, 1994). These students responded to negative academic experiences by trying to gain help that would be instrumental to the achievement of their academic ideals (see also Higgins, Chapter 5, this volume). They "elicited" this help after negative academic experiences through a strategy of contact seeking that entailed studying with friends whom they considered to be "idols" (i.e., "people I would like to be more like"). Like the outcome-focused women, these "improvement-focused" students consolidated academic and social pursuits. Their time spent with friends was also beneficial to their academic pursuit. However, because academic setbacks elicited improvement-focused concerns, their social pursuits were structured differently from those of outcome-focused students. Instead of bringing academics to their social pursuits, these students brought friends to their academic pursuits.

These examples demonstrate that individuals can respond to multiple tasks in ways that minimize role strain. They can prioritize, attending less to those that are less pressing, and they can consolidate, pursuing multiple tasks contemporaneously. Both approaches demonstrate ways of reducing stress that involve conserving energy—either by withdrawing from particular tasks or by streamlining efforts in multiple tasks. However, it should be noted that maintaining multiple and even highly distinct life tasks does not *necessarily* cause elevated role strain. This is because strategic pursuit, even while requiring effort, is at times quite rewarding and energizing (Marks, 1977; Csikszentmihalyi & LeFevre, 1989).

In this vein, a strategy for dealing with stress may be one of *differentiating* life task pursuits—interspersing alternative, energizing pursuits around those requiring a great deal of effort. Rather than pursuing one or two tasks to the point of fatigue, individuals may find it possible to "break up" the day by pursuing other meaningful life tasks. Such a strategy of overcoming stress by taking on more pursuits may sound counterintuitive at first. However, people often experience a re-energization after working on engaging activities, even when doing so requires high levels of effort (Csikszentmihalyi, 1990). Thoits (1983, 1986) makes similar claims when she suggests that accumulating social roles can attenuate daily stress by enriching one's sense of personal identity. Moreover, work by Linville (1987) on self-complexity would suggest that adding pursuits will be particularly effective when each is highly differentiated and thus unlikely to cast a generalized negative pall when task pursuit stumbles (cf. Block, 1961; Donahue, Robins, Robert, & John, 1993).

Indirect empirical evidence for such a differentiation strategy was reported by Bolger and Tordesillias (1993). They investigated a style of activity pursuit that they termed "refreshing," in which individuals with multiple and distinct pursuits found frequent shifts in their daily life activities to be reinvigorating rather than exhausting. Thus, to avoid stress or fatigue in any one pursuit, individuals can reduce the negative impact of competing life tasks either by dropping or consolidating pursuits, or, paradoxically, by maintaining involvement in many distinct and energizing life tasks.

Life Task Interrelations and "Spillover"

Even when an individual has the resources necessary to avoid role strain, difficulties can arise because of the interdependence of particular task pursuits. Life tasks can conflict, such that success in one lowers the ability to succeed at another (Emmons & King, 1988). An example might be an instance when romantic success creates difficulties in the social life task because friends have a lukewarm reaction to a new partner. Such conflicts may result in behavioral inhibition (Emmons & King, 1988), as well as psychological and physical ill-being (Emmons & King, 1988; Van Hook & Higgins, 1988). Moreover, strategies developed as part of ongoing task pursuit in one domain may create difficulties in another. For example, defensive pessimism can have an adverse effect on social pursuits, even when applied solely in the academic domain. Because defensive pessimism necessitates maintenance of an (inappropriately) negative self-view, it is quite possible that academic defensive pessimists will tend to express seemingly unwarranted self-criticism to their friends and acquaintances. Unfortunately, a common result of such remarks is diminished social attractiveness (Powers & Zuroff, 1988), the long-term consequences of which may be a more restricted social network (Cantor & Norem, 1989).

These examples suggest that successful outcomes and strategies in one task domain can have negative consequences for the pursuit of other tasks. This "spillover" differs from role strain in that the negative consequences are the result of specific intertask relations. A task that could otherwise easily be pursued at the same time as some tasks may have detrimental consequences when paired with a particular other task. Conflicts of this sort are perhaps most likely between tasks in which pursuit has been consolidated. For instance, the strategy of seeking academic reassurance that Harlow and Cantor (1994a, 1994b) studied was carried out specifically in the context of social pursuit (which is not necessarily true of defensive pessimism). It should not be surprising, then, that reassurance seeking would have an impact on pursuit of the social life task. In this case, the effect was decidedly negative. Consistent with research showing that support seeking is debilitating to social interactions (Coyne, 1976), strategic reassurance seeking lowered social satisfaction (Harlow & Cantor, 1994a). Thus, for these outcome-focused women, the price for consolidating their academic and social pursuits was paid in the social domain. In effect, they "ruined" their social life by consolidating it with academic pursuit. They turned it into something less like socializing and more like academics. Social pursuit ceased to be a way of making and maintaining friends, and instead turned into a forum for sharing negative academic experiences and thereby eliciting academic reassurances. This is why Harlow and Cantor (1994a) have referred to this strategy as the "social pursuit of academics." Social pursuits were used *for* academics, *at the expense of* the social life task.

These examples highlight the difficulties of pursuing many tasks in concert. However, just as tasks can conflict and create "negative spillover," it is also possible for them to complement one another, in the form of "positive spillover." This would be the case when success in one task furthers efforts in another. Romantic success, for instance, may improve family relations when a new partner is deemed "suitable" by the family. Similarly, strategies for pursuing one task may spill over and have positive consequences on the pursuit of another. Perhaps an example of this can be found in the strategy of the "illusory-glow optimist" (Norem & Cantor, 1986a). This type of optimist responds to academic challenge by setting high expectations and "positively marking" (Langston, 1994) successes with friends and acquaintances. Accordingly, academic optimists may reap benefits in the social domain for exactly the reasons that defensive pessimists may suffer. Unlike pessimists, optimists will be more likely to create an "upbeat" social environment and thereby benefit from their optimism in social as well as in academic tasks. In this way, the optimists' academic strategy can have the pleasant "side effect" of helping out social pursuit.

This latter example hints at the full range of strategies people develop for coordinating multiple pursuits. People do not have to play the role of passive recipients to spillover, but instead can "set up" positive intertask relations by pairing pursuits together in ways that create positive (rather than negative) spillover. Central to this discussion is the concept of "instrumentality"—the idea that people can utilize already positive features of a particular task to address specific obstacles in another life task domain. One possible strategy may be setting up "self-efficacy instrumentality" between two tasks—one that is appraised as threatening and intimidating, and another that is appraised as in control and manageable. For instance, a woman who is a successful corporate executive could draw on the sense of mastery she gets from her work to help her overcome the intimidation she feels in her interactions with her parents. Alternatively, one could think of a person setting up an "esteem instrumentality" relationship between two tasks. An example of this would be the man who draws on the positive regard and feeling of acceptance he gets from his social and family pursuits to help him deal with the depression and self-doubt that accompany his graduate school training.

In both cases, the individual creates an instrumental relationship between two tasks by harnessing what was already positive about one task to address the particular obstacle inherent in another. This is not the case with outcome focus. The outcome-focused women studied by Harlow and Cantor (1994a, 1994b) did not capitalize on *positive* features of socializing, but instead turned socializing into reassurance seeking. Similarly, it should be distinguished from the differentiation strategy discussed earlier. With instrumentality, the "boost" one gets from alternative tasks is the result of particular intertask dynamics. One task helps another because it addresses a particular obstacle. With differentiation, any alternative task can help any other pursuit, insofar as switching attention between tasks and maintaining multiple pursuits is engaging and invigorating, rather than stressful and overly demanding.

In our recent work (Blanton, 1994), we have investigated instrumental relations between academic and social pursuit among college students. We begin this discussion by noting what is already positive about social pursuit. Socializing is considered by most people to be "fun." Scherer, Walbott, and Summerfield (1986) find that socializing is the primary source of positive daily affect, and Morris and Reilly (1987) report that spending time with friends is the most frequently endorsed way of getting out of a bad mood. Thus, one way of using social support to further academic pursuit would be developing a "mood instrumentality" relationship between academic and social pursuits, in which the positive affect gained from social pursuit is utilized for academic pursuit. Such a strategy should not lead to problems in the social domain, because it should be harnessing an already positive aspect of social pursuit.

Our investigation of this strategy began with an assessment of students' self-reported strategies for coordinating social and academic life tasks. We administered a questionnaire that assessed the use of social pursuits as a means of improving mood for academic work. From this, we identified subjects who reported a belief that their social life could be utilized to improve their mood when they were experiencing academic stress, *and* who also showed evidence that negative mood debilitated their ability to work and make progress on academics. Thus, "mood-instrumental" subjects experienced an obstacle in academics that necessitated maintenance of a positive mood, and they held a belief that their social life could improve their mood. As predicted, highly mood-instrumental subjects subsequently responded to difficult academic periods—periods that would easily result in negative mood, were these individuals not willing to counter with a strategic intervention—by increasing the frequency and enjoyment of social pursuit. Like those of the outcome-focused individuals, their responses were contextually patterned. They responded specifically, in periods of academic challenge, by improving the quality of their *social* interactions. It is in this specificity of pairing pleasant social pursuit with academic pressures that we see evidence of strategic instrumentality. In this way, mood-instrumental individuals can be distinguished from people engaging in a strategy of differentiation, in which academic difficulties are broken up with a variety of enjoyable pursuits. However, unlike the outcome-focused reassurance seekers, our mood-instrumental subjects showed no evidence of negative spillover. In fact, highly mood-instrumental subjects responded to obstacles in academics by engaging in more *enjoyable* social pursuits. In this regard, they actually benefited socially from their academic strategy. By coordinating academic and social tasks together, such that positive features of one task spilled over in a positive way for the other, these subjects showed that with a little effort and coordination, they really could have their cake and eat it too.

CONCLUDING COMMENTS

Locating Effort in Life Task Pursuit

In closing, we want to return to our initial characterization of incentive-driven pursuit as spontaneous and life task pursuit as strategic and effortful. Life task pursuit is effortful in that it is patterned—temporally, interpersonally, and situationally—to address particular problematic appraisals of self-at-the-task. Individuals exert this coordinated effort, whether successfully or unsuccessfully, in the face of specific personal task obstacles and multiple task demands that might otherwise result in disengagement or frustration. The extent to which this patterning reflects unique strategies that address specific obstacles can also be illustrated by comparing the alternative strategies in our studies. The defensive pessimist reflects on the self and possible task scenarios before a challenging task, whereas the optimist uses protective attributions afterwards (Norem & Cantor, 1986a). The outcome-focused student seeks reassurance in social situations from confidants and encouragers after academic setbacks; the improvement-focused student also responds to similar setbacks by increasing social contact, but with idols, not encouragers (Harlow & Cantor, 1994a; Cantor, 1994). Some students respond to pressure in one task domain by withdrawing effort in other critical tasks (e.g., Cantor et al., 1992); others find positive ways to increase the time and level of engagement in an alternate task to the advantage of a more taxing one (e.g., Blanton, 1994).

This patterning is noteworthy because it guides behavior even when immediate hedonic fulfillment is unlikely, and sometimes does so in ways that actually reduce opportunities for positive affect. For instance, the defensive pessimist continues to reflect on possible disasters, even though doing so may lead to emotional fatigue (Showers, 1992). This contrasts with incentive-driven motivation, which engages only when the possibility of affective fulfillment is anticipated. In a similar way, the patterning of multiple tasks often operates against hedonic interests, such as when outcome-focused students ruin an otherwise positive social activity by discussing academic setbacks (Harlow & Cantor, 1994a, 1994b).

The "Experience" of Effort: Effortful or Spontaneous?

The fact that strategic behavior is patterned to address particular needs is sufficient to label it "effortful." However, there is an additional place for effort, which, though it is not always present, distinguishes it from the spontaneous action linked to implicit motives. Strategic behavior is effortful because often it is also *experienced* as effortful. This happens, for example, during task pursuit when individuals simultaneously act and also reflect on their action, thus "experiencing" the effort involved in coordinating their own behavior (Johnson, 1991). Examples include defensive pessimists who reflect on themselves as they construct another worst-case scenario; students using social life instrumentally, who become acutely aware of the potential for dysphoric mood as they seek out an uplifting social encounter; and outcome-focused students looking at themselves, perhaps skeptically through the "mind's eye," as they seek reassurance once again after an academic disappointment. As these examples illustrate, sometimes self-reflection can be a quite painful part of strategic action (Kihlstrom, 1987).

When people are aware that they have "chosen" to engage a strategy—that they are making decisions and thus forgoing some opportunities—strategic behavior can be described as phenomenologically quite "effortful." However, it may surprise some that we do not think this characterization is always an accurate one for life task pursuit. To use a common comparison, driving a car requires thoughtful, coordinated, specific responses, even involving rapid adjustments to familiar obstacles in a path. An experienced driver, however, is rarely aware of himself or herself guiding the car and making these adjustments until an unfamiliar, dangerous, surprising, or otherwise "attention-getting" object enters the field (Johnson, 1991). When the driver's attention is captured, then he or she may be acutely aware of the effort that it is taking just to stay on track, keep safe, monitor danger, and anticipate problems.

Where does the experience of life task pursuit typically fall along this continuum from the spontaneous effort of the experienced driver to the painstaking awareness and vigilance of the anxious driver? Often, it will be quite spontaneous. In much the same way as the experienced driver has already "put in place" the necessary skills for reacting with "spontaneous" effort to mundane driving conditions, much of life task pursuit involves highly overlearned and repetitious actions under commonplace conditions. Strategic actions can become scripted responses in specific task conditions (Nasby & Kihlstrom, 1986), as Linville and Clark (1989) demonstrated in describing a possible production system for defensive pessimism. Even a strategy that directly involves as much complex self-reflection as the defensive pessimist's weighing of alternative future task scenarios may be *experienced* as being spontaneously evoked in a particular context. Nevertheless, even when strategic behavior is scripted, evidence that it was patterned to address the particulars of task demands reveals coordinated effort; and, as the strategic response unfolds, the participant may become aware of this effort—as do most defensive pessimists (Showers, 1992).

In our system, patterning equals effort. The phenomenal experience of this type of effort, however, may vary considerably. Strategic behavior ranges from a routine drive in the park to an emergency maneuver on an icy highway. To the extent that life task pursuit involves unpredictable obstacles in the environment, some novelty in the task conditions, component projects that are hard to accomplish, and/or long periods of commitment, task pursuit may be experienced as effortful. Moreover, when the individuals involved have particular, well-elaborated anxieties and concerns about performing a task, then even a seemingly routine, time-limited, straightforward project can be experienced as personally threatening and demanding of active coping. After all, students take exams all the time, but sometimes, for some people, these are exhausting events (Folkman & Lazarus, 1985). Furthermore, some people develop strategies that, however unnecessarily burdensome they seem to others, routinely involve extended introspection into their own efforts. The defensive pessimist has a distinct penchant for such self-reflection in preparation for task pursuit, as taxing and tiring as that may be (Showers, 1992).

As Johnson and Reeder (1993) suggest, the "conscious" experience of thinking and behaving can vary a great deal—from the smoothness and spontaneity of drinking a fine wine with a close friend, to the agonizing slow motion of struggling to meet a self-imposed deadline. Strategic behavior will often look and feel like the latter situation, with constant monitoring and deliberate self-reflection guiding responses to each new obstacle. However, even when strategic behavior is like enjoying wine with a friend, effort is very much present. It is important to remember that friends and good wine do not spontaneously co-occur. Arranging this situation requires coordinated effort. This takes the form of picking the right grape and year to go with the meal (perhaps correcting somewhat for the tastes of the guest), presenting the wine at just the right time in appropriate glasses, and pouring it only after it has had time to "breathe." Producing the perfect wine (and friend) for this evening takes a great deal of effort. However, at the time, with the aroma of good food and the atmosphere created by pleasant conversation, nothing could seem easier. At least, until the friend calls for a toast. . . .

REFERENCES

Atkinson, J. W., & Litwin, C. H. (1960). Achievement motive and test anxiety conceived as motive to approach success and motive to avoid failure. *Journal of Abnormal and Social Psychology, 60,* 52–63.

Bandura, A. (1986). *Social foundations of thought and action: A social cognitive theory.* Englewood Cliffs, NJ: Prentice-Hall.

Blanton, H. (1994). *Mood regulation through affiliation: The case of social instrumentality.* Unpublished doctoral dissertation, Princeton University, Princeton, NJ.

Block, J. (1961). Ego-identity, role variability, and adjustment. *Journal of Consulting and Clinical Psychology, 25,* 392–397.

Bolger, N., & Tordesillias, R. (1993). *Multiple roles and multiple identities in daily life.* Paper presented at the Third Annual Conference of the Society for Personality and Social Psychology, Chicago.

Bumpass, L. (1994). *A social map of midlife: Family and work over the middle life course* (Technical Report to MIDMAC). Vero Beach, FL: MacArthur Foundation Research Network on Successful Midlife Development.

Butler, R. B. (1992). What young people want to know when: Effects of mastery and ability goals on interest in different kinds of social comparison. *Journal of Personality and Social Psychology, 62,* 934–943.

Butler, R. B. (1993). Effects of task- and ego-achievement goals on information seeking during task engagement. *Journal of Personality and Social Psychology, 65,* 18–31.

Cantor, N. (1990). From thought to behavior: "Having" and "doing" in the study of personality and cognition. *American Psychologist, 45,* 735–750.

Cantor, N. (1994). Life task problem solving: Situational affordances and personal needs (Division Eight Presidential Address, 1993). *Personality and Social Psychology Bulletin, 20*(3), 235–243.

Cantor, N., Acker, M., & Cook-Flannagan, C. (1992). Conflict and preoccupation in the intimacy life task. *Journal of Personality and Social Psychology, 63*(4), 644–655.

Cantor, N., & Fleeson, W. (1991). Life tasks and self-regulatory processes. In M. Maehr & P. Pintrich (Eds.), *Advances in motivation and achievement* (Vol. 7, pp. 327–369). Greenwich, CT: JAI Press.

Cantor, N., & Fleeson, W. (1994). Social intelligence and intelligent goal pursuit: A cognitive slice of motivation. In W. Spaulding (Ed.), *Nebraska Symposium on Motivation: Vol. 41. Integrative views of motivation, cognition, and emotion* (pp. 125–179). Lincoln: University of Nebraska Press.

Cantor, N., & Harlow, R. E. (1994). Personality, strategic behavior and daily life problem-solving. *Current Directions in Psychological Science, 3*(6), 169–172.

Cantor, N., & Kihlstrom, J. F. (1987). *Personality and social intelligence.* Englewood Cliffs, NJ: Prentice-Hall.

Cantor, N., & Malley, J. (1991). Life tasks, personal needs, and close relationships. In G. J. O. Fletcher & F. D. Fincham (Eds.), *Cognition in close relationships* (pp. 101–125). Hillsdale, NJ: Erlbaum.

Cantor, N., Markus, H., Niedenthal, P., & Nurius, P. (1986). On motivation and the self-concept. In R. M. Sorrentino & E. T. Higgins (Eds.), *Handbook of motivation and cognition: Foundations of social behavior* (Vol. 1, pp. 96–121). New York: Guilford Press.

Cantor, N., & Norem, J. K. (1989). Defensive pessimism and stress and coping. *Social Cognition, 7*(2), 92–112.

Cantor, N., Norem, J. K., Niedenthal, P. M., Langston, C. A., & Brower, A. M. (1987). Life tasks, self-concept ideals, and cognitive strategies in a life transition. *Journal of Personality and Social Psychology, 53*(6), 1178–1191.

Coyne, J. C. (1976). Depression and the responses of others. *Journal of Abnormal Psychology, 85*(2), 186–193.

Csikszentmihalyi, M. (1990). *Flow: The psychology of optimal experience.* New York: Harper & Row.

Csikszentmihalyi, M., & LeFevre, J. (1989). Optimal experience in work and leisure. *Journal of Personality and Social Psychology, 56*(5), 815–822.

Deci, E. L., & Ryan, R. M. (1985). *Intrinsic motivation and self-determination in human behavior.* New York: Plenum.

Donahue, E. M., Robins, R. W., Roberts, B. W., & John, O. (1993). The divided self: Concurrent and longitudinal effects of psychological adjustment and social roles on self-concept differentiation. *Journal of Personality and Social Psychology, 64*(5), 834–846.

Dweck, C. S., & Leggett, E. L. (1988). A social-cognitive approach to personality and motivation. *Psychological Review, 95,* 256–273.

Emmons, R. A., & King, L. A. (1988). Conflict among personal strivings: Immediate and long-term implications for psychological and physical well-being. *Journal of Personality and Social Psychology, 56*(6), 1040–1048.

Emmons, R. A., & McAdams, D. P. (1991). Personal strivings and motive dispositions: Exploring the links. *Personality and Social Psychology Bulletin, 17*(6), 648–654.

Erikson, E. H. (1950). *Childhood and society.* New York: Norton.

Erikson, E. H. (1980). Themes of adulthood in the Freud–Jung correspondence. In N. J. Smelser & E. H. Erikson (Eds.), *Themes of work and love in adulthood* (pp. 43–74). Cambridge, MA: Harvard University Press.

Fleeson, W. (1992). *Life tasks, implicit motives, and self-regulation in daily life.* Unpublished doctoral dissertation, University of Michigan.

Folkman, S., & Lazarus, R. S. (1985). If it changes it must be a process: Study of emotion and coping during three stages of a college examination. *Journal of Personality and Social Psychology, 48,* 150–170.

Gollwitzer, P. (1993). Goal achievement: The role of intentions. In W. Stroebe & M. Hewstone (Eds.), *European review of social psychology* (Vol. 4, pp. 141–185). Chichester, England: Wiley.

Goode, W. J. (1960). A theory of role strain. *American Sociological Review, 25,* 483–496.

Harlow, R. E., & Cantor, N. (1994a). The social pursuit of academics: Side-effects and "spillover" of strategic reassurance seeking. *Journal of Personality and Social Psychology, 66,* 386–397.

Harlow, R. E., & Cantor, N. (1995). To whom do people turn when things go poorly? *Journal of Personality and Social Psychology, 69,* 329–340.

Harlow, R. E., & Cantor, N. (1994b) Overcoming a lack of self-assurance in an achievement domain: Creating agency in daily life. In M. Kernis (Ed.), *Efficacy, agency, and self-esteem* (pp. 171–194). New York: Plenum.

Havighurst, R. J. (1953). *Human development and education.* New York: Longmans, Green.

Havighurst, R. J. (1972). *Developmental tasks and education* (3rd ed.). New York: David McKay.

Heyman, G. D., Dweck, C. S., & Cain, K. M. (1992). Young children's vulnerability to self-blame and helplessness: Relationship to beliefs about goodness. *Child Development, 63*(2), 401–415.

Higgins, E. T. (1987). Self-discrepancy: A theory relating self and affect. *Psychological Review, 94*(3), 319–340.

Higgins, E. T., & Parsons, J. E. (1983). Social cognition and the social life of the child: Stages as subcultures. In E. T. Higgins, D. N. Ruble, & W. W. Hartup (Eds.), *Social cognition and social development: A sociocultural perspective* (pp. 15–62). New York: Cambridge University Press.

Hobfoll, S. E. (1989). Conservation of resources: A new attempt at conceptualizing stress. *American Psychologist, 44*(3), 513–524.

Hooker, K., Kaus, C., & Morfei, E. (1993). *The function of possible selves in linking personal goals to developmental tasks.* Paper presented at the 46th Annual Scientific Meetings of the Genrontological Society of America, New Orleans.

Johnson, M. K. (1991). Reflection, reality-monitoring, and the self. In R. Kunzendorf (Ed.), *Mental imagery* (pp. 3–16). New York: Plenum.

Johnson, M. K., & Reeder, J. A. (1993). *Consciousness as meta-processing.* Paper presented at the 25th Carnegie Symposium on Cognition, Scientific Approaches to the Question of Consciousness, Pittsburgh.

Kandel, D. B., Davies, M., & Raveis, V. H. (1985). The stressfulness of daily social roles for women: Marital, occupational and household roles. *Journal of Health and Social Behavior, 26,* 64–78.

Kihlstrom, J. F. (1987). The cognitive unconscious. *Science, 237,* 1445–1452.

Klinger, E. (1975). Consequences of commitment to and disengagement from incentives. *Psychological Review, 82,* 1–25.

Koestner, R., Weinberger, J., & McClelland, D. C. (1991). Task-intrinsic and social-extrinsic sources of arousal for motives assessed in fantasy and self-report. *Journal of Personality, 59,* 57–82.

Kuhl, J. (1985). Volitional mediators of cognition-behavior consistency: Self-regulatory processes and action versus state orientation. In J. Kuhl & J. Beckmann (Eds.), *Action control from cognition to behavior* (pp. 101–128). Berlin: Springer-Verlag.

Langsson, C. A. (1994). Capitalizing upon and coping with daily-life events: Expressive responses to positive events. *Journal of Personality and Social Psychology, 67,* 1112–1125.

Linville, P. W. (1987). Self-complexity as a cognitive buffer against stress-related illness and depression. *Journal of Personality and Social Psychology, 52*(4), 663–676.

Linville, P. W., & Clark, L. F. (1989). Production systems and social problem solving: Specificity, flexibility, and expertise. In R. S. Wyer & T. K. Srull (Eds.), *Advances in social cognition* (Vol. 2, pp. 131–152). Hillsdale, NJ: Erlbaum.

Little, B. R. (1989). Personal projects analysis: Trivial pursuits, magnificent obsessions and the search for coherence. In D. M. Buss & N. Cantor (Eds.), *Personality psychology: Recent trends and emerging directions* (pp. 15–31). New York: Springer-Verlag.

Marks, S. (1977). Multiple roles and role strain: Some notes on human energy, time, and commitment. *American Sociological Review, 42,* 921–936.

Markus, H., & Nurius, P. (1986). Possible selves. *American Psychologist, 41*(9), 954–969.

McClelland, D. C. (1985). *Human motivation.* Glenview, IL: Scott, Foresman.

McClelland, D. C., Koestner, R., & Weinberger, J. (1989). How do self-attributed and implicit motives differ? *Psychological Review, 96,* 690–702.

Merton, R. K. (1957). *Social theory and social structure* (rev. ed.). New York: Free Press.

Morris, W. N., & Reilly, N. P. (1987). Toward the self-regulation of mood: Theory and research. *Motivation and Emotion, 11*(3), 215–249.

Nasby, W., & Kihlstrom, J. F. (1986). Cognitive assessment of personality and psychopathology. In R. E. Ingram (Ed.), *Information-processing approaches to psychopathology and clinical psychology* (pp. 217–239). New York: Academic Press.

Norem, J. K. (1989). Cognitive strategies as personality: Effectiveness, specificity, flexibility, and change. In D. M. Buss & N. Cantor (Eds.), *Personality psychology: Recent trends and emerging directions* (pp. 45–60). New York: Springer-Verlag.

Norem, J. K., & Cantor, N. (1986a). Anticipatory and post hoc cushioning strategies: Optimism and defensive pessimism in "risky" situations. *Cognitive Therapy and Research, 10*(3), 347–362.

Norem, J. K., & Cantor, N. (1986b). Defensive pessimism: "Harnessing" anxiety as motivation. *Journal of Personality and Social Psychology, 55*(6), 1208–1217.

Norem, J. K., & Illingworth, K. S. (1993). Strategy-dependent effects of reflecting on self and tasks: Some implications of optimism and defensive pessimism. *Journal of Personality and Social Psychology, 65*(4), 822–835.

Parsons, J. E., Adler, T. G., & Kaczala, C. (1982). Socialization of achievement attitudes and beliefs: Parental influences. *Child Development, 53,* 310–321.

Parsons, J. E., Kaczala, C., & Meece, J. (1982). Socialization of achievement attitudes and beliefs: Teacher influences. *Child Development, 53,* 322–339.

Pervin, L. (Ed.). (1989). *Goal concepts in personality and social psychology.* Hillsdale, NJ: Erlbaum.

Phillips, D. A. (1987). Socialization of perceived academic competence among highly competent children. *Child Development, 58,* 1308–1320.

Phillips, D. A., & Zimmerman, M. (1990). The developmental course of perceived competence and incompetence among competent children. In R. J. Sternberg & J. K. Kolligan, Jr. (Eds.), *Competence considered.* New Haven, CT: Yale University Press.

Powers, T. A., & Zuroff, D. C. (1988). Interpersonal consequences of overt self-criticism: A comparison with neutral and self-enhancing presentations of self. *Journal of Personality and Social Psychology, 54*(6), 1054–1062.

Read, S. J., & Miller, L. C. (1989). Interpersonalism: Towards a goal-based theory of persons and relationships. In L. Pervin (Ed.), *Goal concepts in personality and social psychology* (pp. 413–472). Hillsdale, NJ: Erlbaum.

Sarbin, T. R., & Allen, V. L. (1968). Role theory. In G. Lindsey & E. Aronson (Eds.), *The handbook of social psychology* (2nd ed., Vol. 1, pp. 97–115). Reading, MA: Addison-Wesley.

Scherer, K. R., Walbott, H. S., & Summerfield, A. B. (1986). *Experiencing emotion.* Cambridge, England: Cambridge University Press.

Showers, C. (1992). The motivational and emotional consequences of considering positive or negative possibilities for an upcoming event. *Journal of Personality and Social Psychology, 63*(3), 474–484.

Stewart, A. J. (1989). Social intelligence and adaptation to life changes. In R. S. Wyer & T. K. Srull (Eds.), *Advances in social cognition* (Vol. 2, pp. 187–196). Hillsdale, NJ: Erlbaum.

Thoits, P. A. (1983). Multiple identities and psychological well-being: A reformulation and test of the social isolation hypothesis. *American Sociological Review, 48,* 174–187.

Thoits, P. A. (1986). Multiple identities: Examining gender and marital status differences in distress. *American Sociological Review, 51,* 259–272.

Van Hook, E., & Higgins, E. T. (1988). Self-related problems beyond the self-concept: Motivational consequences of discrepant self-guides. *Journal of Personality and Social Psychology, 55*(4), 625–633.

Verbrugge, L. M. (1983). Multiple roles and physical health of women and men. *Journal of Health and Social Behavior, 24,* 16–30.

Veroff, J. (1983). Contextual determinants of personality. *Personality and Social Psychology Bulletin, 9,* 331–344.

Weinberger, J., & McClelland, D. C. (1990). Cognitive versus traditional motivational models: Irreconcilable or complementary? In E. T. Higgins & R. M. Sorrentino (Eds.), *Handbook of motivation and cognition: Foundations of social behavior* (Vol. 2, pp. 562–597). New York: Guilford Press.

Weiner, B. (1986). *An attribution theory of motivation and emotion.* New York: Springer-Verlag.

Wright, R. A., & Brehm, J. W. (1989). Energization and goal attractiveness. In L. A. Pervin (Ed.), *Goal concepts in personality and social psychology* (pp. 169–210). Hillsdale, NJ: Erlbaum.

Zeldow, P. B., Daugherty, S. R., & McAdams, D. P. (1988). Intimacy, power, and psychological health. *Journal of Nervous and Mental Disease, 176*(3), 182–187.

Zirkel, S. A. (1992). Developing independence in a life transition: Investing the self in the concerns of the day. *Journal of Personality and Social Psychology, 62*(3), 506–521.

Zirkel, S. A., & Cantor, N. (1990). Personal construal of life tasks: Those who struggle for independence. *Journal of Personality and Social Psychology, 58*(1), 172–185.

PART IV

Effortful Control of Action

Most theorizing on the control of action is based on the premise that goal-directed action is effortful. This view extends to all phases of goal pursuit, from the origins of goal pursuit (i.e., goal setting) to its conclusion (i.e., the sucessful implementation of the goal). Goal setting necessitates controlled and effortful deliberation of one's wishes and desires. Goal implementation, on the other hand, is furthered by choosing appropriate implementational strategies, mobilizing effort in the face of obstacles, and holding up persistence until the goal is reached. Part IV concerns these issues.

Locke and Kristof (Chapter 16) see the course of goal pursuit as a string of consecutive choices to be made by the striving individual. At the start, choices between values are prevalent, but later on, choices between implementational strategies need to be made. Ajzen (Chapter 17) focuses on the role of attitudes and—based on his theories of reasoned action and planned behavior—suggests that people's effortful deliberation of their beliefs about the likely consequences of possible behaviors has an important influence on their behavioral intentions and subsequent behaviors. Kanfer (Chapter 18) points out that the effectiveness of implementational strategy choices (e.g., setting of specific goals, emotion control, or motivation control) is dependent on an individual's ability level and the intellectual demands of the tasks the individual tries to achieve. Finally, Wright (Chapter 19) explores the question of how much effort a person is willing to exert, given a certain difficulty of the task at hand and a certain amount of potential motivation.

Locke and Kristof begin by discussing Ayn Rand's theory of volition. This leads them to conclude that a person's freedom of action is the indirect result of the freedom to think about whatever one wants to focus on. Through this volitional focus, one can choose what values one wants to achieve and reflect on the means of achieving them. Goals are thought to link values and action, as they are applications of values to specific situations. Goals are set and pursued by making choices. This applies to the goal content, to the various features of the goal (e.g., its difficulty, its specificity, and the strength of commitment to it), and to the implementation of the goal (e.g., choices between different plans and methods, possible solutions to goal conflict, and ways of dealing with obstacles and failures). This theoretical perspective on goal pursuit raises the quesion of what types of choices are most effective. Locke and Latham's goal-setting theory and the research stimulated by it provides some decisive answers. For instance, setting oneself specific and difficult goals leads to higher performance than setting goals that are vague or specific but easy. In the present chapter, Locke and Kristof report data on law school students who set themselves the goal of achieving a certain exam grade. Goal level (in terms of the minimum grade they would be satisfied with) turned out to be a good predictor of exam performance. This effect was mediated by the choices students made in terms of studying plans and methods, ways of dealing with potential goal conflicts, strategies of overcoming obstacles or coping with failure, and strategies of intensifying their commitment. These findings lead Locke and Kristof to conclude that goal pursuits are best understood as a string of choices, and that willpower should be viewed as nothing more than making clever choices.

Ajzen discusses the directive influences of attitudes and intentions on behavior. Presenting the results of various meta-analyses on findings generated by his theories of reasoned action and planned behavior, he concludes that attitudes and behavioral intentions are good predictors of behavior, as long as the principle of compatibility (i.e., the notion that attitudes, intentions, and behaviors should be measured at the same level of generality or specificity) is respected. Concerning how attitudes affect behavior, Ajzen holds a model of effortful information processing. In his view, attitudes enter the stage of a person's conscious thoughts at crucial decision-making times. When confronted with the need to decide on a course of action, the person deliberates the likely consequences of available alternatives, weighs the normative expectations of relevant others, and considers required resources and potential obstacles. These considerations result in the formation of attitudes toward the behavior of interest, subjective norms with respect to the behavior, and perceived behavioral control, respectively. On the basis of these insights, the individual is expected to form behavioral intentions that qualify as the immediate determinants of behavior. This model implies that the principle of compatibility actually refers to compatibility of salient beliefs that determine attitudes, subjective norms, perceived behavioral control, and intentions. High attitude–behavior consistency is expected when the same or similar beliefs are salient at the time and place of attitude formation and at the time and place of the execution of behavior. Ajzen argues that the careful considerations taking place in a deliberative mode (i.e., effortful information processing) are likely to bring to mind the most relevant beliefs. Therefore, congruency of the deliberative mode at the time of attitude formation and the later expression of behavior should enhance attitude–behavior consistency. More problematic is the effect of attitudes on behavior when people are either not sufficiently motivated or incapable of engaging in careful deliberation. If this more spontaneous mode of action predominates, behavior is controlled by whatever beliefs are salient at the moment. As a result, an individual's reasoned attitudes should no longer control the individual's behaviors.

Kanfer studies the effortful implementation of goals in the context of skill acquisition. According to the integrated resource allocation model of skill acquisition proposed by Kanfer and Ackerman as a theoretical starting point, the effects of effortful self-regulatory strategies on task performance are expected to interact with the individual's level of cognitive ability and the cognitive demands of the task at hand. More specifically, it is postulated that cognitive ability determines the upper limit of attentional resources an individual may allocate to a given task. Because applying self-regulation strategies also demands a certain amount of attention, these strategies have either positive or negative effects on task performance, depending on their attentional costs relative to the attentional demands of the task and the individual's cognitive ability. This was observed when subjects were trained to perform a task that simulates the work of air traffic controllers. The self-regulation strategy of setting oneself specific and challenging goals hindered task performance for low-ability subjects when task demands were high, but helped low-ability subjects when task demands were low. The notion that the potential benefits of self-regulatory strategies critically depend on resource availability is also supported by the finding that the goal-setting strategy leads to better performance under spaced practice (i.e., frequent breaks) than under massed practice (i.e., no breaks). Finally, Kanfer treats various self-regulation strategies as individual-difference variables. In particular, she considers emotion control and motivation control. The former relates to a person's skills in coping with emotional responses to failures during skill acquisition; the latter relates to maintaining motivation when performing the task gets boring. Again, these self-regulation strategies affect task performance in interaction with the individual's ability level and the demands of the task at hand. When task demands are high (i.e., at the first few trials), emotion control is particularly beneficial for low-ability individuals, whereas motivation control is particularly beneficial for high-ability individuals at later practice trials (i.e., when task demand is low). Throughout her chapter, Kanfer emphasizes the variable influences of effortful self-regulation on task performance, depending upon the attentional demands of the task, individual differences in cognitive abilities, and the nature of the self-regulation processes involved.

Wright outlines a model that describes the determinants of a person's readiness to mobilize effort at a chosen task. The model is based on Brehm's theory of motivation, and it is argued that the potential motivation to engage in task activity depends on a person's need, the incentive value of the anticipated outcomes, and the instrumentality of the activity with respect to achieving these outcomes. But potential motivation is not directly related to a person's readiness to exert effort; rather, it only sets the upper limit to effort mobilization (i.e., determines potential motivation). What affects effort more directly is the individual's perception of how difficult it is to exert the activity. More specifically, effort is expected to become mobilized in line with perceived increases in task difficulty—up to the limit set by potential motivation. Beyond the upper limit of what the individual is potentially motivated to do, effort expenditure is expected to drop to zero. Wright finds ample support for this model of effort in numerous experiments assessing effort mobilization by employing physiological measures (in particular, systolic blood pressure). The typical experimental design manipulates the level of potential motivation by varying either perceived behavioral instrumentality, incentive value, or need. In addition, various levels of task difficulty are established (i.e., low, medium, high, impossible). The results of these studies strongly suggest that the positive relation between difficulty and effort mobilization is moderated by potential motivation, as the latter determines whether effort mobilization is still justified at higher levels of task difficulty. More recently, Wright has focused on how perceived ability modifies effort mobilization. At an easy task, low-ability individuals consistently exert greater effort than high-ability individuals, whereas at a moderately difficult task, the reverse holds true. This pattern of results again suggests that effort mobilization finds an upper limit in a person's potential motivation. Low-ability individuals reach this limit at a lower difficulty level than high-ability individuals. For the former, the moderately difficult task requires an amount of effort mobilization that they are not willing (or motivated) to exert.

CHAPTER 16

Volitional Choices in the Goal Achievement Process

Edwin A. Locke
Amy L. Kristof

In this chapter, we would like to accomplish four things: (1) to present, in summary form, Ayn Rand's theory of volition and the arguments for it; (2) to link volition to goal-setting theory by showing how volition applies to the process of setting and achieving goals; (3) to apply this analysis to the role of student; and (4) to present some preliminary data illustrating these ideas.

AYN RAND'S THEORY OF VOLITION

The issue of volition or free will versus its opposite, psychological determinism, has been debated by philosophers for centuries. The three key issues in the debate are these: (1) Do people possess free will? (2) If they do, of what does it consist? (3) How can it be validated? The doctrine of free will asserts that in some respect, a person's thoughts or actions or beliefs or desires are chosen by that person and not necessitated by antecedent causes. The doctrine of determinism, in contrast, asserts that whatever a person thinks, does, believes, or feels is outside personal control and necessitated by the sum of the forces acting upon the person, whether these be genetic, environmental, or a combination thereof.

Ayn Rand has presented an original theory of the nature of free will and a unique method of validating it (Rand, 1964; Binswanger, 1991; Peikoff, 1991). This theory has already been presented in some detail in the organizational psychology/organizational behavior literature by Binswanger (1991); thus we only present the highlights here.

Before summarizing this theory, we want to discuss briefly two traditional views of the nature of free will. The doctrine of "freedom of action" asserts that people have direct freedom to choose one action as opposed to another. The typical example used to illustrate this is the choice of whether or not to raise your arm. If someone asks you if you can choose to raise your arm, you will routinely say "Yes," and will then raise your arm to prove it.

This example is misleading, however, because there is nothing at stake in the action; raising your arm has only marginal value significance. You are simply showing that you can make a trivial motion. But consider a different example. If someone asks you whether you can, this minute, run to the top of a tall building and jump off, you would think about this question seriously for a few seconds and say "No." If you were then asked, "What would you have to do first before you could jump?", the honest answer would be this, "Convince myself that life is not worth living." In other words, the action could not be taken unless you were first thinking in a certain way. The same principle applies to raising your arm, but the need for a prior thought process is less obvious. Thus, freedom of action is not direct, but indirect; it depends upon your thinking.

A second common theory of the nature of free will is the doctrine of "freedom of choice between desires." This doctrine argues that, just as you have the power to raise your arm, you have the power to choose between competing action impulses or wants. But, again, on what basis do you make such choices? Desires and emotions are not psychological primaries; they depend on your ideas, including your subconscious beliefs and values (Rand, 1964; see also Locke & Latham, 1990; Packer, 1985–1986). Thus a clash of desires means a clash between ideas. How it is resolved will depend on the nature of your thinking process in response to the clash.

Thus, to identify the root of free will, we must go deeper than the level of actions and desires; we must go to the thinking behind them. Ayn Rand argues that free will, at root, consists of the choice to think or not to think (Rand, 1964). To understand what she means by this, we first have to understand the nature of consciousness.

"Consciousness" is the faculty for perceiving reality; its ultimate biological function is the regulation of action. "Consciousness—for those living organisms which possess it—is the basic means of survival" (Rand, 1964, p. 18). Fundamentally, consciousness exists on two levels: the sensory-perceptual level and the conceptual or rational level. The sensory-perceptual level, present in both the lower animals and humans, has two key features: It operates automatically, and it is not subject to error. You do not have to choose to see; you simply have to open your eyes. (How you interpret what you see, of course, depends on your conceptual knowledge.)

The conceptual level of awareness or reason, which is unique to humans, is different. The conceptual level involves integrating sensory material to form concepts, integrating concepts to form propositions, and so forth. Unlike sense perception, reasoning or conceptual thinking does not occur automatically, but has to be done by choice; and it can be wrong—that is, mistaken.

Let us first consider the aspect of choice. A good example is that of reading a textbook that presents material with which you are not familiar. To understand what you are reading, you have to choose to understand what the new concepts presented mean. You have to choose to see the relationship between these new concepts and the facts on which they were based. You have to choose to see how the different concepts relate to one another. You have to choose to identify the implications and applications of the concepts.

Ayn Rand uses the term "focus" to describe the process of raising one's mind to the fully conceptual level of awareness. If you do not focus when you are reading, for example, your mind may drift back to the sensory-perceptual level; you will see the shapes of the letters on the page, but will have no idea what they mean. Or you may grasp the individual words but not their relationship to each other.

Conceptualizing, then, is an active, not a passive process. To quote Ayn Rand (1964, p. 20):

> The process of concept-formation does not consist merely of grasping a few simple abstractions, such as "chair," "table," "hot," "cold," and of learning to speak. It consists of a method of using one's consciousness, best designated by the term "conceptualizing." It is not a passive state of registering random impressions. It is an actively sustained process of identifying one's impressions in conceptual terms, of integrating every event and every observation into a conceptual context, of grasping relationships, differences, similarities in one's perceptual material and of abstracting them into new concepts, of drawing inferences, of making deductions, or reaching conclusions, of asking new questions and discovering new answers and expanding one's knowledge into an ever-growing sum. The faculty that directs this process, the faculty that works by means of concepts is: *reason.* The process is *thinking.*

To focus means to focus on reality, not fantasy; to distinguish between the objective (reason) and the subjective (feelings); to adhere to logic; and to hold context (Binswanger, 1991). A student, for example, who daydreams about how nice it would be to get an A rather than concentrating on the text material is not in focus. A student who feels, on no rational basis, that the concepts on page 32 can be ignored because they are complicated is not in focus. A student who memorizes two inconsistent propositions and treats them both as true is not in focus.

We now give you a favorite example of failure to hold a context (nonintegration). We choose this particular example because the debate is probably familiar to all of our readers. Starting in about the 1960s, some psychologists began to claim, on the basis of alleged research findings, that lower animal species such as chimpanzees could grasp human sign language—meaning that they could grasp human concepts. These researchers' results and conclusions were widely accepted until one of their own, Herb Terrace (1979), concluded on the basis of a long and intensive research project that these conclusions were wrong; these chimps did not really understand the meaning of the signs they were using. Terrace's results came as a shock to many psychologists.

These results would not have been surprising if psychologists had held the full context of their knowledge. Let us just consider two generally known facts. First, chimpanzees have been on earth for several million years, and during that time have not developed even the rudiments of a quasi-human culture. Second, the existence of even a limited conceptual capacity would give any species that possessed it an enormous advantage in terms of survival over species that did not possess it; yet at no time did chimps show evidence of dominating the earth or even small parts of it. How are we to reconcile these facts with the claims of the animal experimenters about the mental capacity of these primates? At a minimum, it would have to make us suspicious of the experiments—which indeed turned out to be flawed (Terrace, 1979).

Because conceptualizing or reasoning is not an automatic process like perception, conceptual conclusions have to be validated. Validation is achieved by means of using proper procedures for gaining knowledge—specifically logic. Logic includes tracing concepts to their roots in sense perception, understanding the hierarchical relationship among concepts, and integrating one's knowledge into a noncontradictory whole (Peikoff, 1991).

Why should we believe that Ayn Rand's theory of volition is valid? After all, many theories of free will have been offered by philosophers in the past, and all have been cogently attacked—not only by those advocating determinism, but also by those advocating alternative theories of free will. Ayn Rand argues that free will or volition holds the status of an axiom, and therefore is not proven, but antecedes any attempts at proof. What then is an "axiom," or more properly for our purposes, an "axiomatic concept"? To quote Rand (1990, p. 55):

> An axiomatic concept is the identification of a primary fact of reality, which cannot be analyzed, i.e., reduced to other facts or broken into component parts. It is implicit in all facts and in all knowledge. It is the fundamentally given and directly perceived or experienced, which requires no proof or explanation, but on which all proofs and explanations rest.

And Binswanger (1991, p. 173) adds:

> A philosophic axiom cannot be proved precisely because it is presupposed by all proof; hence any attempt at proof would beg the question. . . . Valid axioms need not be proven because they are formulations of the *self-evident*. To be self-evident means to be available to direct observation, without the need of inference.

Ayn Rand's three primary axioms are existence (reality), identity (everything is something particular or is what it is), and consciousness (awareness). Volition is an aspect of the axiom of consciousness. Therefore, Ayn Rand suggests that the validation of volition, like other axioms, is achieved by means of direct observation. Direct observation in the case of volition means introspection. You can observe directly that you can choose to focus your mind, or to allow your mind to remain at or regress to the sensory-perceptual level of awareness. You can also observe that you have the power to actively choose *not* to focus—to evade reality, facts, reason, and logic.

One might protest that introspection is fallible, and therefore that what may seem to be self-evident is not. However, this argument does not refute volition. Addition can be done incorrectly, but that does not invalidate mathematics or accounting. In order to invalidate volition, one would have to show that introspection is wrong on this particular issue. To date, no such argument has been offered. It is questionable whether one could be offered; Binswanger (1991) shows that challenging volition would in the end be self-refuting. To quote Binswanger (1991, p. 174),

> A volitionally self-regulating mind has the power to control itself; it can choose to focus on the factual evidence and to check the validity of its conclusions against the facts, applying the canons of logic. But a determined mind would not be free to do this and would be incapable of judging objectively its own "output."

He is arguing that if determinism were true, all assertions of conceptual knowledge would be invalidated, *including* all assertions of determinists. Therefore, determinists could not logically claim that their doctrines were true, but merely that they were forced by heredity and/or environment to emit certain verbal statements.

Showing the self-contradiction entailed in determinism is not a "back door" proof of the existence of volition. As Ayn Rand suggests, volition can be validated only by direct observation of one's consciousness, not by a process of deduction. She argues that it is axiomatic, because it is directly perceived and presupposed by all attempts at proof and at gaining further knowledge.

It should also be noted that the suggested existence of volition is not a contradiction of the law of causality, as determinists claim. Not all causality is mechanical causality, in which *A* necessarily leads to *B*, which necessarily leads to *C*, and so on. Human nature allows for the possibility of choice—the choice to focus one's mind or not (assuming a normal brain state). Such a choice is not necessitated by any prior event; it is an irreducible primary. Strictly speaking, each individual is the cause of his or her own choice to think; the possession of such a choice is part of a human (rational) being's nature. Experience, environment, genetics, and life circumstances may make thinking easier or harder, but they cannot determine the choice to think or not to think.

Before we turn to volition and the goal-setting process, let us return to the two popular theories of free will that were discussed earlier: the doctrines of freedom of action and of freedom of choice between desires. There is an element of truth in these views, the error being that freedom of action and freedom of choice between desires are *indirect* rather than direct.

Freedom of action is the indirect result of the freedom to think or not to think. Through volitional focus one can choose what values one wants to achieve, discover the means by which one can achieve them, and apply those values and that knowledge to specific situations. To change one's course of action requires that one change values, knowledge, or the application of these to one's life circumstances.

Volition, of course, does not mean omniscience or omnipotence. One's thinking is limited in terms of what it can achieve by one's intelligence and the information available. One's actions are limited by political circumstances, wealth, strength, intellect, and the ability to persuade others to cooperate on a course of action.

Freedom to choose between desires is also indirect. First, emotions are the result of one's conscious and subconscious ideas (Rand, 1964; see also Packer, 1985–1986). Thus, to change a desire or emotion, one has to change the premises behind it. Second, through rational thought, one has the power to ignore the desires of the moment and act in pursuit of long-range values, even though such action may not feel good at the time. We have more to say about both these issues in the next section.

Before proceeding, we want to briefly discuss the role of the subconscious in action. By the "subconscious," we refer to that part of consciousness which is not at a given moment in focal awareness. At any given moment, very little (at most, only about seven disconnected objects) can be held in conscious, focal awareness. Everything else—all of one's prior knowledge and experiences—resides in the subconscious. However, there is a constant interplay between the conscious and the subconscious, with one's perceptions and conscious purposes automatically pulling up or drawing out relevant material.

The operation of the subconscious is not directly volitional; it operates automatically, including in emotion. Emotions are the form in which one experiences one's automatized value judgments (Rand, 1964). The subconscious consists not only of stored knowledge and values, but also of acquired mental habits. Thus, people can take actions based on automatic mechanisms (knowledge, motives, values, emotions, habits) without conscious thought. One cannot achieve long-range goals by going solely on "automatic pilot," but one may make specific choices and respond to particular situations without consciously analyzing them. What is important to recognize is that one has the capacity to observe these automatic responses or habits in action and to modify them either directly or indirectly. For example, one may reprogram an irrational emotion by changing the thinking behind it and reautomatizing one's reaction. One may act against a desire by questioning whether the desire should be acted upon, and convincing oneself that a different action would be more in one's self-interest. One may also act to uncover a repressed desire by discovering through introspection what one really wants, and convincing oneself that the desired action is both possible and morally desirable. Only in the case of severe mental illness is one constrained in managing one's subconscious.

VOLITION, VALUES, AND GOALS

Our next task is to show how we get from volition to action. Broadly speaking, two things are required: the acquisition of knowledge, and the acquisition of values. For a purposeful human being, the first question to ask is "What exists (and how do I know it)?" The second is "What do I want to achieve?" We focus on the second here. It involves the process of pursuing values, or "valuing."

We begin our discussion of valuing from a developmental perspective. Children first come to know about valuing through the sensory experiences of pleasure, which is the result of need fulfillment, and pain, which is the result of need frustration or deprivation. These are, if you like, experiences that happen to them. Pleasure to a child is automatically valued, and pain is automatically disvalued. These sensations are built into the nervous system, and the child has no choice about feeling them or about what conditions cause them. Over time children learn that other people, such as their parents, can take actions (such as feeding them) that produce pleasure, or actions (such as spanking them) that produce pain. About the same time or soon after, they learn that they can influence these other people—at first by crying, later by talking (e.g., demanding, politely asking, or rationally persuading). They eventually learn that they can take actions themselves to get what they want and avoid what they do not want.

As their conceptual faculties develop, children acquire the capacity to integrate percepts into concepts and to integrate concepts into propositions. In the evaluative realm, they acquire the capacity to go beyond sensory pleasures and to pursue objects and activities whose value significance is not builtin biologically; that is, they acquire values. Ultimately they learn that they have the power to choose their values, to plan them, and to execute the actions needed to achieve them (e.g., to save money in order to buy a new bicycle). They can do this passively, by accepting values that everyone around them has chosen or what other people tell them to choose, or actively, by deciding what they want for themselves.

The discovery that they can choose values confronts children with the issue of moral values. They learn that there are things that they should not do, such as steal money or hit their siblings, and things that they should do, such as keep their rooms neat and do their homework. They are eventually confronted by the issue of whether they should pursue their own values (e.g., spend their hard-earned money on the new bicycle) or sacrifice their values for others (e.g., give the money to a poor person they have never met).

As children grow, they are increasingly able to learn to think in terms of moral principles (e.g., honesty is right and dishonesty is wrong) and increasingly able to think and act on a long-range basis. This gives them the capacity to plan their lives—that is, to set long-range purposes and act to achieve them.

They also learn that there exists a wide range of options within the category of moral choices. For example, they can aspire to be doctors, lawyers, professors, cabinetmakers, computer operators, or librarians. In part, their choices are constrained by their intelligence and other facts (e.g., family income), but this still leaves open many possibilities that can be properly chosen on their basis of their personal desires—that is, their personal values.

The final step is to go from values to action. This requires setting of goals. *Goals are the link between values and action, in that they are applications of values (which are general) to specific situations.* The major theory in the United States concerned with goals has been goal-setting theory (Locke & Latham, 1990), which we briefly summarize here.

1. *Volition.* Goal-setting theory asserts that human action is naturally but not automatically goal-directed; goals have to be set and pursued by choice, as noted above.

2. *Goal attributes.* Goals have two main attributes: "content" and "intensity." Goal content pertains to the nature of the object or aim one is pursuing. Goals may differ in degree of specificity (e.g., "Do the best you can to sell" vs. "Increase sales by 5% in the next 6 months") and difficulty ("Increase sales by 3%" vs. "Increase sales by 15%"). Studies show consistently that goals that are both specific and difficult lead to higher performance than do vague goals or goals that are specific but easy (Locke & Latham, 1990). This has been found in over 400 (mostly experimental) studies, using more than 88 different tasks and data from over 40,000 subjects in eight countries. These studies have taken place in both laboratory and field settings; have covered time spans from 1 minute to 25 years; and have used many different types of dependent measures, including productivity, quality, behavior on the job, managerial performance, sports achievement, health-promoting behavior, and research productivity. Meta-analyses reveal average effect sizes between .42 and .82.

3. *Moderators.* Goal setting works most effectively when there is feedback showing performance or progress in relation to the goal sought and commitment to the goal in question. Commitment is highest when people believe that goal achievement is important (because of perceived links to important values, fostered by inspirational leadership, convincing rationales, attractive role models, competition, rewards, etc.) and that the goal or substantial progress toward it is attainable (because of high ability, good training, past success, etc.).

4. *Role of self-efficacy.* "Self-efficacy" refers to task-specific self-confidence (Bandura, 1986) and ties into goal-setting theory in numerous ways. People with high, as opposed to low, self-efficacy perform better independently of goals; choose higher goals; are more committed to high goals; choose better task strategies; and respond more energetically and positively to negative feedback.

5. *Mediators.* There are four mediators or mechanisms by which goals affect performance. First, they direct attention and effort toward goal rele-

vant activities (assuming task-relevant knowledge); second, they arouse effort expenditure to the level required by the task; third, they encourage persistence until the goal is accomplished; and, finally they promote the search for relevant action plans or task strategies. The final mediator is especially important when tasks are new and complex, because attention and effort alone will typically not be sufficient to attain high goals on such tasks. (Specific, high goals do not always lead to the discovery of the best strategies on complex tasks, and sometimes lead to the use of inferior strategies. This issue is the subject of ongoing research.)

6. *Group goals.* Group goals have been less intensively studied than individual goals, but thus far the results appear to be similar to those for individual goal setting (Weldon & Weingart, 1993).

7. *Goals and affect.* Goals are not only outcomes to shoot for, but standards by which to evaluate one's performance (Bandura, 1986). Goals serve as value standards in that when goals are exceeded satisfaction is experienced, and when goals are not achieved dissatisfaction is felt. In fact, the answer to the question "What is the lowest level of performance you would be satisfied with?" is a good measure of a person's performance goal on a task (Mento, Locke, & Klein, 1992), and asking this question yields the same results as asking "What is your goal?" The degree of affect experienced after success and failure depends on many factors, including the importance of the value at stake; the perceived causes of the outcome (self vs. other); the future implications of success and failure; and the degree of success or failure attained.

APPLICATIONS TO THE ROLE OF STUDENT

Let us now apply the concepts of volition and goal setting to the realm of students pursuing grades in college courses. Consider an 18-year-old male who has just entered college. Let us say that he has some inkling that he would like to be a lawyer but is not sure. He is faced with several important choices.

Goal Specificity

One of the student's first choices is the degree of specificity of the goals he will pursue. He can have a firm minimum below which he will not allow himself to go, or he can hold his goals in a vague form, such as "I'll do my best." He can also set goals in the form of wishes and hopes rather than true aspirations. Finally, he has the option of setting no goal other than "to graduate."

Goal Level

Another choice faced by the student involves what level of grade goals to set for his courses. Such a choice requires applying his values to this specific context. What values could come into play here? One is his long-range goal; if he decides to become a lawyer, he will need to get admitted to law school, which will require good grades. A second value is his desire to graduate. Certain majors have minimum requirements for graduation. A third value is his self-image or self-concept. What kind of student does he desire to be? One who performs well across the board? One who performs well but only if the course is interesting? One who just wants to get by with the minimum amount of work possible?

A student without firm, independent values, who wants to be "one of the boys" and "get along," may set as a goal merely to get the sort of grades his fraternity brothers get. One who sees himself as "an obedient child" will most likely set goals to please his parents.

Study Planning and Methods

Once he has chosen his goals, the student then has the option of planning how to achieve them (Locke, 1975). He may not plan at all, may have general plans, or may have detailed plans. Detailed plans (which, for a student with a history of high performance, often consist of well-developed habits) may involve class attendance, the timing of homework, procedures for highlighting the text, note-taking methods, exam study techniques, study location, methods for getting useful information from the professor, and allocation of study time.

One aspect of study planning concerns what to do during class periods. The choices (assuming that the student attends class at all) can range from daydreaming the whole time, to listening for snatches of information at random, to trying to grasp each main point, to trying to connect the points together into an organized and coherent whole. Locke (1977) found a significant relationship between the completeness of the notes students took and course grades. This applied only to material that was *not* written on the blackboard. Almost all students copied the material on the blackboard into their notes, but such information constituted only a small portion of the significant lecture material.

A second aspect of planning involves how to study for exams. We will not make belittling remarks about cramming; almost every student does it, and, besides, it does work to some extent! More important, however, is what is done during the time spent studying. The two keys, we believe, are organizing the material and programming it into memory. The student can choose to organize the material logically, with major categories and subcategories and their interrelationships specified, or can do it haphazardly by composing a long list of disconnected points. (We should add that the typical textbook does not help here, because it too is often just a list of disconnected points). As for programming material into memory, most students try to short-cut memorization by simply rereading the material; however, this is typically an ineffective procedure (Locke, 1975). To be effective, memorization must be done purposefully—that is, by studying and then testing oneself repeatedly until one can recite the material without looking.

Commitment

The next type of choice the student has to make is how to maintain commitment to his grade goal. It is easy to set a goal and not follow through on it (i.e., to have "good intentions"). A key to maintaining commitment is to hold in awareness the reasons for setting and pursuing the goal in the first place. These can first be divided into short-term benefits and long-term benefits. The short-term benefits for our student may involve: winning and keeping a scholarship, being accepted into his chosen major, being able to graduate, and so on. Long-term benefits may include getting a job or admission to law school. Another aspect of commitment is self-concept, the person's desired self. Some students see themselves as "A," "B," or "C" students for whatever reasons, and they try to act accordance with that image. Alternatively, they may see the issue in terms of being "responsible" versus "irresponsible" students. Still others may view themselves as athletes more than as students. In order to sustain his self-concept, our student must keep it in focus when he decides upon a course of action.

Conflict

Once the student has committed himself to a certain grade goal and begins to work toward it, it is inevitable that a certain degree of conflict will arise. This conflict will involve pursuing his chosen goal versus being diverted by other possible goals, activities, and temptations. Such conflicts are inevitable for several reasons. First, studying, at least in most courses, is hard work; expending mental effort may be experienced as unpleasant. Second, the student may find studying for some courses boring and tedious because of his lack of interest in the content. Third, the alternative activities may entail genuine values (e.g., going out on a date with his girlfriend, seeing a new movie, going to a party with friends, watching a favorite TV show). Usually these are short-term values, which, to some extent, have to be given up or postponed in order to attain long-term values.

To overcome these conflicts and temptations, the student has to keep in focal awareness the nature and significance of his chosen goal in the face of these other alternatives. There are a number of ways he can do this, including reminding himself continually of what his goal is and the reasons for it; reminding himself of the self-image to which he aspires; and reminding himself of his promises to himself. On the other side of the coin, it may be easy for him to let the goal slip away by *not* focusing on his goal and not keeping it in focal awareness at the time of action.

A philosophical point needs to be made here. From the time of the ancient Greeks, philosophers have puzzled over the issue of how a person can act against personal knowledge (or, more specifically, knowledge of the good). The answer is that, literally speaking, one cannot. If one *fully* knows what the good is, has no unresolved subconscious conflicts or contradictions concerning it, and keeps this knowledge in mind at the time of action, one cannot act against this knowledge. One can only act against it by not focusing at the time of action (Binswanger, 1991), thus allowing other, contradictory, often subconscious ideas to come into play.

Failure and Frustration

Finally, even when the student sets clear goals, plans how to achieve them, and commits to them in action, there will be times—due to error, lack of knowledge, or factors outside his control—when the results do not come out as well as he had wished. This can involve poorer than desired course performance (failure) and/or frustration over a poor or unfair teacher. Since a single failure or frustration rarely destroys one's long-term or even short-term chances for success, how one deals with temporary setbacks can have a vital influence subsequent on goal-related performance. This relates to the issue of coping, since the failure to achieve a value may be perceived as threatening and therefore may be experienced as stressful (Locke & Taylor, 1990).

A number of studies have shown that indulging emotions in response to stress is not an effective method of coping. For example, if our student gets a low grade on a midterm exam and then wallows in self-pity and self-doubt, he will be unlikely to perform any better on the next exam; indeed, he will probably perform more poorly. Similarly, if the student chooses not to think about a failure at all, he will be unlikely to improve. If the student gets angry (especially at himself), he may perform adequately later, but only if the anger is translated into productive action.

What would productive action consist of in this situation? First, the student would have to identify the causes of the poor performance. These causes might involve failure to study enough, failure to study the right material, failure to anticipate the type of exam to be given, or failure to use proper study methods (e.g., failure to program the material into memory). Going to see the course instructor is often helpful in diagnosing poor performance. Second, the student would have to formulate a plan of action based on the diagnostic information obtained. Finally, the student would have to carry out this plan as intended.

If these procedures failed to work even when applied diligently, the student would need to consider whether he had sufficient ability to do as well as he aspired to in the course (and perhaps curriculum) in question. He could then take further action, such as lowering his aspirations or changing fields of study.

SOME EMPIRICAL DATA

The exploratory research we report in this section had three purposes: (1) to determine whether students could report their own cognitive processes and related actions accurately enough to show some relation to performance; (2) to determine whether the types of goal-relevant choices and actions we had hypothesized as being pertinent to goal achievement were related to performance; and (3) to determine whether these choices and action plans mediated the relationship of goals to performance. The finding of a full mediation effect would indicate that goals lead to goal-relevant performance only if and to the degree that they lead to the choice and implementation of suitable mental and physical actions.

Subjects

The subjects for the first part of the study were 98 undergraduate students in four summer school classes: Introduction to Management (two sections), Organizational Behavior, and Human Resource Management (HRM). The students in each class were given two questionnaires to complete. The first was concerned with overall grade point average (GPA) in college. The questionnaire asked about the typical choices they made when they studied and their current GPAs. This questionnaire was given to the students during the first 2 weeks of classes. The design for this part of the study was concurrent, as both the GPA and questionnaire data were gathered at the same time.

The second questionnaire was given to the same students (except for those in the HRM class, which did not have any exams) after they had gotten their first hourly exams back but before the next exam. It was handed out 1 week before the second exam and was returned on the day of that exam. On this second questionnaire, the students reported choices they had made with respect to their second exam. Thus, the design of this part of the study was predictive, in that the questionnaire data were gathered before the second exam was taken. The total number of subjects for this second part of the study (due to the loss of the HRM students, who did not have exams) was 64.

Questionnaires

The questionnaires were parallel in construction except that the first one focused on college work in general and the second focused only on the second exam, as noted above. GPAs were self-reported. We also asked for high school GPAs as a partial control for ability. The scores on the second exam were taken from professors' class records. Since the three classes had different content and exam questions, we converted the second-exam scores to z scores within each course and used the z scores as the dependent variable.

The content of the questionnaire covered the six choice categories discussed previously. All items, except those concerning grades and one yes–no item, were answered on an 11-point scale. Below we give sample items from each of the six categories, abbreviating the wording of the items in the interests of space.

1. *Goal specificity*
   a. Did you have a specific, minimum goal [yes–no]?
2. *Goal level and goal choice*
   a. What was your minimum goal [for GPA, to two decimal places; for second exam, A to D]?
   b. Was your goal choice determined by the requirements of your major?
   c. Your self-image?
   d. The requirements of graduate school?
   e. Your parents' expectations?
   f. Your friends' or peers' performance?
3. *Study methods/plans*
   a. Do you have/use specific study plans?
   b. Do you have/use specific study methods?
   c. Do your methods include attending every class?
   d. Do your methods include programming material into memory?
   e. Do your methods include doing homework when it is assigned?
   f. Do your methods include paying full attention to what is said in class?
   g. Do your methods include tying together the individual points made in lectures?
   h. Do your methods include relating points made in class to the reading and to other classes?
   i. Do you listen to the points made in class basically at random?
4. *Attaining commitment*
   a. I commit myself to my goal by thinking of the short-term benefits of goal attainment.
   b. I commit myself to my goal by thinking of the long-term benefits.
   c. I commit myself to my goal by relating it to my self-concept.
5. *Dealing with conflict*
   a. When my goal conflicts with having fun, I keep the goal in the forefront of awareness.
   b. When my goal conflicts with having fun, I remind myself of the kind of person I am.
   c. When my goal conflicts with having fun, I focus on the pleasure of having fun but not the benefits of study.
   d. When my goal conflicts with having fun, I let the goal slip from my mind until it is forgotten.

6. *Dealing with failure and frustration*
   a. If the course is boring or confusing, I write it off and do not try.
   b. If the course is boring or confusing, I stop going to class.
   c. If the course is boring or confusing, I spend less time on the homework.
   d. If the course is boring or confusing, I study very little for the exams.
   e. If the course is boring or confusing, I remind myself of the importance of a good grade and keep working hard.
   f. If I do poorly on an exam, I wallow in self-pity.
   g. If I do poorly on an exam, I feel anger.
   h. If I do poorly on an exam, I seek information about how to do better.
   i. If I do poorly on an exam, I think up a strategy I can use to attain my goal.
   j. If I do poorly on an exam, I put in extra work.
   k. If I do poorly on an exam, I feel self-doubt.
   l. If I do poorly on an exam, I try not to think about it.

A note on items 6f, 6g, and 6k above is in order. We have stated earlier that emotions, as such, are automatic and not volitional. However, our focus in this research was on passively accepting one's emotions versus taking active steps to change the conditions that brought them about. The distinction between emotion-focused and action-focused coping is well established in the stress literature (Locke & Taylor, 1990).

Results

Significant correlations between specific items in the first questionnaire and GPA are shown in the first column of Table 16.1. Significant correlations between items in the second questionnaire and grades on the second exam are shown in the second column of Table 16.1. A considerable number of significant correlations were found in both parts of the study, although there were only eight instances where the same items were significant in both parts. (Two items yielding counterintuitive results were omitted.)

The items significantly correlated with the dependent measures in both parts of the study were as follows: level of minimum grade goals; not basing goals on the requirements on one's major; paying full attention in class; relating points made in class to the reading and other classes; committing oneself to one's goal through tying performance to one's self-concept; not doing less homework in response to frustration; and not focusing on self-doubt and anger after failure.

Other items significantly correlated with GPA included using specific methods of study; doing all work when assigned; programming memory; tying lecture points together; keeping the goal in focus in the face of conflict and

TABLE 16.1. Items Significantly Correlated with GPA or Exam Grade

Item	GPA	Exam 2 grade
Goal level		
Minimum goal	.68	.31
Goal choice		
Requirement of my major	−.20	−.29
Self-image, self-concept		.27
Need for graduate school admission		−.22
Parental expectations		−.42
What friends are getting		−.20
Study methods/plans		
Use specific study methods	.21	
Do all work when assigned	.17	
Program material into memory	.20	
Pay full attention	.18	.22
Tie lecture points together in mind	.20	
Tie lecture points to reading and to other classes	.26	.21
Listen in class at random		−.21
Attaining commitment		
Tie goal to my self-concept	.20	.21
Dealing with conflict		
Keep goal in forefront of mind	.22	
Let goal slip from awareness	−.23	
Focus on pleasure of other activity, not study	−.31	
Remind self of kind of person I am		.21
Dealing with failures and frustration		
If boring/confusing, stop trying	−.37	
If boring/confusing, stop attending class	−.31	
If boring/confusing, spend less time on homework	−.19	−.21
If boring/confusing, study little for exams	−.26	
If boring/confusing, remind self that need a good grade and work hard	.31	
In the face of failure, I feel self-doubt	−.19	−.32
In the face of failure, I wallow in self-pity		−.22
In the face of failure, I feel anger	−.19	−.32
In the face of failure, I seek more information	.24	
In the face of failure, I think of new study strategies	.28	
In the face of failure, I do extra work	.20	
In the face of failure, I try not to think about it		−.21

Note. All items were significant at $p < .05$ (one-tailed test).

not letting it slip from awareness; not reducing effort, attendance, and study in the face of frustration; reminding oneself of the importance of the grade; seeking more information about how to do better; thinking of new study strategies; and doing extra work.

For the second exam, additional items that predicted performance included basing one's grade goal on one's self-image; not basing it on what others expect; not listening at random in class; reminding oneself, when in conflict, of the type of person one is; not indulging in self-pity after failure; and not refusing to think about a failure.

In order to see whether the various strategy choices students made mediated the degree to which their goals were translated into action, we performed two sets of hierarchical regressions. The first pertained to overall GPA. High school rank was entered first to control for ability. Minimum grade goals were entered second. The sums of the choice items that were significantly related to GPA (with negatively correlated items being reverse-scored) were entered third. These sums were the sums of all items shown in Table 16.1 (relevant to each criterion, respectively) *except* for the items pertaining to goal choice (which would logically precede goal choice and therefore would not properly be categorized as plans for attaining the goal). This regression was then repeated, entering the sums of the choice items second and minimum GPA goals third. The results are shown in Table 16.2 (Regressions A and B). A parallel set of regressions was run, using grades on the second exam as the dependent measure. These results are also shown in Table 16.2 (Regressions C and D).

The results for GPA reveal that when goals were entered before the choice processes (Regression A), the latter did not add significant incremental variance. When choice processes were entered before goals (Regression B), the strength of the goal effect was reduced by about one-third, indicating partial mediation. The strong goal effect, of course, may have been partly artifactual, since the students could have rationalized their goals to be compatible with the GPAs they had already attained.

In the case of performance on the second exam, when the goals were entered before the choice processes (Regression C), the choice increment was still significant. But when the choice processes were entered before goals, the goal effect was no longer significant (Regression D), indicating complete mediation.

DISCUSSION

Our results show, first, that students' self-reports can provide useful information regarding the choices they make with respect to the goals they set. Second, in line with goal-setting theory, the results show that goal level is positively related to level of performance (Locke & Latham, 1990). Third,

TABLE 16.2. Hierarchical Regressions for the Dependent Variables of Current College GPA and Exam 2 Performance

Current college GPA[a]	R^2	δR^2	p	Exam 2 performance[b]	R^2	δR^2	p
Regression A				*Regression C*			
High school GPA	.0498	.0498	n.s.	High school GPA	.0794	.0794	n.s.
Minimum GPA goal	.5136	.4637	<.001	Minimum exam goal	.1710	.0917	<.05
Choice processes	.5378	.0243	n.s.	Choice processes	.3120	.1410	<.01
Regression B				*Regression D*			
High school GPA	.0498	.0498	n.s.	High school GPA	.0794	.0794	n.s.
Choice processes	.2241	.1743	<.001	Choice processes	.3033	.2240	<.001
Minimum GPA goal	.5378	.3137	<.001	Minimum exam goal	.3120	.0087	n.s.

Note. Pairwise deletion of missing variables was used.
[a]Regressions A and B (n = 67).
[b]Regressions C and D (n = 47).

our findings suggest that the factors hypothesized to influence goal choice and the actions taken after the goal has been set play a crucial role in goal achievement. In the case of grade goals, these choices include what study methods are employed; what the student does mentally in class; what methods the student uses to sustain goal commitment; how the student deals with conflicting desires; and how the student copes with obstacles, frustrations, and failures.

It was especially striking in the second part of the study (performance on the second exam) that three of the significant items pertained to the students' self-concept (see Table 16.1). Thus high-performing students seem to be guided by an independent, internal frame of reference focused around the type of person they want to be, rather than by an external frame of reference focused around what others expect (parents, peers, etc.). One might have expected an item like "requirements of my major" to be positively rather than negatively associated with performance, but this is probably because such requirements are usually quite low and indicate the *minimum* standard needed to graduate. High-performing students want instead to exceed this minimum; they are driven by an internalized ambition.

Two other attributes of high-performing students are keeping the goal or end in focal awareness in the face of temptations and not wallowing in negative emotions in the face of setbacks. We could describe this pattern as one of giving primacy to reason (thought) over emotion.

Our results help to give real meaning to the term "willpower." Willpower is usually viewed as a separate faculty (the "will") that directly overwhelms or outmuscles reason and/or conflicting desires in order to attain some end. In contrast, we view reason as the source of will (Rand, 1964). We would view willpower as *the choice to use one's rational faculty to select goals, to identify the means to achieve them, and to keep one's goals and the reasons and plans for pursuing them in focal awareness at the time of action in the face of contrary thoughts and emotions.* Willpower is volition (focus) put to use—that is, put into action.

It is worth comparing the present theory and findings to those of Gollwitzer (1993) and his colleagues. Gollwitzer identifies four phases in the goal-setting process: (1) setting the goal or formulating the intention; (2) planning; (3) taking relevant action to implement the plan; and (4) evaluation of performance. Gollwitzer (1993) reports a series of experiments relevant mainly to the second and third phases. Those studies found that intentions were far more likely to be carried out if an individual formulated implementation intentions that specified when and where the planned action would be implemented than if an intention was formulated in the absence of any implementation intention. In this respect, Gollwitzer's (1993) results fit in very nicely with ours, although our planning items focused more on "how" and "what" than on "when" and "where."

On the other hand, Gollwitzer (1993) stresses the *automatic* effect of intentions, especially on cognitive functions such as memory, distraction of attention, perception, speed of processing, and associations made to subthreshold stimuli. We have no argument with such results. We believe that goals and intentions can entail both volitional and not directly volitional (subconscious, automatic) processes. The types of action Gollwitzer (1993) has described as automatic effects of intentions tend to be short-term, simple cognitive functions, whereas the actions we focused on were longer-term actions requiring more conceptual thinking processes. We believe that there is a constant interplay between the conscious and the subconscious, and that any complete explanation of human action will have to understand and measure both.

Gollwitzer's work is part of the German "action theory" approach to human motivation (Frese & Zapf, 1994). This approach has much in common with goal-setting theory, and in fact shares many of its concepts (goal attributes such as specificity and difficulty; feedback; planning; and the role of the subconscious). Action theory also recognizes volition, although it includes no validated theory of volition. We do, however, take issue with the term "action theory." Frese and Zapf (1994) claim that action is the starting point of the German approach. Although it is true that thinking without (eventual) action is useless, action cannot be the starting point for a theory of motivation. Thinking precedes action and is the guide to action and the cause of action. Action theory recognizes this in practice, but we do find the label incongruous.

In conclusion, we must stress that the current study was not intended as a definitive investigation of the topic of volitional choice, but rather as an exploratory venture into the goal seeking process. In any evaluation of our quantitative results, several limitations should be kept in mind. First, the initial part of the study, involving GPA goals, followed a concurrent design. Therefore, it does not have the strength of statistical inference contained in the predictive design of the part of the study involving exam goals. As noted earlier, the latter design may have exaggerated the goal effect at the expense of the strategy choice effect. Second, the items found to be significant were not cross-validated on an independent sample; thus, the correlations may be inflated by chance results. A third limitation is the bias that may have resulted from combining classes in the second part of the study, despite the use of z scores. This would have been a conservative bias, however, as it would have served to work against finding significant results. Fourth, the sample size, especially in the second part of the study, may have reduced the statistical power of the analyses. Fifth, it is likely that the self-reports were not fully accurate. Finally, our questionnaire did not measure subconscious motives. The last two limitations also would tend to reduce the strength of the results. Clearly, further, more definitive studies are needed.

REFERENCES

Bandura, A. (1986). *Social foundations of thought and action.* Englewood Cliffs, NJ: Prentice-Hall.

Binswanger, H. (1991). Volition as cognitive self-regulation. *Organizational Behavior and Human Decision Processes, 50,* 154–178.

Frese, M., & Zapf, D. (1994). Action as the core of work psychology: A German approach. In M. Dunnette & L. Hough (Eds.), *Handbook of industrial and organizational psychology.* Palo Alto, CA: Consulting Psychologists Press.

Gollwitzer, P. (1993). Goal achievement: The role of intentions. In W. Stroebe & M. Hewstone (Eds.), *European review of social psychology* (Vol. 4). Chichester, England: Wiley.

Locke, E. A. (1975). *A guide to effective study.* New York: Springer.

Locke, E. A. (1977). An empirical study of lecture note taking among college students. *Journal of Educational Research, 71*(2), 93–99.

Locke, E. A., & Latham, G. P. (1990). *A theory of goal setting and task performance.* Englewood Cliffs, NJ: Prentice-Hall.

Locke, E. A., & Taylor, S. (1990). Stress, coping and the meaning of work. In A. Brief & W. Nord (Eds.), *Meanings of occupational work.* Lexington, MA: Lexington Books.

Mento, T., Locke, E., & Klein, H. (1992). Relationship of goal level to valence and instrumentality. *Journal of Applied Psychology, 77,* 395–405.

Packer, E. (1985–1986). The art of introspection. *The Objectivist Forum, 6*(6), 1–10; 7(1), 1–8.

Peikoff, L. (1991). *Objectivism: The philosophy of Ayn Rand.* New York: Dutton.

Rand, A. (1964). The objectivist ethics. In *The virtue of selfishness.* New York: Signet.

Rand, A. (1990). *Introduction to objectivist epistemology.* New York: New American Library.

Terrace, H. S. (1979). *Nim.* New York: Washington Square Press.

Weldon, E., & Weingart, L. (1993). Group goals and performance. *British Journal of Social Psychology, 32,* 307–334.

CHAPTER 17

The Directive Influence of Attitudes on Behavior

Icek Ajzen

Work on the relation between attitudes and behavior has seen much progress in the past 25 years. Pessimistic conclusions regarding the predictive validity of attitudes, which in the late 1960s culminated in calls to abandon the attitude construct (e.g., Wicker, 1969), have given way to the recognition that attitudes, properly assessed, can and do predict behavior. One of the foremost contributions to this effort was the formulation of the principle of correspondence or compatibility (Ajzen & Fishbein, 1977; Ajzen, 1988; Fishbein & Ajzen, 1975). Numerous investigations have supported this principle by showing that attitudes correlate strongly with behavior when they are assessed at the same level of generality or specificity as the behavioral criterion in terms of action, target, context, and time elements (for reviews, see Ajzen, 1988; Kraus, 1995; van den Putte, 1991). The principle of compatibility is now widely accepted by attitude theorists (see Eagly & Chaiken, 1993), if not always heeded in empirical research.

An example from my own research program may be instructive. The research in question dealt with the problem of assigning monetary values to goods and services that are not traded in the marketplace. A typical study in this domain describes a good or service and asks respondents to rate how much money they would be willing to pay for it—a procedure known as "contingent valuation" (see Mitchell & Carson, 1989, for a review). In one of our investigations (Ajzen & Driver, 1992a), we assessed attitudes and intentions with respect to engaging in each of five leisure activities: mountain climbing, jogging/running, boating, spending time at the beach, and biking. The college students in the study were also asked to indicate how often they had participated in each of the activities in the preceding 12 months, and to rate how much money (in the form of a user fee) they would be willing to pay for engaging in each activity on a single occasion.

The top part of Table 17.1, which presents mean within-subjects correlations (across activities), shows that the amount of money respondents were willing to pay for the different leisure activities was largely unrelated to their

TABLE 17.1. Prediction of Willingness to Pay a User Fee for Leisure Activities: Mean Within-Subjects Correlations

Predictor	r
Incompatible predictors	
Attitude toward engaging in the leisure activities	.21
Intention to engage in the leisure activities	.04
Past participation in the leisure activities	−.21
Compatible predictors	
Attitude toward paying a user fee	.74
Intention to pay a user fee	.76

Note. The data are taken from Ajzen and Driver (1992a).

attitudes toward the activities, their intentions, or their interest in the activities as expressed in past participation. Our initial surprise at these findings soon gave way to the realization that engaging in an activity such as mountain climbing is not the same as paying a user fee for doing so. The target is the same, but the action elements differ.

The disappointing findings in the top part of Table 17.1 contrast sharply with the results for a set of measures that are more closely compatible with the willingness to pay criterion. In another section of the survey, participants were asked to indicate their attitudes and intentions with respect to paying a user fee to engage in each of the five leisure activities. The second part of Table 17.1 shows that these measures were highly predictive of the amount of money the respondents were willing to pay.

MODELS OF THE ATTITUDE–BEHAVIOR RELATION

After resolving the controversy surrounding the predictive validity of attitudes, investigators turned to theoretically more interesting questions concerning the cognitive processes and other mediators responsible for attitude–behavior correspondence. In his influential definition of the attitude construct, Allport (1935) emphasized the "directive or dynamic influence" that attitudes exert on responses to the attitude object. Indeed, most theorists assume that attitudes not only summarize past experience with the attitude object (Campbell, 1963), but play a causal role in determining future behavior. This role is usually viewed not so much as one of motivating action—a role typically reserved for such constructs as needs or goals—but rather as a role of directing or guiding human behavior in one direction or another. Attitudes may thus be considered to enter into the picture at crucial decision junctions (see Abelson, 1981). A great deal of work in the last two decades has been devoted to the exploration and description of the ways in which attitudes may provide this guide to behavior.

Controlled-Process Models

The Theories of Reasoned Action and Planned Behavior

One major line of work has been based on the assumption that the processes involved are of a rather careful, deliberate, and controlled character (e.g., Bagozzi & Warshaw, 1990; Bentler & Speckart, 1979; Kuhl, 1985; Locke & Latham, 1990; Triandis, 1980; see Eagly & Chaiken, 1993, for a review). Much of this work has been stimulated by the "theory of reasoned action" (Ajzen & Fishbein, 1980; Fishbein & Ajzen, 1975) and its successor, the "theory of planned behavior" (Ajzen, 1988, 1991). Very briefly, the theory of planned behavior stipulates that when confronted with the need to decide on a course of action, people consider the likely consequences of available alternatives; they weigh the normative expectations of important reference individuals or groups; and they consider required resources and potential impediments or obstacles. These considerations or beliefs result, respectively, in the formation of attitudes toward the behavior of interest, subjective norms with respect to the behavior, and perceived behavioral control. Expectancy–value formulations are used to describe the ways in which salient beliefs combine to produce the more general constructs. It is assumed that people form behavioral intentions based on their attitudes, subjective norms, and perceptions of behavioral control, and that these intentions, together with behavioral control, are the immediate determinants of behavior. The theory of reasoned action can be viewed as a special case of the theory of planned behavior, applicable to situations in which behavioral control is high and can thus be disregarded (Ajzen, 1985).

It can be seen that the theory of planned behavior assumes a series of processes that are largely of a controlled nature. Salient beliefs (i.e., beliefs available to conscious introspection) determine attitudes, subjective norms, perceptions of behavioral control, and intentions. To the extent that the same or similar beliefs are also salient at the time and place of the behavior, accurate prediction is expected. The principle of compatibility that assures strong attitude–behavior relations can be explained in terms of the compatibility of salient beliefs. Measuring attitudes and behavior at compatible levels of generality increases the likelihood that the same set of salient beliefs will be activated (i.e., that expressions of attitude and performance of behavior will be guided by the same set of considerations), and it is for this reason that strong correlations are observed.

Research on the Theories

A recent survey of the literature has revealed in excess of 250 empirical investigations based explicitly on the theories of reasoned action and planned behavior (Fishbein & Ajzen, 1993). Table 17.2 provides a partial listing of the behaviors to which the models have been applied. By and large, the the-

TABLE 17.2. Behaviors Investigated in Tests of the Theories of Reasoned Action and Planned Behavior

Leisure and recreation	Working after childbirth
Voting behavior	Occupational choice
Use of motorcycle safety helmets	Physician prescribing behavior
Eating at fast-food restaurants	Tax evasion
Risky sexual behavior	Breast self-examination
Limiting infants' sugar intake	Occupational turnover
Cheating, lying, shoplifting	Re-enlistment in the military
Marijuana use	Conserving water
Consumer choice/buying behavior	Abortion
Living kidney donation	Recycling
Energy conservation	Charitable behavior
Using generic prescription drugs	Television viewing behavior
Testicular self-examinations	Lamaze childbirth
Using smokeless tobacco	Choice of infant feeding method
Drinking alcohol	Living with child and partner
Cigarette smoking	Dental care
Seat belt use	Adherence to medical regimen
Contraceptive behavior	Mammography participation
Drug use	Committing driving violations
Using innovative teaching methods	Losing weight
Accepting computer technology	Nurses' charting behavior
Reporting a rape	Salt intake
Class/training session attendance	Fat consumption
Behavior toward the handicapped	Coupon usage
Exercising	Job-seeking behavior
Using infant seats in cars	Aggression

oretical models have been well supported whenever their constructs were carefully operationalized (Eagly & Chaiken, 1993). The results of a meta-analysis of research related to the theory of reasoned action (van den Putte, 1991) are summarized in Table 17.3. The analysis shown in Table 17.3 is based on 150 data sets published in 113 articles between 1969 and 1989, and it includes all studies regardless of the quality of their measures. It can be seen that intentions are generally good predictors of behavior, and that the other relations specified in the model are also quite strong.

Empirical support is also available for the extension of the model embodied in the theory of planned behavior. Perceived behavioral control was added to the theory of reasoned action in an attempt to extend its applicability to behaviors that are not completely under volitional control. Over the past few years, at least two dozen studies have tested the expanded model in a variety of applications. In virtually every case, inclusion of perceived behavioral control is found to improve prediction of intentions, and in many instances it is also found to improve prediction of behavior (e.g., Ajzen & Madden, 1986; Beale & Manstead, 1991; Beck & Ajzen, 1991; Doll & Ajzen, 1992; Godin, Valois, Lepage, & Desharnais, 1992; Madden, Ellen, & Ajzen, 1992; Netemeyer, Burton, & Johnston, 1991; Parker, Manstead, Stradling, &

TABLE 17.3. Meta-Analysis of Research on the Theory of Reasoned Action: Mean Correlations Based on 150 Data Sets Published between 1969 and 1989

Correlation	r or R
Intention–behavior (n = 58)	.62
Attitude–intention (n = 88)	.60
Subjective norm–intention (n = 57)	.42
Multiple R (n = 70)	.68
Attitude–$\Sigma b_i e_i$ (n = 40)	.53
Subjective norm–$\Sigma b_i m_i$ (n = 37)	.54

Note. $\Sigma b_i e_i$ and $\Sigma b_i m_i$ are the expectancy–value summations of salient beliefs underlying attitudes and subjective norms, respectively. The data are taken from van den Putte (1991).

Reason, 1992; Schifter & Ajzen, 1985; Schlegel, d'Avernas, Zanna, DeCourville, & Manske, 1992; Van Ryn & Vinokur, 1992).

A recent study from my own research program may serve as an illustration. The study dealt again with the five leisure activities mentioned earlier in connection with contingent valuation: mountain climbing, jogging/running, boating, spending time at the beach, and biking (Ajzen & Driver, 1992b). With respect to engaging in each activity, college students expressed their attitudes, subjective norms, perceptions of behavioral control, and intentions. One year later they were recontacted and asked to report how often they had engaged in each activity in the preceding 12 months. The results of a within-subjects path analysis are shown in Figure 17.1. The theory of planned behavior accounted for substantial proportions of variance in leisure intentions as well as leisure behavior, and perceived behavioral control made significant contributions to both predictions.

Stability of Predictors

Before I conclude the discussion of research on the theory of planned behavior, it is important to emphasize two preconditions for accurate prediction. First, all terms in the theory must be assessed in strict accordance with the principle of compatibility. That is, intentions, attitudes, subjective norms, and perceived behavioral control must all deal with the same target and action, performed in the same context as the behavior. More important for the discussion below, to obtain accurate prediction of behavior, intentions and perceptions of behavioral control must remain reasonably stable over time until the behavior is performed. Clearly, if changes occur in these factors after they have been assessed, the available measures will no longer permit accurate prediction of later behavior. In the leisure domain, intentions and perceptions of behavioral control appear to remain quite stable over a 1-year time period, as suggested by the prospective study reported earlier.

The stability of the predictor variables in the theory of planned behavior

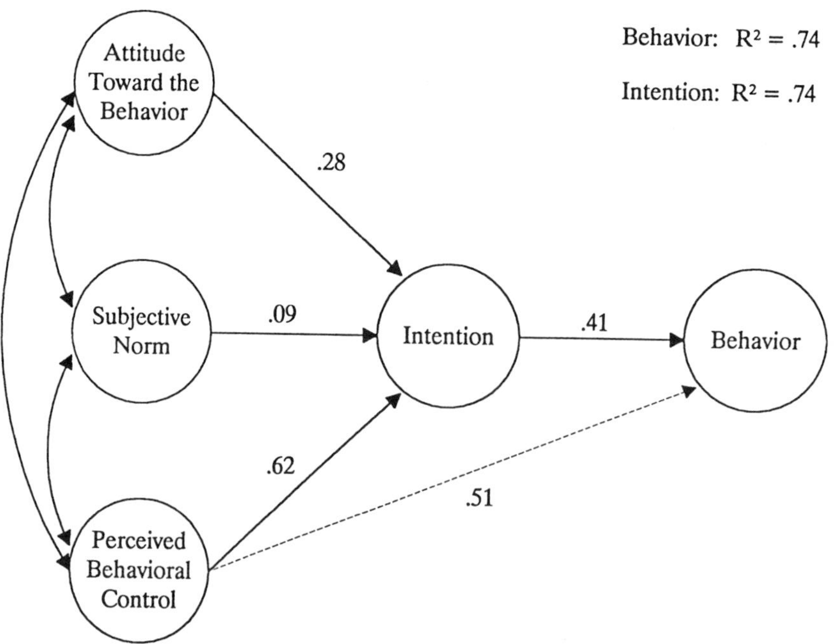

FIGURE 17.1. Path coefficients for the theory of planned behavior applied to leisure choice.

was found to be much lower in an ongoing, as yet unpublished study on sexual behavior among a representative sample of young people conducted in Germany (Schmidt, Reinecke, & Ajzen, in press). The relatively low temporal stabilities of the predictors led to a concomitant reduction in predictive validity. Attitudes, subjective norms, and perceptions of behavioral control were each assessed on the basis of a set of relevant salient beliefs, while a direct measure was obtained with respect to behavioral intentions. For the topic of condom use with new sex partners, the stability coefficients over a 1-year period ranged from .23 to .49. Clearly, the beliefs about using condoms with new sex partners that were salient at the second assessment differed considerable from the beliefs that had been salient 1 year earlier.

Figure 17.2 presents the results of a structural-equation analysis using LISREL 8. Overall, the structural model was well supported, with a goodness-of-fit index close to 1.00. Prediction of intentions to use condoms with new sexual partners was quite accurate, accounting for 82% of the variance. All variables involved in this part of the model (attitudes, subjective norms, perceptions of behavioral control, and intentions) were assessed in the same survey, before any changes could take place. In contrast, only 14% of the variance in behavior could be accounted for. Self-reported use of condoms with new sexual partners was predicted from intentions and perceptions of behavioral control measured 1 year earlier. Apparently, the changes that had taken place over the 1-year period made accurate behavioral prediction impossible. Note also that the contribution of perceived behavioral control was significant for the prediction of intentions; it was slightly negative but not significant for the prediction of behavior.

Automatic-Process Models

The controlled mode of operation described in the theory of planned behavior can be contrasted with more automatic processes, defined as processes that operate without much cognitive effort and that are usually unintentional (cf. Bargh, 1989). Work in social cognition over the past two decades has led to increased understanding of automatic processes in social judgments and decisions. Some of the insights derived from this research have been applied to the relation between attitudes and behavior. Perhaps the best-known effort in this regard is the work by Russell Fazio and his associates (Fazio, 1990; Fazio, Powell, & Herr, 1983; Fazio & Williams, 1986; Fazio & Zanna, 1978). Fazio's (1990) MODE model acknowledges a controlled or deliberative mode of operation, but much of the work related to the model has focused on the alternative mode—the automatic or spontaneous mode. Attitudes are assumed to guide behavior in a spontaneous fashion when people are either not sufficiently motivated to engage in extensive deliberations, or are incapable of doing so.

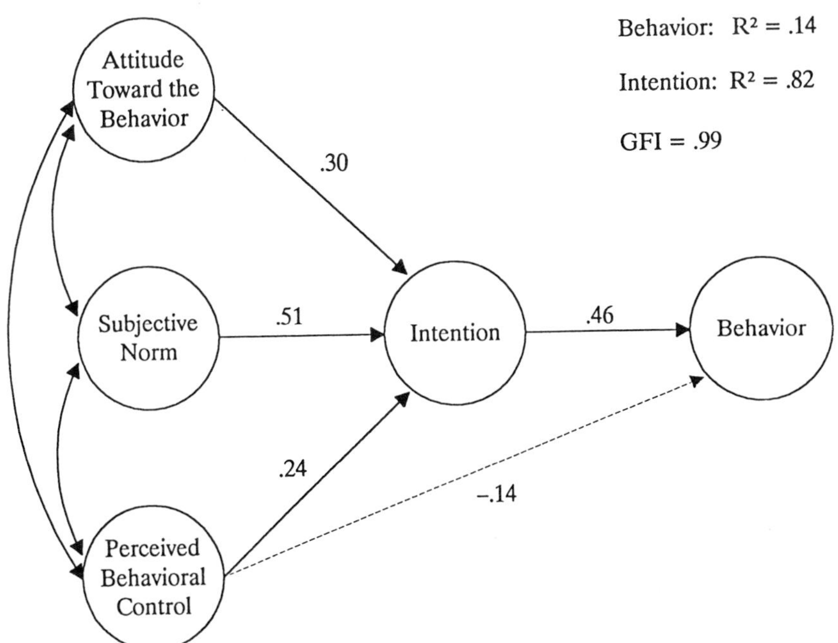

FIGURE 17.2. Path coefficients for the theory of planned behavior applied to condom use with new sexual partners. GFI, goodness-of-fit index.

Spontaneous influence of attitudes on behavior is said to involve a sequence of steps. At the point of behavior, the attitude must be automatically activated, thus becoming available to guide action. Automatic activation depends on attitude strength. Strong attitudes have a well-established object–evaluation link and are assumed to be chronically accessible in memory. Consequently, they are automatically activated in the presence of the object. Once activated, the attitude is said to influence perception or construction of the situation in a manner consistent with the positive or negative evaluation; as a result, the attitude influences behavior toward the object. If the attitude is too weak to be automatically activated, behavior is assumed to be determined by nonattitudinal aspects of the situation that happen to be salient at the moment (Fazio, 1990).

It can be seen that the spontaneous part of the MODE model involves a mixture of automatic and controlled aspects. Under conditions of low motivation or opportunity, chronically accessible attitudes become automatically activated, and they also bias perception of the situation in an automatic manner. However, for attitudes to guide behavior, they must become accessible to conscious introspection. Without it, behavior is guided by features of the situation unrelated to attitude.[1]

Efforts to test the spontaneous-action part of the MODE model fall into two categories. The first approach assesses response latency as an indicator of accessibility in memory. Studies using this operational definition of accessibility have shown that attitudes with relatively fast response times predict behavior better than attitudes with relatively slow response times (Fazio, Powell, & Williams, 1989; Fazio & Williams, 1986). The second approach examines the influence on the attitude–behavior relation of variables likely to influence attitude accessibility. Specifically, it has been shown that past direct experience with the behavior, and repeated expressions of the attitude, tend to lower response latencies and to improve attitudinal prediction of behavior (Fazio, Chen, McDonel, & Sherman, 1982; Houston & Fazio, 1989; Powell & Fazio, 1984; Regan & Fazio, 1977). Recent analysis and empirical research, however, have questioned the proposition that only highly accessible attitudes are automatically activated (Bargh, Chaiken, Govender, & Pratto, 1992). By showing that attitudes with relatively slow response times can also be automatically activated, this research challenges one of the fundamental assumptions of the MODE model. (For a discussion of this issue, see the exchange between Fazio, 1993, and Chaiken & Bargh, 1993.)

THE MODE MODEL VERSUS THE THEORY OF PLANNED BEHAVIOR

Work on the spontaneous influence of attitudes raises two issues for the theory of planned behavior. The first concerns the ways in which attitudes guide the formulation of intentions, plans, or decisions; the second has to do with the effect of attitudes on behavior. With respect to both issues, the current analysis focuses on the role of salient beliefs. To the extent that the beliefs salient at the time of attitude assessment are also salient when plans are formulated or executed, strong attitude–intention and attitude–behavior correlations are expected. Conversely, attitudes will tend to be poor predictors of intentions and actions if the context in which plans are made or executed evokes beliefs that differ substantially from the beliefs that were salient when the attitudes were assessed.

Belief Equivalence versus Mode Congruence

The requirement that salient beliefs be equivalent should not be confused with mode congruence. Depending on motivation and ability, respondents may be either in a controlled, reasoned mode of operation or in an automatic, spontaneous mode. "Mode congruence" refers to the case in which the predictor variables and the criterion are assessed when the respondents are in the same mode of operation (i.e., both are assessed in a controlled mode or both are assessed in an automatic mode). "Mode incongruence" occurs if respondents are in one mode of operation when the predictors are assessed and in the other mode when the criterion is measured.

Generally speaking, attitude–intention and attitude–behavior relations will tend to be relatively weak under conditions of mode incongruence. The reason for this expectation is that different beliefs are likely to be salient in the automatic mode and in the controlled mode. However, a congruent mode of operation does not assure equivalence of salient beliefs. This is especially true for congruence in the automatic or spontaneous mode. In this mode, people are highly susceptible to situational forces, and these of course differ from situation to situation. The particular context in which predictors and criteria are assessed can thus have a strong impact on the beliefs that become salient in the automatic mode. Equivalence of salient beliefs is more likely under conditions of congruence in the controlled or reasoned mode. The careful deliberations that take place in this mode are likely to bring to mind all relevant salient beliefs, thus influencing attitudes, intentions, and actual behavior in the same way. The particular context in which these variables are assessed should thus make relatively little difference in the controlled mode.

From Attitudes to Intentions

The MODE model deals with the effect of attitudes on intentions in the same way that it approaches the attitude–behavior relation. To guide the formulation of intentions or plans of behavior, attitudes must be activated. In the absence of strong motivation or ability to enter the deliberative mode, automatic activation must occur, and this depends on attitude strength. Like the attitude–behavior relation, the attitude–intention relation should thus be a function of attitude accessibility and should be affected by such factors as direct experience and repeated attitude expression.

In the theory of planned behavior, automatic activation of attitudes is neither contemplated nor deemed necessary. Intentions are expected to be consistent with attitudes, subjective norms, and perceptions of behavioral control to the extent that predictors and criterion are measured at compatible levels of generality, and to the extent that the predictors have remained stable prior to assessment of the intention. In most instances, attitudes and intentions are assessed in the same context, making it likely that the considerations that are salient at the time of attitude measurement are also salient at the time that intentions are expressed. Moreover, attitudes and intentions can be assessed in close temporal proximity, assuring that attitudes will not have changed prior to the expression of intentions. We would thus expect good prediction of intentions, whether attitudinal responses show short or long response latencies, whether attitudes have been expressed repeatedly or only once, and whether attitudes are based on direct or indirect experience (Ajzen & Fishbein, 1980).

Sherman et al. (1982) tested the effect of past experience on the ability of attitudes to predict smoking intentions among adolescents. The results showed a somewhat stronger attitude–intention correlation among respondents who reported having more information about cigarette smoking. Statistically significant because of the large sample sizes (n = 1,496 and n = 1,733 in two samples), the effect accounted for only a tiny proportion of the variance (.005 and .003 in the two samples). Although they had no measure of response latency or any other measure of attitude accessibility, the investigators interpreted their findings as support for the effect of attitude accessibility on the attitude–behavior relation. However, alternative interpretations for the results of this correlational study can easily be found. For example, the range of attitudes and intentions may have been lower among respondents who were less knowledgeable about smoking. This restriction of range would produce weaker attitude–intention correlations. No comparisons of means and variances were reported.

Several studies conducted in our laboratory over the past few years have found virtually no support for the predictions of the MODE model concerning the spontaneous effects of attitudes on intentions. In one of our studies (Doll & Ajzen, 1992), fashioned after that of Regan and Fazio (1977), college students were given either direct experience or secondhand information about six computer games, and then expressed their attitudes and intentions with respect to playing each game. Although the attitudinal responses of participants in the direct-experience condition had significantly lower latencies than had the responses of participants in the indirect-experience condition, there was no significant difference in the attitude–intention correlation. In a within subjects analysis, the mean attitude–intention correlation was .92 under direct experience and .93 under indirect experience.

We also examined the role of attitude accessibility more directly by dividing participants into high- versus low-response-latency subgroups, independent of their experimental conditions. There were again no significant differences in attitude–intention correlations.

A second study again directly examined the effect of attitude accessibility on the prediction of intentions (Ajzen & Stanat, 1993). Participants first expressed their attitudes toward capital punishment or toward euthanasia, and later indicated their willingness to sign a petition in favor of the policy in question. Respondents were divided into high- and low-accessibility subgroups on the basis of the latencies of their attitudinal responses. The relation between attitudes and intentions was found to be about the same in the two groups.

A final set of data on the attitude–intention relation comes from a study on the effects of repeated attitude expressions (Rosenthal & Ajzen, 1993). College students were given information about six programs at the university dedicated to different recreational activities: mountain climbing, weight lifting, animal watching, jogging, water aerobics, and figure skating. In one condition of the experiment, subjects were asked to indicate their attitudes toward each program on five evaluative scales prior to responding to a critical attitude item; in a second condition, participants were given no opportunity for prior attitude expression. From 2 to 4 weeks later, all participants were contacted by telephone and asked to indicate their willingness to join each of the programs. Within-subjects correlations revealed no significant difference between the conditions of repeated and single attitude expression; the mean attitude–intention correlation was .60 in the former condition and .66 in the latter.

Although it is difficult to prove the null hypothesis that attitude accessibility has no effect on the attitude–intention relation, the accumulation of negative evidence is consistent with predictions derived from the theory of planned behavior. Attitude–intention correlations appear to be largely unaffected by latency of attitudinal responses, by the nature of prior experience, or by repeated attitude expressions.

From Attitudes to Behavior

In a typical study, attitudes and intentions are assessed at the same time and in the same context. The same beliefs are thus likely to be salient, and there is little danger that attitudes will have changed prior to assessment of intentions. Consistent with these considerations, attitude–intention correlations are generally found to be strong. This is not always the case for the prediction of behavior. The study on condom use (Schmidt et al., in press) showed how changes over time in the theory's constructs made it difficult to secure accurate prediction of behavior. As a general rule, strong correlations with behavior are expected only when the situation in which attitudes, subjective norms, and perceived behavioral control are assessed elicits the same considerations as does the situation in which the behavior occurs. New information that becomes available in the interim or at the time that the behavior is performed will tend to raise new issues and may lead to changes in beliefs about the behavior's consequences, about the expectations of other people, or about the resources required to perform the behavior. As a result, the prediction of behavior will tend to deteriorate.

The computer game study considered earlier (Doll & Ajzen, 1992) tested the proposition that the amount of prior direct experience with a behavior influences attitude–behavior consistency because of its effect on the attitude's stability. As mentioned earlier, the experiment manipulated the nature of prior experience by allowing some participants to try each of the computer games while giving others indirect information about them. We argued that attitudes expressed after direct behavioral experience would be based on a more realistic appreciation of the behavior than would attitudes based on indirect or secondhand information. Because participants in the direct-experience condition had performed the behavior before, little information of a novel nature would be likely to become available during later behavior. In contrast, new experiences and unexpected difficulties might become apparent to participants who had initially received only secondhand information.

To test this explanation of the role of direct experience, we assessed attitudes, perceptions of behavioral control, and intentions to play each of the six computer games before and after a free-play period. The stability of these variables was assessed by computing within-subjects correlations between measures obtained before and after the free-play period. To be able to compare the mediating function of stability to that of attitude accessibility, we also measured response latencies. As expected, both the stabilities of the predictor variables and their accessibilities (as measured by response latencies) were significantly greater in the direct experience than in the indirect-experience condition.

The prediction of behavior was consistent with these effects. Amount of time spent playing with each game correlated significantly better with attitudes, perceived behavioral control, and intentions following direct experience (mean r = .39 to .68) than following indirect experience (mean r = .26 to .51). Explanations of this effect were tested by means of hierarchical regression analyses in which either stabilities or latencies were statistically controlled. Table 17.4 shows that the effects of type of experience on the attitude–behavior and on the intention–behavior correlations remained strong and significant even after response latencies were held constant. In contrast, the effects of type of experience were reduced to nonsignificance when stability was treated as the mediating variable.

REASONED VERSUS SPONTANEOUS PROCESSES

The empirical research discussed in the preceding section has shown that we can go from attitudes to intentions and from attitudes to behavior without

TABLE 17.4. Regression Coefficients and *t* Tests for the Effect of Type of Experience on the Prediction of Game Behavior from Attitudes, Perceived Behavioral Control, and Intention

	Without mediator		Latency as mediator		Stability as mediator	
Correlation	*b*	*t*	*b*	*t*	*b*	*t*
Attitude–behavior	.24	2.12[a]	.31	2.81[b]	.09	0.87
Control–behavior	.15	1.30	.18	1.52	−.03	−0.33
Intention–behavior	.23	2.02[a]	.25	2.17[b]	.18	1.68

Note. The data are taken from Doll and Ajzen (1992).
[a] $p < .05$.
[b] $p < .01$.

making the assumption that attitudes are automatically activated.[2] Direct experience and repeated attitude expression may well reduce response latencies to attitudinal inquiries, but this may not be the important mediating process. Instead, I have argued that attitudes correlate strongly with intentions and behavior when the considerations salient at the time that intentions are formed or behaviors are executed are similar to the considerations that were salient when the attitudes were assessed. Past experience with a behavior tends to ensure the stability of these considerations over time, thus permitting more accurate prediction of behavior. It thus appears that attitude stability may be a better indicator of an attitude's strength than is latency of responses to attitudinal inquiries (see also Higgins, in press).

It should be noted, however, that the theory of planned behavior need not be limited to highly reasoned forms of action. First, routine and well-practiced behaviors do not require extensive deliberation. Attitudes, subjective norms, perceptions of behavioral control, and intentions formed in the past can be directly retrieved from memory. Second, consistent with various dual-process models of attitudes and social cognition, such as the elaboration likelihood model (Petty & Cacioppo, 1986), the heuristic–systematic model (Chaiken, 1980, 1987), the continuum model (Fiske & Neuberg, 1990), and the MODE model (Fazio, 1990), we can postulate that degree of deliberation is likely to be influenced by motivation and ability to process. Although the theory of planned behavior has usually been discussed and applied in the context of reasoned action, we can perhaps better conceive of behavior as ranging from highly reasoned at one extreme to nonreasoned or spontaneous at the other. The reasoned mode is likely to be taken when people are sufficiently motivated and when they have the required time and resources. In this mode, beliefs and attitudes are expressed after relatively careful deliberation, and behavior follows reasonably from these considerations.

In the absence of sufficient motivation or ability to process, the spontaneous mode of action predominates. Here beliefs and attitudes may be formed without extensive deliberations, based on only a few salient considerations. But when confronted with the need to perform a behavior, people may become motivated to evaluate the behavior in a more systematic manner, especially if the behavior is of personal significance. If new considerations become salient as a result of these deliberations, or as a result of early behavioral feedback, then the previously measured beliefs and attitudes will no longer permit accurate prediction of behavior. Generally speaking, therefore, attitudes should predict behavior better in the reasoned than in the spontaneous mode of action.

Intentions may in this regard fall between attitudes and behavior. Formulation of an intention may sometimes engender more deliberation than formation of beliefs or attitudes, but less so than actually engaging in the behavior. The fact that most studies have found attitudes to be good predictors of intentions would suggest, however, that formation of intentions rarely results in more thorough deliberation than does formation of attitude.

A study on willingness to pay for public and private goods (Ajzen, Brown, & Rosenthal, in press) provides indirect support for some of these ideas. College students read persuasive communications designed to influence their attitudes toward construction of a campus movie theater and toward a fictitious noise filter ostensibly under development. Motivation to deliberate was manipulated by making the product appear personally relevant or irrelevant for the subject population. The campus movie theater was described as being planned in time for use by current students or planned to be ready only after current students had left, and the noise filter was described as designed to help college students study in noisy dormitories or to help factory workers to concentrate in a noisy work environment. The issue of paying for the movie theater (in the form of student fees) or for the noise filter was then introduced, and respondents expressed their attitudes toward paying for the product and their intentions to pay. Finally, they indicated the amount of money they would be willing to pay. Although willingness to pay is not a behavior, it does involve considerations that differ from those that underlie attitudes and intentions to pay. These latter measures refer mainly to a preference for or against paying for the product in question, although the strength of this preference varies. The willingness-to-pay measures required that respondents decide on a dollar amount (i.e., that they consider how much money the product is worth to them).

Table 17.5 shows correlations for the prediction of intentions and amount willing to pay under the high- and low-relevance conditions. It can be seen that attitudes predicted intentions equally well in the two relevance conditions; the prediction of willingness to pay, however, was significantly more accurate under high relevance. These results are consistent with the following interpretation. In the high-relevance condition, systematic deliberations occurred at all stages of measurement, assuring strong correlations for the prediction of willingness to pay as well as for the prediction of intentions. In the low-relevance condition, however, respondents engaged in relatively little deliberation when expressing their attitudes, and whatever

TABLE 17.5. Prediction of Intentions to Pay and Amount Willing to Pay from Attitude toward Paying under Conditions of High and Low Relevance

	Intention to pay		Amount willing to pay	
	Relevant	Irrelevant	Relevant	Irrelevant
Movie theater	.73	.66	.50	.29[a]
Noise filter	.82	.86	.61	.44[a]

Note. The data are taken from Ajzen, Brown, and Rosenthal (1993). All correlations are significant at $p < .01$.
[a]Significant difference ($p < .05$) between relevant and irrelevant conditions.

considerations went into expressing an intention toward paying (without specifying a dollar amount) were largely consistent with the attitude. In contrast, when asked to indicate a dollar amount, respondents became more motivated to consider the pros and cons, resulting in an estimate that was only moderately consistent with previously expressed attitudes.

The difference between the current ideas and the MODE model can be illustrated by considering the effect of direct experience on the attitude–behavior relation. According to the MODE model, type of experience should have little effect on predictive accuracy in the reasoned mode of processing. Attitudes should always be activated as a result of the systematic deliberations that occur in this mode, whether the attitudes were formed on the basis of direct or indirect experience. Type of experience is expected to moderate accuracy of prediction primarily in the spontaneous mode of processing. It is here that strong attitudes produced by direct experience become automatically activated, whereas weak attitudes based on secondhand information are not activated.

The present analysis makes very different predictions. In the reasoned mode of action, attitudes are based on systematic deliberations and take into consideration all available information, whether the information is secondhand or obtained through direct experience. The advantage of direct experience is that, in comparison to indirect experience, it provides more realistic information about the behavior's likely consequences, about the expectations of important others, and about the difficulties of performing the behavior. Salient beliefs, and attitudes based on these beliefs, are thus likely to remain unchanged when the behavior is performed again. In contrast, even if expressed after careful deliberation in the reasoned mode of action, salient beliefs and attitudes that are not based on direct experience are likely to change in the face of new information that becomes available while performing the behavior. As a result, reasoned attitudes based on secondhand information should be less predictive of later behavior than reasoned attitudes based on direct experience.

The effect of direct experience on the attitude–behavior relation should be less pronounced in the spontaneous mode of processing. Because individuals in this mode engage in a minimum of systematic information processing, there is little advantage to direct experience. Although direct experience may produce somewhat more stable beliefs and attitudes, prediction of behavior should be relatively poor following either type of experience. In this view, past experiments that have shown a significant advantage of direct experience (e.g., Doll & Ajzen, 1992; Regan & Fazio, 1977) were conducted in situations that promoted reasoned action.

CONCLUSIONS

More than two decades of research have confirmed the idea that attitudes exert a directive influence on behavior. This influence is quite pronounced when attitudes and behaviors follow careful deliberation. In the reasoned mode of action, attitudes toward the behavior, subjective norms, and perceived behavioral control are good predictors of intentions; and behavior is influenced by intentions and perceived behavioral control.

More controversial is the effect of attitudes on behavior when people are either not sufficiently motivated to engage in careful deliberations, or when they are incapable of doing so. The theory of planned behavior suggests that even in this spontaneous mode of action, behavior is based on whatever beliefs are salient at the time, even if only a small number of beliefs are salient in this mode. Good prediction of behavior depends on these same beliefs also being salient when attitudes and intentions are assessed. If, as is likely to be true in many situations, performance of the behavior comes after more careful deliberation than expression of attitudes and intentions, accuracy of prediction will deteriorate. The reasoned mode of action in the theory of planned behavior has been studied extensively, with good results. Research is needed to explore the theory of planned behavior in a more spontaneous mode of action.

NOTES

1. In a recent paper, Greenwald and Banaji (1995) have gone futher to argue that attitudes can guide behavior without conscious awareness of any kind.

2. The discussion in this scetion refers only to the relation between attitudes on one hand and intentions and behaviors on the other. However, the same considerations also apply to the effects of subjective norms and perceived behavioral control on intentions and actions.

REFERENCES

Abelson, R. P. (1981). Psychological status of the script concept. *American Psychologist, 36,* 715–729.

Ajzen, I. (1985). From intentions to actions: A theory of planned behavior. In J. Kuhl

& J. Beckmann (Eds.), *Action control: From cognition to behavior* (pp. 11–39). Heidelberg: Springer-Verlag.

Ajzen, I. (1988). *Attitudes, personality, and behavior.* Chicago: Dorsey Press.

Ajzen, I. (1991). The theory of planned behavior. *Organizational Behavior and Human Decision Processes, 50,* 179–211.

Ajzen, I., Brown, T. C., & Rosenthal, L. H. (in press).. Information bias in contingent valuation: Effects of personal relevance, quality of information, and motivational orientation. *Journal of Environmental Economics and Management.*

Ajzen, I., & Driver, B. L. (1992a). Contingent value measurement: On the nature and meaning of willingness to pay. *Journal of Consumer Psychology, 1,* 297–316.

Ajzen, I., & Driver, B. L. (1992b). Application of the theory of planned behavior to leisure choice. *Journal of Leisure Research, 24,* 207–224.

Ajzen, I., & Fishbein, M. (1977). Attitude–behavior relations: A theoretical analysis and review of empirical research. *Psychological Bulletin, 84,* 888–918.

Ajzen, I., & Fishbein, M. (1980). *Understanding attitudes and predicting social behavior.* Englewood Cliffs, NJ: Prentice-Hall.

Ajzen, I., & Madden, T. J. (1986). Prediction of goal-directed behavior: Attitudes, intentions, and perceived behavioral control. *Journal of Experimental Social Psychology, 22,* 453–474.

Ajzen, I., & Stanat, P. (1993). *Affective and cognitive predictors of intentions.* Manuscript in preparation, University of Massachusetts at Amherst.

Allport, G. W. (1935). Attitudes. In C. Murchinson (Ed.), *A handbook of social psychology* (pp. 798–844). Worchester, MA: Clark University Press.

Bagozzi, R. P., & Warshaw, P. R. (1990). Trying to consume. *Journal of Consumer Research, 17,* 127–140.

Bargh, J. A. (1989). Conditional automaticity: Varieties of automatic influence in social perception and cognition. In J. S. Uleman & J. A. Bargh (Eds.), *Unintended thought* (pp. 3–51). New York: Guilford Press.

Bargh, J. A., Chaiken, S., Govender, R., & Pratto, F. (1992). The generality of the automatic attitude activation effect. *Journal of Personality and Social Psychology, 62,* 389–912.

Beale, D. A., & Manstead, A. S. R. (1991). Predicting mothers' intentions to limit frequency of infants' sugar intake: Testing the theory of planned behavior. *Journal of Applied Social Psychology, 21,* 409–431.

Beck, L., & Ajzen, I. (1991). Predicting dishonest actions using the theory of planned behavior. *Journal of Research in Personality, 25,* 285–301.

Bentler, P. M., & Speckart, G. (1979). Models of attitude–behavior relations. *Psychological Review, 86,* 452–464.

Campbell, D. T. (1963). Social attitudes and other acquired behavioral dispositions. In S. Koch (Ed.), *Psychology: A study of a science* (Vol. 6, pp. 94–172). New York: McGraw-Hill.

Chaiken, S. (1980). Heuristic versus systematic information processing and the use of source versus message cues in persuasion. *Journal of Personality and Social Psychology, 39,* 752–766.

Chaiken, S. (1987). The heuristic model of persuasion. In M. P. Zanna, J. M. Olson, & C. P. Herman (Eds.), *Social influence: The Ontario Symposium* (Vol. 5, pp. 3–39). Hillsdale, NJ: Erlbaum.

Chaiken, S., & Bargh, J. A. (1993). Occurrence versus moderation in the automatic attitude activation effect: Reply to Fazio. *Journal of Personality and Social Psychology, 64,* 759–765.

Doll, J., & Ajzen, I. (1992). Accessibility and stability of predictors in the theory of planned behavior. *Journal of Personality and Social Psychology, 63,* 754–765.

Eagly, A. H., & Chaiken, S. (1993). *The psychology of attitudes.* Fort Worth, TX: Harcourt Brace Jovanovich.

Fazio, R. H. (1990). Multiple processes by which attitudes guide behavior: The MODE model as an integrative framework. In M. P. Zanna (Ed.), *Advances in experimental social psychology* (Vol. 23, pp. 75–109). San Diego, CA: Academic Press.

Fazio, R. H. (1993). Variability in the likelihood of automatic attitude activation: Data reanalysis and commentary on Bargh, Chaiken, Govender, and Pratto (1992). *Journal of Personality and Social Psychology, 64,* 753–758.

Fazio, R. H., Chen, J., McDonel, E. C., & Sherman, S. J. (1982). Attitude accessibility, attitude–behavior consistency, and the strength of the object–evaluation association. *Journal of Experimental Social Psychology, 18,* 339–357.

Fazio, R. H., Powell, M. C., & Herr, P. M. (1983). Toward a process model of the attitude–behavior relation: Accessing one's attitude upon mere observation of the attitude object. *Journal of Personality and Social Psychology, 44,* 723–735.

Fazio, R. H., Powell, M. C., & Williams, C. J. (1989). The role of attitude accessibility in the attitude to behavior process. *Journal of Consumer Research, 16,* 280–288.

Fazio, R. H., & Williams, C. J. (1986). Attitude accessibility as a moderator of the attitude–perception and attitude–behavior relations: An investigation of the 1984 presidential election. *Journal of Personality and Social Psychology, 51,* 505–514.

Fazio, R. H., & Zanna, M. (1978). Attitudinal qualities relating to the strength of the attitude–behavior relationship. *Journal of Experimental Social Psychology, 14,* 398–408.

Fishbein, M., & Ajzen, I. (1975). *Belief, attitude, intention, and behavior: An introduction to theory and research.* Reading, MA: Addison-Wesley.

Fishbein, M., & Ajzen, I. (1993). *Research based on the theories of reasoned action and planned behavior: A bibliography.* Unpublished manuscript, University of Massachusetts at Amherst.

Fiske, S. T., & Neuberg, S. L. (1990). A continuum of impression formation, from category-based to individuating processes: Influences of information and motivation on attention and interpretation. In M. P. Zanna (Ed.), *Advances in experimental social psychology* (Vol. 23, pp. 1–74). San Diego, CA: Academic Press.

Godin, G., Valois, P., LePage, L., & Desharnais, R. (1992). Prediction of smoking behavior: An application of Ajzen's theory of planned behavior. *British Journal of Addiction, 87,* 1335–1343.

Greenwald, A. G., & Banaji, M. R. (1995). Implicit social cognition: Attitudes, self-esteem, and stereotypes. *Psychological Review, 102,* 4–27.

Higgins, E. T. (in press). Knowledge activation: Accessibility, applicability, and salience. In E. T. Higgins & A. W. Kruglanski (Eds.), *Social psychology: Handbook of basic principles.* New York: Guilford Press.

Houston, D. A., & Fazio, R. H. (1989). Biased processing as a function of attitude accessibility: Making objective judgments subjectively. *Social Cognition, 7,* 51–66.

Kraus, S. J. (1995). Attitudes and the prediction of behavior: A meta analysis of the empirical literature. *Personality and Social Psychology Bulletin, 21,* 58–75.

Kuhl, J. (1985). Volitional aspect of achievement motivation and learned helplessness: Toward a comprehensive theory of action control. In B. A. Maher (Ed.), *Progress in experimental personality research* (Vol. 13, pp. 99–171). New York: Academic Press.

Locke, E. A., & Latham, G. P. (1990). *A theory of goal setting and task performance.* Englewood Cliffs, NJ: Prentice-Hall.

Madden, T. J., Ellen, P. S., & Ajzen, I. (1992). A comparison of the theory of planned behavior and the theory of reasoned action. *Personality and Social Psychology Bulletin, 18,* 3–9.

Mitchell, R. C., & Carson, R. T. (1989). *Using surveys to value public goods: The contingent valuation method.* Washington, DC: Resources for the Future.

Netemeyer, R. G., Burton, S., & Johnston, M. (1991). A comparison of two models for the prediction of volitional and goal-directed behaviors: A confirmatory analysis approach. *Social Psychology Quarterly, 54*(2), 87–100.

Parker, D., Manstead, A. S. R., Stradling, S. G., & Reason, J. T. (1992). Intention to commit driving violations: An applications of the theory of planned behavior. *Journal of Applied Psychology, 77,* 94–101.

Petty, R. E., & Cacioppo, J. T. (1986). The elaboration likelihood model of persuasion. In L. Berkowitz (Ed.), *Advances in experimental social psychology* (Vol. 19, pp. 123–205). New York: Academic Press.

Powell, M. C., & Fazio, R. H. (1984). Attitude accessibility as a function of repeated attitudinal expression. *Personality and Social Psychology Bulletin, 10,* 139–148.

Regan, D. T., & Fazio, R. H. (1977). On the consistency between attitudes and behavior: Look to the method of attitude formation. *Journal of Experimental Social Psychology, 13,* 38–45.

Rosenthal, L. H., & Ajzen, I. (1993). *Effect of repeated attitude expression: Attitude accessibility versus stability.* Manuscript in preparation, University of Massachusetts at Amherst.

Schifter, D. B., & Ajzen, I. (1985). Intention, perceived control, and weight loss: An application of the theory of planned behavior. *Journal of Personality and Social Psychology, 49,* 843–851.

Schlegel, R. P., d'Avernas, J. R., Zanna, M. P., DeCourville, N. H., & Manske, S. R. (1992). Problem drinking: A problem for the theory of reasoned action? *Journal of Applied Social Psychology, 22,* 358–385.

Schmidt, P., Reinecke, J., & Ajzen, I. (in press). Application of the theory of planned behavior to adolescents' condom use: A panel study. *Journal of Applied Social Psychology.*

Sherman, S. J., Presson, C. C., Chassin, L., Bensenberg, M., Corty, E., & Olshavsky, R. W. (1982). Smoking intentions in adolescents: Direct experience and predictability. *Personality and Social Psychology Bulletin, 8,* 376–383.

Triandis, H. C. (1980). Values, attitudes, and interpersonal behavior. In H. E. Howe, Jr., & M. M. Page (Eds.), *Nebraska Symposium on Motivation* (Vol. 27, pp. 195–259). Lincoln: University of Nebraska Press.

van den Putte, B. (1991). *Twenty years of the theory of reasoned action of Fishbein and Ajzen: A meta analysis.* Unpublished manuscript, University of Amsterdam, The Netherlands.

Van Ryn, M., & Vinokur, A. D. (1992). How did it work? An examination of the mechanisms through which a community intervention influenced job-search behavior among an unemployed sample. *American Journal of Community Psychology, 5,* 557–597.

Wicker, A. W. (1969). Attitudes versus actions: The relationship of verbal and overt behavioral responses to attitude objects. *Journal of Social Issues, 25,* 41–78.

CHAPTER 18

Self-Regulatory and Other Non-Ability Determinants of Skill Acquisition

Ruth Kanfer

During the past decade or so, interest in understanding the role of motivation during learning and skill acquisition has burgeoned. Theoretical advances in motivational psychology have focused increasing attention on the volitional or self-regulatory processes that take place during implementation of goals (see, e.g., Bandura, 1986; Dweck & Leggett, 1988; F. Kanfer & Hagerman, 1981; Kanfer, 1987, 1990a, 1990b; Kuhl & Beckmann, 1985). Learning contexts that permit observation of these goal-striving activities have become the paradigms of choice in motivational research (e.g., see Boggiano & Pittman, 1992; Corno & Kanfer, 1993; Wood & Locke, 1990). In the applied domain, recent demographic changes in the composition of the work force and technological changes in the way that work is performed have led to emphasis on skill training (as opposed to selection), and to consideration of how various instructional interventions may maximize learning outcomes (cf. Goldstein & Gilliam, 1990). These recent developments have served to re-establish motivation as a topic of considerable importance in both basic and applied psychology.

This chapter describes a continuing program of research specifically aimed at investigating determinants and consequences of motivation during skill acquisition. This research adopts both experimental and correlational perspectives, and it builds upon contemporary developments in multiple areas, including motivational, cognitive, information-processing, and differential psychology. The first section of this chapter overviews key characteristics of the skill-learning context that have implications for motivation research. The next section describes the basic elements of a dynamic resource allocation model of performance that permits assessment of motivational processes in the context of skill training. Subsequent sections review the model's implications with respect to the effects of self-regulatory activities on learning and performance, as well as the results of two series of studies derived from the model. The final section highlights continuing issues and implications for applied settings.

THE CONTEXT OF SKILL ACQUISITION

When goals can be accomplished without task learning, the influence of motivation on behavior is often largely a matter of choice. For example, the decision about which of two job offers to accept depends primarily on the individual's evaluation of the costs and benefits associated with each offer. Once a decision is made, however, the actions involved in implementing the goal of accepting the job are straightforward. Barring other circumstances that may alter commitment to the goal, accepting the job is an action that can typically be carried out swiftly and without difficulty.

However, such is *not* the case in skill acquisition. During skill training, goal accomplishment proceeds slowly, as the individual develops an understanding of the task and proficiency in skills relevant to performance. Goals pertaining to the development of skills, such as typing or word processing, often involve frustrations and failures, particularly during the early stage of learning. In short, initial performance is typically slow and error-prone. Continued task practice (i.e., persistence) is necessary to yield improvements in task performance. But for practice to have a positive effect on performance, additional motivational mechanisms are required to sustain attention and effort over time and in the face of difficulties and failures. This aspect of motivation—namely, self-regulation—pertains to the mechanisms that operate during skill acquisition or goal implementation. In skill training, where trainees often hold similar skill-learning and performance goals, self-regulatory processes take on special significance as key motivational determinants of learning and performance.

A second point about investigating motivation in skill training pertains to the dynamic changes in task demands that occur when people are learning difficult tasks, such as word processing or air traffic control. Theory and research by Shiffrin and Schneider (1977) and Fisk and Schneider (1983) indicate that the attentional demands imposed by such consistent information-processing tasks decline with practice. During the early phase of skill training, the task demands substantial cognitive resources, and most trainees must devote a substantial proportion of their attentional effort toward the task. As task demands on attentional effort decline with practice, fewer resources are required for sustaining performance at current levels. At this point, performance is generally faster and less error-prone. For *continued* performance improvement, however, it is essential that individuals redirect "spare" attentional resources to the task (Woodworth, 1938).

A dynamic perspective on task demands in skill learning has an important implication for motivation research. Specifically, this perspective suggests that the effectiveness of particular motivational processes in enhancing learning and performance may vary, depending on the phase of skill acquisition (for a review, see Kanfer & Ackerman, 1989). For example, in the early phase of learning, when task demands on attention are the highest, self-regulatory activities that divert attention from the task are likely to impede performance. In contrast, during later phases of training, when attentional demands of the task decline, self-regulatory activities may enhance performance by redirecting spare attentional resources toward task learning.

A final point about skill training pertains to the critical role of individual differences in general cognitive ability in predicting performance. Individual differences in general cognitive ability play a key role in predicting performance and typically account for substantial variance in performance, particularly during the early stage of skill learning (see, e.g., Ackerman, 1987; Fleishman, 1972). Higher-ability trainees generally outperform lower-ability trainees during the early stage of training and often throughout training, since attentional resource demands imposed by the task decline (over practice) more rapidly for higher-ability than for lower-ability trainees. In many tasks, however, performance differences between higher- and lower-ability trainees attenuate with practice (see, e.g., Ackerman, 1987, 1988). That is, over the course of practice, motivational processes may importantly affect the extent to which lower- and higher-ability trainees sustain performance improvements. These results suggest that motivational effects on skill learning cannot be evaluated without consideration of both basic learning phenomena and individual differences in abilities.

In summary, understanding the role of motivational processes in the context of skill training provides a unique opportunity for the study of self-regulatory activities. In skill training, trainees are expressly engaged in goal-directed purposive behaviors (i.e., goal implementation). Such an environment minimizes motivational influences associated with the initial decision to pursue a goal, and permits a more refined investigation of how self-regulatory processes operate to affect action during goal implementation.

However, nonmotivational factors also exert a strong influence on the criteria typically used to index motivational effects in skill learning. A large body of research attests to the influences of individual differences in abilities and changing task demands on learning and performance (see, e.g., Ackerman, 1987, 1988; Fleishman, 1972). Higher-ability individuals tend to outperform lower-ability individuals at the onset of training, although performance differences often attenuate with practice. To demonstrate the role of motivation and self-regulation in skill acquisition, it is essential to develop a unified framework that permits consideration of the independent and joint effects of these motivational and nonmotivational influences.

OVERVIEW OF THE INTEGRATED RESOURCE ALLOCATION MODEL

Drawing from advances in motivation, ability, and information-processing theories, my colleagues and I have developed a model of attention and performance during skill acquisition that provides theoretical linkages among individual differences in cognitive ability, motivation, and task demands—with particular attention to the role of self-regulatory processes and mechanisms as they influence complex skill learning. This section summarizes the basic elements of this model (see Figure 18.1; see also Kanfer & Ackerman, 1989).

The integrated model of resource allocation utilizes the construct of attentional resources as the common theoretical linkage among individual differences in ability, motivation, and task demands. Drawing upon Kahneman's (1973) model of attentional resources, our model posits that individuals have a pool of attentional capacity from which attentional resources are allocated to various activities at two different points—distally, in terms of the proportion of total resources allocated, and proximally, in terms of suballocations of the initial allocation. In the Kahneman (1973) model, task performance is related to the extent to which attentional resources are devoted to the task.

More recently, theory and research by Ackerman (1987, 1988) on the

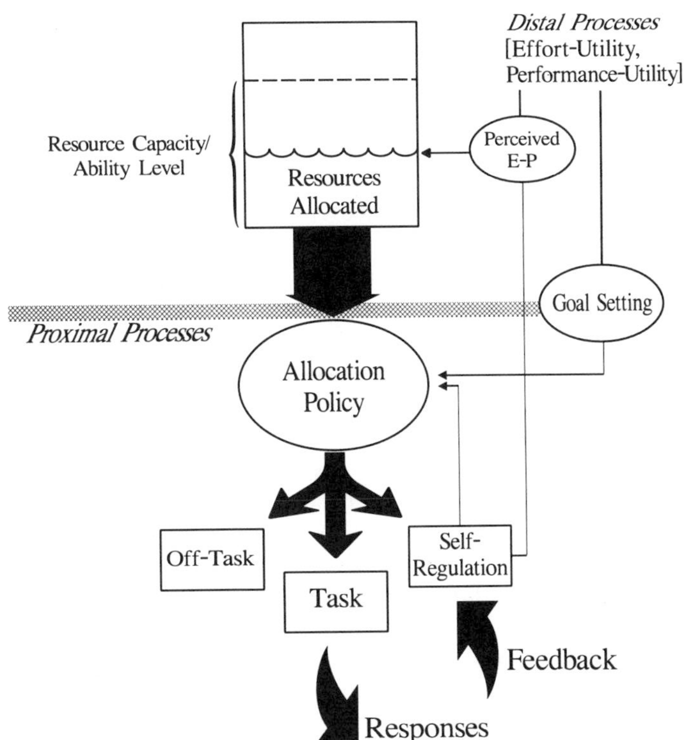

FIGURE 18.1. An integrated resource allocation model depicting ability–motivation interactions for attentional effort. From Kanfer and Ackerman (1989). Copyright 1989 by the American Psychological Association. Reprinted by permission.

relation between attentional resources and individual differences in abilities has shown that individual differences in total attentional capacity can be related to individual differences in general cognitive ability. As such, in the integrated resource allocation model, measures of individual differences in general cognitive ability provide assessment of the upper limit on the availability of attentional resources for task performance. In essence, individual differences in general cognitive ability index how much attention an individual has to give to a task.

In contrast, motivational processes are the mechanisms by which attentional resources are allocated to tasks. That is, motivational processes influence the direction in which available attentional resources are allocated. Corresponding to the distinction between choice motivation and self-regulation, motivational processes are posited to affect allocation of attentional resources at two distinct points. In the integrated model, the first point at which motivation is posited to affect attentional resource allocation policies is in the determination of the proportion of an individual's total attentional capacity that will be directed toward goal accomplishment. As such, this motivational influence sets the stage for subsequent learning and performance. In the context of skill acquisition, this influence is termed "distal," since this decision typically occurs outside the context of task engagement and is not posited to draw attentional resources away from the task during practice. In performance contexts in which the task is well learned and the goal is executed quickly, no further motivational influences may come into play.

However, in the context of skill acquisition, additional motivational influences operate during task engagement. In the model, this is represented by the second allocation process, in which resources are suballocated to various activities during task engagement. In contrast to the distal mechanism, this process is termed "proximal," since it occurs during task engagement and represents information-processing strategies that may facilitate or impede goal-directed behavior. At this stage, attentional resources are posited to be allocated among three broad classes of activities: on-task, off-task, and self-regulatory. Allocation of attentional resources to the task is hypothesized to exert a direct positive influence on performance. Allocation of resources to off-task activities, such as daydreaming, is expected to exert a direct negative influence on task performance. Allocation of resources to self-regulatory strategies, however, may exert positive or negative effects on task performance, depending upon their attentional costs relative to the attentional demands of the task.

Self-regulation is an essential mechanism for bringing about changes in both distal and proximal allocation policies as attentional demands of the task change during skill acquisition. Ideally, self-regulatory activities enable individuals to adjust allocation policies effectively as conditions change. For example, as individuals gain proficiency at the task and attentional demands associated with performance decline, self-regulatory strategies may be used to increase goal commitment (i.e., the proportion of resources devoted to the task) or to reduce daydreaming (i.e., the proportion of resources allocated to off-task activities).

In summary, the integrated model proposes that when abilities and motivation are mapped to a common metric, any individual's performance may be represented as a joint function of the individual's relative attentional capacity (i.e., cognitive ability) and the proportion of the individual's total capacity actually devoted to the task through various motivational processes. During skill acquisition, self-regulatory activities serve as the primary determinant in modifying policies of attentional resource allocation.

IMPLICATIONS OF THE INTEGRATED RESOURCE ALLOCATION MODEL

In complex skill-learning situations, trainees typically commit substantial effort to the task during the initial phase of skill acquisition. The commitment of a substantial proportion of total attentional capacity to the task, and the allocation of this effort to on-task activities, are consistent with the high demands imposed by the task in the early phase of skill learning. At this stage of skill acquisition, individuals must devote as much effort as possible to understanding and mastering basic elements of the task, regardless of their level of general cognitive ability.

The integrated model suggests that popular motivational interventions (such as goal setting) that emphasize performance accomplishments can be expected to have few positive effects or even negative effects on performance at this phase of skill training. In goal-setting interventions, for example, individuals are assigned specific and difficult performance goals. A large number of studies show positive effects on performance for this motivational intervention on well-learned or simple tasks (see, e.g., Locke & Latham, 1990). According to the goal-setting conceptualization, goal assignments facilitate performance in part by mobilizing on-task effort. In the context of skill acquisition, however, individuals are already likely to be putting forth substantial on-task effort. In this situation, the model suggests that performance goal assignments early in skill training may have the opposite of their intended effect, as the goal instruction focuses attentional resources on self-evaluation at the time when the attentional resource demands of the task are at their highest.

In contrast, during later phases of skill acquisition, the attentional demands of the task decline as performance improves. During these phases, individuals have spare attentional resources that may be redirected to the task. As a result, at this point in training, goal assignments that promote self-evaluative activities are unlikely to divert critical resources from the task. Furthermore, in contrast to the early phase of skill learning, where task comprehension and performance are poor, self-evaluative processing during later phases of skill learning will be less likely to generate strong (resource-consumptive) negative affective reactions. During later phases of skill training, then, performance goal assignments are expected to facilitate performance through activation of self-regulatory activities that emphasize redirection of spare attentional resources to the task.

Finally, the integrated model also implies that motivational interventions, such as goal setting, during skill acquisition will have a greater impact on trainees of lower general cognitive ability than on persons of higher general cognitive ability. Assume, for example, that both a higher- and a lower-ability trainee commit 80% of their attentional resources to task performance. Since differences in general cognitive ability place an upper limit on total attentional capacity, the lower-ability trainee would have fewer attentional resources committed to the task than would the higher-ability trainee. Because the attentional demands of the task remain fixed, regardless of ability level, diversion of committed attentional resources by goal assignments is predicted to have a stronger negative impact on the performance of the lower-ability trainee than on that of the higher-ability trainee. Similarly, since the lower-ability trainee is likely to take longer to achieve an asymptotic level of performance than the higher-ability trainee, the lower-ability trainee will benefit more from sustained on-task effort over practice than the higher-ability trainee. As such, the provision of a goal assignment late in training is expected to have a more pronounced positive effect on the performance of lower-ability trainees than on that of higher-ability trainees.

EMPIRICAL TESTS OF THE INTEGRATED RESOURCE ALLOCATION MODEL

Over the past several years, we have conducted a series of studies investigating the viability of the integrated of resource allocation model (see Ackerman & Kanfer, 1993; Kanfer & Ackerman, 1989, 1990; Kanfer, Ackerman, Murtha, Dugdale, & Nelson, 1994). As a first step, however, it was necessary to construct an experimental task that was sufficiently difficult to permit display of individual differences in cognitive and motivational aptitudes, yet allowed for learning to occur with practice. In this section, I describe the task used and summarize the results of several studies that provided empirical evidence for implications derived from the integrated model.

The Kanfer–Ackerman Air Traffic Controller Task

The Kanfer–Ackerman Air Traffic Controller (KA-ATC) task is a rule-based, real-time computerized task that simulates some of the activities performed by air traffic controllers. In essence, the task requires trainees to accept incoming planes into their airspace, to move planes within a three-level hold pattern, and to land planes on a set of runways as quickly and accurately as possible (see Figure 18.2 for an example of the KA-ATC task display screen).

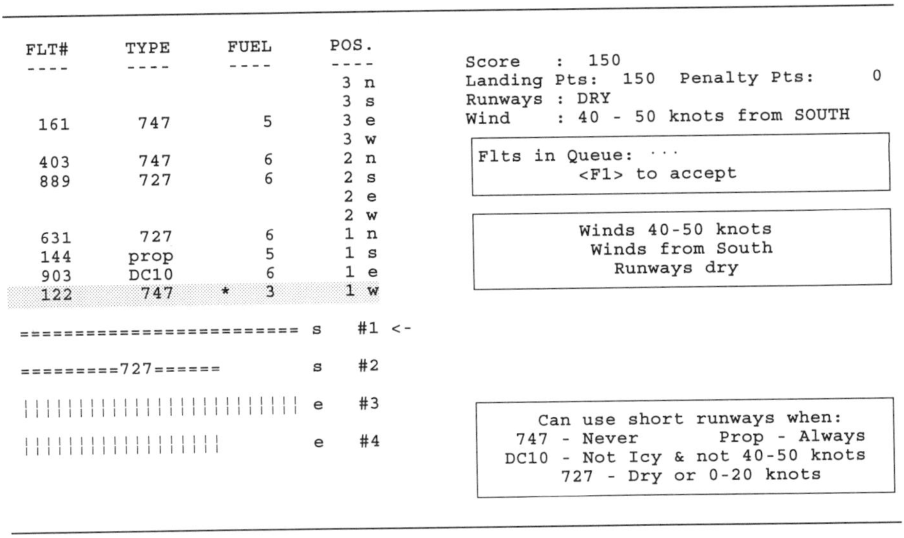

```
FLT#      TYPE      FUEL      POS.
----      ----      ----      ----      Score    :  150
                              3 n       Landing Pts:  150   Penalty Pts:     0
                              3 s       Runways  : DRY
 161       747         5      3 e       Wind     : 40 - 50 knots from SOUTH
                              3 w
 403       747         6      2 n       Flts in Queue: ...
 889       727         6      2 s              <F1> to accept
                              2 e
                              2 w
 631       727         6      1 n              Winds 40-50 knots
 144      prop         5      1 s               Winds from South
 903      DC10         6      1 e                Runways dry
 122       747    *    3      1 w

========================= s    #1 <-

=========727======        s    #2

|||||||||||||||||||||||||  e    #3         Can use short runways when:
                                        747 - Never         Prop - Always
|||||||||||||||||          e    #4      DC10 - Not Icy & not 40-50 knots
                                           727 - Dry or 0-20 knots
```

FIGURE 18.2. The Kanfer–Ackerman Air Traffic Controller (KA-ATC) task. The figure is a literal static representation of the real-time display. From Kanfer and Ackerman (1989). Copyright 1989 by the American Psychological Association. Reprinted by permission.

Trainees receive points for each plane successfully landed and lose points for rule-based errors. Rules governing task performance address which movements of planes are permissible within the hold pattern, when planes must be landed, and which plane types may land on which runways under which weather conditions.

The Effects of Goal Setting

The first results obtained using the KA-ATC task stem from a larger set of experiments conducted with over 1,000 U.S. Air Force basic trainees (see Kanfer & Ackerman, 1989). For purposes of brevity, discussion is limited here to the results obtained from the final experiment in this series. In that study, we examined the interactive effects of ability and motivation on performance following a part-task training procedure designed to differentially influence the cognitive demands imposed by the full KA-ATC task.

Trainees were assigned to either a "procedural" or a "declarative" part-task training procedure. Trainees in the procedural part-task training condition were given training designed to enhance motor skills without reducing cognitive demands associated with learning the rules governing task performance. In contrast, trainees assigned to the declarative part-task training condition were given practice designed to enhance declarative understanding of the rules governing task performance. After training, all trainees performed six full KA-ATC task trials.

To stimulate self-regulatory activities during skill acquisition, half of the trainees in each training condition were assigned difficult and specific performance goals (e.g., reaching a cumulative performance score of 2,100 points by the end of the trial) for each of the full KA-ATC task trials. Trainees in the control condition were instructed to "do your best."

Results obtained in this experiment provide support for several tenets of the integrated resource allocation model. As shown in the upper panel of Figure 18.3 (depicting final full KA-ATC task trial landing score performance), goal assignments made during the early, cognitively demanding phase of performance exerted an overall detrimental effect on performance among trainees provided with the procedural part-task training. Moreover, the cognitive costs of such activities were greater for lower-ability trainees than for higher-ability trainees. Such an effect was expected, given the no-

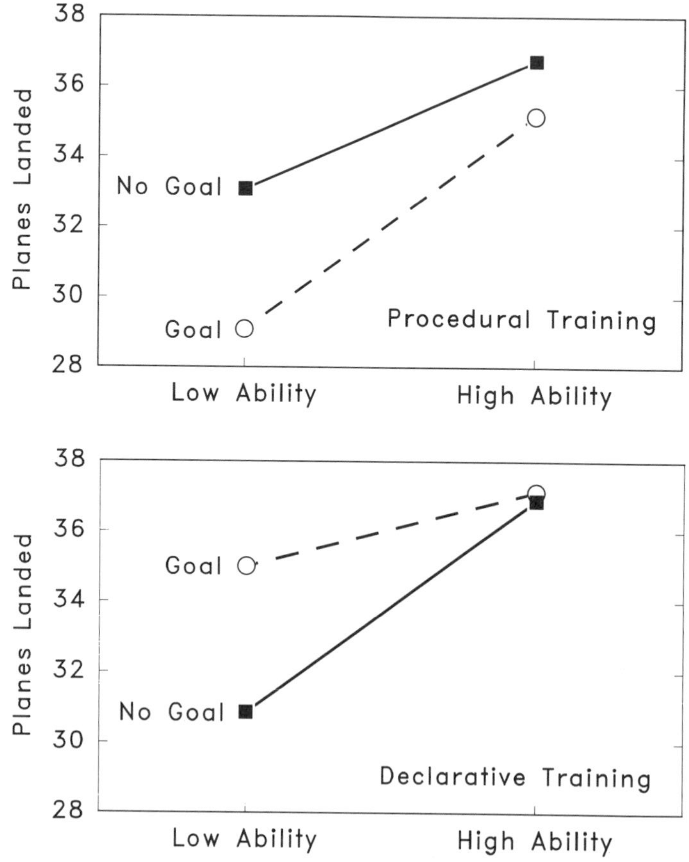

FIGURE 18.3. Number of planes landed on the final KA-ATC task trial, by part-task training condition and ability group. (No-goal conditions are shown in solid lines and filled squares; goal conditions are shown in dashed lines and open circles.) From Kanfer and Ackerman (1989). Copyright 1989 by the American Psychological Association. Reprinted by permission.

tion that self-regulatory processing associated with goal setting would divert a proportionately greater amount of attentional resources among lower-ability trainees than among higher-ability trainees. Consistent with these performance data, trainees in the goal condition reported greater frequency of off-task cognitions and negative affective self-reactions compared to trainees in the control ("do your best") condition.

Among trainees provided with the declarative part-task training, a contrasting pattern of results was obtained (see lower panel of Figure 18.3). It was expected that providing trainees with part-task training aimed at reducing the cognitive demands associated with subsequent full KA-ATC task performance would result in spare attentional resources that the trainees could devote to self-regulation. In the declarative training conditions, goal assignments exerted a significant beneficial effect, with a greater benefit accruing to lower-ability trainees than to higher-ability trainees.

These findings suggest that self-regulation mechanisms may help or hinder task performance. The interaction between goals and general cognitive ability is consistent with the notion that the costs and benefits of self-regulatory processes depends on the availability of spare attentional resources. When cognitive demands imposed by the task are high, trainees with less attentional capacity appear to be hurt more by explicit goal setting than trainees with greater attentional capacity. In contrast, goal setting helped lower-ability trainees more than higher-ability trainees when task demands were lessened.

The Effects of Conditions on Practice

In the experiment just described, limitations on resource availability were attributable to phase of skill acquisition. In a further attempt to test basic tenets of the integrated resource allocation model, we again examined the influence of goal setting (as a means of inducing self-regulatory activities) on performance, but this time under conditions where limitations on resource availability stemmed from the structure of training rather than from the phase of skill acquisition.

In most skill training programs, task practice is rarely continuous. Task performance is typically alternated with rest intervals, though the frequency and duration of rest intervals may vary widely, depending on external factors (e.g., the availability of equipment). Though a number of studies suggest that spaced practice may be more effective than massed practice in enhancing performance, the findings are inconsistent and appear related to the characteristics of the skill to be acquired as well as the performance criteria adopted (see Kanfer, Ackerman, et al., 1994).

The integrated resource allocation perspective suggests that the superiority of spaced practice in a skill learning context may stem in part from the fact that the rest interval frees attentional resources that may be unavailable during task engagement. During a rest interval, these attentional resources may then be used for self-regulatory activity. In the absence of other strong demands on cognitive resources, self-regulatory processing during the rest interval should benefit subsequent on-task performance (e.g., by stimulating covert rehearsal). In contrast, goal assignments in a massed-practice paradigm should exacerbate the conflict between task demands on attentional effort and attentional demands imposed by self-regulatory activities. In this context, as in the previous experiment, goal assignments early in skill acquisition should result in lower levels of performance.

To investigate this hypothesis, 203 trainees completed a series of KA-ATC task trials under one of four training conditions: (1) massed practice, control ("do your best" goal); (2) massed practice, goal; (3) spaced practice, control; and (4) spaced practice, goal. Trainees in the massed-practice conditions performed a series of fourteen 10-minute KA-ATC task trials with approximately 15-second intertrial intervals (i.e., 140 minutes of on-task practice). Trainees in the spaced-practice conditions performed ten 10-minute KA-ATC task trials with a computer-timed 4-minute break between each trial (i.e., 100 minutes of on-task practice); these trainees were instructed to sit quietly at their work station between breaks. Trainees in the goal conditions were assigned specific and difficult performance score goals for each trial throughout the training session. Again, trainees in the control conditions were instructed to "do your best."

Results obtained in this experiment provided further support for the notion that the potential benefits of self-regulation depend critically on resource availability. A repeated-measure analysis of variance on landing score performance indicated an interaction of goal × type of practice. Figure 18.4 displays this interaction in terms of the number of planes landed after all trainees had completed 100 minutes of time-on-task. As shown, with similar amounts of on-task practice, trainees in the spaced-practice/goal condition landed more planes than did trainees in the massed-practice/goal condition. In addition, as expected, trainees in the massed-practice/goal condition performed more poorly than trainees in the massed-practice/control condition. The difference in performance obtained in the two massed-practice conditions suggests that task fatigue alone cannot account for these results, but rather that the goal assignments diverted attention from on-task processing. That is, the advantage conferred by massed practice appears to have been attenuated when self-regulatory processing was stimulated via goal setting. In contrast, however, goal assignments facilitated performance among trainees in the spaced-practice condition.

EXTENDING THE MODEL: A SKILLS PERSPECTIVE

Results obtained in the studies described above indicate that self-regulatory activities do affect on-task utilization of attentional resources. In addition, the findings also indicate that such activities may help or hinder skill learning, depending on the demands of the task and on individual differences in general cognitive ability. Instigation of specific and difficult goal assign-

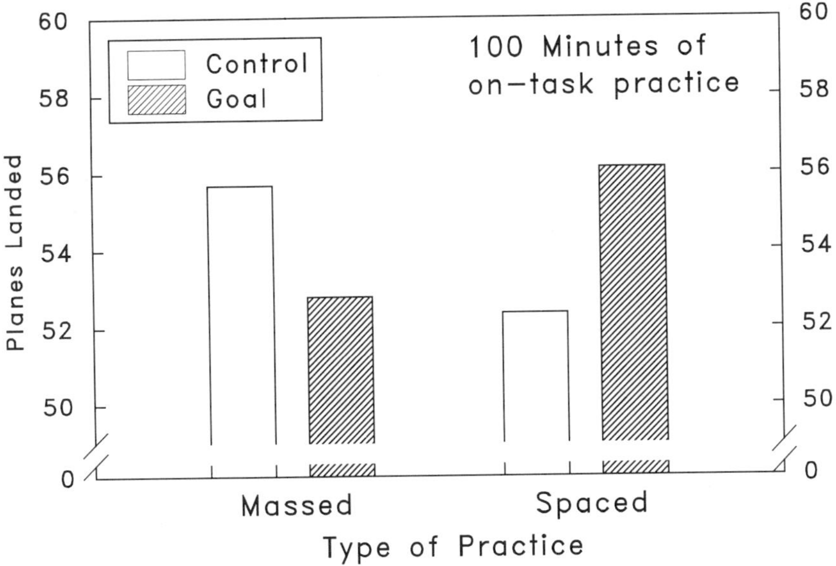

FIGURE 18.4. Number of planes landed at 100 minutes of time on the KA-ATC task (KA-ATC task trial 10 for both massed- and spaced-practice conditions). From Kanfer, Ackerman, Murtha, Dugdale, and Nelson (1994). Copyright 1994 by the American Psychological Association. Reprinted by permission.

ments during the early, resource-intensive phase of learning hindered performance in these studies, whereas instigation of assignments during later or less resource-demanding phases of skill acquisition facilitated performance, particularly among lower-ability trainees.

We also noted a striking regularity in our results across studies with respect to the frequency of negative affective self-reactions reported by trainees during the early phase of learning. This led us to further consider the possibility that patterns of self-regulatory activity reported to occur during learning might be more effectively conceptualized in terms of skills that persons develop, modify, and use during skill acquisition, *regardless* of their current performance level. In the studies described below, we extended the integrated model, using an individual-differences perspective to consider the self-regulation component more precisely. In contrast to the previously described work highlighting the attentional costs associated with self-regulatory activities per se, the aim of the work described in the following section was to investigate the feasibility of adopting an individual-differences or "motivational-skills" perspective to predicting the effects of motivational processes on skill learning.

The motivational-skills perspective is consistent with recent work by Kuhl (1985) and others (e.g., Dweck & Leggett, 1988; see Kanfer, Ackerman, Murtha, & Goff, 1995) emphasizing the role of individual differences in specific self-regulatory activities. Looking back at our earlier research using the KA-ATC task, we noted that poorer-performing trainees reported a much higher level of off-task cognitions than did higher-performing trainees. Many of the thoughts reported had a basis in negative emotions and represented distracting intrusions into task concentration. Examples included reports of thinking about doing more poorly than others on the task, dissatisfaction and anger with oneself for making mistakes, feelings of unhappiness, and so on. In contrast, higher-performing trainees reported having significantly fewer of these thoughts during task engagement. We hypothesized that one fundamental group of self-regulatory skills pertains to inhibiting worry and avoiding intrusion of emotion-based, off-task thoughts. This set of skills, which we have termed "emotion control" (after Kuhl, 1985) emphasizes the use of self-regulatory processes to keep performance anxiety and other negative emotional distractions at bay during task engagement.

Our review of previous ATC trainees' self-reports also indicated that task interest and commitment often declined during later stages of practice, particularly among higher-performing trainees. For many tasks, the early phase of skill acquisition is often both the most demanding and rewarding. Devoting attention and effort to the task at this point in training typically yields readily visible improvements in performance. But as task proficiency develops, these big gains in performance diminish. Performance improvements continue, but at a less impressive rate, in accord with the "power law of practice" (Newell & Rosenbloom, 1981). Concomitant with performance improvements over practice, task demands on attention for sustaining current performance levels attenuate. That is, people can perform the task at current performance levels with less effort—and often do. From a motivational perspective, these characteristics of later phases of skill training are potentially quite detrimental. The task no longer demands effort, and intrinsic rewards associated with readily observed performance improvements are gone. As many athletes report, the most effective self-regulatory skills at this point pertain to processes that bolster motivation to perform and further increase on-task effort (see Sonnichsen, 1994, for a review). Examples include goal setting, creating imaginary and contrived consequences for performance outcomes, and other practices aimed at the maintenance of high levels of attention and effort toward task performance. Consistent with Kuhl's (1985) theorizing, we consider these to be examples of "motivation control" skills—that is, self-regulatory activities aimed at keeping attention and effort on the task, despite boredom and general satisfaction with current performance.

Motivational Skills as a Predictor of Skill Acquisition

Overall, then, the motivational-skills perspective states that individuals may differ in terms of their development and use of two basic self-regulatory sets of skills: emotion control and motivation control. Whereas individual differences in abilities are relatively fixed, motivational skills are assumed to develop in complex task learning.

The first step in investigating this extension of the model with respect to skill acquisition was to construct an individual-differences measure that would provide a reliable historical account of the use of these self-regulatory skills, and then to ascertain whether such knowledge about an individual's skills would aid in the prediction of training performance.

After developing a brief (18-item) self-report measure of motivational skills in the context of air traffic control, we conducted two predictive validity studies (one laboratory and one field study) to assess the extent to which individual differences in such skills aid in predicting air traffic controller training performance (see Ackerman & Kanfer, 1993). In the laboratory study, 118 students completed a multitest battery, including the motivational-skills test, prior to 15 hours of terminal radar approach control (TRACON) training. In contrast to the KA-ATC task, the TRACON task is a high-fidelity, real-time computerized air traffic controller simulation task that involves the use of a radar screen and is considerably more complex. As in the KA-ATC task, the goals of training are to maneuver and land planes safely and efficiently within the assigned airspace. To accomplish these goals, trainees must learn the rules governing airplane movement in the airspace and handoffs for landing.

In the laboratory study, we modified the TRACON task to provide standardization of each 30-minute TRACON trial and to enable trainees to learn the task sufficiently to permit performance after a 1-hour videotape training session. Figure 18.5 provides a static display of the TRACON stimulus screen. In this TRACON study, trainees completed about 15 hours of task training. Acquiring proficiency in this simplified task version may take 20 or more hours of training. (In the field, acquiring proficiency in this job typically takes 2 or more years.) Overall success in TRACON training, presented here in terms of the average number of planes successfully handled, was used as the criterion measure.

Findings obtained in the lab study showed a substantial correlation between the motivational skills measure and final TRACON performance (r = .422). Not surprisingly, of course, so did the ability battery (R = .686). Most important, however, was the significant incremental contribution of the motivational-skills measure to prediction of TRACON performance, over and above that predicted by individual differences in ability (R = .718). That is, knowing the subject's level of motivational skills explained approximately 4% of performance variance not explained by individual differences in cognitive abilities.

In the field study, we administered the test battery to 206 Federal Aviation Administration (FAA) air traffic controller trainees at the onset of their training. At the time, the FAA training program consisted of an 8½-week nonradar program. Trainees who scored above a certain cutoff on standardized tests continued with air traffic controller training; those who failed

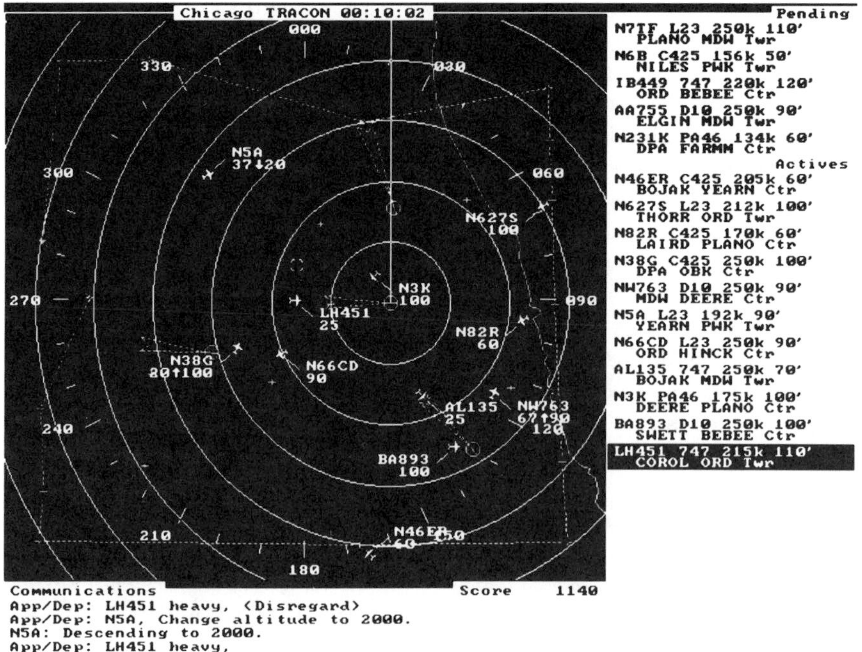

FIGURE 18.5. Static copy of the terminal radar approach control (TRACON) screen. From Ackerman and Kanfer (1993). Copyright 1993 by the American Psychological Association. Reprinted by permission.

were dropped from the training program and employment. Results obtained in the field study were remarkably similar to those obtained in the laboratory study. Again, motivational skills correlated with training outcome (r = .323), and, again, ability explained the greatest part of variance in training outcome (R = .545). Nonetheless, individual differences in level of motivational skills significantly added to the prediction of training success (R = .595), again explaining approximately 4% of the variance in performance not explained by ability.

These findings were quite encouraging. Our next step was to examine more precisely the role of each motivational skill and its malleability in the training context.

Motivational-Skills Training

In the context of skill acquisition, emotion control skills are likely to be most important early in training—when task demands on attention are highest. Early in training, people often experience failures and displeasure with their behavior and performance. Emotion control skills help to keep such off-task concerns and emotions from diverting attention from the task. For lower-ability trainees, emotion control skills are particularly important, since these are the individuals who are most likely to experience difficulty early in training.

Late in training, the frequency of failures declines as performance improves. But at this point, different potential motivational impediments to performance come into play. Trainees may become bored with the task and fail to exert the effort needed to improve their performance further. Motivation control skills enable individuals to sustain on-task attention and effort. In the standard training environment, motivation control skills are likely to be most important for higher-ability trainees—that is, those who most quickly reach a less effortful, but suboptimal, level of task proficiency.

We conducted two air traffic controller training studies to examine whether explicit instruction and training in emotion control skills and motivation control skills might indeed facilitate performance (see Kanfer & Ackerman, 1990). In the first study, 237 U.S. Air Force basic trainees performed nine 10-minute KA-ATC task trials in one of two randomly assigned motivational-skill instruction conditions: emotion control or motivation control. Prior to initial task performance and during the intertrial intervals, half of the trainees received instructions to control the occurrence of negative emotions (e.g., worry or upset following errors) during KA-ATC task performance. The remaining trainees received motivation control instructions. These instructions directed trainees to control and further increase the amount of effort they devoted to the task at all times during the performance trial.

The results, shown in Figure 18.6, indicate that provision of motivation and emotion skills instruction during training had significantly different effects on performance among lower-ability trainees, but not higher-ability trainees. Among lower-ability trainees, those in the emotion control condition made significantly fewer errors than those in the motivation control condition. As shown in Figure 18.6, this effect occurred early in practice and was sustained throughout practice. Consistent with these results, lower-ability trainees instructed to implement emotion control skills during task performance reported significantly fewer negative affective self-reactions or attempts to monitor their performance score than did lower-ability trainees in the motivation control condition.

In the second study, we again provided training in either emotion control or motivation control skills, but this time in the context of a part-task training module that trainees completed before performing the full KA-ATC task. The use of this part-task training module permitted investigation of later phases of skill acquisition; it also made it feasible to provide training in emotion control and motivation control skills outside the regular KA-ATC practice context. Results from this study replicated the beneficial effect of emotion control skills training for lower-ability trainees found in the previous study. In addition, however, motivation control skills training was also found to reduce errors later in KA-ATC practice among higher-ability trainees.

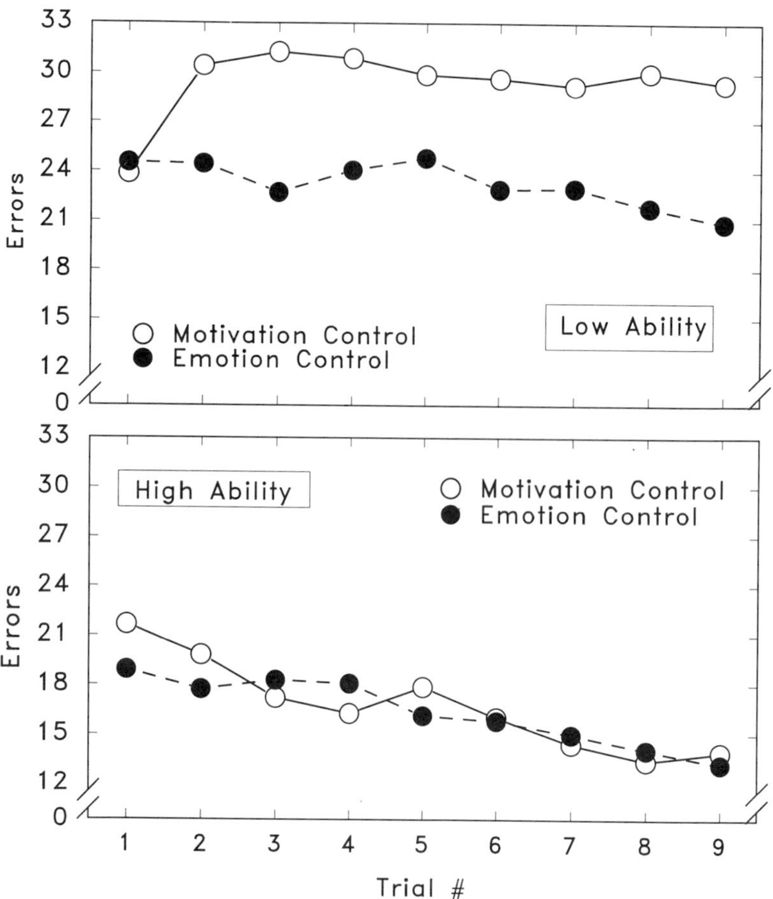

FIGURE 18.6. Frequency of errors across KA-ATC task trials by instructional condition and ability group. (Motivation control condition is shown in solid lines and open circles; emotion control condition is shown in dashed lines and filled circles.) From Kanfer and Ackerman (1990).

Overall, then, the findings obtained in the studies just described indicate that the influence of self-regulation processes on learning and performance can be profitably studied from a motivational-skills perspective. Individual differences in motivational skills reflect historical accounts of skill development, and add something distinct from individual differences in ability to the prediction of performance. That these skills may be modifiable with direct instruction or training is not at all inconsistent with a differential approach; rather, it suggests that motivational processes, like other attributes of the individual, are changed slowly and with experience.

SUMMARY

The integrated resource allocation perspective has proved quite useful as a starting point for demonstrating the operation of motivation processes in complex skill learning. From a practical standpoint, our findings show that proximal motivation processes exert a variable influence on learning outcomes, depending upon the attentional demands of the task, individual differences in cognitive abilities, and the nature of self-regulatory processes engaged. The model provides a theoretically-based explanation for past inconsistencies in research investigating the benefits of goal-setting assignments, and suggests that future research on goal–performance relations must take into account the information-processing demands of the task, as well as potential individual differences in self-regulatory processing during task performance.

At a broader theoretical level, our program of research is quite consistent with the perspectives taken by researchers emphasizing the importance of implementational processes (e.g., Carver & Scheier, 1990; Gollwitzer, 1990). Our conceptualization of emotional processes in terms of their attentional costs, and our treatment of only a narrow range of emotions to date, may be dissatisfying for some emotion theorists. On the other hand, the results we have obtained using the integrated resource model provide a clear demonstration of the role of affective reactions in cognitive processing, and also serve to complement theory and research on the role of affect and emotion in achievement-related action.

Our more recent work investigating the feasibility of an individual-differences approach to proximal motivational skills has implications for both theory and practice. Our findings demonstrate the existence of important individual differences in proximal motivation processing, and suggest that continued work from a differential perspective is useful. However, it is also clear that the measurement and detection of such differences will require further elaboration on the goals or context in which action is situated. For example, our findings on the development of non-ability measures of self-regulatory activities and tryouts in both field and laboratory training environments indicated that self-report measures of related non-ability constructs (e.g., action control) were not predictive of performance or self-regulatory activities when assessed independently of the context or an articulated goal (Kanfer, Dugdale, & McDonald, 1994). However, when we assessed motivational skills in a task-related context, in which the goal of action was at least implicit, we found significant incremental predictive validity for performance in both the laboratory and the field (Ackerman & Kanfer, 1993).

During the past two decades, motivation research has broadened in myriad ways, including growing emphases on biological, psychophysiological, emotional, and unconscious determinants of action. The research program described in this chapter attempts to integrate recent developments in the field by explicitly considering the role of interindividual differences in motivation and cognitive abilities during skill learning.

ACKNOWLEDGMENTS

Portions of the research reported here were supported by grants to Ruth Kanfer and to Phillip L. Ackerman from the U.S. Air Force Office of Scientific Research (Nos. AFOSR 87-0234, AFOSR 89-0242, and AFOSR F49620-93-1-0206) and the Office of Naval Research (Contract No. N00014-91-J-4159). This research program is also supported in part by a grant to Ruth Kanfer from the National Science Foundation (No. NSF/SBR-9223357).

REFERENCES

Ackerman, P. L. (1987). Individual differences in skill learning: An integration of psychometric and information processing perspectives. *Psychological Bulletin, 102,* 3–27.

Ackerman, P. L. (1988). Determinants of individual differences during skill acquisition: Cognitive abilities and information processing. *Journal of Experimental Psychology: General, 117,* 288–318.

Ackerman, P. L., & Kanfer, R. (1993). Integrating laboratory and field study for improving selection: Development of a battery for predicting air traffic controller success. *Journal of Applied Psychology, 78,* 413–432.

Bandura, A. (1986). *Social foundations of thought and action.* Englewood Cliffs, NJ: Prentice-Hall.

Boggiano, A. K., & Pittman, T. S. (Eds.). (1992). *Achievement and motivation: A social-developmental perspective.* New York: Cambridge University Press.

Carver, C. S., & Scheier, M. F. (1990). Principles of self-regulation: Action and emotion. In E. T. Higgins & R. M. Sorrentino (Eds.), *Handbook of motivation and cognition: Foundations of social behavior* (Vol. 2, pp. 3–52). New York: Guilford Press.

Corno, L., & Kanfer, R. (1993). The role of volition in learning and performance. In L. Darling-Hammond (Ed.), *Review of research in education* (Vol. 21, pp. 301–341). Itasca, IL: F. E. Peacock.

Dweck, C. S., & Leggett, E. L. (1988). A social-cognitive approach to motivation and personality. *Psychological Review, 95,* 256–273.

Fisk, A. D., & Schneider, W. (1983). Category and word search: Generalizing search principles to complex processing. *Journal of Experimental Psychology: Learning, Memory, and Cognition, 10,* 177–195.

Fleishman, E. A. (1972). On the relation between abilities, learning, and human performance. *American Psychologist, 27*(11), 1017–1032.

Goldstein, I. L., & Gilliam, P. (1990). Training system issues in the year 2000. *American Psychologist, 45,* 134–143.

Gollwitzer, P. M. (1990). Action phases and mind-sets. In E. T. Higgins & R. M. Sorrentino (Eds.), *Handbook of motivation and cognition: Foundations of social behavior* (Vol. 2, pp. 53–92). New York: Guilford Press.

Kahneman, D. (1973). *Attention and effort.* Englewood Cliffs, NJ: Prentice-Hall.

Kanfer, F. H., & Hagerman, S. M. (1981). The role of self-regulation. In L. P.

Rehm (Ed.), *Behavior therapy for depression* (pp. 143–179). New York: Academic Press.

Kanfer, R. (1987). Task-specific motivation: An integrative approach to issues of measurement, mechanisms, processes, and determinants. *Journal of Social and Clinical Psychology, 5,* 237–264.

Kanfer, R. (1990a). Motivation and individual differences in learning: An integration of developmental, differential, and cognitive perspectives. *Learning and Individual Differences, 2,* 221–239.

Kanfer, R. (1990b). Motivation theory and industrial/organizational psychology. In M. D. Dunnette & L. Hough (Eds.), *Handbook of industrial and organizational psychology: Vol. 1. Theory in industrial and organizational psychology* (pp. 75–170). Palo Alto, CA: Consulting Psychologists Press.

Kanfer, R., & Ackerman, P. L. (1989). Motivation and cognitive abilities: An integrative/aptitude-treatment interaction approach to skill acquisition [Monograph]. *Journal of Applied Psychology, 74,* 657–690.

Kanfer, R., & Ackerman, P. L. (1990). *Ability and metacognitive determinants of skill acquisition and transfer* (Air Force Office of Scientific Research Final Report). Minneapolis: University of Minnesota.

Kanfer, R., Ackerman, P. L., Murtha, T. C., Dugdale, B., & Nelson, L. (1994). Goal setting, conditions of practice, and task performance: A resource allocation perspective. *Journal of Applied Psychology, 79,* 825–835.

Kanfer, R., Ackerman, P. L., Murtha, T., & Goff, M. (1995). Personality and intelligence in industrial and organizational psychology. In D. H. Saklofske & M. Zeidner (Eds.), *International handbook of personality and intelligence* (pp. 577–602). New York: Plenum.

Kanfer, R., Dugdale, B., & McDonald, B. (1994). Empirical findings on the Action Control Scale in the context of complex skill acquisition. In J. Kuhl & J. Beckmann (Eds.), *Volition and personality: Action- and state-oriented modes of control* (pp. 61–77). Göttingen, Germany: Hogrefe & Huber.

Kuhl, J. (1985). Volitional mediators of cognition–behavior consistency: Self-regulatory processes and action versus state orientation. In J. Kuhl & J. Beckmann (Eds.), *Action control: From cognition to behavior* (pp. 101–128). New York: Springer-Verlag.

Kuhl, J., & Beckmann, J. (Eds.). (1985). *Action control: From cognition to behavior.* New York: Springer-Verlag.

Locke, E. A., & Latham, G. P. (1990). *A theory of goal setting and task performance.* Englewood Cliffs, NJ: Prentice-Hall.

Newell, A., & Rosenbloom, P. S. (1981). Mechanisms of skill acquisition and the law of practice. In J. R. Anderson (Ed.), *Cognitive skills and their acquisition* (pp. 1–55). Hillsdale, NJ: Erlbaum.

Shiffrin, R. M., & Schneider, W. (1977). Controlled and automatic human information processing: II. Perceptual learning, automatic attending, and a general theory. *Psychological Review, 84,* 127–190.

Sonnichsen, J. E. (1994). *Motivational strategy use in a sports setting: A coaches' perspective.* Unpublished manuscript, University of Minnesota.

Wood, R. E., & Locke, E. A. (1990). Goal setting and strategy effects on complex tasks. In B. M. Staw & L. L. Cummings (Eds.), *Research in organizational behavior* (Vol. 12, pp. 73–109). Greenwich, CT: JAI Press.

Woodworth, R. S. (1938). *Experimental psychology.* New York: Holt.

CHAPTER 19

Brehm's Theory of Motivation as a Model of Effort and Cardiovascular Response

Rex A. Wright

Well over a decade has passed now since I joined a small cadre of students at the University of Kansas conducting studies related to a theory being developed by our graduate advisor, Jack Brehm. At the time I joined, core members of the research group were Tom Pyszczynski, Linda Silka, Sheldon Solomon, and Challenger Vought. At later stages in my training, the group included Paul Biner, Jeff Greenberg, Tom Hill, Bruce Roberson, and Miho Toi.

The theory we investigated was one of motivation. Its central focus was "motivational intensity," or the magnitude of effort (task engagement) at a particular point in time; however, it had implications for other outcomes thought to be associated with that dimension of behavior. Most notably, the formulation made predictions about the conditions under which individuals (1) should be more and less motivationally aroused (i.e., energy mobilized for action), and (2) should appraise potential positive and negative incentives as more and less valent (i.e., attractive or repellent). Underlying assumptions were that energization is at least partially a function of engagement and that incentive appraisals are partially a function of energization.

My earliest involvement was in studies that examined effects of theoretically relevant variables on incentive appraisals (e.g., Brehm, Wright, Solomon, Silka, & Greenberg, 1983; Wright & Brehm, 1984), but over time I became increasingly interested in evaluating effects of these variables on physiological responses. The interest in physiological responses derived from both theoretical and practical considerations. For one thing, there was only limited physiological evidence relevant to implications of Brehm's analysis with respect to motivational arousal. This was particularly worrisome, in view of the fact that our interpretation of early appraisal effects assumed that those effects were accompanied by underlying energization effects. For another, it was widely recognized that performance outcomes and effort ratings provide, at best, only limited indication of actual engagement levels; therefore, it seemed that physiological indices could be useful for revealing the extent to which individuals are task-engaged. Finally, there was growing evidence implicating certain physiological responses in the etiology of negative health outcomes, and hence there was interest in factors that influence those responses. Insofar as the motivation model could uniquely account for one or more of these responses, it would have the potential to elucidate research findings and to suggest strategies for reducing responsivity and health risk.

Our initial forays into the physiological realm were unsophisticated in some respects. On the other hand, they were sufficiently informed to be guided by two assumptions that continue to appear reasonable. One was that effort effects are likely to be manifested within a system whose function is directly related to the energy mobilization process. This, along with a concern for health, led me and a few others of our team to study the cardiovascular system, which functions chiefly to convey oxygen and nutrients to tissue and to remove metabolic waste. In theory, cardiovascular adjustment occurs to maintain a rate of flow to tissue that accords with (tissue) need (Papillo & Shapiro, 1990); consequently, it would be expected to be more revealing with respect to motivation than would adjustment in some alternative system whose function is not clearly relevant to the mobilization process (e.g., the electrodermal system; see Dawson, Schell, & Filion, 1990).

The second assumption was that effort effects are probably mediated via activity in the sympathetic branch of the autonomic nervous system. Although we did not realize it early on, this is significant because it implies that engagement is more likely to affect some cardiovascular responses than others. Our thinking in this regard was originally based on classic conceptions (now known to be oversimplified) that associated the sympathetic branch with activation and the contrasting parasympathetic branch with deactivation (Andreassi, 1989). Later, it was based on emerging findings in the field of psychophysiology, which documented a link between effort (termed "active coping") and sympathetic influence on the heart and vasculature (e.g., Obrist, 1976; Obrist et al., 1978).

Postdoctoral work at SUNY–Stony Brook provided specialized training in cardiovascular psychophysiology. Thanks largely to the counsel and patience of individuals such as David Glass, Bernard Tursky, Larry Jamner, Jim Papillo, and particularly Richard Contrada, I gained greater insight into the complexities of cardiovascular function and became better positioned to carry out the full program of investigations I viewed as being suggested by the motivational model. Ensuing years have yielded progress in this regard, but have also made it apparent that implications of the model are broader than I first understood them to be. Thus, although advances have been made, my students and I see ourselves as far from a point of final accounting. The main objective of this chapter is to present an overview of what we have done and found to date. Following the overview, I comment on the findings and suggest some directions for future research.

SOME BACKGROUND

Before describing Brehm's theory and studies we have carried out, I should say something about the measures we have examined and their determinants. In all but a few investigations, we have assessed heart rate, systolic blood pressure, and diastolic blood pressure. "Heart rate" refers to the pace at which the heart pumps. "Systolic blood pressure" is the maximum pressure exerted by the blood against vessel walls following a heartbeat (the pressure at the peak of a pulse). "Diastolic blood pressure" is the minimum pressure exerted against vessel walls following a heartbeat (the pressure between pulses).

As noted above, our assumption is that engagement effects cardiovascular adjustment via the sympathetic nervous system. An increase in sympathetic activity has the potential to induce simultaneous elevations in heart rate, systolic blood pressure, and diastolic blood pressure (for a possible example, see Smith, Baldwin, & Christenson, 1990). However, it should not necessarily do so, because the three outcomes result from a complex of underlying events. Heart rate is affected not only by sympathetic activity, but also by parasympathetic activity (e.g., Berntson, Cacioppo, & Quigley, 1993). The impact of sympathetic outflow on heart rate is accelerative; the impact of parasympathetic (vagal) outflow on rate is decelerative. Although sympathetic and parasympathetic influences can be reciprocal (i.e., activity in one can decrease as activity in the other increases), they are not always. Indeed, they are sometimes antagonistic. Of particular relevance to our studies is evidence that vagal influence tends to dominate at low to moderate levels of task demand (Obrist, 1981). Thus, even with a modest increase in sympathetic arousal, heart rate can remain relatively constant.

Systolic pressure is a function of peripheral resistance and of myocardial contractility (Obrist, 1981). "Peripheral resistance" refers to the degree of resistance to flow in the circulatory system. It is produced by the state of constriction of vessels in the system. "Myocardial contractility" refers to the force of contraction in the left ventricle, the chamber of the heart that ejects blood into systemic circulation. An increase in sympathetic excitation can both enhance and diminish the caliber of blood vessels by stimulating sympathetic (adrenergic) receptors on vessel walls. A detailed account of receptor types and the manner in which they are stimulated is beyond the scope of this chapter. For present purposes, it is sufficient to understand that peripheral resistance reflects the *balance* of constrictive and dilative effects in the vasculature, and that as a result it can increase, show no change, or decrease in response to a sympathetic discharge.

Sympathetic arousal potentiates myocardial contractility; furthermore, it appears to be the main, if not sole, autonomic influence on that response (Berne & Levy, 1977). Because the relation between sympathetic activation and contractility is reasonably direct, sympathetic outflow is generally expected to increase systolic blood pressure. One exception would be when the outflow yields a decrease in peripheral resistance that is substantial enough to offset a contractility effect. Another might be when sympathetic activity is so low that its impact on contractility can be masked by some countervailing nonautonomic influence, such as that of baroreceptors, which sense vessel wall extension and reflexively reduce contractility in response to a pressure increase (Papillo & Shapiro, 1990). Even there, a systolic effect would be in evidence if resistance increased to a sufficient degree.

Diastolic pressure varies chiefly as a function of peripheral resistance. It also can be affected by heart rate, in that the pace of pumping determines the time available for pressure to drop following a pulse (Obrist, 1981). However, the effect of heart rate is likely to be minimal until a marked rate increase has been achieved. Up to a point, there can be acceleration and still an adequate interval between pulses for pressure to fall to the nadir set by the level of resistance.

The foregoing considerations, along with data from early studies of effort correlates (e.g., Obrist et al., 1978), have led us to expect systolic pressure to be the most sensitive of the responses we investigate to group differences in engagement. Systolic reactivity (elevation above baseline) should increase with effort unless (1) the induced sympathetic discharge yields a profound decrease in resistance, or (2) the sympathetic effect on contractility is slight and a contrary nonautonomic influence is powerful enough to offset any increase in resistance. We have expected heart rate to be sensitive to effort as well, but less so than systolic pressure, because the sympathetic effect on rate is likely to be masked when engagement is modest. Because diastolic pressure should be a simple function of peripheral resistance in the absence of substantial heart rate acceleration, we have expected it to be the least sensitive of our measures to engagement effects.

BREHM'S THEORY

The field of motivation is concerned with what makes an organism go. Generally speaking, motivational theories offer explanations for why organisms approach or avoid some outcomes rather than others, why they do so more or less persistently, and why they do so more or less vigorously (intensively). To the degree that traditional conceptions address the intensity aspect of motivated behavior, they suggest that it should be determined by the significance of the outcome driving behavior (see Heckhausen, 1989/1991; Weiner, 1992). Outcome significance is usually assumed to be a function of the state of the organism (need) and the character or quality of the outcome (incentive value). Thus, for example, food (an attractive incentive) should seem more significant to, and produce more vigorous behavior in, individuals who have not eaten in a while than individuals who have. Similarly, electric shock (an aversive incentive) should seem more significant and generate more vigor if it is severe than if it is mild.

Value–expectancy theories (e.g., Atkinson & Birch, 1970) highlight a third variable relevant to motivational intensity—the perceived probability of motive satisfaction (i.e., outcome attainment or avoidance). This actually constitutes an integration of at least two subperceptions: (1) that of the probability that an instrumental task may be successfully executed, and (2) that of the probability that a motive will be satisfied upon task completion. There is not complete agreement concerning the effect of the first subperception on intensity; however, most theorists agree that intensity should increase with the second. Stated differently, intensity generally is expected to increase with the perceived efficacy, or "instrumentality" (Vroom, 1964), of available behavior.

Brehm's theory of motivation (Brehm & Self, 1989; Brehm et al., 1983; Wright & Brehm, 1989) concurs with the classic and value–expectancy views insofar as it assumes that needs, incentives, and instrumentality appraisals play a role in determining the intensity of motivation. However, it differs from those views in terms of the role it proposes them to play. Brehm observes that the function of effort is not to obtain and avoid outcomes per se, but rather to carry out instrumental activity. Instrumental task demand varies independently of need, incentive value, and behavioral instrumentality; consequently, it makes little sense that the latter variables would determine effort directly. A more reasonable proposition is that they exert an indirect influence by setting the upper limit of motivation, or the peak of what individuals would be *willing* to do in the service of motive satisfaction. What should directly determine effort is what individuals believe they *must* do to satisfy a motive (i.e., the perceived difficulty of instrumental behavior). When an instrumental task is viewed as possible, engagement should be proportional to task difficulty so long as individuals are willing to invest the effort required to succeed (so long as their upper limit—or level of *potential* motivation—is not exceeded). Beyond the upper limit of what individuals are willing to do, engagement should be uniformly low. Engagement also should be low when an instrumental task is viewed as impossible or is simply unavailable. Even though there might be considerable potential for energy expenditure in such circumstances, that potential should not be realized because effort would be futile.

The essence of the preceding logic is portrayed in the panels of Figure 19.1. In the upper panel, engagement is shown to increase with task demand up to the point at which potential motivation is reached. In the lower panel, engagement is shown to increase with demand to the point at which success is perceived as impossible.

RESEARCH

The cardiovascular studies we have carried out have examined two implications that derive directly from Brehm's model and one that derives from a simple extrapolation from the model. Our first experiments were concerned

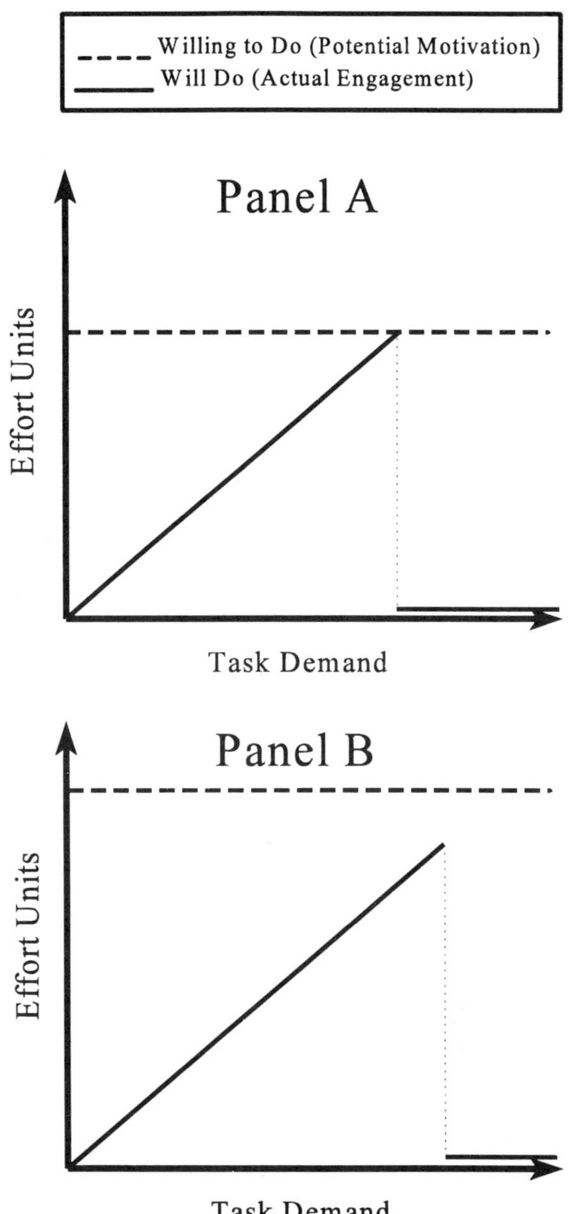

FIGURE 19.1. Effort as a function of difficulty at two levels of potential motivation.

with simple difficulty effects—that is, with the implication that effort and thus reactivity on at least some response dimensions should be greater when instrumental behavior is moderately difficult than when such behavior is easy, extremely difficult, or unavailable. More recent investigations have been concerned with the implication that the effects of difficulty and potential motivation should be interactional. This refers to the suggestion that individuals' effort and cardiovascular response to a possible behavioral challenge (potential stimulus to action) should depend not only on the difficulty of the challenge, but also on their level of potential motivation. If potential motivation is not surpassed, engagement and sympathetically mediated effects should be proportional to task difficulty (i.e., low if the challenge is mild and high if the challenge is substantial). However, if potential motivation is surpassed, engagement and reactivity should be low regardless of task demand.

Our most recent studies have examined the role perceptions of ability play in determining individuals' responses to tasks that are more and less difficult. Expectations have been predicated on the assumption that difficulty appraisals are determined not only by characteristics of a task, but also by ability perceptions with respect to the task (Ford & Brehm, 1987; Kukla, 1972, 1974; Meyer, 1987; Smith & Pope, 1992). Individuals who view themselves as having low ability should perceive the task as more difficult than should individuals who view themselves as having high ability. If Brehm's notions are correct, one suggestion is that low-ability individuals should be more engaged and manifest greater cardiovascular responsivity than should high-ability individuals, so long as both groups perceive success as possible and worthwhile. A further suggestion is that low ability-individuals should abandon their efforts to succeed more readily than high-ability individuals, because low-ability individuals should conclude at a lower (objective) difficulty level that success is too costly or impossible. Thus, where demand is high, those who see themselves as incapable should sometimes be less engaged and evince less responsivity than those who see themselves as capable. The essence of this reasoning is depicted in Figure 19.2.

In the subsections that follow, I review studies of each type in turn. Readers should understand that these are not the only implications pertaining to motivational intensity. Moreover, they should be reminded that Brehm's theory has implications for outcomes other than effort and arousal. Those interested in a more complete presentation of the model and evidence relevant to it are referred to Brehm and Self (1989) and Wright and Brehm (1989).

Simple Difficulty Effects

Not long after deciding to investigate cardiovascular responses, my coworkers and I became aware that considerable ground had already been covered with respect to simple difficulty effects. That is, various investigators, including Elliott (1969), Johnson (1963), and Obrist (e.g., Obrist et al., 1978), had

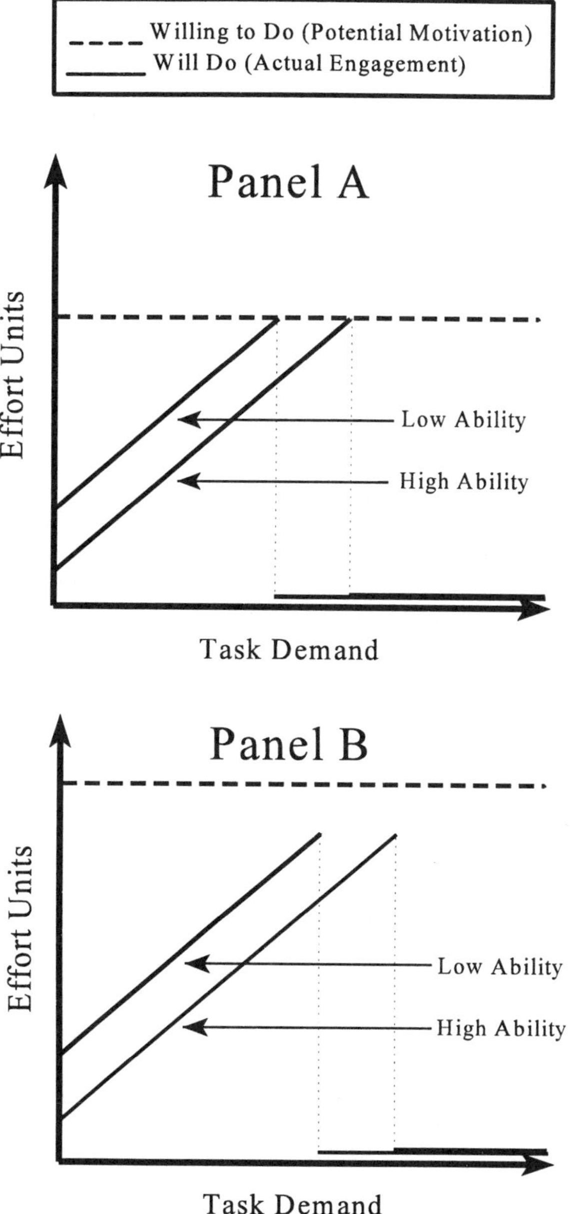

FIGURE 19.2. Effort–difficulty relation at two levels of potential motivation for individuals with low and high perceived ability.

already obtained evidence that certain responses vary nonmonotonically with the difficulty of instrumental behavior. Elliott (1969, Experiment 2), for example, gave subjects the chance to earn a monetary incentive by performing a tone discrimination task. Some subjects learned over time that the task was easy; others learned that the task was moderately difficult; and still others learned that the task was extremely difficult. Results revealed that heart rate increased over trials when demand was moderate, but decreased over trials when demand was low and when demand was extreme.

Data such as these clearly accord with Brehm's analysis (for more recent examples, see Light & Obrist, 1980, 1983; Scher, Furedy, & Heslegrave, 1984; Smith et al., 1990). However, what they reflect is how people respond when behavior is ongoing, and a major concern of ours was how people respond when behavior is imminent. This concern stemmed mainly from a desire to document as directly as possible the assumption that incentive appraisal effects are accompanied by underlying energization effects (see the introduction to this chapter). Typically, incentive appraisals were assessed just prior to task performance; hence, it was important to know whether anticipatory cardiovascular responses vary with task demand in the same fashion that performance responses appeared to vary. The issue also had some functional import. That is, if difficulty effects are anticipatory, the suggestion is that cardiovascular adjustment occurs not only to sustain behavior, but also to prepare individuals for impending action.

One of the first anticipatory studies (Wright, 1984) was one in which subjects were told either (1) that they would avoid a "learning session" involving electric shock if they successfully performed a motor task (avoidance conditions), or (2) that they were in a control group that would not have the chance to avoid the session (no-avoidance condition). For half of the avoidance subjects, the task was to flip a toggle switch, and therefore easy; for the rest, it was to make a powerful dynamometer grip, and therefore difficult. Measures of heart rate and finger pulse volume (an index of digital blood flow) were taken during the 30 seconds prior to the point at which subjects were either to perform their task (avoidance) or to pause for further instructions (no avoidance). These indicated greater anticipatory responsiveness when avoidance was to be difficult than when avoidance was to be easy and when avoidance was impossible (see Figure 19.3).[1]

Subsequent investigations conceptually replicated these effects with different tasks and incentives. In one, we (Wright, Brehm, & Bushman, 1989) varied the difficulty and availability of a cognitive avoidance task. Some subjects (easy avoidance) learned that they could prevent exposure to an aversive noise by memorizing a single nonsense trigram (e.g., "AED") in 2 minutes. Others (difficult avoidance) learned they could prevent exposure by memorizing seven trigrams in 2 minutes. For a final group (no avoidance), instructions made no mention of avoidant activity; rather, they indicated that this was a control condition in which participants would be exposed to aversive noise. Once they understood the instructions, subjects pressed a call button

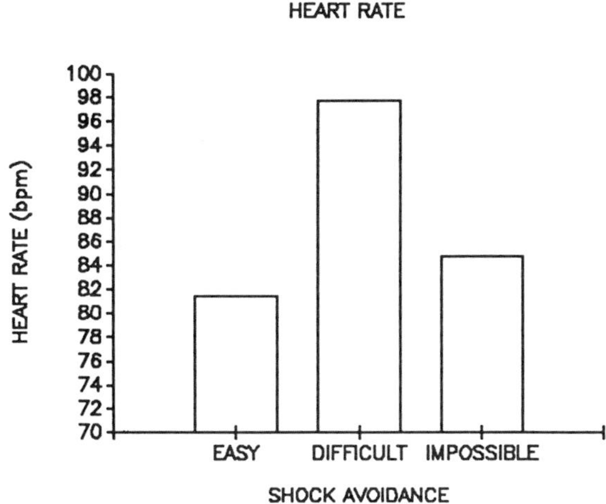

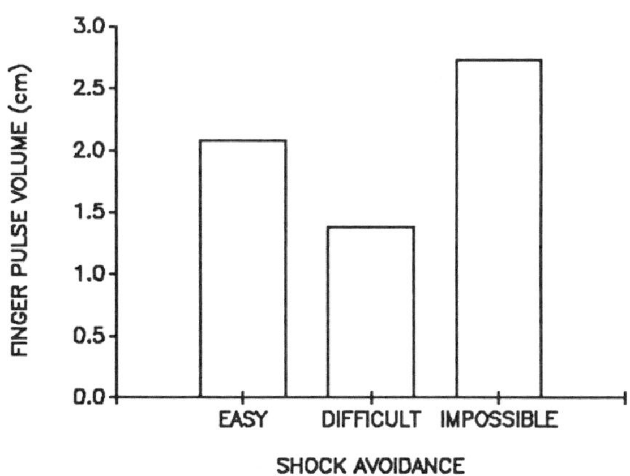

FIGURE 19.3. Anticipatory heart rate and finger pulse volume for avoidance and no-avoidance subjects. Values are residualized with respect to baseline. Adapted from Wright (1984). Copyright 1984 by the American Psychological Association. Adapted by permission.

on an intercom to indicate they were ready. Those in the conditions where avoidance was possible expected a brief (30- to 40-second) pause and then a signal to begin work. Those in the no-avoidance condition also expected a pause and signal, but were told that the signal would not apply to them. After 2 minutes, the noise was simply to come on. Measures taken after the button press indicated greater systolic and heart rate reactivity in the difficult-avoidance condition than in the easy-avoidance and no-avoidance conditions.

Diastolic responsiveness decreased as the difficulty of avoidance increased, which may be interpreted to suggest that the sympathetic discharge in the difficult-avoidance condition yielded a drop in peripheral resistance. The fact that difficult-avoidance subjects manifested respectable systolic increases ($M = +11.04$ mm Hg) implies that the drop was not great enough to offset the effect of a coincidental increase in contractility.

In another study, we (Wright, Brehm, Crutcher, Evans, & Jones, 1990, Experiment 2) also used a noise threat and a cognitive avoidance task. However, this experiment (1) included a no-avoidance condition in which a task was impossible, instead of unavailable; and (2) made cardiovascular assessments during as well as before the performance period. Instructions simply informed subjects they could avoid noise by memorizing 2 (easy task), 8 (difficult task), or 20 (impossible task) nonsense trigrams in 3 minutes. Immediately prior to performance, systolic responsivity was found to be nonmonotonically related to avoidant task demand; that is, it was greater in the difficult condition than in the easy and impossible conditions. During performance, the nonmonotonic pattern was observed for heart rate as well as systolic pressure.

Two studies examined anticipatory effects in an appetitive, rather than an avoidant, context. In one (Contrada, Wright, & Glass, 1984), subjects were offered $3.00 for solving 8 out of 10 (mental) math problems in 5 minutes. Half received problems that were easy, and half received problems that were moderately difficult. Measures taken just before the work period indicated more pronounced systolic responses among those in the latter group than among those in the former group. The other experiment (Wright, Contrada, & Patane, 1986) changed the task and added a third difficulty condition. Subjects learned that they could earn a small prize (their choice of several pens) by memorizing 2 (easy task), 6 (difficult task), or 20 (impossible task) nonsense trigrams in 2 minutes. Once again, measures of blood pressure and heart rate were taken just prior to work. Results showed greater systolic responsiveness when the task was to be difficult than when the task was to be easy or impossible.

Together, studies that have examined anticipatory effects and studies that have examined effects during the performance period strongly support the suggestion that engagement and sympathetically-mediated cardiovascular effects are a nonmonotonic function of difficulty when instrumental behavior is available and low when instrumental behavior is unavailable. On the other hand, they do not address the central suggestion of Brehm's analysis—that needs, incentives, and instrumentality appraisals do not affect effort and reactivity directly, but rather do so indirectly by setting the upper bound of what people are willing to do. In view of these studies, one could maintain that difficulty is simply one of many factors that exerts a direct effect. It is largely for this reason that the experiments described in the next subsection are critical.

Interactional Influences

The implication from Brehm's model is that potential motivation should moderate the relation between difficulty and cardiovascular response. So long as success is viewed as possible and worthwhile, effort and reactivity should be proportional to task demand. However, when the difficulty of a possible task surpasses potential motivation, effort and reactivity should be low.

Some evidence comes from a well-known investigation by Manuck, Harvey, Lecheiter, and Neal (1978), in which subjects performed easy or difficult concept formation problems with instructions that success either would (control) or would not (no control) prevent an unpleasant noise. Systolic elevations during performance were found to be proportional to task demand for control subjects, but low in both task conditions for no-control subjects. These findings can be interpreted to indicate that the effort required by the difficult task was perceived as warranted when instrumentality was high (i.e., when there was a 100% chance that success would prevent noise), but not when instrumentality was low (i.e., when there was a 0% chance that success would prevent noise). Unfortunately, because performance consequences were certain, the data are open to other interpretations as well. For example, it could be that they provide another demonstration of how individuals respond when it is easy, difficult, and impossible to avoid an unpleasant outcome. Better evidence comes from studies we have conducted, which included explicit manipulations of behavioral instrumentality, incentive value, and need.

Instrumentality

The earliest instrumentality experiment (Wright & Gregorich, 1989) provided subjects the opportunity to earn either a high or a low chance of winning a prize by succeeding on an easy or a moderately difficult memorization task. More specifically, subjects were assigned either two or five nonsense trigrams to memorize in 2 minutes, and were told that if they succeeded, the experimenter would draw from a deck of cards numbered from 1 to 15. Those in the high-instrumentality conditions were informed that they would be given a spiral notebook if the experimenter drew anything but the 15. Those in the low-instrumentality conditions were informed that they would be given the notebook if the experimenter drew the 15. Analysis revealed greater anticipatory systolic responsivity in the moderately difficult than in the easy condition only when the probabilistic link between success and motive satisfaction was strong (i.e., when success earned a high chance of winning the prize). When the link was weak, anticipatory systolic responsivity was low regardless of task demand (see Figure 19.4).

Later experiments examined interactional effects in avoidance and al-

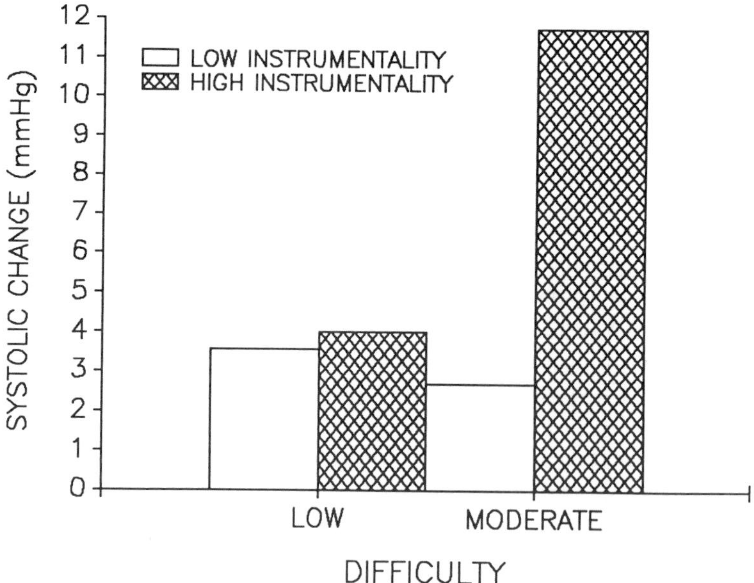

FIGURE 19.4. Systolic change scores for low- and high-instrumentality subjects under easy and moderately difficult task conditions. Adapted from Wright and Gregorich (1989). Copyright 1989 by the Society for Psychophysiological Research. Adapted by permission.

leviation contexts. In one, we (Wright, Williams, & Dill, 1992) presented subjects with computer-generated trials of an easy or moderately difficult digit recognition task. On each trial, the computer presented a string of either three (easy) or seven (moderately difficult) digits, went blank for a brief period, and then produced a question asking whether a particular digit had been in the preceding string. If the digit had been, subjects were to press a button on a keypad with which the computer had been equipped; if the digit had not been, subjects were to press another keypad button. Half of the participants were told that a good performance (90% success rate) would ensure a high (19/20) chance of avoiding noise at the end of the work period, whereas the rest were told that a good performance would ensure a low (1/19) chance of avoiding noise at the end of the period. Measures taken during work indicated that systolic and heart rate responses were proportional to difficulty when behavioral instrumentality was high, but low under easy and difficult conditions when behavioral instrumentality was low.

In another study, we (Murray, Wright, & Williams, 1993) used a similar procedure; however, we (1) presented strings of letters instead of strings of digits, (2) exposed subjects to intermittent noise during the task period, and (3) told the subjects they could earn a high or low chance of turning the noise off by performing well. The situation was considered analogous to a variety of real-life circumstances in which individuals have the chance to gain relief from physical or psychic discomfort by adhering to some therapeutic regimen (which may be more or less difficult and may be perceived as more or less efficacious). Results showed the expected interactive pattern for systolic responsivity.

Incentive Value

To date, two studies have examined interactional effects of difficulty and incentive value. The first operationalized value in terms of the noxiousness of a noise that could be avoided (Wright, Shaw, & Jones, 1990, Experiment 1). Subjects were assigned an easy or a moderately difficult (trigram) memorization task and were led to believe that they could prevent a mild blast (low incentive value) or a severe blast (high incentive value) by doing well. Cardiovascular measures were taken immediately prior to and during a brief performance period. Difficulty was found to potentiate systolic and heart rate responses when the noise was presented as severe; by contrast, it had a slight attenuating effect on these responses when the noise was presented as mild (see Figure 19.5).

The other study of this type operationalized value in a less traditional manner, in terms of the potential for social evaluation (Wright, Tunstall, Williams, Goodwin, & Harmon-Jones, 1995, Experiment 1). Conventional conceptions in social psychology assume that social evaluation enhances physiological activation, either inherently (Zajonc, 1965, 1980) or through some secondary process such as anxiety production (Cottrell, 1972; Cottrell, Wack, Sekerak, & Rittle, 1968) or distraction (Baron, 1986; Sanders, 1981). Our engagement research does not necessarily dispute this, but does present the possibilities that cardiovascular effects of social evaluation may be at least partially mediated by effort, and, insofar as they are, may be manifested only under certain conditions. From the current perspective, a publicity manipulation frequently constitutes a manipulation of incentive value, because evaluated subjects often have greater reason to try than unevaluated subjects (Geen, 1991; Geen & Bushman, 1989). To the degree that publicity increases the subjective significance of success, it would be expected to increase the peak of what subjects would be willing to do (potential motivation), but not actual effort and reactivity. What should determine effort and reactivity is the difficulty of the task with which subjects are confronted. When a possible task is easy, these should be low regardless of the potential for evaluation. On the other hand, when a possible task is difficult, effort requirements should sometimes be viewed as worthwhile only if an audience is present. In such circumstances, effort and reactivity would be expected to be relatively great under public conditions, but low under private conditions.

Subjects performed trials of an easy or moderately difficult version of a recognition memory task similar to the one used in the Murray et al. (1993) study. Instructions indicated that the study was a pilot study and therefore that responses would not be permanently recorded. In half of the cases (no-

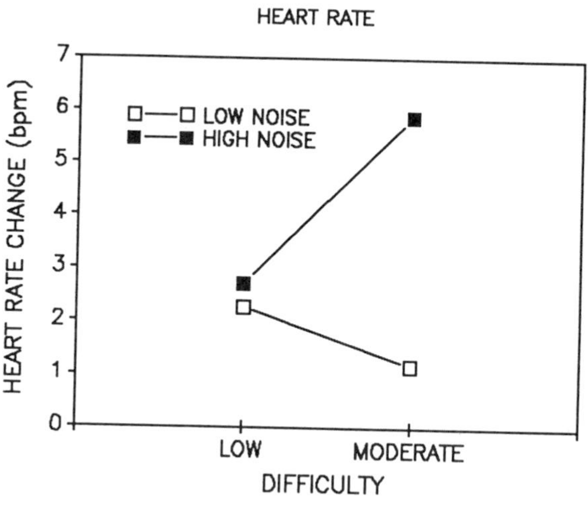

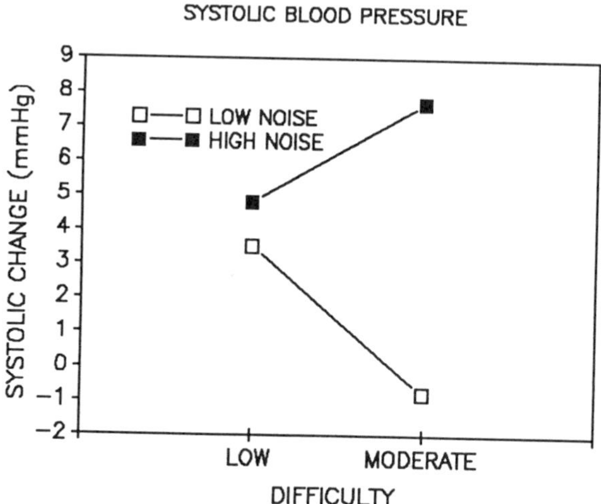

FIGURE 19.5. Heart rate and systolic change scores for low- and high-noise (incentive value) subjects under easy and moderately difficult task conditions. Adapted from Wright, Shaw, and Jones (1990, Experiment 1). Copyright 1990 by the American Psychological Association. Adapted by permission.

audience conditions), the instructions went on to say that because responses would not be recorded, people in an adjacent control room would have no way of knowing how well subjects performed. In the remaining cases (audience conditions), they went on the say that although responses would not be recorded, people in the control room could observe the session on a remote monitor and determine how well subjects performed. Systolic responses for females confirmed expectations (Figure 19.6). When the task was easy, both the audience and no-audience groups manifested little systolic reactivity; by contrast, when the task was difficult, audience subjects had substantial systolic elevations, whereas no-audience subjects showed little systolic responsiveness. Systolic elevations for males were uniformly modest and thus did not conform to expectations. Although the reason is not certain, a possibility is that males were less concerned with impressing the primary evaluative audience (an undergraduate assistant) than were the females. If they

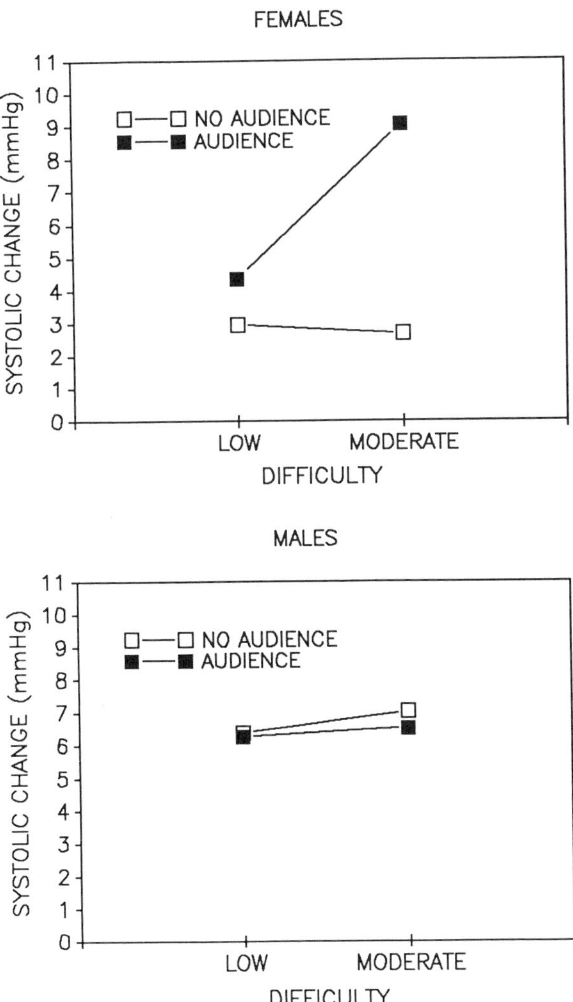

FIGURE 19.6. Systolic change scores for female and males who performed the easy and moderately difficult versions of the memory task under private (no-audience) and public (audience) conditions. Adapted from Wright, Tunstall, Williams, Goodwin, and Harmon-Jones (1995). Copyright 1995 by the American Psychological Association. Adapted by permission.

were, their potential motivation might have been low enough that the effort required by the more difficult task was not perceived as warranted.

Need

We also conducted two investigations that examined interactional effects of difficulty and need. The earlier of the two was unconventional, in that its aim was to alter potential motivation by affecting subjects' inclination to benefit another person (Wright, Shaw, & Jones, 1990, Experiment 2). Subjects were assigned an easy or moderately difficult (trigram) memorization task and told that if they succeeded, they would earn a donation for a woman with various personal problems (Toi & Batson, 1982). Half had listened earlier to an audiotape describing the woman's plight, with instructions to imagine how she must feel; the rest had listened with instructions to attend to technical aspects of the presentation. On the basis of research and theory implicating empathy in the activation of altruistic motives (e.g., see Batson, 1987), it was assumed that the need to help would be greater in subjects who took the victim's perspective than in subjects who took the technical perspective. Consequently, it was predicted that reactivity would be a function of task demand among victim-perspective subjects, but not among technical-perspective subjects. Systolic responses assessed just prior to performance supported this prediction. For those with a high need to help, responsivity was greater in the moderately difficult than in the easy condition; for those with a low need to help, responsivity was low regardless of the task assigned.

In the later study, we (Storey, Wright, & Williams, 1995) took a more conventional tack, but obtained less typical results. In this case, need was operationalized in terms of fluid deprivation. Subjects who either had (dehydrated) or had not (hydrated) refrained from drinking for a relatively extended period were given the chance to earn a choice of beverages by doing well on trials of the computer recognition memory task (e.g., Murray et al., 1993). For half the trials were easy, and for half they were moderately difficult. Analysis indicated that difficulty and need (deprivation) interacted to determine diastolic responsivity during the work period. Whereas diastolic responses were more pronounced under moderately difficult than under easy conditions for dehydrated subjects, they were slightly (not reliably) lower under moderately difficult than under easy conditions for hydrated subjects (Figure 19.7).

The interactive pattern observed for diastolic responsivity suggests that engagement effects were present and were manifested in terms of an increase in vascular resistance. The absence of systolic and heart rate effects was not expected; however, it might be explained in terms of the observation that heart rate reactivity was low ($M = +1.55$ beats per minute) and blood pressure reactivity was modest (systolic $M = +6.85$ mm Hg, diastolic $M = +5.92$ mm Hg) even when effort was expected to be the greatest (difficult/dehydrated condition). This suggests that the procedure may have elicited less engage-

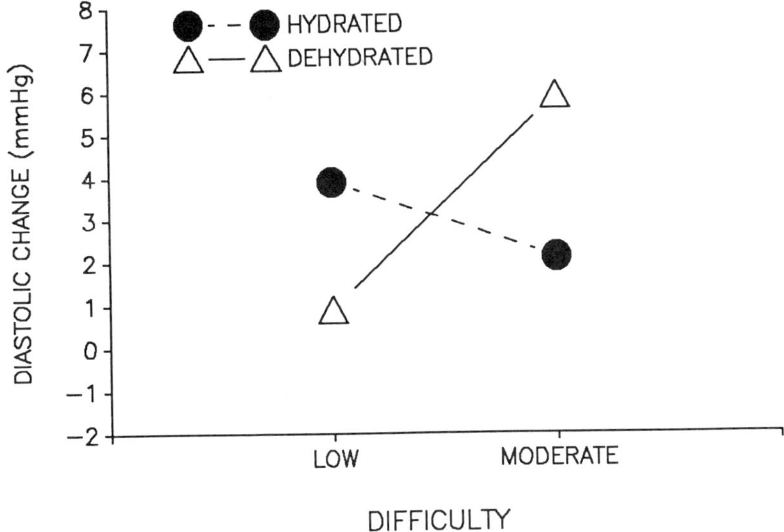

FIGURE 19.7. Diastolic change scores for hydrated and dehydrated subjects under easy and (moderately) difficult task conditions. Adapted from Storey, Wright, and Williams (1995).

ment than other procedures have, possibly because of the energy-deleting effects of fluid deprivation. If engagement was limited, the effect of sympathetic activity on rate could have been neutralized by the countervailing effect of parasympathetic activity. Furthermore, sympathetic influence on contractility could have been so slight as to be offset by a contrary nonautonomic influence.

Summary

A total of seven experiments have crossed difficulty manipulations with explicit manipulations of potential motivation. The findings support the suggestion that potential motivation moderates the relation between difficulty on the one hand, and effort and reactivity on the other. Potential motivation has been operationalized in terms of all three variables specified by Brehm's model—need, incentive value, and behavioral instrumentality. In no instance did these affect cardiovascular responses directly. Instead, they did so indirectly, apparently by determining whether effort requirements were justified.

Role of Perceived Ability

The third line of investigation we have pursued is that concerned with ability perceptions. Predictions have been based on the assumption that tasks appear more difficult to individuals who feel incapable with respect to them than to individuals who feel capable with respect to them. In combination with Brehm's reasoning, this suggests that effort and reactivity should be a conjoint function of perceived ability and objective task demand. Effort and reactivity should be greater for those with low perceived ability than for those with high perceived ability, so long as both groups view success as possible and worthwhile. However, low-ability individuals should abandon their efforts to succeed more readily than high-ability individuals; thus, where objective demand is high, effort and reactivity should sometimes be *lower* in the former group than in the latter group.

The first experiment had subjects do their best on a scanning task and then provided them with feedback that they had done either well (high ability) or poorly (low ability) in comparison to others (Wright & Dill, 1993). Later, subjects performed a similar task with the chance to win a prize if they attained a low or a high performance standard. Measurements before and during the performance period indicated that blood pressure (systolic and diastolic) reactivity was greater under high-standard than low-standard conditions for high ability subjects, but somewhat (not reliably) lower under high-standard than low-standard conditions for low-ability subjects. Moreover, whereas blood pressure responses tended to be greater for low-ability than high-ability subjects when the standard was low, they were greater for high-ability than low-ability subjects when the standard was high.

We (Wright, Wadley, Pharr, & Butler, 1994) later extended this study by examining anticipatory responses evoked (1) in an avoidant (instead of an appetitive) context, and (2) by naturally occurring (instead of experimentally manipulated) ability perceptions. Subjects who reported in a screening session that they were good or bad at math were told that they could avoid noise by solving math problems described as easy, difficult, or extremely difficult. As expected, the relation between difficulty and anticipatory systolic responsivity differed between the ability groups. High-ability subjects tended to evince greater responsivity as the challenge became greater (linear trend, $p < .10$); by contrast, low-ability subjects manifested greater responsiveness in the difficult condition than in the easy or extremely difficult conditions (quadratic trend, $p < .05$). Comparisons within difficulty conditions indicated that whereas low-ability subjects tended to show more elevated responses than high-ability subjects when avoidance was easy, and did show such responses more than high-ability subjects when avoidance was difficult, they tended to respond less than high-ability subjects when avoidance was extremely difficult.

In another study, we (Wright & Dismukes, 1995) also examined responses in an avoidant context. However, we manipulated ability perceptions experimentally and evaluated effects when behavior was ongoing instead of imminent. As in the Wright and Dill (1993) investigation, subjects performed a scanning task and received feedback indicating that they had low or high scanning ability. They then were exposed to a noxious noise sample and were told that they could avoid extended exposure to the noise by attaining a low (easy) or high (difficult) standard on a second task similar to the first. Analysis revealed that ability interacted with standard to determine systolic, diastolic, and heart rate responsiveness during the performance period (see Table 19.1). The expected crossover pattern was strongest in the case of heart rate. Heart rate responses were more pronounced in the difficult than in the easy condition for high-ability subjects, but less pronounced in the difficult than in the easy condition for low-ability subjects. Moreover, they were more pronounced for low-ability than high-ability subjects when the standard was objectively easy ($p < .06$), but less pronounced for low-ability than high-ability subjects when the standard was objectively difficult. Patterns were generally the same for systolic and diastolic reactivity; however, pairwise comparisons in those cases were less consistently reliable.

The most recent study of this type (Murray, 1994) was conducted to investigate the possibility that the ability analysis may shed light on reported gender differences in cardiovascular responsivity (Stoney, Davis, & Matthews, 1987). Most often, men show greater responsivity than women; however, in some studies the opposite has been found (e.g., Liberson & Liberson, 1975). A popular conjecture is that men try harder and evince more pronounced responses on "masculine" tasks, whereas women try harder and evince more pronounced responses on "feminine" tasks (Lash, Gillespie, Eisler, & Southard, 1991; Matthews, Davis, Stoney, Owens, & Caggiula, 1991). Typically, masculine tasks are considered to be those in regard to which males are socialized to feel competent, and feminine tasks are considered to be those in regard to which females are socialized to feel competent. Although this popular gender-relevance hypothesis is not unreasonable, it assumes that engagement is proportional to perceived competence within a performance domain. The present reasoning, of course, implies something different. It suggests that members of the gender socialized to feel more capable should try harder and show greater reactivity than members of the other gender only at comparatively high levels of objective demand. At lower levels of demand—where individuals in both gender groups view success as possible and worthwhile—the relation between gender on the one hand, and effort and reactivity, on the other, should be reversed.

TABLE 19.1. Blood Pressure and Heart Rate Change as a Function of Perceived Ability and Objective Task Demand

	Low ability		High ability	
	Easy	Difficult	Easy	Difficult
Systolic blood pressure (mm Hg)	11.2	7.7	10.6	12.7
Diastolic blood pressure (mm Hg)	12.3	5.0	9.9	10.0
Heart rate (bpm)	11.0	4.5	5.8	12.7

Note. Adapted from Wright and Dismukes (1995). Copyright 1995 by the Society for Psychophysiological Research. Adapted by permission.

Murray (1994) evaluated this application in an experiment that led subjects to believe a version of the computer recognition memory task was something on which females consistently excelled (feminine task) or males consistently excelled (masculine task). Instructions in each case indicated that the gender gap was substantial and apparently attributable to a difference in ability rather than a difference in effort. Shortly after receiving the information about gender relevance, subjects performed the task with the opportunity to avoid an unpleasant noise by obtaining either a low or a high performance standard. Analysis of systolic responses assessed during the performance period revealed a gender × gender relevance × standard interaction (Figure 19.8). When the task was identified as feminine, males demonstrated greater reactivity than females under easy conditions, but slightly (not reliably) less reactivity than females under difficult conditions. When the task was identified as masculine, males demonstrated less reactivity than females under easy conditions, but slightly (not reliably) greater reactivity than females under difficult conditions. Similar effects were observed for heart rate, although the three-way interaction in that case only approached significance.

In sum, four studies have examined factorially the effects of perceived ability and objective demand. Overall, results support the suggestion that effort and reactivity will be greater for low-ability than high ability individuals when objective demand is low, but will tend to be lower for low-ability than high-ability individuals when objective demand is high. Ability has been studied both as an experimental variable and as a quasi-experimental variable. In no instance did ability have a main effect on responsivity. Instead, its influence was found to be reversed at one level of difficulty relative to another or others.

SOME OBSERVATIONS

I suggested at the beginning of this chapter that I began to study physiological responses with several purposes in mind. One was to investigate implications of Brehm's analysis with respect to motivational arousal, with an eye toward anticipatory responses because of their special relevance to studies that have assessed incentive appraisals just prior to performance. Another was to attempt to identify a response or set of responses that provides information about the extent to which individuals are task-engaged. A third was to determine whether Brehm's model is uniquely predictive with respect to potentially pathological physiological responses, and thus might serve as a framework for interpreting effects and developing interventions aimed at reducing responsivity and health risk. Findings presented in the preceding section indicate that some degree of success has been achieved with respect to each of these purposes.

Regarding the first, my colleagues and I have obtained evidence that

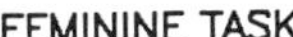

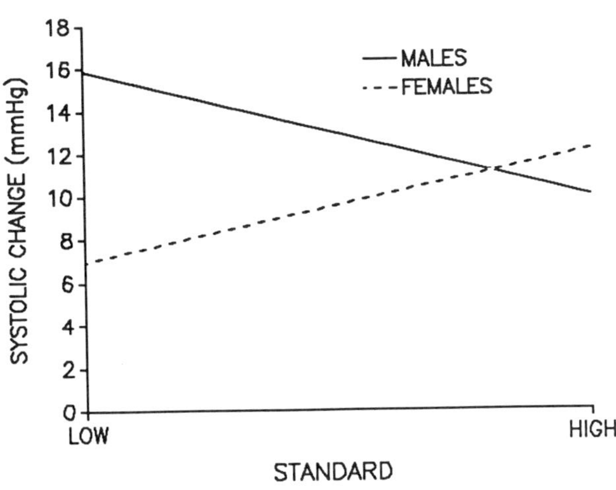

MASCULINE TASK

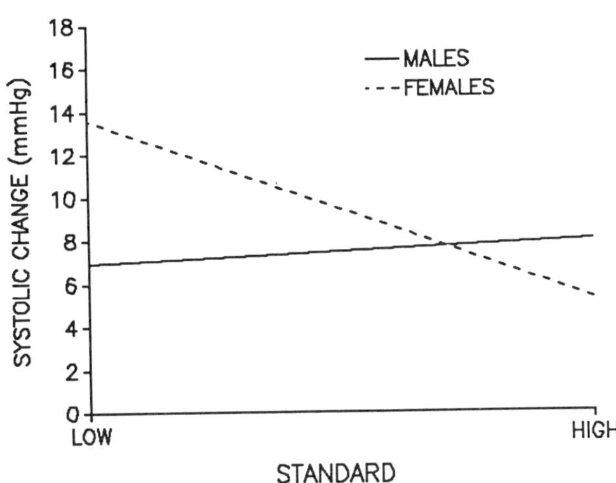

FIGURE 19.8. Systolic change scores for males and females who received low- and high-ability feedback under low- and high-standard conditions. Adapted from Murray (1994). Copyright 1994 by J. B. Murray. Adapted by permission of the author.

cardiovascular adjustment is affected by difficulty and variables associated with potential motivation in the manner predicted by the theory. Cardiovascular adjustment presumably occurs to support behavior; therefore, implications with respect to motivational arousal appear to be borne out. Predictions have been confirmed not only during performance, but also immediately prior to performance. Consequently, the data bolster interpretations of corresponding appraisal effects predicated on the assumption that valence strength varies with energy level (for reviews of appraisal findings, see Brehm & Self, 1989; Wright & Brehm, 1989).

Regarding the second purpose, we have obtained evidence that tonic (relatively long-term) cardiovascular changes in comparison to baseline are informative with respect to task engagement. The most revealing measure we have studied appears to be systolic change. In all but a few experiments, systolic responses were in the pattern predicted for effort. Heart rate change also appears revealing, but less so than systolic change, presumably because rate is under parasympathetic as well as sympathetic control. Diastolic change appears relatively insensitive to group differences in engagement, although in one study it was the only response dimension on which experimental effects were observed. This latter investigation underscores the point that cardiovascular responses are *not* invariant reflections of effort or arousal. Rather, they are indices that must be interpreted cautiously in light of their underlying determinants.

I might note that the potential utility of cardiovascular measures as indices of engagement seems boundless. One circumstance in which they could be of considerable value is in studies of learned helplessness, where poor performance following extended exposure to noncontingency is commonly taken to reflect reduced effort (e.g., Abramson, Seligman, & Teasdale, 1978). Though this appears reasonable, it is not necessarily the case, because the relation between effort and performance is imperfect. An alternative possibility is that failure yields redoubled effort and hence motivational arousal that is great enough to interfere with performance (Ford & Neal, 1985). By including cardiovascular measures in their research, helplessness investigators could facilitate the interpretation of performance deficits.

Cardiovascular measures may also prove useful in studies of persuasion and person perception. In the former domain, there has been the suggestion that people sometimes process messages directly in terms of content, and at other times process them indirectly in terms of secondary presentation features (Chaiken, 1980; Petty & Cacioppo, 1986). Direct processing is thought to be more effortful than indirect processing; thus, research scientists could utilize measures of cardiovascular response to gain information about which type is taking place. In the latter domain, it has been suggested that observers initially make characterological attributions with respect to the behavior of others and then "correct" those attribution to account for situational factors that might have caused the behavior (Gilbert, McNulty, Guiliano, & Benson, 1992). The second step (correction) is seen as harder than the first:

therefore, cardiovascular measures might be used to help determine whether it is being taken.

Regarding the third purpose, we have obtained evidence that Brehm's model not only predicts cardiovascular responses (which have been implicated in the development of heart disease and hypertension; e.g., Turner, 1994), but accounts for them where other conceptions cannot. Two cases in point are situations where (1) avoidant behavior is extremely difficult or unavailable, and (2) success on an instrumental task affects only slightly the likelihood that an aversive outcome will occur. Popular stress and coping models suggest that cardiovascular responses should be pronounced in such circumstances, because control is low and therefore threat is high (Baum, Grunberg, & Singer, 1982). By contrast, Brehm's formulation suggests that reactivity should be low because effort is either futile or not worthwhile. A related case is a situation where perceived ability is low with respect to an objectively difficult avoidant task. Self-efficacy theory (Bandura, 1983, 1991) implies that reactivity should be high, because stress and the physiological stress response are inversely proportional to the perceived capacity to cope. By contrast, our simple extrapolation from the motivation model suggests that reactivity should be low, because those who view themselves as relatively incapable should tend to abandon their efforts to succeed where objective demand is high.

Still another case in point is a situation where difficulty is low and there is a manipulation of need or incentive value. Most general motivational views and at least one (motivationally based) formulation in psychophysiology (Fowles, 1982, 1987) imply that responsivity should be greater as the level of need or value becomes higher. By contrast, Brehm's model indicates that responsivity should be low regardless of need or value, because only a small amount of effort is called for.

Examples of effects that might be illuminated by the model are the gender differences in cardiovascular reactivity discussed earlier. A further example is the limited relationship observed between individuals' physiological responses to one task and their physiological responses to another task (e.g., Kamarck, 1992). This could be partially attributable to subjects' view of themselves as being differentially capable with respect to different types of activities (e.g., quantitative vs. verbal). In theory, ability effects observed with one task ought to generalize only to other tasks in regard to which individuals feel comparably capable.

Insofar as therapeutic intervention is concerned (Jacob & Chesney, 1986), the present reasoning suggests that in general, those interested in reducing reactivity should focus less on threats and challenges per se and more on conditions under which those things translate into an increased intention to try. At a more specific level, it suggests that programs designed to foster perceptions of self-efficacy and thereby reduce responsivity and health risk (e.g., Bandura, 1991) may not always have their intended effect. That is, they may sometimes potentiate responsivity and risk by encouraging effort when demands are extremely difficult or even impossible to meet.

In the broadest sense, findings reviewed in the preceding section clarify how needs and incentives give rise to energy. Collectively, the data make a good case for the argument that they do so indirectly, via perceptions of what is necessary and possible to do in the service of motive satisfaction.

DIRECTIONS FOR FUTURE RESEARCH

Although strides have been made, considerable work remains to be done. One need is for a more complete evaluation of effects of individual-difference dimensions relevant to parameters of the motivation model. We have begun research on one of these, perceived ability. However, there are issues pertaining to this that we have not addressed, and a host of potentially relevant dimensions with which we have not dealt at all. Regarding ability, we have shown interactional effects, but have not demonstrated that responses will be relatively reduced for both low- and high-ability groups if objective demand is sufficiently high. We also have not investigated determinants of ability percepts. Presumably these derive in part from innate capacities (talents), but they also should derive from training (skills) and could derive from moment-to-moment evaluations of energy availability or even mood. Thus, for example, an individual who is exhausted from a day at the office may feel less capable with respect to some tasks than an individual who is rested. And someone who is anxious may feel less capable than someone who is calm.

In regard to other dimensions, it is important to recognize that need may be construed not only narrowly in terms of the state of an individual, but also broadly in terms of differences among individuals. Hence, Type A individuals might be conceived of as having a greater need to satisfy certain motives (e.g., achievement motives; O'Keefe & Smith, 1988) than Type B persons (Matthews, 1982). Similarly, those who are high in hostility might be conceived of as having a greater need to correct injustice than those who are low in hostility (Friedman, 1992). To the degree that these conceptions are appropriate, the implication is that dimension status should combine with the difficulty of satisfying dimension-relevant motives to determine effort and reactivity. A characteristic like optimism is particularly interesting to consider in this connection, because it appears related to more than one parameter of the model. That is, optimistic individuals could have relatively favorable expectancies with respect to their capacity to perform and the likelihood that success will yield desired outcomes (instrumentality; see Scheier & Carver, 1985). This suggests that those who are optimistic may generally view success as easier and may have higher potential motivation than those who are pessimistic.

Other needs are for (1) studies of difficulty effects on physiological outcomes other than those discussed here, and (2) studies of the motivational effects of variables not identified in the model as it is presently specified. Of special interest with respect to the former might be outcomes accessed via a relatively new technique known as "impedence cardiography" (see Papillo & Shapiro, 1990). This permits assessment of underlying cardiovascular responses such as contractility, stroke volume (amount of blood pumped in a cardiac cycle), and cardiac output (heart rate × stroke volume), some of which could prove more closely associated with engagement than blood pressure and heart rate responses are. Of interest with respect to the latter might be the expectancy that an outcome will be attained or avoided in the *absence* of action (e.g., Heckhausen, 1989/1991). This expectancy is not a part of Brehm's analysis, but might reasonably be predicted to diminish potential motivation.

One of the most pressing needs, in my view, is for research aimed at understanding motivational responses in situations where difficulty is not fixed—that is, where individuals are free to expend as much energy as they choose, and potential benefit varies depending on the performance level attained. In such circumstances, individuals should set their own performance standard (difficulty level); furthermore, the standard set should be a function of variables associated with potential motivation (Brehm & Self, 1989). Thus, subjects might be expected to work harder generating uses for a knife if they are paid a dime for each use generated than if they are paid a penny for each use generated. This is interesting because it provides an explanation for why needs and incentives sometimes seem to affect intensity directly. It also is interesting because it offers an account of results in studies that appear to show direct cardiovascular effects of need and incentive value (e.g., Belanger & Feldman, 1962; Fowles, Fisher, & Tranel, 1982). If the present reasoning is correct, these "direct" effects would not have been observed had difficulty been held constant.

NOTE

1. The Wright (1984) investigation was designed in part to distinguish the determinants of motivational intensity from those of anxiety. Manipulations intended to affect the magnitude of anxiety are only marginally relevant to the present discussion and are therefore not presented here.

REFERENCES

Abramson, L. Y., Seligman, M. E. P., & Teasdale, J. D. (1978). Learned helplessness in humans: Critique and reformulation. *Journal of Abnormal Psychology, 87,* 49–74.

Andreassi, J. L. (1989). *Psychophysiology: Human behavior and physiological response* (2nd ed.). Hillsdale, NJ: Erlbaum.

Atkinson, J. W., & Birch, D. A. (1970). *A dynamic theory of action.* New York: Wiley.

Bandura, A. (1983). Self-efficacy determinants of anticipated fears and calamities. *Journal of Personality and Social Psychology, 45,* 464–469.

Bandura, A. (1991). Self-efficacy conception of anxiety. In R. Schwarzer & R. A. Wicklund (Eds.), *Anxiety and self-focused attention* (pp. 89–110). Chur, Switzerland: Harwood.

Baron, R. S. (1986). Distraction–conflict theory: Progress and problems. In L. Berkowitz (Ed.), *Advances in experimental social psychology* (Vol. 19, pp. 1–40). New York: Academic Press.

Batson, C. D. (1987). Prosocial motivation: Is it ever truly altruistic? In L. Berkowitz (Ed.), *Advances in experimental social psychology* (Vol. 20, pp. 65–122). San Diego, CA: Academic Press.

Baum, A., Grunberg, N. E., & Singer, J. E. (1982). The use of psychological and neuroendocrinological measurements in the study of stress. *Health Psychology, 1,* 217–236.

Belanger, D., & Feldman, S. M. (1962). Effects of water deprivation upon heart rate and instrumental activity in the rat. *Journal of Comparative and Physiological Psychology, 55,* 220–225.

Berne, R. M., & Levy, M. N. (1977). *Cardiovascular physiology* (3rd ed.). St. Louis: C. V. Mosby.

Berntson, G. G., Cacioppo, J. T., & Quigley, K. S. (1993). Cardiac psychophysiology and autonomic space in humans: Empirical perspectives and conceptual implications. *Psychological Bulletin, 114,* 296–322.

Brehm, J. W., & Self, E. (1989). The intensity of motivation. *Annual Review of Psychology, 40,* 109–131.

Brehm, J. W., Wright, R. A., Solomon, S., Silka, L., & Greenberg, J. (1983). Perceived difficulty, energization, and the magnitude of goal valence. *Journal of Experimental Social Psychology, 19,* 21–48.

Chaiken, S. (1980). Heuristic versus systematic information processing and the use of source versus message cues in persuasion. *Journal of Personality and Social Psychology, 39,* 752–766.

Contrada, R. J., Wright, R. A., & Glass, D. C. (1984). Task difficulty, Type A behavior pattern, and cardiovascular response. *Psychophysiology, 21,* 638–646.

Cottrell, N. B. (1972). Social facilitation. In C. G. McClintock (Ed.), *Experimental social psychology* (pp. 185–236). New York: Holt.

Cottrell, N. B., Wack, D. L., Sekerak, G. J., & Rittle, R. H. (1968). Social facilitation of dominant responses by the presence of an audience and the mere presence of others. *Journal of Personality and Social Psychology, 9,* 245–250.

Dawson, M. E., Schell, A. M., & Filion, D. L. (1990). The electrodermal system. In J. T. Cacioppo & L. G. Tassinary (Eds.), *Principles of psychophysiology: Psychical, social, and inferential elements* (pp. 295–324). New York: Cambridge University Press.

Elliott, R. (1969). Tonic heart rate: Experiments on the effects of collative variables lead to a hypothesis about its motivational significance. *Journal of Personality and Social Psychology, 12,* 211–228.

Ford, C. E., & Brehm, J. W. (1987). Effort expenditure following failure. In C. R. Snyder & C. E. Ford (Eds.), *Coping with negative life events: Clinical and social psychological perspectives* (pp. 51–79). New York: Plenum.

Ford, C. E., & Neal, J. M. (1985). Learned helplessness and judgments of control. *Journal of Personality and Social Psychology, 49,* 1330–1336.

Fowles, D. C. (1982). Heart rate as an index of anxiety: Failure of a hypothesis. In

J. T. Cacioppo & R. E. Petty (Eds.), *Perspectives in cardiovascular psychophysiology* (pp. 93–126). New York: Guilford Press.

Fowles, D. C. (1987). Psychophysiology and psychopathology: A motivational approach. *Psychophysiology, 25,* 373–391.

Fowles, D. C., Fisher, A. E., & Tranel, D. T. (1982). The heart beats to reward: The effect of monetary incentive on heart rate. *Psychophysiology, 19,* 506–513.

Friedman, H. S. (1992). *Hostility, coping and health.* Washington, DC: American Psychological Association.

Geen, R. G. (1991). Social motivation. *Annual Review of Psychology, 42,* 377–399.

Geen, R. G., & Bushman, B. J. (1989). The arousing effects of social presence. In H. Wagner & A. Manstead (Eds.), *Handbook of social psychophysiology* (pp. 261–281). Chichester, England: Wiley.

Gilbert, D. T., McNulty, S. E., Giuliano, T. A., & Benson, J. E. (1992). Blurry words and fuzzy deeds: The attribution of obscure behavior. *Journal of Personality and Social Psychology, 62,* 18–25.

Heckhausen, H. (1991). *Motivation and action* (P. K. Leppman, Trans.). Berlin: Springer-Verlag. (Original work published 1989)

Jacob, R. G., & Chesney, M. A. (1986). Psychological and behavioral methods to reduce cardiovascular reactivity. In K. A. Matthews, S. M. Weiss, T. Detre, T. M. Dembroski, B. Falkner, S. B. Manuck, & R. B. Williams (Eds.), *Handbook of stress, reactivity, and cardiovascular disease* (pp. 417–457). New York: Wiley.

Johnson, H. J. (1963). Decision making, conflict, and physiological arousal. *Journal of Abnormal and Social Psychology, 2,* 114–124.

Kamarck, T. W. (1992). Recent developments in the study of cardiovascular reactivity: Contributions from psychometric theory and social psychology. *Psychophysiology, 29,* 491–503.

Kukla, A. (1972). Foundations of an attributional theory of performance. *Psychological Review, 79,* 454–470.

Kukla, A. (1974). Performance as a function of resultant achievement motivation (perceived ability) and perceived difficulty. *Journal of Research in Personality, 7,* 374–383.

Lash, S. J., Gillespie, B. L., Eisler, R. M., & Southard, D. R. (1991). Sex differences in cardiovascular reactivity: Effects of gender relevance of the stressor. *Health Psychology, 10,* 392–398.

Liberson, C. W., & Liberson, W. T. (1975). Sex differences in autonomic responses to electric shock. *Psychophysiology, 12,* 182–186.

Light, K. C., & Obrist, P. A. (1980). Cardiovascular response to stress: Effects of the opportunity to avoid shock, shock experience, and performance feedback. *Psychophysiology, 17,* 243–252.

Light, K. C., & Obrist, P. A. (1983). Task difficulty, heart rate reactivity, and cardiovascular responses to an appetitive reaction time task. *Psychophysiology, 20,* 301–312.

Manuck, S. B., Harvey, S. H., Lechleiter, S. L., & Neal, K. S. (1978). Effects of coping on blood pressure responses to threat of aversive stimulation. *Psychophysiology, 15,* 544–549.

Matthews, K. A. (1982). Psychological perspectives on the Type A behavior pattern. *Psychological Bulletin, 91,* 481–489.

Matthews, K. M., Davis, M. C., Stoney, C. M., Owens, J. F., & Caggiula, A. R. (1991). Does the gender relevance of the stressor influence sex differences in psychophysiological responses? *Health Psychology, 10,* 112–120.

Meyer, W. U. (1987). Perceived ability and achievement-related behavior. In F. Halisch & J. Kuhl (Eds.), *Motivation, intention, and volition* (pp. 73–86). Berlin: Springer-Verlag.

Murray, J. B. (1994). *Gender relevant tasks and the elicitation of sex differences in cardiovascular response.* Unpublished doctoral dissertation, University of Alabama at Birmingham.

Murray, J. B., Wright, R. A., & Williams, B. J. (1993). Difficulty as a determinant of cardiovascular response: Moderating effect of instrumentality in an alleviation paradigm. *International Journal of Psychophysiology, 15,* 135–145.

Obrist, P. A. (1976). The cardiovascular–behavioral interaction as it appears today. *Psychophysiology, 13,* 95–107.

Obrist, P. A. (1981). *Cardiovascular psychophysiology: A perspective.* New York: Plenum Press.

Obrist, P. A., Gaebelein, C. J., Teller, E. S., Langer, A. W., Grignolo, A., Light, K. C., & McCubbin, J. A. (1978). The relationship among heart rate, carotid dp/dt, and blood pressure in humans as a function of type of stress. *Psychophysiology, 15,* 102–115.

O'Keefe, J. L., & Smith, T. W. (1988). Self-regulation and Type A behavior. *Journal of Research in Personality, 22,* 232–251.

Papillo, J. F., & Shapiro, D. (1990). The cardiovascular system. In J. T. Cacioppo & L. G. Tassinary (Eds.), *Principles of psychophysiology: Psychical, social, and inferential elements* (pp. 456–512). New York: Cambridge University Press.

Petty, R. E., & Cacioppo, J. T. (1986). The elaboration likelihood model of persuasion. In L. Berkowitz (Ed.), *Advances in experimental social psychology* (Vol. 19, pp. 123–205). New York: Academic Press.

Sanders, G. S. (1981). Driven by distraction: An integrative review of social facilitation theory and research. *Journal of Experimental Social Psychology, 17,* 227–251.

Scheier, M. F., & Carver, C. S. (1985). Optimism, coping, and health: Assessment and implications of generalized outcome expectancies. *Health Psychology, 4,* 219–247.

Scher, H., Furedy, J. J., & Heslegrave, R. J. (1984). Phasic T-wave amplitude and heart rate changes as indices of mental effort and task incentive. *Psychophysiology, 21,* 326–333.

Smith, C. A., & Pope, L. K. (1992). Appraisal and emotion: The interactional contributions of situational and dispositional factors. In M. S. Clark (Ed.), *Review of personality and social psychology: Vol. 14. Emotion and social behavior* (pp. 32–62). Newbury Park, CA: Sage.

Smith, T. W., Baldwin, M., & Christenson, A. J. (1990). Interpersonal influence as active coping: Effects of task difficulty on cardiovascular reactivity. *Psychophysiology, 27,* 429–437.

Stoney, C. M., Davis, M. C., & Matthews, K. A. (1987). Sex difference in physiological responses to stress and in coronary disease: A causal link? *Psychophysiology, 24,* 127–131.

Storey, P. L., Wright, R. A., & Williams, B. J. (1995). *Need as a moderator of the difficulty–cardiovascular response relation: The case of fluid deprivation.* Unpublished manuscript, University of Alabama at Birmingham.

Toi, M., & Batson, C. D. (1982). More evidence that empathy is a source of altruistic motivation. *Journal of Personality and Social Psychology, 43,* 281–292.

Turner, J. R. (1994). *Cardiovascular reactivity and stress: Patterns of physiological response.* New York: Plenum.

Vroom, V. H. (1964). *Work and motivation.* New York: Wiley.
Weiner, B. (1992). *Human motivation: Metaphors, theories, and research.* Newbury Park, CA: Sage.
Wright, R. A. (1984). Motivation, anxiety, and the difficulty of control. *Journal of Personality and Social Psychology, 46,* 1376–1388.
Wright, R. A., & Brehm, J. W. (1984). The impact of task difficulty upon perceptions of arousal and goal attractiveness in an avoidance paradigm. *Motivation and Emotion, 8,* 171–181.
Wright, R. A., & Brehm, J. W. (1989). Energization and goal attractiveness. In L. A. Pervin (Ed.), *Goal concepts in personality and social psychology* (pp. 169–210). Hillsdale, NJ: Erlbaum.
Wright, R. A., Brehm, J. W., & Bushman, B. J. (1989). Cardiovascular responses to threat: Effects of the difficulty and availability of a cognitive avoidant task. *Basic and Applied Social Psychology, 10,* 161–171.
Wright, R. A., Brehm, J. W., Crutcher, W., Evans, M. T., & Jones, A. (1990). Avoidant control difficulty and aversive incentive appraisals: Additional evidence of an energization effect. *Motivation and Emotion, 14,* 5–73.
Wright, R. A., Contrada, R. J., & Patane, M. J. (1986). Task difficulty, cardiovascular response, and the magnitude of goal valence. *Journal of Personality and Social Psychology, 52,* 837–843.
Wright, R. A., & Dill, J. C. (1993). Blood pressure responses and incentive appraisals as a function of perceived ability and objective task demand. *Psychophysiology, 30,* 152–160.
Wright, R. A., & Dismukes, A. (1995). Cardiovascular effects of experimentally-induced efficacy (ability) appraisals at low and high levels of avoidant task demand. *Psychophysiology, 32,* 172–176.
Wright, R. A., & Gregorich, S. (1989). Difficulty and instrumentality of imminent behavior as determinants of cardiovascular response and self-reported energy. *Psychophysiology, 26,* 586–592.
Wright, R. A., Shaw, L. L., & Jones, C. R. (1990). Task demand and cardiovascular response magnitude: Further evidence of the mediating role of success importance. *Journal of Personality and Social Psychology, 59,* 1250–1260.
Wright, R. A., Tunstall, A. M., Williams, B. J., Goodwin, J. S., & Harmon-Jones, E. (1995). Social evaluation and cardiovascular response: An active coping approach. *Journal of Personality and Social Psychology, 69,* 530–543.
Wright, R. A., Wadley, V. G., Pharr, R. P., & Butler, M. (1994). Interactive influence of self-reported ability and avoidant task demand on anticipatory cardiovascular reactivity. *Journal of Research in Personality, 28,* 68–86.
Wright, R. A., Williams, B. J., & Dill, J. C. (1992). Interactive effects of difficulty and instrumentality of avoidant behavior on cardiovascular reactivity. *Psychophysiology, 29,* 677–689.
Zajonc, R. B. (1965). Social facilitation. *Science, 149,* 269–274.
Zajonc, R. B. (1980). Compresence. In P. Paulus (Ed.), *Psychology of group influence* (pp. 35–60). Hillsdale, NJ: Erlbaum.

PART V

Nonconscious Control of Action

Not all action is instigated through conscious, deliberate planning and decision making. The two chapters in this section explore the ways in which action is produced nonconsciously. Whereas Bargh and Barndollar (Chapter 20) focus on the routinization of intentions made consciously and deliberately in the past, Ansfield and Wegner (Chapter 21) describe a cognitive mechanism that produces currently counterintentional actions. Neither Bargh and Barndollar's preconsciously activated motivations nor Ansfield and Wegner's "ironically" instigated counterintentional behaviors are the products of a current conscious intention; they are based on nonconscious sources of action control.

According to the "auto-motive" model discussed by Bargh and Barndollar, a person's chronic motivations and goals are triggered directly by environmental information, entirely without conscious involvement in the choice of action. The nonconsciously activated goals operate to guide relevant behavior. Experimental demonstrations of such nonconsciously activated goals and their resultant behavior are provided in support of this hypothesis of automatic social behavior.

Ansfield and Wegner propose a theory of ironic processes in producing counterintentional behavior—actions that lack the "feeling of doing" associated with the phenomenal will. They argue that often behavioral goals involve avoiding certain actions (i.e., not doing something), as well as specifying desired actions. However, in order not to perform an undesired action one must watch out for it in order to stop it from occurring if it starts to. This vigilance has the drawback of making the idea of the undesired action accessible in the mind, so that if the conscious, intentional (and attention-demanding) process is distracted, the counterintentional behavior itself is often likely to be produced. The authors propose that the operation of such ironic processes accounts for the full range of "automatisms" that have long fascinated us, such as the apparently self-generated movements of a divining rod, the pointer on a Ouija board, and the table at a seance. According to Ansfield and Wegner, these movements, taken by many as evidence of the operation of supernatural forces, are phenomenally effortless products of the very act of trying not to make them.

CHAPTER 20

Automaticity in Action

The Unconscious as Repository of Chronic Goals and Motives

John A. Bargh
Kimberly Barndollar

"In all languages derived from Latin, the word 'reason' (ratio, raison, ragione) *has a double meaning: first, it designates the ability to think, and only second, the cause. Therefore reason in the sense of a cause is always understood as something rational. A reason the rationality of which is not transparent would seem to be incapable of causing an effect. But in German, a reason in the sense of a cause is called* Grund, *a word having nothing to do with the Latin* ratio *and originally meaning 'soil' and later 'basis.'. . Such a* Grund *is inscribed deep in all of us, it is the ever-present cause of our actions, it is the soil from which our fate grows. I am trying to grasp the* Grund *hidden at the bottom of each of my characters, and I am convinced more and more that it has the nature of a metaphor."*

"Your idea escapes me," said Avenarius.

"Too bad. It is the most important thought that ever occurred to me."

—MILAN KUNDERA, *Immortality* (1990, p. 237)

In *The Rediscovery of the Mind,* Searle (1992) argues against those who deny the reality of consciousness and of subjective states because they are not observable to an objective, outside party. The problem, he notes, is that this equates the methodology used to study a phenomenon with the phenomenon itself; in other words, it confuses the epistemology with the ontology. It is of course true that to study the mind scientifically and objectively, as with the scientific study of anything else, we must deal with observables and must separate the act of observation from what is being observed. But both of these methodological principles are impossible to follow in the case of consciousness: It is not observable in another person, only in oneself; and one cannot study it in oneself because one cannot separate the act of observing from what is being observed.

The logical fallacy, Searle argues, is to conclude that because one cannot apply the preferred scientific method to the study of consciousness, it therefore does not exist or is epiphenomenal. It is one thing to wish to study a phenomenon as objectively and reliably as possible (i.e., to measure observables that can be operationally defined). It is quite another to draw the conclusion that phenomena that do not lend themselves to this scientific procedure must not exist.

Searle (1992) gives many examples of the nonsensical consequences of confusing epistemology with ontology. Imagine yourself completely paralyzed but fully aware. You can produce no observable signs of consciousness, and an outside observer would have to conclude that you are not conscious, even though you yourself know you are. Searle also quotes the old joke about the two behaviorists who make love, with one saying to the other afterwards: "It was good for you. How was it for me?"

We do, of course, have subjective states and phenomenal awareness. It is just that we cannot observe them in *other* people. We should not conclude from this that other people do not have subjective states. As Searle cautions us, when we study *him* or *her,* we should keep in mind that we are studying the *me* that is the him or her.

IS THE UNCONSCIOUS JUST A SOURCE OF ERROR AND MISTAKE?

Our claim in this chapter is that a very similar confusion of epistemology and ontology has occurred in the study of the unconscious. At a very deep cultural level, as the quote from Kundera's novel illustrates so well, people have a strong and deep faith in the rationality of consciousness. Therefore, in order to demonstrate the existence of nonconscious or unconscious phenomena, researchers have had to demonstrate irrationality—judgments and behavior that cannot be explained in terms of the conscious goals or intentions of the person.

This trend was given a rousing sendoff by Freud (1901/1965), whose *The Psychopathology of Everyday Life*—subtitled *Forgetting, Slips of the Tongue, Bungled Actions, Superstitions, and Errors*—was a rich compendium of counterintentional mistakes, all attributed to the operation of unconscious forces. The more recent body of cognitive research on nonconsciously determined behavior follows Freud's lead, giving the strong impression that unconscious phenomena are solely irrational in nature. Norman (1981) has catalogued a variety of "action slips" in which intentional action becomes sidetracked when attention is distracted away from its performance. A common example is a person's being deep in thought on some matter and deciding to get something from the other room, walking there, and standing there finally wondering what it was he or she wanted. Another is a city bus driver's taking the family to a shopping mall on a Saturday morning and pulling over at all the bus stops on the way. Without a continual supplying of attentional resources to ongoing behavioral goals, action either ceases or falls into habitual grooves. In any case, the resultant behavior is unintentional—a mistake or "slip."

In another guise, these "slips" have been labeled "mindless" behavioral responses (Langer, 1978; Langer, Blank, & Chanowitz, 1978). Several experimental demonstrations were provided in which subjects acted in a manner that seemed irrational, given the information available in the environment. Again, the key variable that produces such effects is a lack of attention paid to that information, because conscious attention is focused elsewhere. In the absence of noting the presence of a critical detail that might have changed the behavioral response, that response is based on the habitual response to that situation. For instance, when one person asks to cut in front of another in a line, usually the asker gives a good reason for needing to do so. If the person being asked is not paying attention to the actual content of the request, then, as long as the request follows the usual form, that person gives the usual response. Requests that deviate from the usual form do not produce such "mindless" responses, because there is no default habitual response to these unusual, infrequently experienced situations.

Langer et al. (1978) concluded that the source of such behavior in their subjects was nonconscious or "mindless." However, there were no measures taken of awareness or consciousness or memory to substantiate this claim (see Bargh, 1984; Kitayama & Burnstein, 1988). The entire basis for the conclusion that the behavior was not conscious was that it was not *rational:* It did not appear to be the most logical response, based on all of the information present in the situation. But because of the implicit assumption, embedded in our language itself, that what is conscious is rational and what is not conscious is irrational, Langer et al. (1978) concluded that the source of their subjects' behavior was not conscious.

More recently, Wegner's (1994; Ansfield & Wegner, Chapter 21, this volume; Wegner & Erber, 1992; Wegner & Wenzlaff, in press) research on mental control mechanisms has used counterintentional thoughts and acts as the evidence for an unconscious, automatic, ironic process monitor. Intrusions of thoughts one is trying to suppress, or the occurrences of behaviors one is trying to avoid (usually while under attentional load), are typical dependent variables in this research. Jacoby and his colleagues (e.g., Jacoby, 1991; Jacoby, Lindsay, & Toth, 1992) have explicitly played on the assumption of a rational consciousness in their paradigm in order to demonstrate unconscious influences of memory. To the extent that effects occur that are opposite in direction to the subject's conscious intention (as manipulated by experimental instructions)—in other words, errors—one can assume that the effects are unconscious or automatic.[1]

In our view, the unconscious has received a "bad rap." Researchers are forced to study its manifestations in terms of errors, mistakes, and slips in order to convince skeptics that the obtained effects are not attributable to supposedly more rational, conscious processing. In doing so, this body of research has created an illusory data base, as if the only effects of unconscious processing were mistakes or errors. One of the themes of the present chapter is that the unconscious is actually quite adaptive and usually does not produce errors, but instead produces appropriate and rational decisions, choices, and behaviors.

In our own research, we deviate from the usual contemporary practice of relying on errors, slips, or "counterintentional" behaviors as our dependent measures. Instead, we activate different social goals for different subject groups outside of their awareness, and show the corresponding behavioral differences. It is one of our hopes that this methodology will enable the future study of the unconscious to move into realms of normal social functioning instead of focusing exclusively (and, in the long run, misleadingly) on maladaptive miscues.

THE UNCONSCIOUS AS ROUTINIZED CONSCIOUSNESS

Our view of the unconscious is in the spirit of James (1890, Ch. 6), Vera and Simon (1993), Searle (1992, Ch. 7), and others who view it as the as the implicit repository of a person's long-term experience. Any skill—perceptual, motor, or cognitive—requires less and less conscious attention the more frequently and consistently it is engaged in (e.g., Atkinson & Shiffrin, 1968; Newell & Rosenbloom, 1981), and eventually can operate with no conscious attention at all. In social psychology, we have demonstrations of the subsidation of several processes with frequency of use; self-relevant thought (Bargh, 1982; Bargh & Tota, 1988), dispositional attribution (Gilbert, 1989), and trait judgments of others' behavior (Bargh & Thein, 1985; Smith & Lerner, 1986) are the best examples. Smith's research (e.g., Smith, 1994) in particular has documented the decreasing need for conscious guidance of social judgments with increased experience in making them. These are intentional, goal-directed processes, just as are typing and driving a car—those two hackneyed but still useful examples of automatic phenomena. With experience, these processes come to operate autonomously; once started in motion, they interact with the complex environment as automated strategies. The professional tennis player does not consciously decide to run to a certain spot on the court, but moves there "instinctively" on the basis of the relevant cues: the speed of the ball, the angle of the opponent's racket, and expectancies of where the return shot will land (based on considerable experience in that same situation). The experienced automobile driver on a familiar route can drive for miles while daydreaming or participating in an intense conversation.

Vera and Simon (1993, p. 14) have referred to this as the "functional transparency" of the skill. With sufficient experience in the given domain, the relevant information is represented at a highly abstract functional level, so that one does not need to know anything about details. When one is just learning to drive, one must consciously make decisions as minute as when to let go of the steering wheel during a turn. Soon, one no longer needs to make that decision, because it is subsumed under the skill of making a turn; however, one still has to decide consciously to turn the wheel to make the turn. Eventually, on a familiar route, even the decision of making the turn is subsumed—becomes functionally transparent—under the abstract goal of "following the road" or "driving home."

It is important to note that what is running off autonomously and without conscious guidance here is not a static behavioral response, but an automated *strategy* for dealing with the environment to affect a desired goal. The pattern of cars, weather conditions, light, and so on is never the same, no matter how often one drives the same road. What is operating is a mental system that interacts with environmental information; in fact, the system *requires* the input in order to operate. In other words, these skills that operate nonconsciously are not simple, fixed stimulus–response connections, but complex and sophisticated strategies or plans that guide responses according to the information available in the current environment. As Vera and Simon (1993, p. 17) put it, "Plans are not specifications of fixed sequences of actions, but are strategies that determine each successive action as a function of current information about the situation."

Those who tend to view the unconscious as limited or "dumb" (see Bruner, 1992; Greenwald, 1992; Loftus & Klinger, 1992) define it rather restrictively, not allowing for any use of consciously perceived information, and not considering any immediate unconscious (i.e., preconscious) influence beyond perceptual ones. In other words, the unconscious is equated with the subliminal, and because subliminal registration of information is hardly the norm in day-to-day life (see Bargh, 1992) and results in only weak mental activations even then, it is hardly surprising for an "unconscious" so defined to be found to have limited powers. Conscious spatial attention has been found to be necessary for nearly any cognitive effect of interest, including such otherwise automatic and nonconscious effects as the Stroop phenomenon (see Kahneman & Treisman, 1984). Mental processes, not to mention ongoing plans and goals, require informational input to operate; in fact, they *only* operate when they are applicable to the informational input (see Higgins, 1989). To assess the "intelligence" of the unconscious by seeing how it does in the absence of informational input (i.e., by withholding from it any attentionally supplied information) is like taking a fish out of water and concluding from the fact that it just lies there that it is pretty stupid.

THE AUTO-MOTIVE MODEL

It is one thing to hold the position that well-practiced, complex skills can operate autonomously and without conscious guidance. It is quite another to argue that one can engage in these goal-directed actions without consciously intending to do so.

In all of the examples given above—playing tennis, driving a car, making social judgments, engaging in self-relevant thought—the person intends to engage in the activity. Once that conscious act of will takes place, the goal operates interactively with environmental information without the need for conscious guidance; however, the act of will is necessary to start the process in motion. Therefore, one should not—and we certainly do not—construe them as evidence for unconscious behavior (see Logan & Cowan, 1984).

What these examples do show, however, is that the goals that an individual frequently and consistently pursues in a given situation are capable of operating autonomously and without the need for conscious guidance. What starts them in motion? It is the activation of the goal or intention—the "top node" in the goal system under which the substrategies and processes are subsumed.

The "auto-motive" model (Bargh, 1990) makes a fundamental prediction: that this goal or intention itself—this complex strategy of interacting with the world—can be activated or triggered by environmental stimuli. In other words, the environment can directly activate a goal, and this goal can then become operative and guide cognitive and behavioral processes within that environment, all without any need or role for conscious decision-making. Because there is no involvement of conscious processing at any point in the chain from the triggering environmental information to the enactment of goal-directed action, such a phenomenon can accurately be described as "unconsciously motivated" behavior.

Thus, what the auto-motive model adds to the already extant and well-accepted notion of autonomous, well-practiced skills or goals is that the initiating act of will itself can become delegated to the environment. Take again the example of driving (one we have gotten a lot of "mileage" out of in the past). We have argued above that driving is a complex perceptual–motor skill, in which decisions as to how to move the wheel, how hard to push the accelerator, when to be ready to hit the brakes, and so on are guided nonconsciously (in the experienced driver) by environmental information. In other words, these behavioral decisions are activated by the information in the environment relevant to those decision processes. Now recall that those decisions, in the novice and less experienced driver, are at first made *consciously*. Therefore, with experience, decisions that used to have to be made consciously no longer are, and what makes those decisions if conscious processes do not? Those decisions as to what to do next—what subgoal to follow, in other words—are made directly on the basis of the environmental information present. The information itself triggers those goal-directed actions.

Thus, in principle, there is no reason to believe that the goal "to drive," or, to take a more social example, "to be patient," cannot be removed from conscious control and delegated to the environment. This is the key hypothesis of the auto-motive model of unconscious motivations—that conscious intent or will can be bypassed, that the gap between the environment and the autonomous goal can be bridged, making the entire process from start to finish nonconscious.

This position has precedents. James (1890, Ch. 4) described "secondarily automatic" thought and behavior patterns that function as do instincts ("primarily automatic") in most animals, and that develop out of extensive experience and repetition. Jung (1931/1969) also posited that regular and routine patterns of behavior can become "instinctive" and, furthermore, can occur in the absence of a conscious motive: "Instincts are typical modes of action, and wherever we meet with uniform and regularly recurring modes of action and reaction we are dealing with instinct, no matter whether it is associated with a conscious motive or not". Jung went on to note that because the motive for these habitual patterns of behavior may not be accessible to consciousness, the individual will supply a conscious motive or "rationalization" for it nonetheless and experience the action as if it were consciously chosen in the first place:

> We are in a far better position to observe instincts in animals or in primitives than in ourselves. This is due to the fact that we have grown accustomed to scrutinizing our own actions and to seeking rational explanations for them. But it is by no means certain that our explanations will hold water, indeed it is highly unlikely. . . . As a result of our artificial rationalizations it may seem to us that we were actuated not by instinct but by conscious motives. . . . There is no doubt that we have succeeded in enveloping a large number of instincts in rational explanations to the point where we can no longer recognize the original motive behind so many veils. . . . I am therefore inclined to believe that human behavior is influenced by instinct to a far higher degree than is generally supposed, and that we are prone to a great many falsifications of judgment in this respect. . . .

Gazzaniga (1985) has noted the same phenomenon in split-brain or Korsakoff's syndrome patients: A message is flashed to their right brain hemispheres to get up and leave the room (for example), and they do so. When stopped by the experimenter and asked where they are going, the subjects respond nearly immediately with a plausible (conscious) motive, such as "I needed to get a drink of water." And posthypnotic suggestions have the same flavor. A subject is given the command that when she awakens from the trance, she is to crawl around on the floor on her hands and knees. She is awakened; she crawls around on the floor and says, "I think I lost an earring down here" (Hilgard, 1977; see also Searle, 1992, Ch. 7).

The auto-motive model posits that goals and motives can become automatically associated with mental representations of environmental features in the same way that perceptual representations do—through frequent and consistent coactivation (Hebb, 1948; Shiffrin & Schneider, 1977). Perceptual categories (e.g., "tree," "house," "human being," "hat") become strongly tied to their relevant environmental features, so that these categories are activated preconsciously in the presence of the features. By "preconsciously" we mean that the categories are activated immediately and reflexively upon sensory pickup of those features in the environment, with no conscious intent or involvement necessary (Bargh, in press). So too are such more abstract social categories as racial and sex stereotypes (Bargh, 1994; Brewer, 1988; Devine, 1989) in the presence of the corresponding racial or gender features of an individual, and trait categories in the presence of relevant social behavior (Bargh & Thein, 1985; Carlston & Skowronski, 1994; Gilbert, 1989). Goals and motives must be represented mentally, just as are trait concepts and stereotypes (Bargh, 1990; Kruglanski, Chapter 26, this volume), and so in principle, should be just as capable of developing these automatic preconscious links (Bargh, 1990).

Thus, if an individual frequently and consistently chooses the same goal within a given situation, that goal eventually will come to be activated by the features of that situation and will serve to guide behavior, without the individual's consciously intending, choosing, or even being aware of the operation of that goal within the situation.

THE WISE UNCONSCIOUS

We turn next to recent experimental evidence concerning the existence of unconsciously motivated social behavior. But first let us return once more to the issue of whether the unconscious is smart or dumb. If motivations and intentions that have been pursued repeatedly by an individual in a given situation can come to be activated nonconsciously and then guide behavior, the myth of the irrational and counterintentional unconscious would be exploded. The unconscious mind would thus take over control of behavior in situations in which the individual has chronically pursued the same goal in the past. In effect, over time the individual has delegated control over his or her behavior to the environment (Bargh & Gollwitzer, 1994). The system, in other words, recognizes regularities and eventually subsumes them, so that the conscious mind no longer has to make decisions it always makes the same way anyway.

The unconscious can therefore, in principle, be a source of intentions and goals independently from conscious intents and purposes. The unconscious intentions and goals activated by situational features would be the chronic, habitual ones pursued by the individual in that situation, whereas conscious intentions are the momentary, temporary ones that may or may not be the same as the unconsciously activated ones (see Bargh & Gollwitzer, 1994; Gollwitzer, Chapter 13, this volume). That there may be these two independent sources of intentions in any given (frequently experienced) situation fits well with Freud's notion of the society of the mind, in which the conscious and unconscious portions of the ego were said to function as independent agents with their own agendas (see Glymour, 1992). The action slips categorized by Norman (1981) are good examples of these competing chronic and temporary intentions as well; doing something differently from the usual and habitual is possible but requires effort and attention, lest the behavior fall back into the chronic and unconsciously guided path.

But why should we consider the conscious purpose to be necessarily the "intentional" one, so that if behavior falls into the worn unconscious grooves, it is considered necessarily "counterintentional" or a "slip"? To our minds, the unconscious intention is just as "intentional" as—and, we would contend, perhaps even more "rational" than—the momentary conscious goal. For one thing, the unconscious intention reflects the regularities and frequency of past choices. The unconscious intention is to conscious intention as base rates are to single individuating pieces of information in the domain of judgments and decisions (e.g., Nisbett & Ross, 1980). The unconscious intention, which represents the entire history of choices by that individual in that situation, is arguably more stable and rational than the conscious choice that is in conflict with it, especially given the limits and foibles to which spur-of-the-moment conscious choices are prone (Dawes, 1976; Nisbett & Ross, 1980; Wilson & Schooler, 1991).

And why can't the *conscious* choice be the "unintended" one? Imagine that we say or do something based on how we feel at that moment—perhaps while angry, or after a drink or two, or in a very happy, giddy mood—and that it turns out badly. Later on, when we are not in that same momentary state, we regret our statement or action. We plead that what we said or did was not reflecting our true feelings or beliefs, and we point to our long past history of saying or doing something very different as evidence of our "true" beliefs in the matter. The point is that our conscious intentions and choices are always affected and moved around by our current state. Schwarz and Clore (1983; see also Schwarz, 1990) have shown how even our satisfaction with our entire lives is affected by our current, momentary mood state. To have our conscious intentions and decisions pushed around by our current temporary state is to make them much more variable and "noisy" than those based on a long history of choice; the latter must be the more stable.

Of course, there are bad habits as well as good ones. And being flexible enough to do something different from what one usually does in a situation is a critically important human ability. We are not proposing that unconscious intentions and processing are "better" than conscious intentions and processes—only that it is a mistake to equate *either* conscious or unconscious processing with rationality, and the other with irrationality. Conscious processing can be harmful or beneficial, and the same is true for unconscious processing; in other words, the dimensions "conscious–unconscious" and "good–bad" are orthogonal to one another (Higgins & Bargh, 1992).

UNCONSCIOUS INTENTIONS AND AUTOMATIC BEHAVIOR: EXPERIMENTAL EVIDENCE

Research on social perception has documented the existence of preconscious perceptual processes that influence one person's categorization of another's behavior, and consequently the impressions formed of the other person. Trait concepts such as "honesty," "intelligence," and "aggressiveness" can, with frequent use in understanding relevant social behavior, become capable of preconscious automatic activation in the presence of the features of that type of behavior in the environment. This means that the behavior is encoded and categorized in terms of that trait, regardless of the current focus of conscious attention or the current processing goal (Bargh & Pratto, 1986; Bargh & Thein, 1985; Higgins, King, & Mavin, 1982). The corresponding trait category is activated in the course of perceiving the behavior, without conscious intent or awareness of this interpretation of the information.

In the same way, social group stereotypes have been found to be preconsciously activated by the presence of features of the stereotyped group (see review in Bargh, 1994). Thus, complex mental representations of social information such as trait concepts and stereotypes can become so strongly associated with patterns of environmental information that they are activated by these patterns with no conscious involvement necessary.

The auto-motive model assumes that such preconscious effects are not limited to social-perceptual representations, but that all aspects of the psychological situation (Mischel, 1973; Mischel & Shoda, 1995)—evaluations and motivations as well as meanings and beliefs—are capable of preconscious activation (Bargh, in press). The rule in all cases is that the psychological state or representation must be frequently and consistently activated in response to the given environmental situation or event. Thus, if a given goal or motive is chronically chosen and pursued within a given situation, it should eventually come to be preconsciously (i.e., nonconsciously) triggered by the presence of those situational features.

From research on social perception, we know as well that temporarily activated or "primed" trait constructs behave identically to chronically accessible trait constructs (Bargh, Bond, Lombardi, & Tota, 1986; Bargh, Lombardi, & Higgins, 1988). For example, Bargh et al. (1986) found exactly the same biased interpretation of shy or kind behaviors by randomly sampled subjects whose concepts of "shy" or "kind" had been primed as for subjects who possessed a chronically accessible concept of "shy" or "kind" (but who were not primed). Thus, as long as one has independent confirmation that people do possess the mental structure in chronic form, one can simulate the chronic, preconscious effect of the structure in subjects selected at random via the experimental technique of priming.

These same priming techniques should be applicable to the study of whether motivations can also be preconsciously triggered by the environment. In standard priming procedures (e.g., Bargh & Pietromonaco, 1982;

Higgins, Rholes, & Jones, 1977; Srull & Wyer, 1979), informational input relevant to a mental category is presented unobtrusively in the context of a separate first experiment (e.g., synonyms of a trait concept are presented as part of a "language ability test"), and then the influence of the primed category is measured in a second, ostensibly unrelated experiment.

Priming Cognitive Processing Goals

Researchers have already provided tests of the auto-motive model's hypothesis that goals and motives can be triggered nonconsciously (Bargh, 1990) within the domain of cognitive processing motivations. In the first study of this kind, Gollwitzer, Heckhausen, and Steller (1990) showed how a processing goal used in one context can persist in its activation and then carry over to be used in a subsequent context, even though there is no explicit choice of that goal in the second, apparently unrelated context. Subjects were instructed to adopt either a "deliberative" or an "implemental" mind-set in a first experiment, by thinking about a personal problem either in terms of alternative approaches to solving it, or in terms of specific actions they would actually take to solve it. Next, subjects completed a fairy tale after being given only the first few sentences; one example concerned a king who had to go away to war, but did not want to leave his daughter behind unprotected. Subjects who had previously thought in a deliberative mode were more likely to discuss all the possibilities the king was thinking about, whereas subjects who had previously thought in an implemental manner were more likely to complete the story with what the king actually did to solve the problem. Thus, the primed processing goal carried over to influence information processing in a subsequent task without conscious choice or awareness of that goal's operation, just as primed trait constructs carry over to influence subsequent person perception in the absence of choice or awareness of the influence.

More recently, Chaiken and her colleagues (see Chaiken, Giner-Sorolla, & Chen, Chapter 24, this volume) used the unrelated-first-experiment priming technique to activate either an impression or an accuracy motivation on the part of their subjects. Subjects were given scenarios to read and respond to, in which the protagonist either was concerned with being accurate in assessing the situation, or was concerned with making a good impression on another person. Next, in an apparently unrelated second experiment, subjects expected to discuss their opinions on a certain attitude topic with another subject, who was described as holding either favorable or unfavorable opinions on the matter. They then read an essay that contained arguments on both sides of the issue.

Results showed that subjects whose impression management goal had been primed aligned their own attitude position with that of the other subject; accuracy-motivated subjects' attitudes were not affected by the partner's position. Moreover, analysis of subject thought protocols showed that impression-motivated subjects were evaluating the arguments supporting the partner's position more positively while they were reading the essay. Thus, the nonconscious activation of the impression goal changed the way subjects processed the arguments in the essay, in the service of the interpersonal goal to make a good impression on the partner.

Cialdini and his colleagues (Bator, 1994; Cialdini, Trost, & Newsom, 1995) have investigated individual differences in consistency motivation. Bator (1994) used a priming procedure to activate subjects' consistency goals, in order to experimentally manipulate whether consistency motivation was active for the subject or not during a standard cognitive dissonance experiment. The technique used was similar to that used by Chaiken et al. As part of a first experiment, Bator had her subjects read an essay ostensibly from another subject with whom they were going to interact later, after the second experiment was over. This essay indicated that the partner either valued consistency in beliefs and deeds, or did not. In the allegedly unrelated experiment, subjects wrote a counterattitudinal essay in favor of instituting comprehensive examinations at their university, under free-choice or no-choice conditions.

The standard dissonance effect is that final attitude positions in the free-choice group are more favorable toward the essay issue than are attitudes in the no-choice group. This effect was obtained, but only in the condition in which consistency motivation was primed. Subjects in the no-prime condition showed identical final attitude positions, whether they had written the counterattitudinal essay under free-choice or no-choice conditions.

Importantly, both Chaiken et al. in their research on motivated processing of persuasive arguments, and Cialdini and his collaborators in theirs on consistency motivation, also showed similar differences using measures of chronic individual differences in these motivations. Shechter and Chaiken (see Chaiken et al., Chapter 24, this volume) showed that subjects high in self-monitoring were more likely than those low in self-monitoring to have chronic impression motivations in persuasion situations, and to tailor their expressed attitudes to those of their experimental partner. Cialdini et al. (1995) have developed a "preference for consistency" scale that predicts individual differences in responding to classic consistency experimental situations: foot-in-the-door, balance, and dissonance. Results in line with these three effects was obtained only for those subjects who possessed this chronic preference for consistency; at least half of their subjects showed no such intrinsic preference for consistency in those experimental situations.

In other words, these cognitive motivations exist in chronic form as well as in temporarily primed form. And the same results are obtained with priming as are obtained with the chronic measure. This is important because, as stated earlier, priming as an experimental technique can demonstrate the role played by *chronic* motivational tendencies that are activated nonconsciously by features of relevant situations (i.e., situations in which those particular motivations have been frequently and consistently pursued in the past). It is thus critical to show, as the research described above has done, that what is being primed exists in the real world in chronic form.

Priming Social Behavior

Thus far, the evidence indicates that both perceptual and motivational constructs can be activated unobtrusively and can proceed to influence cognitive processing, without the subject's knowledge of this influence (and hence without his or her current intention that it occur). Is it possible that social behavior can be determined automatically as well, by the mere presence of relevant situational features that activate the goal to behave in a certain way?

We (Bargh, Barndollar, & Gollwitzer, 1995; see Bargh & Gollwitzer, 1994) used the Srull and Wyer (1979) "scrambled-sentence test" priming procedure to activate the achievement goal, the affiliation goal, or no goal in subjects in an ostensibly separate "first experiment." We primed subjects with words related to achievement (e.g., "strive," "success") or affiliation (e.g., "friend," "sociable") in an initial "word search" puzzle. Next, subjects were placed in a goal conflict situation, in which the subjects could fulfill either the achievement goal at the expense of the affiliation goal, or the affiliation goal at the expense of the achievement goal. Each subject worked together with another subject (actually a confederate) as a team to find as many words as possible in each of a series of five additional word search puzzles.

This confederate, however, was very bad at the task, and as the experimental session progressed the confederate became more and more humiliated for not doing well. The subject was thus placed in a goal conflict situation where he or she could achieve a high score, but at the cost of hurting the confederate's feelings. Results showed that, as predicted, subjects primed with achievement stimuli found significantly more words on the puzzle than did the other subjects, especially on the early trials of the task. Debriefing of subjects revealed no awareness of the possible influence of the priming manipulation on their performance.

In a second experiment, this procedure was replicated, but we also measured each subject's chronic achievement and affiliation needs, using the Thematic Apperception Test to assess achievement motivation (McClelland, Atkinson, Clark, & Lowell, 1953; Sorrentino & Higgins, 1986) and the Jackson Personality Research Form (Jackson, 1984) to assess affiliation motivation. Again, subjects whose achievement goal had been primed performed at a reliably higher level than did the other subjects on the word search task, but only on the early trials. On the later trials, the temporary goal priming wore off, and now the subjects' chronic motivational tendencies took over. On the later trials, chronically achievement-motivated subjects scored higher than did the chronically affiliation-motivated subjects.

This result is important because it shows that priming of achievement and affiliation goals simulates in the short term the same effects that classical measures of chronic motivational states—achievement and affiliation, in this case—show within the same experiment. Thus our confidence that motivations are being primed with our procedure is increased, because there are alternative interpretations for these findings.

A Nonmotivational Interpretation: The "Behavioral Schema"

Carver, Ganellen, Froming, and Chambers (1983) replicated an experiment by Srull and Wyer (1979) that utilized an unobtrusive priming technique. The concept of hostility was primed for some subjects in an unrelated first experiment. Next, subjects were instructed to shock a "learner" subject. Carver et al. found that those subjects primed with hostility gave longer shocks than did control subjects.

Carver et al. (1983) explained their results in terms of the activation of a "behavioral schema" for hostility. They argued that the mental representation subjects used to perceive hostility in others was likely to share many semantic features with the representation they used to produce hostile behavior themselves, and so activation of the perceptual construct of hostility was likely to spread to the behavioral construct. This would make a hostile response more likely to be consciously chosen by the subjects if such behavior was relevant (applicable) to the situation.

The concept of the behavioral schema has the elegant feature of being able to account for why the same priming manipulation (e.g., the Srull & Wyer [1979] scrambled-sentence test) can produce effects on impression formation in some studies and behavioral effects in others. Because Carver et al. (1983) used the same priming procedure that Srull and Wyer (1979) had shown to influence social perception, the inescapable conclusion is that the preconscious effect of hostile information is *simultaneously* to influence both one's perception of another's behavior and to increase the chances of one behaving the same way oneself.

Are the same mental structures involved in perceiving the behavior of others and in producing that same behavior oneself? This is a long-standing issue within psychology, called the "common-coding hypothesis" (Prinz, 1990). The question is whether perceptual representations and action representations are separate and distinct, requiring some kind of translation of information from one code to the other, or whether the same single code is used both to perceive and to engage in that type of behavior. Especially in the study of imitative behavior, including speech imitation, the controversy has raged for some time as to whether perception and behavior share a common coding system at the symbolic level (e.g., Koffka, 1925; MacKay, Allport, Prinz, & Scheerer, 1987).

The behavioral-schema account of our (Bargh et al., 1995) findings is that our priming manipulation did not activate a motive or goal to achieve or affiliate, but the perceptual representation of one or the other, which then spread to activate the behavioral representation. Thus, the behavioral representation of either achievement or affiliation was primed and more accessible than the other, and when the subjects made a conscious choice as to what to do in the situation, this choice was influenced by the relative accessibility of one behavioral alternative over the other.

The behavioral-schema alternative raises two difficulties for the automotive model. One is that evidence must be acquired to demonstrate that motivational states are being primed, and not merely nonmotivational cognitive representations. The Bargh et al. (1995, Experiment 2) finding that the achievement- and affiliation-priming manipulations simulated the effects of classically measured chronic achievement and affiliation motivations is one piece of evidence that we did in fact prime motivations.

Motivational Qualities of Primed Goal States

In the face of this alternative explanation, we have conducted additional studies to test for the presence of qualities associated with motivational states that are not predicted by any purely cognitive account of our findings. These qualities are (1) persistence on a task in the face of interruptions or obstacles (Lewin, 1926; Ovsiankina, 1928; see also Heckhausen, 1989/1991; Wicklund & Gollwitzer, 1982); and (2) an increase in motivational tendency over time (Atkinson & Birch, 1970), as opposed to the decrease in activation strength over time (or at least no increase) predicted by all cognitive priming accounts (e.g., Higgins, Bargh, & Lombardi, 1985).

We (Bargh et al.. 1995, Experiment 3) found that achievement-primed subjects showed greater persistence on a task in the face of an obstacle than did neutral-primed subjects. Some subjects were primed with achievement-related stimuli, and the remaining subjects with neutral stimuli. Subjects participated three at a time, with partitions between their desk chairs so that they could not see each other. However, all three subjects faced the front of the room, where a hidden video camera recorded them during the experimental session. After completing the priming task under the instructions that it was a separate "language ability" measure, subjects were given a rack of seven Scrabble letter tiles and told to find as many words with those letters as they could in the next 3 minutes, and write each down on the piece of paper provided. The experimenter then explained that she had to leave the room to run another experiment, but that if she could not get back by the end of the 3 minutes, she would give the signal to "stop" over the room's intercom.

Subjects were then told to begin, and the experimenter left the room. At the end of the 3 minutes, subjects were told to stop. The dependent measure was the proportion of subjects who continued to work on finding the words after the signal to stop had been given, as monitored by the experimenter via the hidden camera. The results were as predicted: 55% of the subjects in the achievement priming condition, but only 22% of subjects in the neutral-priming condition, persisted on the task after being told to stop.

In our final experiment (Bargh et al., 1995; Experiment 4), subjects first performed a matrix word search task in which they were primed with achievement-related or neutral stimuli. Next, for half the subjects in each priming condition, a 5-minute delay was interpolated before the dependent measure was assessed; for the other half, no delay was interpolated. Subjects in the delay condition drew their family trees in as much detail as they could. This was a task intended not to satisfy the achievement motive in any way. Next, subjects either read about a target person who behaved in an ambiguously achievement-oriented way (e.g., he crammed for an exam the night before) and then rated the target on achievement-related trait dimensions, or they found as many words as they could in a set of Scrabble letter tiles.

For subjects who performed the impression formation task, those who had been primed on achievement considered the target person to be more of an achiever than did other subjects, but only in the no-delay condition. Importantly, this difference disappeared after the 5-minute delay, replicating previous priming research in social perception. However, on the behavioral task, not only did subjects in the achievement-priming condition outperform the other subjects in both the no-delay and delay conditions; as the motivational interpretation would predict, the performance of the achievement-primed subjects was better after the delay than after no delay.

Another way to put this is that the achievement-priming condition results show a clear dissociation between the behavioral and judgmental effects of priming over time, in that the direction of the effect of delay is reversed between the two dependent measures (Dunn & Kirsner, 1988). Our obtained effect of achievement priming on behavior, in other words, cannot be merely an effect of the activation level of a perceptual or behavioral representation. No model of cognitive activation effects posits an *increase* in activation over time following priming. Only motivational systems show such effects (Atkinson & Birch, 1970).

One additional point to be made in the wake of these results is that it is a goal or strategy that is clearly being activated by our priming manipulation, and not a specific behavioral tendency. If we were just priming a specific behavioral tendency, it would be enacted right away. Instead, the activated goal follows the principle of "applicability" (Higgins, 1989): An accessible representation does not operate on its own, in the absence of relevant input, but only in the presence of environmental information for which it is applicable. Notably, Ach (1935) defined intentional states in a similar way; according to this early theorist of the conscious will, it is usually not the case that one begins acting immediately upon the activation of a motivational tendency. Rather, one waits for the opportune moment in time—the occurrence of situational events that give one the chance to attain the goal (see also Vera & Simon, 1993).

Goals Can Operate without Conscious Consent

The second objection that could be raised by proponents of the nonmotivational, behavioral-schema model is that our studies thus far do not rule out the involvement of conscious intention or choice in producing the achievement or affiliation behavior. The strong form of the auto-motive hypothesis is that the entire sequence from triggering environmental information to enactment of goal-directed action requires no conscious intervention. Without evidence that goals can be activated and operate without conscious choice, what we are left with is evidence for a weak form of the auto-motive hypothesis: that the environment can trigger goals and motives, and make them more accessible, but that conscious choice of those goals is nonetheless needed for action to result.

However, recent studies argue against the necessity of a conscious choice point. We find it implausible, for example, that subjects in the consistency-priming condition of the Bator (1994) dissonance study described above consciously chose the goal of preserving consistency between their attitude and their behavior, and therefore changed their attitude as a result. Equally unlikely in our view is that subjects in the Gollwitzer et al. (1990) study consciously chose the primed implemental or deliberative goal when asked to complete the fairy tale. And in the experiments (Bargh et al., 1995, Experiments 3 and 4) that documented the motivational qualities of primed goal states, our findings of greater persistence, and especially the increase in unconscious motivational tendency with increased time since priming, speak against the role of conscious choice as well. In these studies, the dependent measure was not the *choice* of behavior among possible alternatives, as in the previous studies, but the presence of heightened goal desire and increasing effort over time. It is difficult to see how these effects are somehow a matter of deliberate choice.

As discussed earlier, the standard method for demonstrating that an effect is unconscious and not attributable to conscious intent is to show that it is different from what subjects would do when that unconscious influence is not operating (Jacoby, 1991). Accordingly, in order to demonstrate that activated goals operate without the need for conscious selection of them, an experiment was conducted to show the counterintentional effects of an activated processing goal.

Bargh and Green (1995) showed subjects a videotaped conversation between two men, from the vantage point of behind one man and looking over his shoulder toward the other. Subjects were told either that the conversation was between two acquaintances who had not seen each other for a while, that the situation was a job interview for the position of investigative crime reporter for a city newspaper, or that it was a job interview for a restaurant waiter position. The conversation condition was intended as a control condition in which no explicit evaluative goal was given to subjects. The reporter and waiter conditions were designed on the basis of pretesting, which showed that the qualities the pretest subjects felt would make a good reporter (e.g., tough, aggressive, dominant) were the opposite of those that would make a good waiter (e.g., friendly, acquiescent), and vice versa. The scripted conversation subjects saw on the videotape was the same for all three conditions, and was ambiguous enough that each of the three cover stories was plausible.

The critical experimental manipulation came about halfway through the tape, in which another male knocked on the door, entered the room, and inquired of the interviewer whether he was ready for their lunch date. The interviewer expressed regret that he was busy at the moment with an interview. At this point, in one condition the interrupter ("Mike") became testy and reminded the interviewer that his (Mike's) time was very short that day and that they would have to leave right at noon. When the interviewer persisted in his position that he could not leave in the middle of the interview, Mike also persisted in his position that he could not wait and they would have to make it another time. In the other tape condition, Mike apologized for having interrupted.

Our hypothesis was that even though subjects were not intending to evaluate Mike (their attention was focused on the interview), they would do so in line with the goal that was currently operating for the interview itself. Immediately after the tape had finished, we informed subjects that we were actually interested in their opinion of Mike, the person who interrupted about the lunch date, and asked subjects to rate Mike's likeability. As expected, subjects in the control condition did like the polite Mike better than the assertive Mike. More importantly, this difference was stronger in the waiter condition, and was actually reversed in the reporter condition. Subjects who were considering the interviewee for the crime reporter position liked the assertive Mike reliably better than the polite Mike.

Importantly, auxiliary trait ratings of Mike by subjects showed that the obtained likeability effect was not attributable to subjects' interpreting Mike's behavior differently on the basis of their particular processing goal. Subjects in the reporter condition rated Mike as more rude and stubborn, and less agreeable, cheerful, and polite, than did the subjects in the waiter or control conditions; subjects in the latter two groups rated Mike as less adventurous, aggressive, and persistent than did the reporter subjects. In other words, subjects in the reporter condition liked the interrupting Mike better, *despite* having accurately perceived him as behaving badly.

Left to their own devices, subjects in this experiment showed a clear preference for the polite, apologetic version of Mike. When a goal was operating, however, it operated on all available information for which it was applicable, regardless of whether the individual intended it to. Operating goals are autonomous in that respect. Moreover, judgments were made that were clearly counter to what the subjects would make normally. One can imagine asking control subjects whether they would want the interrupting Mike as a friend, and their emphatic negative answer. Yet subjects in the reporter condition, if asked to choose between the two versions of Mike, would—based on their comparative likeability ratings—choose interrupting Mike. And real-life versions of this effect are not hard to imagine either: A person working all day in a cutthroat, competitive atmosphere, where being hard-nosed and tough-minded are highly valued traits, might well choose a romantic partner with the same qualities (with potentially disastrous results), whereas asking him or her about the ideal mate might result in quite a different description.

Summary

Taken as a whole, these studies show that behavioral as well as cognitive goals can be activated directly by the environment without conscious choice or awareness of the activation; that the goals, once activated, direct information processing and social behavior; that the state activated by the priming manipulations in these studies has demonstrable motivational qualities; that the states achieved by priming in these studies also exist in chronic form; that there are individual differences in these chronic motivations; and that the activated goals operate autonomously, bypassing the need for any conscious selection or choice of them, and even producing outcomes different from what the individual would choose if the goal were not primed. In short, every postulate of the auto-motive model (Bargh, 1990) has been supported by these studies, demonstrating that the entire sequence from environmental information to goal and motivation, and then to judgment and action can and does transpire automatically and unconsciously.

CONCLUSIONS

We have argued for the existence of unconsciously generated motivations and automatic action—for a conception of the unconscious as an implicit repository of a person's long-term experience and history of past choices. We have disputed the traditional view of the unconscious as the source of the irrational, in contrast to a presumably rational consciousness. Instead, just as Bayesian norms of decision making call for substantial weight to be placed on long-term frequencies or base rates of events, relative to single recent occurrences (e.g., Kahneman & Tversky, 1973; Nisbett & Ross, 1980), it may often be more rational to base one's decisions and preferences on unconscious rather than conscious information processing (see also Wilson & Schooler, 1991). In any case, we have attempted to show that the unconscious is not limited to brief and relatively uninteresting perceptual effects (see Greenwald, 1992), but plays a important and determining role in the creation of all aspects of the psychological situation, from perception to evaluation (Bargh, in press) to motivations and behavior.

The central proposition of the auto-motive model that guided the research discussed above—that automatic links exist between specific sets of situational features and behavioral goals—is quite consistent with recent research and models of the conditions under which people actually do behave consistently. Ajzen and Fishbein (1977; see also Ajzen, Chapter 17, this volume), for example, argued that attitudes and behavior correlate poorly because attitudes are assessed too generally in relation to the specificity of behavior. Their review showed that the correlation between attitude and behavior increases when a more specific attitude is assessed, that toward performing the behavior in question. In other words, consistency is not found so much over broader domains of attitude-related behaviors, but is found when attitudes toward more specific behaviors are measured.

The auto-motive model is also quite compatible with Mischel and Shoda's (1995) model of personality coherence. They have shown that evidence for the existence of personality as a consistent pattern of behavior is quite weak when behavior is averaged across different situations thought by the experimenter to be similar, but that when behavior within specific situations is examined, consistency is actually quite high (Shoda, Mischel, & Wright, 1995). In other words, it is the psychological situation for the individual that matters, and this may vary for the individual within apparently similar objective situations. Most importantly, when the situation is defined at the level of a specific set of features, a much greater degree of behavioral consistency is found over time. If an individual's chronic goals and motivations are tied to specific sets of situational features, as the auto-motive hypothesis holds, these unconsciously activated and operating goals would be expected to produce the high degree of behavioral consistency that Mischel and Shoda (1995) have uncovered.

William James could think of no better advice for the young than to develop good social and interpersonal habits, so that their behavior would be guided by these habits for the rest of their lives:

> We must make automatic and habitual, as early as possible, as many useful actions as we can, and guard against the growing into ways that are likely to be disadvantageous to us, as we should guard against the plague. The more of the details of our daily life we can hand over to the effortless custody of automatism, the more our higher powers of mind will be set free for their own proper work. There is no more miserable human being than one in whom nothing is habitual but indecision. . . . Full half the time of such a man goes to the deciding, or regretting, of matters which ought to be so ingrained in him as practically not to exist for his consciousness at all. (1890, Vol. 1, p. 122)

The grooves into which social behavior falls, for the most part, are laid down by the decisions we make in those particular circumstances in the past. The automation of those decisions of the past, as James noted, results in their being made for us nonconsciously in the present. The automation of the goals we pursue in each of the wide variety of social situations we frequently encounter enables us to deal effectively or ineffectively with the world; they produce either satisfaction or hardship, friends or enemies. Regardless of how adaptive and functional the particular unconscious goals in a person's repertoire may be, in our view they are the *Grund* of that individual's personality and true self.

ACKNOWLEDGMENTS

The research described in this chapter and its preparation were supported in part by Grant No. SBR-9409448 from the National Science Foundation. The development of several of the ideas presented in the chapter profited from discussions with Peter Gollwitzer and Joseph LeDoux.

NOTE

1. That a given researcher uses counterintentional behavior to document the existence of nonconscious influences does not mean necessarily that he or she personally holds the view that the unconscious is only a source of error or mistake. Our point here is merely that the evidentiary basis for the existence of the unconscious is heavily skewed in the direction of error and mistake, giving a potentially misleading impression as to the actual capabilities and usual functioning of the unconscious.

REFERENCES

Ach, N. (1935). Analyse des Willens. In E. Abderhalden (Ed.), *Handbuch der biologishen Arbeitsmethoden* (Vol. 6, Part E). Berlin: Urban & Schwarzenberg.

Ajzen, I., & Fishbein, M. (1977). Attitude–behavior relations: A theoretical analysis and review of empirical research. *Psychological Bulletin, 84,* 888–918.

Atkinson, J. W., & Birch, D. (1970). *A dynamic theory of action.* New York: Wiley.

Atkinson, R. C., & Shiffrin, R. M. (1968). Human memory: A proposed system and its control process. *Psychology of Learning and Motivation, 2,* 89–195.

Bargh, J. A. (1982). Attention and automaticity in the processing of self-relevant information. *Journal of Personality and Social Psychology, 43,* 425–436.

Bargh, J. A. (1984). Automatic and conscious processing of social information. In R. S. Wyer, Jr., & T. K. Srull (Eds.), *Handbook of social cognition* (Vol. 3, pp. 1–43). Hillsdale, NJ: Erlbaum.

Bargh, J. A. (1990). Auto-motives: Preconscious determinants of thought and behavior. In E. T. Higgins & R. M. Sorrentino (Eds.), *Handbook of motivation and cognition: Foundations of social behavior* (Vol. 2, pp. 93–130). New York: Guilford Press.

Bargh, J. A. (1992). Does subliminality matter to social psychology? Awareness of the stimulus versus awareness of its influence. In R. Bornstein & T. Pittman (Eds.), *Perception without awareness* (pp. 236–255). New York: Guilford Press.

Bargh, J. A. (1994). The Four Horsemen of automaticity: Awareness, intention, efficiency, and control in social cognition. In R. S. Wyer, Jr., & T. K. Srull (Eds.), *Handbook of social cognition* (2nd ed., pp. 1–40). Hillsdale, NJ: Erlbaum.

Bargh, J. A. (in press). The automaticity of everyday life. In R. S. Wyer, Jr. (Ed.), *Advances in experimental social cognition* (Vol. 10). Hillsdale, NJ: Erlbaum.

Bargh, J. A., Barndollar, K., & Gollwitzer, P. M. (1995). *Social ignition: Automatic activation of motivational states.* Manuscript submitted for publication.

Bargh, J. A., Bond, R. N., Lombardi, W. J., & Tota, M. E. (1986). The additive nature of chronic and temporary sources of construct accessibility. *Journal of Personality and Social Psychology, 50,* 869–878.

Bargh, J. A., & Gollwitzer, P. M. (1994). Environmental control of goal-directed action: Automatic and strategic contingencies between situations and behavior. In W. D. Spaulding (Ed.), *Nebraska Symposium on Motivation: Vol. 41. Integrative views of motivation, cognition, and emotion* (pp. 71–124). Lincoln: University of Nebraska Press.

Bargh, J. A., & Green, M. (1995). *Unintended consequences of intentional information processing.* Manuscript submitted for publication.

Bargh, J. A., Lombardi, W. J., & Higgins, E. T. (1988). Automaticity of person × situation effects on impression formation: It's just a matter of time. *Journal of Personality and Social Psychology, 55,* 599–605.

Bargh, J. A., & Pietromonaco, P. (1982). Automatic information processing and social perception: The influence of trait information presented outside of conscious awareness on impression formation. *Journal of Personality and Social Psychology, 43,* 437–449.

Bargh, J. A., & Pratto, F. (1986). Individual construct accessibility and perceptual selection. *Journal of Experimental Social Psychology, 22,* 293–311.

Bargh, J. A., & Thein, R. D. (1985). Individual construct accessibility, person memory, and the recall–judgment link: The case of information overload. *Journal of Personality and Social Psychology, 49,* 1129–1146.

Bargh, J. A., & Tota, M. E. (1988). Context-dependent automatic processing in depression: Accessibility of negative constructs with regard to self but not others. *Journal of Personality and Social Psychology, 54,* 925–939.

Bator, R. J. (1994). *Priming a consistency motivation enhances cognitive dissonance effects.* Unpublished master's thesis, Arizona State University.

Brewer, M. B. (1988). A dual process model of impression formation. In T. K. Srull & R. S. Wyer, Jr. (Eds.), *Advances in social cognition* (Vol. 1, pp. 1–36). Hillsdale, NJ: Erlbaum.

Bruner, J. S. (1992). New Look I revisited. *American Psychologist, 47,* 780–783.

Carlston, D. E., & Skowronski, J. J. (1994). Savings in the relearning of trait information as evidence for spontaneous inference generation. *Journal of Personality and Social Psychology, 66,* 840–856.

Carver, C. S., Ganellen, R. J., Froming, W. J., & Chambers, W. (1983). Modeling: An analysis in terms of category accessibility. *Journal of Experimental Social Psychology, 19,* 403–421.

Cialdini, R. B., Trost, M. R., & Newsom, J. T. (1995). Preference for consistency: The development of a valid measure and the discovery of surprising behavioral implications. *Journal of Personality and Social Psychology, 69.*

Dawes, R. (1976). Shallow psychology. In J. Carroll & R. Payne (Eds.), *Cognition and social behavior.* Hillsdale, NJ: Erlbaum.

Devine, P. G. (1989). Stereotypes and prejudice: Their automatic and controlled components. *Journal of Personality and Social Psychology, 56,* 680–690.

Dunn, J. C., & Kirsner, K. (1988). Discovering functionally independent mental processes: The principle of reversed association. *Psychological Review, 95,* 91–101.

Freud, S. (1965). *The psychopathology of everyday life* (J. Strachey, Ed. & Trans.). New York: Norton. (Original work published 1901)

Gazzaniga, M. (1984). *The social brain.* New York: Basic Books.

Gilbert, D. T. (1989). Thinking lightly about others: Automatic components of the social inference process. In J. S. Uleman & J. A. Bargh (Eds.), *Unintended thought* (pp. 189–211). New York: Guilford Press.

Glymour, C. (1992). Freud's androids. In J. Neu (Ed.), *The Cambridge companion to Freud* (pp. 44–85). New York: Cambridge University Press.

Gollwitzer, P. M., Heckhausen, H., & Steller, B. (1990). Deliberative and implemental mind-sets: Cognitive tuning toward congruous thoughts and information. *Journal of Personality and Social Psychology, 59,* 1119–1127.

Greenwald, A. G. (1992). New Look 3: Unconscious cognition reclaimed. *American Psychologist, 47,* 766–779.

Hebb, D. O. (1948). *Organization of behavior.* New York: Wiley.

Heckhausen, H. (1991). *Motivation and action* (P. K. Leppmann, Trans.). Berlin: Springer-Verlag. (Original work published 1989)

Higgins, E. T. (1989). Knowledge accessibility and activation: Subjectivity and suffering from unconscious sources. In J. S. Uleman & J. A. Bargh (Eds.), *Unintended thought* (pp. 75–123). New York: Guilford Press.

Higgins, E. T., & Bargh, J. A. (1992). Unconscious sources of subjectivity and suffering: Is consciousness the solution? In L. L. Martin & A. Tesser (Eds.), *The construction of social judgments* (pp. 67–103). Hillsdale, NJ: Erlbaum.

Higgins, E. T., Bargh, J. A., & Lombardi, W. (1985). Nature of priming effects on categorization. *Journal of Experimental Psychology: Learning, Memory, and Cognition, 11,* 59–69.

Higgins, E. T., King, G. A., & Mavin, G. H. (1982). Individual construct accessibility and subjective impressions and recall. *Journal of Personality and Social Psychology, 43,* 35–47.

Higgins, E. T., Rholes, W. S., & Jones, C. R. (1977). Category accessibility and impression formation. *Journal of Experimental Social Psychology, 13,* 141–154.

Hilgard, E. R. (1977). *Divided consciousness.* New York: Wiley.

Jackson, D. N. (1984). *Personality Research Form manual.* Port Huron, MI: Research Psychologists Press.

Jacoby, L. L. (1991). A process dissociation framework: Separating automatic from intentional uses of memory. *Journal of Memory and Language, 30,* 513–541.

Jacoby, L. L., Lindsay, D. S., & Toth, J. P. (1992). Unconscious influences revealed: Attention, awareness, and control. *American Psychologist, 47,* 802–809.

James, W. (1890). *Principles of psychology* (2 vols.). New York: Holt.

Jung, C. G. (1969). The structure of the psyche (R. F. C. Hull, Trans.). In H. Read, M. Fordham, & G. Adler (Eds.), *The collected works of C. G. Jung* (Vol. 8, pp. 283–342). Princeton, NJ: Princeton University Press. (Original work published 1931)

Kahneman, D., & Treisman, A. (1984). Changing views of attention and automaticity. In R. Parasuraman (Ed.), *Varieties of attention.* New York: Academic Press.

Kahneman, D., & Tversky, A. (1973). On the psychology of prediction. *Psychological Review, 80,* 237–251.

Kitayama, S., & Burnstein, E. (1988). Automaticity in conversations: A reexamination of the mindlessness hypothesis. *Journal of Personality and Social Psychology, 54,* 219–224.

Koffka, K. (1925). *Die Grundlagen der psychischen Entwicklung.* Osterwieck, Germany: Zickfeldt.

Langer, E. J. (1978). Rethinking the role of thought in social interaction. In J. H. Harvey, W. I. Ickes, & R. F. Kidd (Eds.), *New directions in attribution research* (Vol. 2, pp. 35–58). Hillsdale, NJ: Erlbaum.

Langer, E. J., Blank, A., & Chanowitz, B. (1978). The mindlessness of ostensibly thoughtful action: The role of "placebic" information in interpersonal interaction. *Journal of Personality and Social Psychology, 36,* 635–642.

Lewin, K. (1926). Vorsatz, Wille und Bedürfnis. *Psychologische Forschung, 7,* 330–385.

Loftus, E. F., & Klinger, M. R. (1992). Is the unconscious smart or dumb? *American Psychologist, 47,* 761–765.

Logan, G. D., & Cowan, W. (1984). On ability to inhibit thought and action: A theory of an act of control. *Psychological Review, 91,* 295–327.

MacKay, D. G., Allport, A., Prinz, W., & Scheerer, E. (1987). Relationships and modules within language perception–production: An introduction. In A. Allport, D. G. MacKay, W. Prinz, & E. Scheerer (Eds.), *Language perception and production.* Orlando, FL: Academic Press.

McClelland, D. C., Atkinson, J. W., Clark, R. A., & Lowell, E. L. (1953). *The achievement motive.* New York: Appleton-Century-Crofts.

Mischel, W. (1973). Toward a cognitive social learning reconceptualization of personality. *Psychological Review, 80,* 252–283.

Mischel, W., & Shoda, Y. (1995). A cognitive–affective system theory of personality: Reconceptualizing situations, dispositions, dynamics and invariance in personality structure. *Psychological Review, 102,* 246–268,

Nisbett, R. E., & Ross, L. (1980). *Human inference: Strategies and shortcomings.* Englewood Cliffs, NJ: Prentice-Hall.

Newell, A., & Rosenbloom, P. S. (1981). Mechanisms of skill acquisition and the law of practice. In J. R. Anderson (Ed.), *Cognitive skills and their acquisition* (pp. 1–55). Hillsdale, NJ: Erlbaum.

Norman, D. A. (1981). Categorization of action slips. *Psychological Review, 88,* 1–15.

Ovsiankina, M. (1928). Die Wiederaufnahme unterbrochener Handlungen [The resumption of interrupted goals]. *Psychologische Forschung, 11, 302*–379.

Prinz, W. (1990). A common coding approach to perception and action. In O. Neumann & W. Prinz (Eds.), *Relationships between perception and action* (pp. 167–201). Heidelberg: Springer-Verlag.

Schwarz, N. (1990). Feelings as information: Informational and motivational functions of affective states. In E. T. Higgins & R. M. Sorrentino (Eds.), *Handbook of motivation and cognition: Foundations of social behavior* (Vol. 2, pp. 527–561). New York: Guilford Press.

Schwarz, N., & Clore, G. L. (1983). Mood, misattribution, and judgments of well-being: Informative and directive functions of affective states. *Journal of Personality and Social Psychology, 45,* 513–523.

Searle, J. R. (1992). *The rediscovery of the mind.* Cambridge, MA: MIT Press.

Shiffrin, R. M., & Schneider, W. (1977). Controlled and automatic human information processing: II. Perceptual learning, automatic attending, and a general theory. *Psychological Review, 84,* 127–190.

Shoda, Y., Mischel, W., & Wright, J. C. (1994). Intra-individual stability in the organization and patterning of behavior: Incorporating psychological situations into the idiographic analysis of personality. *Journal of Personality and Social Psychology, 67,* 674–687.

Smith, E. R. (1994). Procedural knowledge and processing strategies in social cognition. In R. S. Wyer, Jr., & T. K. Srull (Eds.), *Handbook of social cognition* (2nd ed., pp. 99–151). Hillsdale, NJ: Erlbaum.

Smith, E. R., & Lerner, M. (1986). Development of automatism of social judgments. *Journal of Personality and Social Psychology, 50,* 246–259.

Sorrentino, R. M., & Higgins, E. T. (1986). Motivation and cognition: Warming up to synergism. In R. M. Sorrentino & E. T. Higgins (Eds.), *Handbook of motivation and cognition: Foundation of social behavior* (Vol. 1, pp. 3–19). New York: Guilford Press.

Srull, T. K., & Wyer, R. S., Jr. (1979). The role of category accessibility in the interpretation of information about persons: Some determinants and implications. *Journal of Personality and Social Psychology, 37,* 1660–1672.

Vera, A. H., & Simon, H. A. (1993). Situated action: A symbolic interpretation. *Cognitive Science, 17,* 7–48.

Wegner, D. M. (1994). Ironic processes of mental control. *Psychological Review, 101,* 34–52.

Wegner, D. M., & Erber, R. (1992). The hyperaccessibility of suppressed throughts. *Journal of Personality and Social Psychology, 63,* 903–912.

Wegner, D. M., & Wenzlaff, R. M. (in press). Mental control. In E. T. Higgins & A. W. Kruglanski (Eds.), *Social psychology: Handbook of basic principles.* New York: Guilford Press.

Wicklund, R. A., & Gollwitzer, P. M. (1982). *Symbolic self-completion.* Hillsdale, NJ: Erlbaum.

Wilson, T. D., & Schooler, J. W. (1991). Thinking too much: Introspection can reduce the quality of preferences and decisions. *Journal of Personality and Social Psychology, 60,* 181–192.

CHAPTER 21 The Feeling of Doing

Matthew E. Ansfield
Daniel M. Wegner

We all know what it is like to do something. It is not just that we know in advance what we will do or when we will do it. It is that when we do it, we *feel* we are doing it. Some sort of sensation, an internal "oomph," goes with the effort of doing, and it is this feeling that certifies that we know we are acting. The feeling is not there when we simply think about an action, when we are physically forced to perform an action, or when our bodies do something (such as hiccuping) that we wouldn't call an action. Nor is this just the feeling we get back from our bodies as a result of having done something. That sort of feedback occurs even with a hiccup, and proprioception of this kind is not the topic of this chapter. The feeling of doing occurs just when we do something voluntarily. It is this feeling, a sort of "phenomenal will," that is special to the experience of intended behavior—the conscious sense of acting.

The question of interest in the study of this feeling is whether it is indeed always present during intentional action. There are a number of important anomalies, cases in which phenomenal will does not seem to accompany behavior that otherwise qualifies as sentient and seemingly will-relevant. This chapter is about these cases. It is an exploration of the psychological processes accompanying activity that is disavowed. Our goal is to create a starting point for understanding these instances—first by examining cases of "automatisms," actions that occur without the feeling of doing. Next, we review the major psychological explanations that have been proffered for these cases and discuss their relative merits. This background will allow us to introduce, then, a theory that is relevant to the phenomenal will—the theory of ironic processes of mental control (Wegner, 1994). This theory has stimulated us to conduct some research that shows how the feeling of doing can be subverted under certain conditions when people are specifically trying *not* to do something. As we shall see, some proportion of the things people do unintentionally may in fact be *counter*intentional, deriving from processes that ironically oppose the phenomenal will.

A CATALOG OF AUTOMATISMS

Automatisms are actions that are so remarkably divorced from a feeling of doing that they have become widely celebrated and studied—and often attributed to the doings of supernatural forces. The heyday for the discovery of automatisms was the spiritualist fad of the late 19th century, when automatic writing, table turning, and the like were the focus of tremendous popular attention. Many North Americans and Europeans of that time amused themselves in their homes by arranging circumstances in such a fashion that they might do things they did not intend. Several of these curious phenomena eventually found use as measures of suggestibility (e.g., Eysenck & Furneaux, 1945), and others have now been added to the list by contemporary observers. As a first step in understanding when phenomenal will may be absent, it is useful to review a range of these oddities.

Chevreul's Pendulum Illusion

People have long been fascinated by the ostensibly magical properties of the hand-held pendulum, and it has been ascribed many powers (Easton & Shor, 1976). There are superstitions that the swing pattern of a pendulum held over a pregnant woman's tummy, for example, will foretell the sex of the child, and there once were very elaborate expectations of how a pendulum held over ore samples would swing to indicate their metallic content. Such occult properties of the pendulum's swing were dispelled by Michel Chevreul (1833), a chemist whose research showed that the action of the pendulum was entirely dependent on the psychological involvement of the person holding it. For the pendulum to "work," the holder had to be looking at it, and indeed suspending it from a hand or arm in such a manner that muscular movement could influence the swing. Still, even when people are aware of this connection, there is a sense in which the pendulum movement is unintentional. Just thinking about a circular or left-to-right swing pattern, for example, seems to be sufficient for many people to have that pattern occur (Easton & Shor, 1975, 1976, 1977). W. G. Carpenter (1884) and William James (1904/1986) both observed that when a person is thinking about the hour of the day and swings a ring by a thread inside a glass, it often strikes the hour even while the person has no conscious sense of doing this on purpose.

Automatic Writing

There have been many claims of writing that is automatic or otherwise not intentional or voluntary (Koutstaal, 1992). Automatic writing was associated by early theorists with hypnotic states or cases of hysterical neurosis (Binet, 1905; Janet, 1889), and also with claims of spirit mediumship. William James made notes on cases of automatic writing (1889/1986) and automatic drawing (1904/1986), and estimated that "in twenty persons taken at random an automatic writer of some degree can always be found" (1904/1986, p. 221). The production of such writing often occurs with the aid of a "planchette"—a device for frictionless writing, consisting of a three-cornered pen mount with the pen as one corner and gliding ball-bearings or the like as the other two. Solomons and Stein (1896) studied their own abilities with a planchette, and found that they came with practice to perform repetitive actions (such as figure-eights) and to write some letters or forms without the feeling of doing so. There is a colorful historical literature of apparently far more complex writings performed by individuals who report no feeling of voluntary action at all. Most radical perhaps are cases in which individuals claim to have written volumes of prose or poetry, or to have written script that appears backward, upside down, or in a foreign language they profess not to know (James, 1904/1986; Sidis, 1906).

Ouija Board Spelling

The familiar household Ouija board has an alphabet and numbers printed on it, and one touches a three-legged pointer or a planchette with one's fingertips in the attempt to spell out messages. The modern version is registered by Parker Brothers, even though the idea is apparently traceable to antiquity (Hunt, 1985). Usually billed as a way ostensibly to communicate with the dead or the spirit world, Ouija board spelling is reported to involve little phenomenal will, especially when the pointer is operated by more than one person. Although there may be some feeling of doing associated with the production of movement per se, this phenomenal will does not always extend to the specific letters or words that are found with the pointer.

Table Turning, Tilting, and Tapping

Another lapse in the feeling of doing can happen when a number of individuals are seated around a table on which they place their hands, with the idea impressed on their minds that the table will rotate, tilt, or rise and fall so as to tap on the floor. The party sits, often for a long time, in a state of expectation that the table will move in the specified direction, with their full attention aimed toward the first sign of the anticipated motion. Generally one or two slight changes in the desired direction foreshadow the approaching movement. As Carpenter (1884) observed, "All this is done, not merely without the least consciousness on the part of the performers that they are exercising any force of their own, but for the most part under the full conviction that they are not" (pp. 292–293). Yet in many cases, the table will eventually perform just as expected. In fact, a rotating table may eventually have the participants running rapidly to keep up, and a tapping table may be so active that it can be used to answer questions posed by members of the group in an agreed-upon code. Chemist and physicist Michael Faraday debunked claims of supernatural sources of table turning in 1853 by observing that force measurement devices placed between subjects' hands and the table showed that the source of movement was their hands and not the table (Carpenter, 1884).

Dowsing or Divining

The movement of a forked stick, angle rod, or other hand-held instrument purportedly in response to underground water is another case of action that may occur without phenomenal will. Typically, the dowser holds the forked ends of a stick in the hands palm upright, and walks about while waiting for the tip of the stick to move. Volumes have been written about the "correct" way to dowse (e.g., Bird, 1979; Graves, 1986), but the research literature evaluating its effectiveness shows that there really is no correct way because it does not work (e.g., Vogt & Hyman, 1959). Because the rod is held in an awkward and unstable position, often for long periods as the dowser walks the terrain, a combination of fatigue and minor jostling creates the "dip"—and water is found no more often than it would be by chance. What is intriguing about this activity is the great faith dowsers exhibit in their judgment that they do not move the divining rod. Without the feeling of doing, they maintain that the rod's affinity for water is what makes the movement occur.

Facilitated Communication

"Facilitated communication" is a technique recently advocated for use with individuals who have impaired communication abilities (Crossley & Remington-Gurney, 1992). A trained "facilitator" typically supports the pointing finger or hand of the "communicator" during the attempt to help the communicator spell out words on a keyboard or other template. The function of the facilitator is to assist the muscular control of the communicator by holding the communicator's arm steady, and yet to be uninfluential so that the communicator will "get his or her own words out" (Biklen, 1991). Initial results were reported that verged on the miraculous, as even autistic communicators who had never shown any verbal expression or comprehension were evidently answering questions in grammatical sentences. Some such communicators even took this new opportunity to report that they had been sexually abused (Hostler, Allair, & Christoph, 1993). As it turns out, however, the communications garnered in this way are often entirely traceable to the facilitators and may be counted as another form of automatism (Mulick, Jacobson, & Kobe, 1993).

Wheeler, Jacobson, Paglieri, and Schwartz (1993), for example, ran a study for which 12 autistic participants consented (via facilitated communication!). They were shown pictures of familiar objects, and were asked to report the names of the objects under several conditions. On those trials in which communicators and facilitators were shown different pictures, the only correct identifications were for the pictures shown to the facilitators and not those shown to the communicators. Wheeler et al. (1993) concluded from these findings that facilitated communication is really only communication by the facilitator. The facilitators in these circumstances are often caring and involved individuals who, far from being actively duplicitous, are genuinely convinced that the communicators—and not they themselves—are responsible for the communications. This, then, is a situation that can produce quite dramatic lapses in the feeling of doing on the part of facilitators.

Hypnosis

One of the key phenomena of modern hypnosis is the hypnotic subject's experience of *involuntariness* of action. When subjects are given the suggestion "Your arm is feeling very light, so light it is rising up," for example, a proportion of subjects indeed do lift their arms, and many of those who do so report later that they felt their motion was involuntary (e.g., Spanos & Barber, 1972). There is a substantial literature on this effect—more than we can treat here—but the general finding is that the experience of involuntariness in hypnosis is associated with hypnotic susceptibility and with the tendency for behavior to occur as suggested (e.g., Gorassini & Perlini, 1988; Lynn, Rhue, & Weekes, 1990; Spanos & Katsanis, 1989; Spanos, Rivers, & Ross, 1977).

Trance States

Various trance states experienced by individuals contain important elements of the loss of phenomenal will (Hughes, 1991; Winkelman, 1986). Spirit possession, channeling, visionary states, ecstatic states, and the like are often conscious and memorable to the performer, and so can yield actions that are later disavowed by the person in the nontrance state. These states are not necessarily pathological, in that they may not be associated with electroencephalographic patterns characteristic of epileptiform disorders (Hughes & Melville, 1990) and may also have no symptomatic similarity to multiple personality disorder (Hughes, 1992). Yet the individual will often disavow actions performed in the trance. Usually this disavowal takes the form of an attribution of responsibility for action to some nonself agent, such as a spirit or entity.

Motor Automatisms

A person's body may move involuntarily under certain conditions. When one stands at the edge of a precipice, for example, it is not uncommon to sense one's body teetering a bit. This tendency has been exploited in the "body sway" test of hypnotic susceptibility introduced by Hull (1933), in which subjects are told to stand still with eyes closed and are given verbal suggestions that they are falling forward. Slight tilts are commonly observed, and from time to time someone falls over completely (Eysenck & Furneaux, 1945). A related effect was described by James (1904/1986) as a motor automatism that occurs in the "willing game." In this game, players lay hands on a blindfolded perceiver who is charged with finding an object hidden by the players in the room. The perceiver often successfully finds the object merely by sensing the involuntary checking and encouraging pressures of the players. The players typically disavow any feeling of doing in this guidance, and may even produce the effect when it is against their monetary self-interest (Kreskin, 1984).

EXISTING ACCOUNTS OF THE AUTOMATISMS

This collection of automatisms, although no doubt incomplete, gives some sense of the range of activities it is popularly acknowledged that normal people may disavow, as well as of the circumstances that accompany such disavowal. The feeling of doing can obviously be disattached from actions that vary from the simple to the highly complex. The whole range of these phenomena seems not to have been explained by any one theory that is widely satisfying, but there do exist several explanations that have important merits and that offer various compelling kinds of evidence. We explore each of these briefly here.

The Imagination Hypothesis

One explanation of automatisms is that action can follow from imagination without intent. This notion of "ideomotor action" was proposed by Carpenter (1884) and elaborated by James (1890) and Arnold (1946). Carpenter suggested that action that occurs without willful intent is generated by "expectant attention," a state of "the whole Mind being 'possessed' with the idea that a certain action will take place, and being eagerly directed (generally with more or less of emotional excitement) towards the indications of its occurrence" (p. 282).

Remarking on the Chevreul pendulum, for example, Carpenter (1884) suggested that the imagination of movement is what creates disavowed movement:

> If "a fragment of anything, of any shape," be suspended from the end of the fore-finger or thumb, and the Attention be intently fixed upon it, regular oscillations will be frequently seen to take place in it.... Now this will occur, notwithstanding the strong Volitional determination of the experimenter to maintain a complete immobility in the suspended finger.... [The] impulse to

> [the movements] is entirely derived by his expectation of the given result. For if he be ignorant of the change which is made in the conditions of the experiment, and should expect or guess something different from that which really exists, the movement will be in accordance with his Idea, not with the reality. (pp. 284–286)

Carpenter went on to describe the pendulum illusion as a "satisfactory example of the general principle, that, in certain individuals, and in a certain state of mental concentration, the expectation of a result is sufficient to determine—without any voluntary effort, and even in opposition to the Will (for this may be honestly exerted in the attempt to keep the hand perfectly unmoved)—the Muscular movements by which it is produced" (1884, p. 287).

Carpenter extended this hypothesis to many of the favorite 19th-century automatisms, as he saw the influence of ideomotor action in the divining rod, table turning and tapping, and automatic writing and drawing. In the case of the divining rod, for example, he suggested that phenomenal will is not present: "For the mere act of holding the rod for some time in the required position, and of attending to its indications, is sufficient to produce a tendency to spasmodic contractions in the grasping muscles, notwithstanding a strong effort of the Will to the contrary" (1984, p. 289).

The imagination hypothesis was elaborated by Arnold (1946) to explain hypnotic suggestion more generally. She argued that the processes involved in imagining an event determine the experience of involuntary action, and she tested this hypothesis in an experiment. Subjects given a body sway test were asked to close their eyes and imagine themselves falling in a certain direction, and the extent of their excursion in this direction was recorded by a pencil fastened to a shoulder stirrup. The main finding of this research was that a combination of visual and kinesthetic imagination resulted in a more pronounced sway than did visual imagination alone. Arnold concluded that the more vivid the imaginative process, the more pronounced the overt movements. She noted:

> In all these cases the supposedly "central" process of thinking or imagining seems to initiate directly certain peripheral changes. Probably because of this direct connection, movements are experienced as different from ordinary "willed" movements. Psychologically speaking, the experience of "effort" or "intent" is absent. Thus executing a movement as the result of imagining it represents a gradual intensification of the minimal motor nerve excitation accompanying the imaginative process. (Arnold, 1946, p. 115)

Modern variations on the imagination hypothesis have emphasized the idea that the mechanism whereby imagination yields action is different in important ways from the mechanism whereby intention yields action. Gordon and Rosenbaum (1984), for example, have suggested that "subconsciously controlled" movements—which are produced by imagination of movement—can be performed more slowly even than intentional movements that occur in response to the instruction to move "as slowly as possible." Their version of the hypothesis anticipates the possibility that imagination produces action through a different psychological pathway than does intention. The nature of this pathway is not clear from these analyses, however, as it is proposed less as a positive alternative than as a default explanation of what must be happening if the feeling of doing is absent.

There are further contemporary expressions of the imagination hypothesis that emphasize the role of imagination in the transformation of intention or motivation. Unlike the early research that focused on bypassing phenomenal will, these studies have attempted to show that imagination can yield new intentions or motives, so as to change the direction of the willed action. Although the feeling of doing has not been measured in this research, it seems unlikely that this feeling would be dispelled under conditions that simply bend intention and do not override it. Still, this research suggests some possible mechanisms for the operation of the imagination hypothesis.

Carver, Ganellen, Froming, and Chambers (1982) observed, for example, that subjects for whom the idea of aggressive action was primed were subsequently likely to behave aggressively. Along the same line, Anderson (1983) had subjects imagine either themselves, a friend, or a disliked acquaintance performing or not performing a series of behaviors (e.g., donating blood). Subjects were asked to sketch a cartoon of the target performing the imagined behavior. It was found that imagining oneself performing (or not performing) a task produced corresponding changes in intentions toward that task (i.e., imagining oneself giving blood made one more likely to intend to give blood) relative to a pretest measure of intention to perform the behavior. In addition, the more frequent the imaginings, the more intention change was produced. These changes only occurred, however, when the target person was the subject himself or herself, and not the friend or disliked acquaintance.

In the same vein (pun unintended), Wilson and Capitman (1982) found evidence that making a behavioral script increasingly available to memory can have influential effects on subsequent social behavior. In a series of studies, subjects read either a story depicting a "boy-meets-girl" scenario or a control story. Afterwards, male subjects were asked to interact with a female confederate while the experimenter left the room. Those subjects who read the boy-meets-girl story behaved in a more friendly manner toward the female confederate (i.e., talked more, smiled more, leaned forward more, gazed more) than those who read the control story. These findings suggest that making a script more available to memory can change subsequent behavior.

The most recent variation on the imagination hypothesis is the body of research and theory on "auto-motives," the generation of actions that occurs when motives are prompted directly by the environment (Bargh, 1990; Bargh & Gollwitzer, 1994). Such activation is said to occur without the person's conscious awareness of the presence of the information in the environment, and the activated motivation subsequently influences the interpretation of behavioral information and the outcome of social judgment processes (e.g., Bargh, Bond, Lombardi, & Tota, 1986; Bargh & Tota, 1988). This activation occurs even under conditions of information overload and even when the subject is actively attempting to prevent it from occurring (Bargh & Pratto, 1986).

In sum, the imagination hypothesis has taken many forms over its history, but its central idea remains: Information suggestive of action can lead to action. In some cases, this process appears to happen without the occurrence of conscious intention, and when this happens the feeling of doing may be sidestepped on the way to action. In other cases, imagination may transform intentions or motives, and so yield action for which the feeling of doing is retained. None of the contemporary experimental work has focused on phenomenal will per se. Thus, there is insufficient evidence currently available to explicate when imagination might operate through intention, when it might create action without the experience of phenomenal will, or when it might not lead to action at all.

The Dissociation Hypothesis

If imagination can make a person act without phenomenal will, perhaps there is a whole psychological system underlying imagination-produced action that is separable from the psychological system underlying intentional action. This is the central idea of theories of dissociation. As originally proposed by Janet (1889), dissociation theory holds that the mind allows divided consciousness, in that separate components of mind may regulate mental functioning without intercommunication. According to this hypothesis, perceptions of involuntariness in hypnosis (or other states) are the result of dissociation between the mental subsystems that cause action and those that allow consciousness. Ideas and their associated actions can be dissociated or "split off" from normal consciousness, so that they no longer allow consciousness of the feeling of doing. Janet pointed out some parallels of hypnotic states and hysterical neuroses, and attempted to explain both by virtue of this theory.

The idea of dissociation was also explored by Sidis (1906), who believed that automatisms could be explained by the specific bifurcation of the individual psyche into two "selves." He maintained that in addition to the normal waking self (the controlled consciousness), each of us has a subconscious self, "a presence within us of a secondary, reflex, subwaking consciousness—the highway of suggestion" (p. 179). Whereas the waking self is responsible for actions that occur with phenomenal intent, the subconscious self produces those actions that occur through suggestion and without the feeling of doing. Sidis described the two selves as expressions in personality of the same intentional and imaginal sources of action with which we are already familiar, but noted that these selves are often in opposition regarding the control of behavior. He explained that the elaborate productions of meaningful material through automatic writing, Ouija boards, and the like are the results of the richness of the subconscious self. He believed the subconscious to be a homuncular entity of the first order, possessing its own form of memory, intelligence, and personality.

The modern version of all this is the neodissociation theory of Hilgard (1986). Like Janet and Sidis, Hilgard has argued that the operation of dissociated cognitive subsystems during hypnosis underlies subjects' diminished control over muscular movements, relative to more conscious, voluntary processes that mediate nonhypnotic, goal-directed experience. Actual conscious control is thus reduced along with the feeling of doing. This theory of divided consciousness holds that certain circumstances alter the integration of action-relevant cognitive structures and their relations to the executive ego (Kihlstrom, 1992). The theory is consistent in approach with recent theories of mind that stress its modular nature (e.g., Fodor, 1983; Gazzaniga, 1985) and the potential separability of conscious and nonconscious functions (Schacter, 1987). According to this viewpoint, then, the feeling of doing is associated specifically with an executive or controlling module of mind. Actions that occur without this feeling are processed through some other mental module, and simply do not contact the part of the mind that feels it does things.

The Social Pressure Hypothesis

Several researchers have campaigned fervently for the idea that people who report the loss of the feeling of doing are responding to social pressures to report such a loss (e.g., Lynn et al., 1990; Spanos, 1986). This work is concentrated on the explanation of hypnosis, but it can profitably be applied to other automatisms as well. In essence, the argument here is that the reported abridgement in the feeling of willful control of behavior that occurs in hypnosis arises not because of any reduction in willed action, but instead as a result of strong social influences that promote the alteration of the report.

The specific locus of this influence has differed for different commentators. Sarbin and Coe (1972) suggested that hypnotized subjects respond according to the scripted role they conceptualize for hypnotic behavior, modifying their own behaviors and reports of internal states strategically to fit the role. Barber, Spanos, and Chaves (1974) also suggest that hypnotic subjects truly do retain control of their actions during hypnosis, but add the idea that reports of involuntariness arise to reflect context-generated interpretations of these goal-directed actions. So, for example, a hypnotist's implication that an action will occur involuntarily (e.g., "Your arm is rising") rather than voluntarily (e.g., "Raise your arm") leads subjects to interpret the action as involuntary, despite its voluntary origin. Unlike the imagination hypothesis, the social pressure hypothesis does not ascribe a causal role to subjects' imaginings. Imaginings instead act to legitimize and reinforce the interpretation that the action occurred without phenomenal will (Lynn et al., 1990).

The social pressure hypothesis is very compelling at one level. This hypothesis emphasizes the observation that hypnotic behaviors (and many other automatisms) have all the properties typically associated with voluntary action, except that they lack the feeling of doing. Hypnotic behaviors appear to occur on purpose, can be changed to suit different situations, can be varied to meet a goal, and appear to consume attentional resources in a manner comparable to that of nonhypnotic performances (Lynn et al., 1990). It makes sense that in the face of strong social pressure to report no feeling of doing in these circumstances, people would indeed succumb and bring to bear various cognitive strategies to bolster their report and try to create an authentic experience in which the feeling of doing is indeed dissipated. This observation also holds for many of the other automatisms, because it could well be that cultural transmission of expectations about them has shaped pressures unique to each.

There is a difficulty with this hypothesis, however, that suggests it must be an incomplete account of automatisms. As Kihlstrom (1986) points out, even if social influences such as compliance, persuasion, self-presentation, and causal attribution do affect the responses of hypnotized subjects, it is not clear what mental mechanisms support these effects. Saying that people will forsake reports of voluntariness under social pressure does not explain what cognitive processes arise to allow this response to social pressure in the first place. Various cognitive processes must operate to enable people to respond to social pressures of any kind (Wegner & Erber, 1993; Wegner & Wenzlaff, in press), and the study of these could offer far more satisfying intrapsychic explanations than the claim that people are only responding to social pressure.

The Automatic-Habit Hypothesis

It has long been recognized that as actions are repeated, they become more automatic (e.g., Bryan & Harter, 1899). One of the concomitants of this effect is that the feeling of doing can abandon the action. Jastrow (1906) commented on the way in which well-learned and habitual actions drop out of conscious attention and lose their feeling of voluntariness: "When these accomplishments are of long standing and deeply ingrained, we call them automatic, and note with what suppressed consciousness and with what slightness of effort they are conducted; if new or of peculiar complexity, or if involving unusual intellectual factors, we observe how they enlarge in the field of our awareness and encroach upon our directive energies" (p. 314).

A particular turn one takes each day on the way home, for example, may begin after many such trips to shed the phenomenal will, so that it eventually has much the same lack of the feeling of doing as would one of the automatisms. It may be the case, of course, that the feeling of doing will return when one's attention is directed to the act of turning—say, by a verbal instruction or a disruption of the act. But in the normal course of making that turn, one may not experience it as phenomenally willed.

A modern version of the habit hypothesis has not been applied to the automatisms, however, because of the absence of practice and/or learning in most instances of such action. Despite a large contemporary literature on automatic processes in cognition and behavior (Bargh, 1984, 1989; Hasher & Zacks, 1979; Logan, 1988; Norman & Shallice, 1986; Posner & Snyder, 1975; Shiffrin & Schneider, 1977; Stelmach & Hughes, 1985; Vallacher & Wegner, 1985), there is no evidence to support the notion that automatisms are automatic behaviors in this fundamental sense. In large part, the automatisms are interesting for the very reason that they have some of the same psychological amorphousness we attribute to activities that recede through habit to the background of our minds.

AN IRONIC PROCESS ACCOUNT

A theory of ironic processes of mental control has recently been proposed to account for the intentional and counterintentional effects of individuals' attempts to control their minds (Wegner, 1994). The theory offers an explanation of the mental processes that foster people's successful control over their thoughts and actions, as well as the circumstances involved when their control efforts fail. This theory suggests a potentially useful approach to the feeling of doing that has not been captured in the prior accounts of automatisms. Specifically, the theory suggests that cases of automatism as well as other involuntary actions may paradoxically be a result of willful attempts to perform or to keep from performing an action. In the case of the divining rod, for example, unintended dips of the rod may result from the holder's constant efforts not to move it purposefully in his or her attempts to find water. The theory suggests that during people's attempts at controlling their actions, counterintentional actions may result as a consequence of the nature of the mental processes responsible for promoting successful control.

Description of the Theory

According to the theory, an attempt to control one's mind (or emotion or action) initiates two cognitive processes, an "intentional operating process" and an "ironic monitoring process." The intentional operating process is the willful probe searching for the mental contents consistent with the desired mental state. In other words, the operating process is the conscious and strategic process involved in mental control attempts. The ironic monitoring process, in contrast, searches for thoughts that indicate a failure to reach the desired state. Both processes increase the cognitive accessibility of the mental contents for which they are searching, and thereby have separate influences on the mind. Whereas the operating process is effortful and consciously guided, however, the monitoring process is unconscious and less demanding of mental effort. Normally, these two processes work together to promote effective control of the mind. The control of anything involves changing it to a certain criterion, after all, and processes are thus needed to provide both the change and the assessment of progress in reaching the criterion. The processes suggested here thus resemble the "operate" and "test" components of any control system (Miller, Galanter, & Pribram, 1960).

Consider how these processes would function when one is trying to control one's laughter at seeing someone slip on a patch of ice. When one resolves not to laugh, the operating process will probably search for thoughts or activities inconsistent with laughter. One may try to think about how much the fall must hurt, or one may look away to find a different focus of attention. These conscious and effortful activities may very well succeed in achieving the avoidance of mirth. The monitoring process is specifically set to detect laughing, however, by searching for thoughts or sensations or activities that are inconsistent with the desired state of impassivity. On encountering the beginnings of a giggle, the monitor indicates that one's control efforts are failing and puts the intentional operating process to work. The operating processes again searches for sensations and thoughts consistent with the desired state (i.e., not laughing). In many cases, the efforts furnished by the intentional operating process are effective, and the person's attention becomes preoccupied by stimuli congruent with the desired state. One politely holds back the hilarity, and perhaps even helps the person to his or her feet.

When attentional resources are limited, however, these efforts can go awry. Because the operating process is effortful, it can be distracted or undermined by any number of other demands on mental resources. When resources are reduced (e.g., by fatigue, time pressure, difficulty, or stress), the search process guided by the intentional operator could fail to increase access to the desired mental contents. Meanwhile, though, the ironic monitoring process will continue to increase accessibility of thoughts, sensations, and activities that indicate failure of the intended operation. It is in this sense that the monitoring process is ironic. When cognitive load exhausts one's attentional capacities, efforts at mental control may liberate the monitoring process to induce just the very state that the intentional efforts have been attempting to avoid. A person who is tired, drunk, or in a hurry, for instance, may find that the attempt to stifle laughter instead produces it.

This theory depends, then, on the idea that mental search processes underlie the production of thought, action, and emotion. Both the operating process and the monitoring process increase the influence of ranges of stimulation that can prompt thoughts, acts, or affects. The processes function by enhancing the likelihood that such stimulation will be selected from preconscious sensory and memory input to influence the production of thought as well as somatic and autonomic activation. The operating process performs this task more effectively and with greater use of cognitive resources than the monitoring process, and is accompanied by the feeling of doing. Even so, the ironic monitoring process can take charge of the inputs that produce thought, action, and emotion when the operating process is distracted. When this happens, the person may do, think, or feel precisely the opposite of what he or she intends to do, think, or feel.

Evidence supporting the theory of ironic processes of mental control has arisen in several domains (Wegner, 1994). The research has uncovered ironic effects of thought suppression and concentration (Wegner & Erber, 1992; Wegner, Erber, & Zanakos, 1993): Under cognitive load, people trying to avoid a thought find it returning to mind more often than a thought on which they are trying to concentrate. There are ironies of mood control (Wegner, Erber, & Zanakos, 1993): Under cognitive load, people trying to be happy become sad—and people trying to be sad get happy. There are also ironic effects of intentional relaxation (Wegner, Broome, & Blumberg, 1993): People trying to relax under load become more anxious than those who are not trying to relax. Intentional sleep induction is another venue for irony (Ansfield, Wegner, & Bowser, 1994): People trying hard to go to sleep under load fall asleep more slowly than those who are not trying. Also, there are ironic effects of intentional stereotype inhibition (Wegner, Erber, & Bowman, 1994): People trying not to be sexist when under cognitive load are more likely to make sexist statements than people who are not attempting to avoid sexism. The general finding in these studies, then, is that when mental control can be exercised successfully in a particular realm, the imposition of a cognitive load during a control attempt typically produces mental and behavioral expressions that represent the ironic opposite of the desired state.

As a rule, the ironic effects that accrue in these circumstances are not embraced as willful or intentional. When a person tries to suppress a thought, for example, and experiences intrusive returns of that thought as the result of the ironic monitoring process, these returns are disavowed and seen as having occurred against the person's will (Wegner, 1992). Indeed, because ironic effects always directly oppose intention, they are wholly divorced from any experience of phenomenal will. How can people have the feeling of doing for a particular behavior or mental event when they are fully devoted to the feeling of doing the opposite?

This reasoning suggests that ironic processes may underlie some of the losses of phenomenal will observed in the automatisms. This idea is bolstered by the recognition that the specific circumstances that produce ironic effects—willful control combined with mental load—are often the precise conditions that appear necessary for the production of automatisms. The attempt *not* to move in a particular way has been mentioned as a precondition for the pendulum illusion (Carpenter, 1884), for motor automatisms such as body sway (Arnold, 1946) and the willing game (Kreskin, 1984); for the rod movement in dowsing (Carpenter, 1884; Vogt & Hyman, 1959); for table turning and tapping (Sidis, 1906); and for some forms of automatic writing and drawing (Koutstaal, 1992). People trying to perform such automatisms are, after all, motivated to gain the benefits of the mystical or otherwise impersonal forces they are summoning in their efforts to create the automatic movement. Any willful initiation of an action consistent with the automatism will undermine their efforts, resulting in a failure to produce the desired automatism.

It seems, then, that some proportion of these automatisms may occur because of ironic effects occuring under conditions of mental load. Some form of mental load, after all, is also mentioned widely in this literature as an important precondition for most of the automatisms, including hypnosis and other trance states (Carpenter, 1884; Sidis, 1906; Jastrow, 1906; Hilgard, 1986). Perhaps the feeling of doing is bypassed primarily by the occurrence of ironic behavioral effects. Automatism may occur without phenomenal will because the person either is trying to do the opposite of the automatism or is specifically trying not to "do" the automatism.

The Pendulum Studies

As a first step in exploring this possibility, we have conducted studies of the ironic effects of movement in the Chevreul pendulum illusion (Wegner & Ansfield, 1995). In our first study, subjects each held a pendulum made of a 2-g crystalline pendant on a 30-cm length of nylon fishing line. All subjects were given the task of attempting to control the movement of the pendulum, by not letting it move in the direction paralleling one axis of two drawn on a sheet of paper over which they held it. Observers recorded the movement of the pendulum, noting the maximum distance (in centimeters) that the point of the bob traveled along the forbidden axis. Also, some subjects were given a mental load during the task of counting backward from 1,000 by sevens. Consistent with the ironic process theory, the subjects who performed the task under high cognitive load exhibited significantly greater movement in the forbidden direction (M = 3.11 cm) than those who were under no cognitive load (M = 2.56 cm), t (17) = 2.40, p = .03. This little experiment lacked an important comparison condition, however: A measure was not made of changes in movement in other, nonforbidden directions.

To examine whether movement in the forbidden direction exceeds movement in other directions, we (Wegner & Ansfield, 1995) performed another study. As in the first, subjects were either asked to control the movement of a pendulum under a high cognitive load (counting backward from 1,000 by sevens) or under no load. Again, some of the subjects were asked to try *not* to allow the pendulum to move in the direction paralleling the x-axis. Other subjects, however, were asked to hold the pendulum as steady as they could, with no forbidden direction stated. The pendulum was held over a glass plate on which a transparent grid with highlighted axis was centered. A videotape record of the pendulum movement was made by a video camera facing upward under the glass plate.

We predicted that subjects would be more likely to produce movement of the pendulum in the forbidden direction when told to try not to let it move in that direction than when asked simply to hold it as steady as they could. The further prediction made by the ironic process model was that this ironic effect would be magnified under a high cognitive load. As an illustration of these expectations, we show in Figure 21.1 the patterns of movement we observed for a pilot subject in this study who was asked to perform each of the tasks in turn. For these drawings, we played back a 30-second video clip in each condition frame by frame, and traced movement onto a transparency fastened to the video screen. The greatest distance of pendulum swing for this subject was 2.5 cm.

When the subject was asked to hold the pendulum as steady as possible (Figure 21.1a), only slight movements occurred in random directions. When the cognitive load was introduced (Figure 21.1b), the subject became less accurate in holding the pendulum steady, but again this movement was not concentrated in any direction. When the subject was told not to allow the pendulum to move in the direction paralleling the *x*-axis (Figure 21.1c), however, movement of the pendulum in just that forbidden direction resulted. And finally, when the subject attempted not to move the pendulum in the direction paralleling the *x*-axis while under the high load (Figure 21.1d), the movement of the pendulum in the forbidden direction was most pronounced.

These observations were mirrored in the aggregate data for the study as a whole (see Figure 21.2). Observers watched the videotapes and counted the number of movements of the pendulum parallel to each of the two axes. We then calculated the ratio of the average number of movements of the pendulum in the (sometimes forbidden) direction parallel to the *x*-axis to

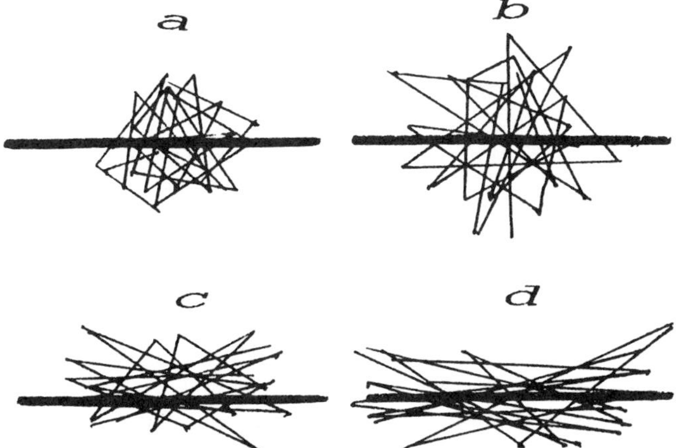

FIGURE 21.1. Pendulum movements for a subject asked (a) to hold the pendulum steady, (b) to hold it steady and to perform a mental task, (c) not to move it along the displayed axis, and (d) not to move it along the axis and to perform a mental task. Based on data from Wegner and Ansfield (1995).

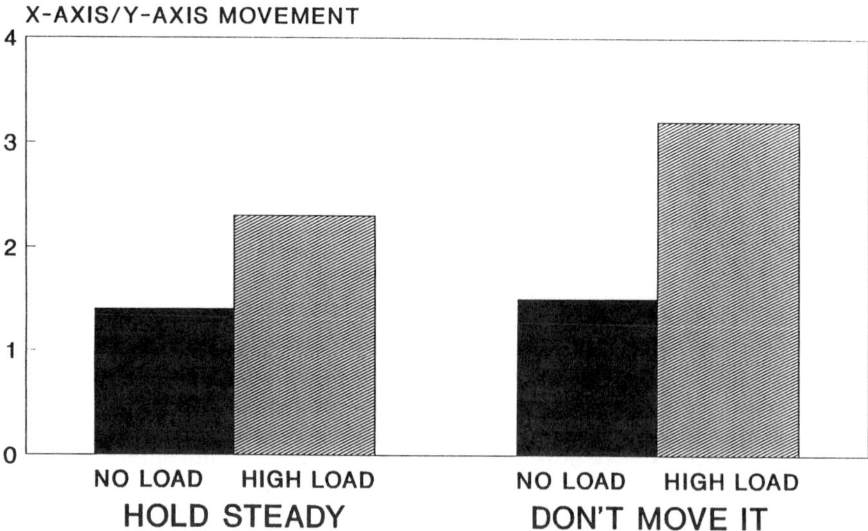

FIGURE 21.2. Mean ratio of *x*-axis pendulum movements to *y*-axis movements under instruction to hold it steady or not to move it on the *x*-axis, and under cognitive load versus no load. Based on data from Wegner and Ansfield (1995).

the average number of movements in the direction paralleling the *y*-axis for five trials over a 5-minute period. Any number greater than 1 illustrates greater pendulum movements in the forbidden direction (paralleling the *x*-axis) than in the direction paralleling the *y*-axis. First, without considering cognitive load, we found that subjects told not to allow the pendulum to move back and forth exhibited more movement in the forbidden direction ($M = 2.67$) than did subjects told to hold the pendulum steady ($M = 1.47$), $F(1, 20) = 6.50$, $p = .02$. Across both levels of load, then, there was an overall tendency for the mentioning of a forbidden direction to induce pendulum movement in that direction.

Cognitive load had the expected magnifying influence on this difference. With no cognitive load, subjects told not to allow movement in the *x*-axis direction ($M = 2.21$) did move it in the forbidden direction more often than did those told to hold the pendulum steady ($M = 1.36$), but not significantly so, $F(1, 20) = 1.64$, n.s. However, there was a significant difference in the measured ratio for subjects under a high cognitive load. Subjects asked not to allow the pendulum to move in the forbidden direction moved the pendulum more often in the forbidden direction ($M = 3.12$) than did those told to hold the pendulum steady ($M = 1.58$), $F(1, 20) = 5.40$, $p = .03$.

We did not interview subjects systematically about the feeling of doing in these experiments, but they frequently mentioned the odd absence of this in their informal comments. Many of them spontaneously reported being aware that the pendulum was moving not only without their phenomenal will, but in fact *against* that will. This, then, indicates one way in which the feeling of doing may be divorced from action in a relatively simple and replicable laboratory situation. It seems that when people are asked not to do something, and are given a taxing mental load at the same time, they find themselves doing that very thing without any feeling that they are doing it.

Ironic Processes and the Automatisms

It is tempting to conclude from these findings, and from findings regarding other manifestations of ironic processes (Wegner, 1994), that the ironic monitoring process might be a key component in an overall account of the automatisms. Clearly, the motor automatisms that involve discrete, simple movements—pendulum movement; dowsing; body sway; the willing game; and table turning, tilting, and tapping—seem readily explainable by this process. It makes sense that people who come to perform these automatisms have some skepticism about their occurrence at the outset, enough to fuel a subtle desire not to have these things happen. Even a desire not to perform a willful act is enough to create this inclination. This motive thus installs an ironic monitoring process that inclines the person toward the unplanned action. Even minimal cognitive load, then, in the form of brief disattention from the operating process that is attempting to forestall the movement, may be sufficient to produce these movements.

This ironic process account goes beyond the imagination hypothesis to suggest that the actions one does not want to have happen are the ones that may be produced by a type of imagination without phenomenal will. The reason why the feeling of doing is absent in these cases, moreover, is that there is indeed no will involved. Counterintentional action is produced by the monitoring process rather than the operating process, and so does not carry the usual portents of will—the consciousness and effortfulness associated with the operating process. The ironic process account is in this sense also consistent with the dissociation hypothesis. Just as dissociation theories would hold that actions can be initiated by cognitive systems that are not conscious or effortful, the ironic process account traces simple automatisms to the ironic monitoring process. This process can increase the cognitive accessibility of a range of mental content without any experience of effort (Wegner & Erber, 1992), and so may qualify as an independent mental module that can control action without the feeling of doing. In a sense, any attempt to control mind or action thus produces a dissociation—between the operating process bent on producing that effect and the monitoring process that ironically enhances the likelihood of opposing effects.

The ironic process account is less compatible with the social pressure hypothesis, at least as it is applied to the simple automatisms. The social pressure account holds that behavioral automatisms accrue from the person's perception of pressure to interpret his or her voluntary actions as involuntary. The ironic movements we have observed in the pendulum studies, however, cannot arise from perceptions of social pressure, because any prevailing pressure in that situation is aimed at influencing the person *not* to produce the automatism. It may be the desire not to perform the automatism, rather than the desire to perform it, that induces the ironic monitoring process to generate the movement. For this reason, any straightforward application of a social pressure account in these sorts of instances must be incorrect.

It is also difficult to assimilate the ironic process account to any standard version of the automatic-habit hypothesis. Clearly, there is no basis for claiming that the ironic movements observed in the pendulum studies are any more habitual or practiced than the intentional movements. Because it is unlikely that repetition plays a role in the production of ironic movements, but these movements still occur without the feeling of doing and without other indications of effortful, conscious activity (Wegner & Erber, 1992), there may be a basis in these findings to suggest that the ironic process model provides a path to automaticity that is very different from the path assumed in the learning or habit account. The simple automatisms may well be automatic, in other words, but not because they are well rehearsed.

Although the ironic process hypothesis thus seems to provide a compelling alternative to prior hypotheses in the case of the simple motor automatisms, it remains to be seen whether it will be equally useful in explaining the more complex automatisms. How could a lengthy bout of automatic writing, for example, be induced by an ironic process? Could the person be specifically hoping not to write what appears to come automatically from the pen? The difficulty with applying the ironic process hypothesis to this case is echoed by similar problems in using it to account for automatisms in hypnosis, Ouija board spelling, facilitated communication, or trance channeling. These protracted performances that occur without phenomenal will seem to be far less amenable to an elementary application of the ironic process theory.

Nonetheless, it may be that the theory opens a small door toward an explanation of these puzzling phenomena. We can speculate on three avenues of explanation. It might be, first, that ironic effects serve as initial pieces of evidence that convince people it is reasonable to interpret their subsequent voluntary actions as arising from involuntary sources. Just as a person who has teetered at the edge of a precipice, for example, may conclude that he or she has had a subconscious impulse to jump, the person who experiences some ironic automatisms may conclude that he or she is capable generally of performing actions without phenomenal will. This interpretive set could operate through mechanisms such as those suggested by the social pressure theorists (Spanos, 1986) to promote long performances that are not automatisms themselves, but are produced by people who have become persuaded by ironic effects that these performances may also be unwilled.

A second way in which ironic processes may be involved in the production of complex automatisms is through the chaining of separate acts that are variously random, willful, or ironic—but that are identified after the fact as unwilled. In the case of the Ouija board, for example, there are points in each performance that might be willed or random or ironic. When one has asked the board "What will I do next summer?" and it has answered "SW______," for example, one may hope it will go on to say "SWIM" rather "SWEAT." The "SW______" may have been produced randomly, and the continuation may occur then in the ironic direction ("E") because the player has specifically entertained the "SWEAT" completion and hoped against it. Finally, the word may be completed willfully ("AT") in the attempt to have it make sense. The entire performance will have a certain unwilled quality, given the contribution of randomness and ironic process, so that overall it may seem reasonable to call it "unwilled." The generation of long or complex acts that occur without the feeling of doing does not require that willful or random subacts *never* occur along the way, but only that the completed act be identified as unwilled at the end. The emergent meaning of an act produced in this way can be far more compelling than the meanings of its components, and it may thus come to seem unwilled as a whole (cf. Wegner, Vallacher, Macomber, Wood, & Arps, 1984).

There is one other way in which ironic processes may help us to understand lengthy sequences of action that occur without phenomenal will. It may be that some form of the mental monitoring process that is enlisted in the pursuit of mental control extends beyond the error-monitoring function it fulfills in ironic process theory. The unconscious and relatively effortless monitoring system that is invoked in mental control may perhaps be recruited in some form for other psychological purposes. Most of the continuous, complex automatisms occur under conditions of attenuated cognitive capacity, and this is precisely when monitoring processes that are not just tuned to catch errors may reach a level of influence over behavior rivaling that of operating processes. There is evidence, for example, that unconscious monitoring systems initiated by conscious choice may be responsible for creative insights (e.g., Bowers, Regehr, Balthazard, & Parker, 1990), memory retrieval (Reason & Lucas, 1984), and many other cognitive processes (Bargh, 1989, 1990). Why shouldn't they create behavior as well? It may be that the more elaborate automatisms arise through a monitoring process that, like the imagination system envisioned by Carpenter (1884), can be initiated through conscious intention, but then exerts its influence on behavior without the feeling of doing. Suffice it to say that at this point, there is evidence of such monitoring-induced behavior for the simple automatisms—but there is only the suggestion that it may be possible to elude the feeling of doing through such monitoring more generally.

Finally, even if ironic monitoring processes do present a useful approach to the understanding of disavowed behavior, we must note that they offer only one facet of a complete analysis of the problem of the feeling of doing. The automatisms include some of the most enigmatic behaviors facing modern psychology, from trance channeling to hypnotic phenomena and beyond, and it is clear that much more remains to be added on the way to a full account of such unusual, apparently unwilled behavior. Many of the automatisms occur under conditions in which the causes of one's own behavior are made murky by the contributions of others, for example, and this source of ambiguity has barely been touched on in the existing literature. For our part, we have tried to use an ironic process approach to organize this unruly set of phenomena in terms of two key variables: the desire to exert mental control, and the presence of mental load. When these are present, ironic behaviors may result that occur without the feeling of doing, and even in spite of the feeling of doing the opposite.

CONCLUSION

In some sense, our theoretical approach to the problem of the feeling of doing is backward. Most commentators who have puzzled over the problems of phenomenal will would conclude that when people do something without feeling they are doing it, there is some difficulty or breakdown in the part of the mind that is responsible for consciousness of action. Some monitoring function appears to be asleep while some operating function is making things happen. Our approach, suggested by the ironic process theory, is the reverse. We believe that the feeling of doing is irrevocably associated with the operating processes that create mental and behavioral changes. Thus, many of the activities of mind or body that ensue without this feeling may be attributable to the monitoring processes. And, as a rule, these monitoring processes create behaviors that are the opposite of those engendered by the operating processes. By and large, then, the feeling of doing is absent when, under conditions of mental load, people find that these monitoring processes take the reins and lead them to do what they least intend.

ACKNOWLEDGMENTS

Research reported in this chapter was supported by Grant No. MH49127 from the National Institute of Mental Health. We thank Robin Vallacher for his helpful comments on an earlier draft.

REFERENCES

Anderson, C. A. (1983). Imagination and expectation: The effect of imagining behavioral scripts on personal influences. *Journal of Personality and Social Psychology, 45,* 293–305.

Ansfield, M., Wegner, D. M., & Bowser, R. (1994). *Ironic effects in sleep and wakefulness.* Manuscript in preparation.

Arnold, M. B. (1946). On the mechanism of suggestion and hypnosis. *Journal of Abnormal and Social Psychology, 41,* 107–128.

Barber, T. X., Spanos, N. P., & Chaves, J. F. (1974). *Hypnosis, imagination, and human potentialities.* Elmsford, NY: Pergamon Press.

Bargh, J. A. (1984). Automatic and conscious processing of social information. In R. S. Wyer, Jr., & T. K. Srull (Eds.), *Handbook of social cognition* (Vol. 3, pp. 1–43). Hillsdale, NJ: Erlbaum.

Bargh, J. A. (1989). Conditional automaticity: Varieties of automatic influence in social perception and cognition. In J. S. Uleman & J. A. Bargh (Eds.), *Unintended thought* (pp. 3–51). New York: Guilford Press.

Bargh, J. A. (1990). Auto-motives: Preconscious determinants of thought and behavior. In E. T. Higgins & R. M. Sorrentino (Eds.), *Handbook of motivation and cognition: Foundation of social behavior* (Vol. 2, pp. 93–130). New York: Guilford Press.

Bargh, J. A., Bond, R. N., Lombardi, W. J., & Tota, M. E. (1986). The additive nature of chronic and temporal sources of construct accessibility. *Journal of Personality and Social Psychology, 50,* 869–878.

Bargh, J. A., & Gollwitzer, P. M. (1994). Environmental control of goal-directed action: Automatic and strategic contingencies between situations and behavior. In W. D. Spaulding (Ed.), *Nebraska Symposium on Motivation: Vol. 41. Integrative views of motivation, cognition, and emotion* (pp. 71–124). Lincoln: University of Nebraska Press.

Bargh, J. A., & Pratto, F. (1986). Individual construct accessibility and perceptual selection. *Journal of Experimental Social Psychology, 22,* 293–311.

Bargh, J. A., & Tota, M. E. (1988). Context-dependent automatic processing in depression: Accessibility of automatic constructs with regard to self but not others. *Journal of Personality and Social Psychology, 54,* 925–939.

Biklen, D. (1991). Communication unbound: Autism and praxis. *Harvard Educational Review, 60,* 291–314.

Binet, A. (1905). *On double consciousness: Experimental psychological studies.* Chicago: Open Court.

Bird, C. (1979). *The divining hand.* New York: Dutton.

Bowers, K. S., Regehr, G., Balthazard, C., & Parker, K. (1990). Intuition in the context of discovery. *Cognitive Psychology, 22,* 72–110.

Bryan, W. L., & Harter, L. (1899). Studies on the telegraphic language: The acquisition of a hierarchy of habits. *Psychological Review, 6,* 345–378.

Carpenter, W. G. (1884). *Principles of mental physiology, with their applications to the training and discipline of the mind and study of its morbid conditions.* New York: Appleton.

Carver, C. S., Ganellen, R. J., Froming, W. J., & Chambers, W. (1983). Modeling: An analysis in terms of category accessibility. *Journal of Experimental Social Psychology, 19,* 403–421.

Chevreul, M. E. (1833). Lettre à M. Ampère sur une classe particulaire. *Review des Deux Mondes, 2,* 258–266.

Crossley, R., & Remington-Gurney, J. (1992). Getting the words out: Facilitated communication training. *Topics in Language Disorders, 12,* 29–45.

Easton, R. D., & Shor, R. E. (1975). Information processing analysis of the Chevreul pendulum illusion. *Journal of Experimental Psychology: Human Perception and Performance, 1,* 231–236.

Easton, R. D., & Shor, R. E. (1976). An experimental analysis of the Chevreul pendulum illusion. *Journal of General Psychology, 95,* 111–125.

Easton, R. D., & Shor, R. E. (1977). Augmented and delayed feedback in the Chevreul pendulum illusion. *Journal of General Psychology, 97,* 167–177.

Eysenck, H. J., & Furneaux, W. D. (1945). Primary and secondary suggestibility: An experimental and statistical study. *Journal of Experimental Psychology, 35,* 485–503.

Fodor, J. A. (1983). *The modularity of mind.* Cambridge, MA: MIT Press.

Gazzaniga, M. S. (1985). *The social brain.* New York: Basic Books.

Gorassini, D. R., & Perlini, A. H. (1988). Making suggested responses seem involuntary: Experience structuring by hypnotic and nonhypnotic subjects. *Journal of Research in Personality, 22,* 213–231.

Gordon, A. M., & Rosenbaum, D. A. (1984). Conscious and subconscious arm movements: Application of signal detection theory to motor control. *Bulletin of the Psychonomic Society, 22,* 214–216.

Graves, T. (1986). *The diviner's handbook.* New York: Destiny.

Hasher, L., & Zacks, R. T. (1979). Automatic and effortful processes in memory. *Journal of Experimental Psychology: General, 108,* 356–388.

Hilgard, E. R. (1986). *Divided consciousness: Multiple controls in human thought and action* (expanded ed.). New York: Wiley-Interscience.

Hostler, S. L., Allaire, J. H., & Christoph, R. A. (1993). Childhood sexual abuse reported by facilitated communication. *Pediatrics, 91,* 1190–1192.

Hughes, D. J. (1991). Blending with an other: An analysis of trance channeling in the United States. *Ethos, 19,* 161–184.

Hughes, D. J. (1992). Differences between trance channeling and multiple personality disorder on structured interview. *Journal of Transpersonal Psychology, 24,* 181–192.

Hughes, D. J., & Melville, N. T. (1990). Changes in brainwave activity during trance channeling: A pilot study. *Journal of Transpersonal Psychology, 22,* 175–189.

Hull, C. (1933). *Hypnosis and suggestibility.* New York: Appleton-Century.

Hunt, S. (1985). *Ouija: The most dangerous game.* New York: Harper & Row.

James, W. (1890). *Principles of psychology* (2 vols.). New York: Holt.

James, W. (1986). Notes on automatic writing. In *The works of William James: Essays in psychical research* (pp. 37–55). Cambridge, MA: Harvard University Press. (Original work published 1889)

James, W. (1986). A case of automatic drawing. In *The works of William James: Essays in psychical research* (pp. 220–228). Cambridge, MA: Harvard University Press. (Original work published 1889)

Janet, P. (1889). *L'automatisme psychologique.* Paris: Félix Alcan.

Jastrow, J. (1906). *The subconscious.* Boston: Houghton Mifflin.

Kihlstrom, J. F. (1986). Strong inferences about hypnosis. *Behavioral and Brain Sciences, 9,* 474–475.

Kihlstrom, J. F. (1992). Dissociation and dissociations: A comment on consciousness and cognition. *Consciousness and Cognition, 1,* 47–53.

Koutstaal, W. (1992). Skirting the abyss: A history of experimental explorations of automatic writing in psychology. *Journal of the History of the Behavioral Sciences, 28,* 5–27.

Kreskin. (1984). *Secrets of the Amazing Kreskin.* Buffalo, NY: Prometheus Books.

Logan, G. D. (1988). Toward an instance theory of automatization. *Psychological Review, 95,* 492–527.

Lynn, S. J., Rhue, J. W., & Weekes, J. R. (1990). Hypnotic involuntariness: A social cognitive analysis. *Psychological Review, 97,* 169–184.

Miller, G. A., Galanter, E., & Pribram, K. H. (1960). *Plans and the structure of behavior.* New York: Holt.

Mulick, J. A., Jacobson, J. W., & Kobe, F. H. (1993). Anguished silence and helping hands: Autism and facilitated communication. *Skeptical Inquirer, 17,* 270–280.

Norman, D. A., & Shallice, T. (1986). Attention to action: Willed and automatic control of behavior. In R. J. Davidson, G. E. Schwartz, & D. Shapiro (Eds.), *Consciousness and self-regulation* (Vol. 4, pp. 1–18). New York: Plenum.

Posner, M. I., & Snyder, C. R. R. (1975). Attention and cognitive control. In R. L. Solso (Ed.), *Information processing and cognition* (pp. 55–85). Hillsdale, NJ: Erlbaum.

Reason, J., & Lucas, D. (1984). Using cognitive diaries to investigate naturally occurring memory blocks. In J. E. Harris & P. E. Morris (Eds.), *Everyday memory, actions, and absent-mindedness* (pp. 53–70). London: Academic Press.

Sarbin, T. R., & Coe, W. C. (1972). *Hypnosis: A social psychological analysis of influence communication.* New York: Holt, Rinehart & Winston.

Schacter, D. L. (1987). Implicit memory: History and current status. *Journal of Experimental Psychology: Learning, Memory, and Cognition, 13,* 501–518.

Sidis, B. (1906). *The psychology of suggestion.* New York: Appleton.

Shiffrin, R. M., & Schneider, W. (1977). Controlled and automatic human information processing: II. Perceptual learning, automatic attending, and a general theory. *Psychological Review, 84,* 127–190.

Solomons, L. M. & Stein, G. (1896). Studies from the psychological laboratory of Harvard University: II. Normal motor automatism. *Psychological Review, 3,* 492–512.

Spanos, N. P. (1986). Hypnotic behavior: A social-psychological interpretation of amnesia, analgesia, and "trance logic." *Behavioral and Brain Sciences, 9,* 449–502.

Spanos, N. P., & Barber, T. X. (1972). Cognitive activity during "hypnotic" suggestibility: Goal-directed fantasy and the experience of nonvolition. *Journal of Personality, 40,* 510–524.

Spanos, N. P., & Katsanis, J. (1989). Effects of instructional set on attributions of nonvolition during hypnotic and nonhypnotic analgesia. *Journal of Personality and Social Psychology, 56,* 182–188.

Spanos, N. P., Rivers, S. M., & Ross, S. (1977). Experienced involuntariness and response to hypnotic suggestions. *Annals of the New York Academy of Sciences, 296,* 208–221.

Stelmach, G. E., & Hughes, B. G. (1985). *Attention, motor control, and automaticity* (ASHA Report No. 15). Rockville, MD: American Speech–Language–Hearing Association.

Vallacher, R. R., & Wegner, D. M. (1985). *A theory of action identification.* Hillsdale, NJ: Erlbaum.

Vogt, E. Z., & Hyman, R. (1959). *Water witching U.S.A.* Chicago: University of Chicago Press.

Wegner, D. M. (1992). You can't always think what you want: Problems in the suppression of unwanted thoughts. In M. Zanna (Ed.), *Advances in experimental social psychology* (Vol. 25, pp. 193–225). San Diego, CA: Academic Press.

Wegner, D. M. (1994). Ironic processes of mental control. *Psychological Review, 101,* 34–52.

Wegner, D. M., & Ansfield, M. (1995). *Magnification of the Chevreul pendulum illusion under mental load.* Manuscript in preparation.

Wegner, D. M., Broome, A., & Blumberg, S. (1993). *When trying to relax makes you nervous: Electrodermal evidence of ironic effects of intentional relaxation.* Manuscript in preparation.

Wegner, D. M., & Erber, R. (1992). The hyperaccessibility of suppressed thoughts. *Journal of Personality and Social Psychology, 63,* 903–912.

Wegner, D. M., & Erber, R. (1993). Social foundations of mental control. In D. M. Wegner & J. W. Pennebaker (Eds.), *Handbook of mental control* (pp. 36–56). Englewood Cliffs, NJ: Prentice-Hall.

Wegner, D. M., Erber, R., & Bowman, R. E. (1994). *On trying not to be sexist.* Manuscript in preparation.

Wegner, D. M., Erber, R., & Zanakos, S. (1993). Ironic processes in the mental control of mood and mood-related thought. *Journal of Personality and Social Psychology, 65,* 1093–1104.

Wegner, D. M., Vallacher, R. R., Macomber, G., Wood, R., & Arps, K. (1984). The emergence of action. *Journal of Personality and Social Psychology, 46,* 269–279.

Wegner, D. M., & Wenzlaff, R. M. (in press). Mental control. In E. T. Higgins & A. W. Kruglanski (Eds.), *Social psychology: Handbook of basic principles.* New York: Guilford Press.

Wheeler, D. L., Jacobson, J. W., Paglieri, R. A., & Schwartz, A. A. (1993). An experimental assessment of facilitated communication. *Mental Retardation, 31,* 49–60.

Wilson, T. D., & Capitman, J. A. (1982). Effects of script availability on social behavior. *Personality and Social Psychology Bulletin, 8,* 11–20.

Winkelman, M. (1986). Trance states: A theoretical model and cross-cultural analysis. *Ethos, 14,* 174–204.

PART VI

Goal Influences on Social Interaction

Goals and motives can also affect behavior through their effects on social perception. One's current purposes determine in large part the way one conceptualizes or understands the behavior of those with whom one is interacting. And subsequent behavior towards those persons will be based on those categorizations. The chapters in Part VI demonstrate the many ways in which social perception mediates the motivation-behavior link.

Wicklund and Steins (Chapter 22) point out some important negative consequences of goal orientation. That is, the current press or dominant motive of the individual can determine the perception of others, inasmuch as those others are relevant to the achievement of that motive. In the example the authors give, as restaurant customers grow hungrier and hungrier waiting for their food to arrive, their perception of the waitress changes from an understanding of her as a complete person to one as a food deliverer and finally as a person who is thwarting their need for sustenance. In other words, the stronger the press operating on individuals, the more their perception and understanding of other people are reduced to the relevance and significance to that press. The larger point is that people are never motivated merely to form accurate and individuating impressions of others (such as when their outcomes depend on them); they are motivated to form impressions of others in terms of their utility to the satisfaction of the perceivers' important goals (i.e., egocentric perceptions).

Neuberg (Chapter 23) and Chaiken, Giner-Sorolla, and Chen (Chapter 24) highlight the importance of the individual's current goal for the outcome of person perception and persuasion attempts. Neuberg provides a cogent analysis of the motivational and cognitive variables that moderate the influence of expectancies on perception and behavior (i.e., the expectancy confirmation process). Neuberg argues that in social interaction a person can have any of a variety of motivations—from that of forming an accurate impression of the other person, to getting the other to like him or her, to being deferential to the other. This current goal influences whether one's initial expectancy of the other person is confirmed with little scrutiny, confirmed because of biased information-gathering strategies and selective attention, or confirmed or disconfirmed after an objective search for individuating information about the target. Neuberg emphasizes the importance of the outcome of this person perception process as a basis for how the perceiver then behaves toward the target (or avoids him or her entirely).

Chaiken and her colleagues also discuss the role of varying motivations—to hold accurate beliefs about the world, to hold beliefs consistent with existing attitudes and beliefs important to the self-concept, and to enjoy smooth and congenial social interactions—for the outcome of judgments and decisions. Specifically, the authors propose two basic modes of processing, heuristic and systematic. The former is characterized by a reliance on simple decision rules (e.g., bigger is better), and the latter is a more cognitively effortful analysis of the information. Which of these modes will be relied upon primarily is said to be a function of the level of confidence a person wants to have in his or her resultant opinion; the mode that achieves a sufficient amount of confidence will be employed. The importance of this sufficiency principle is therefore that it allows one to predict not simply whether the individual will engage in effortful information processing or not—in other words, engage in piecemeal versus stereotypic processing—but how much effort the individual will engage in to process the information. Moreover, Chaiken et al. show experimentally that which motivation a person has within the situation determines both how much effort is expended, and also (largely) the outcome of the judgment process.

Strack and Hannover (Chapter 25) are concerned with correction processes in judgment. Under what conditions do people attempt to correct judgments they have already made; when are they motivated to do so; and how do they go about it? The authors raise a very telling point at the outset: Exactly what does it mean to hold an accurate, unbiased belief? This is a critical issue for models (such as these described in Neuberg's and in Chaiken et al.'s chapters) that posit a motivation to hold accurate beliefs. Strack and Hannover note that "accuracy" can be defined by the individual in several ways: a judgment free of presumed bias, but perhaps also one that conforms to contemporaneous social norms as to appropriate beliefs to hold (viz., political correctness of beliefs). In other words, an important theoretical and research issue for those concerned with accuracy motivation is that of the definition and standards of accuracy as held by the individual.

Strack and Hannover continue by discussing the circumstances under which a person is motivated to correct a judgment. One critical precondition is the individual's being aware of an unwanted influence, such as perhaps being biased by a cultural or personally held stereotype. Even with this awareness, however, it is necessary to understand why the individual would be motivated to adjust a belief when it is understood as having been influenced by a stereotype or other false information. The authors proceed to analyze the epistemic and social motivations the individual may have for correction (such as a desire to hold valid beliefs), as well as the potential interpersonal costs of holding socially undesirable opinions.

CHAPTER 22 Person Perception under Pressure

When Motivation Brings About Egocentrism

Robert A. Wicklund
Gisela Steins

WHAT (WHO) IS THE PERSON IN PERSON PERCEPTION?

When psychology speaks of "perception of persons," the object of study is more often than not the physical being and that being's overt behaviors. Research is devoted to skin color, gender, facial characteristics, age, clothing, and other permanent, highly physical or material, visible features of people. Similarly, the focus of person perception research and theory is on the overt actions of people. How loudly do they speak? How many gestures do they make? How much smiling or grimacing do they engage in? How many intelligent-appearing answers to tests do they give? Not content to count up such physical and behavioral instances, the person perception literature devotes its attention especially to summary statements of such behavior (cf. Buss & Craik, 1983), in the form of terms that psychology often refers to as "behavioral dispositions" (e.g., "cheerful," "generous," "bad-tempered"). The *person,* then, for the psychology of person perception, is a physical event—one that is reduced to its overt expressions (i.e., the manifestation of "dispositions") and to physical characteristics such as gender, weight, height, or hair color.

If a perceiver (e.g., a respondent in a person perception study) ascribes the terms "aggressive" or "happy" to someone, the psychologist's interpretation is usually that the perceiver is inferring some sort of internal mental state (Benenson & Dweck, 1986). There is, however, no reason to impute such higher-order thinking processes to observers generally, given that the use of "aggressive" and so forth can easily be nothing more than a direct reference to the person's emitting aggressive or damaging behaviors, as observed by Buss and Craik (1983) in their reworking of the trait concept. It is interesting that the ascription of such terms (e.g., "She is loyal") also denotes a certain permanence.

In short, the person perceived in the person perception literature—at least as treated by the research psychologist—is to date a highly physicalistic entity, composed of overt physical characteristics (e.g., Cunningham, 1986; Dion, Berscheid, & Walster, 1972) and of permanent behavioral repertoires (Hamilton, 1979). In line with this existing movement or research enterprise, it seems clear that the respondents or perceivers can easily be judged for accuracy, in that all of what they are supposed to be perceiving has to do with physical, directly observable facts. But should we be content to leave this realm as the ultimate or sole definition of person perception? There may be more to the person, especially if we take a careful look at the perspective of the perceived.

PERSON PERCEPTION VIA INFERENCES

A study by White and Younger (1988) is instructive here. Requested to describe themselves, respondents referred frequently to emotions, attitudes, individual thoughts, or cognitions, and comparatively seldom to their own physical features or long-term behavioral tendencies (i.e., habits or so-called "dispositions"). Perceptions, apperceptions, motives, emotions, and attitudes—none of these is directly (visually or auditorily) perceivable by the external perceiver. These are elements residing inside the person, perhaps mysterious "phantoms" for many psychologists who prefer the route of physicalism, positivism, peripheralism, radical behaviorism, and the like (cf. Murray, 1938). For the hard-headed, positivistic observer, talking about someone else's emotions, motives, or thoughts is a wild process of inferences, guesswork, and unjustified imputations, unless, of course, the referent for the perceiver is the physical/behavioral fact. To be sure, this *is* the referent for many psychological theorists and researchers, in that the so-called "construct" is made equivalent to observable facts such as physical characteristics, overt behavior, or especially questionnaire responses, which are assumed to bear a one-to-one correspondence to fixed behavior patterns.

A Parallel between Person Perceivers in General and Psychologists as Person Perceivers

Cronbach and Meehl (1955) and Campbell and Fiske (1959) attempted to educate their readers in matters of psychological constructs. A "construct" is a construction made up or implemented by the observer to characterize a process that must be taking place in the thoughts, cognitions, emotions, and so forth of the perceived—but, at the same time, a process that cannot be touched, seen, or smelled directly. According to these authors' argumentation (which should not surprise readers as something new), the psychological observer makes inferences on the basis of multiple cues as to the inner state. For example, the inference of an anxious state can be made on the basis of answers to a standardized test (Taylor, 1952), as well as on the basis of facial expressions, the basis of escape behavior, and/or others.

If readers would like to appeal to logic to appreciate these points, then Feigl's (1958) idea of "triangulation" will be a comfortable one. Scientific concepts, whether in psychology or elsewhere, are said by Feigl to be "fixed" by triangulation in logical space. A parallel triangulation concept, but with respect to the search for causality, is to be found in Heider (1958). Other ways of referring to the same inference process are the terms "convergent operationalism" (Garner, Hake, & Eriksen, 1956) and "methodological triangulation" (Campbell & Fiske, 1959).

It is no different with person perception more generally. A person is confronted with wanting to make a statement about the inner psychological condition of the observed, but can arrive at "knowledge" of this condition only in the form of an inference. A good example, primarily as applied to children, is the privileged-information paradigm of Flavell, Botkin, Fry, Wright, and Jarvis (1968). Subjects are asked implicitly to make a judgment about another's knowledge state. In order to do this, the observer (perceiver) has to think about whether the perceived person was present in a setting in which the information was first made available. Not all respondents draw on this source of information, but if they do so they realize that the perceived was not present for the full story, and thus would be thinking in terms of a quite different version of the story. The Flavell et al. (1968) example is a crucial one for the psychology of person perception, in that it indicates that "knowledge" about another's knowledge or other experiential state cannot always be based on direct perceptions. In this case, the inference is based on the perceiver's knowledge of the target person's exposure.

More generally, if a perceiver is oriented toward uncovering another person's inner psychological condition, it is necessary to draw on multiple cues and to draw inferences from a combination of these cues. The construction or inference ("The child is tired," "The old man is hungry," "The workers are angry") is of course often mistrusted, both by positivistically thinking psychologists and by "normal" humans who want some kind of definitive evidence.

The Construct: Free and Uncertain

The difficulty that such constructs (constructions or inferences) pose for so many person perceivers is that they are indefinite. They are based on the accumulation of cues from different sources (e.g., self-reports, childhood events, and particular situations) and the placing together of these cues (i.e., drawing an inference based on them, which is necessarily an uncertain matter). The perceiver, when pressed for the "absolute correctness" of the inference, must admit that the subjective probability of such correctness is only 50%, or 20%, or 85%—in other words, that the inference is necessarily a construction, built around a psychological condition that *must* be in the perceived person's mind.

The person perception of which we are speaking here, involving the perceiver's building a construction with respect to inner events in the perceived person, stands in contrast to the usual person perception paradigms in psychology. For instance, the psychologist who is working with a thesis of visual salience (Hamilton, 1979; McArthur & Post, 1977) begins with the physical presence of the perceived person (the intensity of that presence is the independent variable), and then assesses the perception of some physicalistic aspects of the target person, such as the extremity of the person's behavioral inclinations. Or when person perception research steps into the realm of national stereotypes, as in a study by Katz and Braly (1933), the dimensions are (1) 5 traits from a list of 84 traits that are typical for nationality *X*, and (2) nationality. Each of these elements is purely physicalistic; the trait represents an assumed behavioral readiness (e.g., "friendly and open"), and the naming of a nation refers strictly to a geographical fact. In the course of such research, there is no inference of psychological events in the perceived person's mind.

When the perceived person is regarded as reducible to tangibles, then the perceiver, as well as the psychological investigator, gains a definite control over the perceived. Nothing about that which is perceived is free to vary without the perceiver's knowledge, since the perceived aspects are up front, not constituted by inferences.

In this respect, the inferred construction (construct) allows the perceived person a certain freedom. One should never be surprised when the other manifests signs of psychological states that are different from or even opposite to the inferred one. After all, the inference, in not reducing the perceived to a single-minded, physical state of affairs such as skin color or constant aggressiveness, automatically opens the way for degrees of freedom in the perceived person's thoughts or mental states. The inference is thus the product of a perceiver who is in a tolerant frame of mind—one who can at least for the moment live with uncertainties, and one whose world view is not shocked by the perceived person's occasionally disconfirming the inference. In the language of Garner et al. (1956), the inference of a psychological event is never certain, since it entails the triangulation of several pertinent cues. And if the correlation among those cues were perfect, then the inference would lose its status as a construct (Campbell & Fiske, 1959).

IS THERE A "MOTIVE" TO PUT TOGETHER CONSTRUCTS ABOUT OTHERS?

The existence of another is a potential stimulus to curiosity. If we follow the thoughts of Berlyne (1960), Harlow (1950), McClelland (1961), or Peak

(1955), we find a construct-building motive that works in the direction of openness in perceptions, exploring what is not obvious and delving into the intangible. Berlyne (1960) has employed such concepts as "preference for complexity" and "preference for surprise" in studies with adults. Cohen, Stotland, and Wolfe (1955) have looked at deprivation from cognitive complexity as a stimulus to seeking out complexity. Montgomery (1954) speaks of "exploratory drive," Berlyne (1960) of "curiosity," and Harlow (1950) of "manipulative motives."

Somewhat related are the hedonic or activation theories of motivation (see Cofer & Appley, 1964). They all postulate that positive affect comes from a moderate deviation from adaptation level (Engel, 1928; Hebb, 1949; Helson, 1964; McClelland, Atkinson, Clark, & Lowell, 1953). All of these theories—whether they are explicitly about curiosity, about orienting toward the unknown, or about gaining positive affect from moderate departures from adaptation level—lead in the direction of a person's enjoying, creating, seeking out nonclosure, and playing with cognitive risks. These notions imply a person's preferring that a construct not be anchored 100% in a single physical event. Although none of this research (i.e., that of Berlyne, Harlow, and others) deals directly with our issue of constructs, the point is very clear. Human beings enjoy a moderate discrepancy from what they are accustomed to, and thus will tolerate and seek out uncertainty.

WHAT ARE THE CHARACTERISTICS OF INFERENCE AND CONSTRUCT BUILDING?

In moving toward a moderate degree of uncertainty, in which a seemingly uncertain inference is drawn on the basis of cues that scarcely relate to one another, the person perceiver is taking a chance. This first characteristic of an orientation toward construct building can be called *the less than perfect probability that the construct is "right."* If there is only one cue, such as a score on a personality test, obvious conformity pressure, or past behavior, the perceiver is then inclined to reduce the "construct" to that one element. As such, the construct is then equivalent to that element, and we no longer have an inference (Campbell & Fiske, 1959). The second characteristic is as follows: *The perceived person is free to move away from the inferred state,* not being totally fixed to a given cue or singular physical definition. If a perceiver analyzes a Russian's behavior in terms of "It's obvious—every Russian would do that," then the perceiver has "explained" that behavior totally. The statement, based on an assumed fixed relation between nationality and a certain habit, reduces the person to a fixed physical entity. There is no inference as to mental events. But as soon as further elements enter the picture, the perceiver then uses the cues to estimate and infer some process. None of the cues can operate to the exclusion of the others, meaning that they all contribute to some grander conclusion, and none of them singularly defines the person's physical essence. Rather, their entirety triangulates on an inferred psychological event—a construct.

PRESS, CONFLICT, AND CONTROL MOTIVATION

But openness to constructs is challenged occasionally by counterforces. Openness assumes that the perceiver is ready to adapt to the person-field that is given; to explore its contours; and to imagine the underlying, hidden "phantoms" that are interesting in and of themselves, and that help explain the target person's fluctuations and habits. What, then, do these counterforces look like?

First, a challenge or counterforce can only loom as significant when the target person has some strong motivational meaning for the perceiver, meaning that the target person engenders a strong press (Steins & Wicklund, 1993a). The term "press," first used by Murray (1938), signifies the individual's subjective sense of having to take action and/or direct thought in regard to some event. When this term is used specifically within a person perception context, it means that the perceiver, with respect to a given target person, can experience various strengths of impulses to act toward that person. The determinants of the strength of press lie in such variables as the extent to which the target is bound up with the perceiver's need states; the target's prestige; the perceiver's commitment to the target; or the figural prominence of the target. For instance, the target may be a partner in a firm, a family member, an immediate neighbor, or a private detective. Such a person, prominent in one's sensory fields, does not automatically pose a counterforce to openness, but a substantial press is the first prerequisite, the starting point.

The critical element is conflict (Steins & Wicklund, 1993a). A subjectively realized conflict with the other person (i.e., the perceived other) exists when the relation with that other does not flow dynamically. The other poses a stumbling block, and at the moment—maybe even for a second—the perceiver wants either (1) to eliminate or avoid the other, or (2) to change the other to suit the perceiver's own sense of what needs to be accomplished. If press is high, in the sense of the other's being psychologically present, then only the second possibility is pertinent. That is, the perceiver wishes to change the other—the other's opinions (which are a nuisance and a hindrance), the other's habits (which get in the perceiver's way), or the other's physical position (which renders one's own movements difficult). This wanting to transform the other, as a result of some subjectively realized obstacle posed by the other, is labeled "conflict" (Steins & Wicklund, 1993a).

Although common sense and even reinforcement analyses (Thibaut & Kelley, 1959) might argue that exploring the inner world of the other would be especially noticeable given high press and conflict, our assumption is quite the opposite. As soon as a person has a need that directly involves having to influence another, then that other's role in this motive moves to the perceptual foreground. The other is then perceptually transformed into an element that is bound up in the perceiver's reaching a desired state of affairs. The stronger the motive (e.g., to win a court case, to get hired, to pass a crucial test), the more the other person who poses a motive-relevant conflict will be perceptually reduced.

HOW TO RECOGNIZE PERCEPTUAL REDUCTION

The Construct Is Eliminated

Once the other is perceptually transformed into a "blockade" and an "object of influence," perceived as a concrete hindrance with respect to the perceiver's own progress, then the other can no longer exist in one's perceptions as a construct that is pieced together on the basis of a multiplicity of cues. This means that the cues will no longer be acted upon or acknowledged; the perceiver will devote less energy to drawing inferences; and there will be no correspondence between the other's actual perceptions or other inner states and the perceiver's construal of the other. The other will instead be reduced to the perceiver's own goal-oriented concerns, and will be regarded as an element to be physically influenced or altered.

Perspective Taking Collapses

The elimination of the readiness to infer a construct implies directly that perspective taking, in the sense of drawing an inference on the basis of cues (Flavell et al., 1968; Piaget & Inhelder, 1947), will collapse. In fact, perspective-taking performance should do more than collapse. A mere collapse would mean that the other is no longer noticed. The perception of the other person, given high press and conflict, is now an *active* transformation of the other. This means that instead of perspective taking's simply falling to zero (as would be the case under highly distracting conditions, or among very young children with a complex perspective-taking task), the perspective of the other will be transformed into one's own thoughts or wishes. For example, the highly motivated perceiver will do more than just neglect the cues in making an inference. An "anti"-inference will be drawn, in that the perceiver's own preoccupations will be projected into the thoughts of the other. This is the "egocentrism" that Piaget was referring to; in this case, it is the actual injection of one's own mental state into the other, or reduction of the other to one's own concerns.

AN ILLUSTRATION OF THE MOVEMENT FROM CONSTRUCT BUILDING TO EGOCENTRISM

Several people are sitting in a new foreign restaurant. The waitress comes, gives them the menu, chats with them a minute, and then leaves the table while they decide what to order. The people at the table attend especially to three cues. First, the waitress responds to their questions as though she is highly unfamiliar with the menu; second, she barely communicates in the local language, which is Spanish; and third, as she walks away from the table, she limps.

The guests begin discussing the waitress, since she dominates their perceptual field at the moment. She is highly salient, and certainly she engages their curiosity, this being the only Croatian restaurant in town. Piecing the cues together and correcting one another, they come to the hypothesis that she is a refuguee who has been suffering a great deal, and who has had to leave her home country under duress. They proceed to refine the hypothesis further, all the time focusing on what she has experienced, on how she feels in this strange new place, and on how she is dealing with her first days on the job.

Twenty minutes pass and the food doesn't come. A couple of the people at the table start referring to their hunger; the others insist that food preparation naturally takes longer in a good Croatian restaurant. After 30 minutes, the need is stronger and more dominant for all four of the guests. They seem to have turned their attention from the inner states and background of the waitress to their own hunger state. And now a conflict begins to enter—certainly not an open conflict or strife with the waitress, but a contradiction between the multifacetedness of the person of the waitress and the guests' getting their evening meal. The waitress is not bringing the food, and the guests' attention to her has suddenly acquired a goal-oriented quality. They are now regarding her as a "food provider." As the delay grows longer still, they begin to think of her as "the person who is ruining our evening" or "the woman who is wrecking our first fair-minded attempt to eat Croatian cooking."

The waitress is thus reduced, in their perceptions, thoughts, and communications, to the person who is nothing more than an interference with their desire to eat something different and enjoy the evening. As the guests talk about her after 40 minutes of waiting, all of the remarks have to do with her lateness. "Has she forgotten us?" "Doesn't she like us?" "Does she have something against Spanish people?" "Why doesn't she tell the cook to get our meals ready?" In short, they have reduced her thinking, her whole being, to that of a person who hinders.

The construct building, acting on multiple cues, has now vanished. Instead, the guests' perception of the waitress's inner states, her behavioral readiness, is determined by their own conflict with her. Perceptions of her have been reduced to the food-is-late issue.

WHEN CUES TO INNER STATES ARE NOT ACTED UPON: THE ROLE OF PRESS

Let's deal with a highly simplified construct-building setting, adopted from Piaget's (1924/1966) examples. Hass (1979, 1984) developed a straightforward test of visual perspective taking that we have adapted for our research (Steins & Wicklund, in press). The Hass technique works as follows: Confronted face-to-face with a target person, subjects are requested to write a letter of the alphabet on a card that they hold against their foreheads. If the letter is written so as to correspond to the other's perspective, then it appears, of course, as an "E" to the other. If written egocentrically, thus disregarding the other's visual orientation, then it appears as "Ǝ."

The cue as to the other's mental state—in this case, to the other's perceptions of the stimulus figure ("E")—is simply the fact of the other's sitting at a 180-degree angle to the subject. The perceiver must take this difference into account in order to infer correctly how an "E" or "Ǝ" will be registered in the other's perceptions. There is of course no absolute, objective certainty that an "E" will be encoded better than an "Ǝ," but in this paradigm, averaging across all possible stimulus persons, the subjective probability that an "E" will register better is rather substantial.

Here is a parallel (if somewhat unusual) example. Suppose that it is the subject's task to present a number of words, including "parlor" and "color," to the stimulus person who sits opposite the subject. In each of these cases, the subject must not only decide in which order the letters must be presented (i.e., "color" or "roloc"), but must also consider whether the words might possibly acquire an additional "u" (i.e., the British "colour" and "parlour"). The subjective issue remains the same: Is the perceiver prepared to incorporate available cues as to the target's probable subjective state—in this case, the target's quick encoding of the presentation? Obviously, the subject in such an experiment must consider not only the fact of sitting at a 180-degree angle to the other, but also the question of whether the other is from Great Britain or the United States.

Now to the issue of conflict and press. Provided that the perceiving person has no conflict with the other, and thus no particular concentration on controlling and changing the other, then the perceiver's attention should be free to grasp the divergent perspectives offered by the other. Under these circumstances, an increase in subjective press—a general motivation to notice and react to the other—should lead to increments in perspective taking. But once the perceiver's attention toward the other becomes channeled in the direction of a dominant conflict, then increments in press should work to intensify the conflict and the associated desire to bring the conflict (i.e., the other) under control. Given a conflict, press should be negatively related to perspective-taking performance.

Press can be determined by numerous motivation-instigating facets of the perceiver and of the person perception setting. Interesting for the present example is press as set off by a general proclivity of some perceivers to take interpersonal problems up into their own thoughts, and to experience the negative emotions that are presented in the setting. Such people can be regarded as experiencing high press with respect to those problem settings. Exactly how such individuals are selected out for study is an issue of finding the right methods. As we describe below, we have used items from a standard "empathy" scale to locate individuals who are especially sensitive to conflict with others. Such individuals, confronted with a target person within a conflict-provoking context, should then manifest lessened perspective-taking performance for that same target.

In one study (Steins & Wicklund, 1992), we measured this tendency of individuals to transform others' thoughts into their own problems with a scale developed by Mehrabian and Epstein (1972), labeled by them a measure of emotional empathy. The scale items (e.g., "I tend to get emotionally involved with a friend's problems") point toward an attunement to single characteristics (usually problematic ones) of another person. Furthermore, the items point simultaneously to becoming absorbed in those characteristics oneself.

Our hypothesis was the following: Given that subjects are confronted with a potential conflict person, for whom interaction-relevant cues are ambiguous, then high press should lead to decrements in perspective taking. Subjects expected an interview with a high-prestige unknown person. After the measurement of subjective press (empathy), the target was introduced in such a manner that subjects' relative feelings of competence with regard to a forthcoming interaction should have been threatened. The character of the interaction was purposely left highly ambiguous, and there was no contact with the person prior to the expected interaction.

Once these expectations were set up, perspective-taking performance was measured with the Hass technique. The instruction accompanying the task was this: "Now concentrate on the window of the side room, where your interaction partner is sitting, and draw the letter 'E' (as well as 'L' and 'Z') on your forehead as fast as possible." In line with the hypothesis, the subjects with high empathy scores manifested poorer perspective taking. The overall correlation between scale score (the press variable) and correctness of perspective taking was $-.38$ ($p < .05$, two-tailed).

An assumption underlying this study was that subjects with higher empathy scores would become more fully absorbed in the partner, with whom a conversation of unstructured quality was expected. This implies, for instance, that the high-press subjects should have evidenced more motivation with respect to the forthcoming interaction. Evidence for this point is seen in the correlation between press and the item "excited to begin" ($r = .37$, $p < .05$), such that the high-press subjects (i.e., the "empathic" subjects) evidenced more desire to begin the interaction. Also pertinent to the strength of motivation was the relationship between the press variable (empathy score) and the importance of making a favorable impression during the discussion

($r = .41, p < .05$). The very subjects who wanted most to impress the partner showed the lowest perspective-taking performance. This study thus shows how motivation (press) changes the character of person perception.

On the other hand, it is not all so simple. If we return to our guesswork about the elements that bring forth construct building, then a certain press must be present for that to happen. But this is press without conflict—without the perceiver's regarding the perceived person (object) as an element that stands in the way. In this case, the other is not a source of uncertainty for the perceiver's behavioral directions.

We conducted two more studies, again employing our simplified letter-drawing index of egocentrism versus perspective taking. The first of these studies examined a setting in which conflict was explicitly eliminated, and thus where subjects' possible reactions to the other were clear and unambiguous (Steins & Wicklund, in press). There was no possibility of incompetence or conflict in reacting. It was hypothesized, therefore, that increased subjectively felt press would enhance taking the other's perspective. Each subject came individually to two sessions. The first session was for the measurement of press as well as other pertinent variables. Subjects were informed that the study would research the way in which people transmit private information to an unknown other. Press was measured in this case by a single concrete question that tapped into subjects' motivation to communicate effectively to the interviewer (a therapist). Subjects were to return after 2 weeks to a second session, expecting an interview with the therapist about private matters.

The second session involved the subject's being interviewed, in a very direct and simple manner, by an ostensible psychologist. The central dependent variable consisted of subjects' taking the psychologist's visual perspective, using the letter-drawing technique of Hass (1979, 1984). The press variable, owing to the distribution of the scores, organized itself into a tripartite measure: Subjects were partitioned into those with low, medium, and high press to communicate effectively to the therapist.

The analysis showed an overall effect of press on correctness of perspective taking. The low-press group was significantly worse than the high-press group, and the medium-press group fell in the middle. The latency of letter drawing was also measured; there was an overall effect of press on latency, in that subjects in the high-press group were faster than subjects in the low-press group. The findings fit with the assumption that increments in subjectively perceived press are associated with improved perspective taking, given a situation in which the stimulus person does not pose significant conflicts for the subject.

The relationship between press and perspective taking is thus clear: The higher the press, the better the perspective taking, provided that no conflict dominates the setting. However, once conflict enters, the relationship between press and perspective taking should be more complex. First, it should be the case that with a strong conflict (i.e., an intrapsychic conflict involving another person), increasing press will lead to further reduction of the other to one's own preoccupations. This directly implies a collapse of openness to constructs in person perception, and of course a collapse of perspective taking.

On the other hand, Piaget (1924/1966) has argued that a certain level of conflict is necessary for perspective-taking to occur at all. Thus it is conceivable, when we add this consideration to our theoretical notion, that conflict in the absence of substantial press would benefit perspective taking, relative to conditions of no conflict (and no press).

We (Steins & Wicklund, 1993b) therefore conducted another experiment in order to investigate the press and conflict factors and their possible interaction. Male subjects came individually to a study that was said to involve the exchange of private information with a female subject. Early in the session half of the subjects (high-conflict condition) were induced to insult the woman (a confederate); the other half (low-conflict condition) made no insult. Our reasoning, drawn from equity theory (Adams, 1965; Adams & Freedman, 1976; Walster, Berscheid, & Walster, 1976), was that inequity that was disadvantageous for the other would arouse guilt in the subject. If the harm could not be directly compensated for, then the subject would be laden with a conflict: the relationship was supposed to proceed normally, but the subject could not reinstate equity or normality.

Press was varied by presenting the confederate in an anonymous manner in one condition (low press), whereas in another condition she was cast as having a multifaceted childhood, and details of her childhood experiences were made salient. It was assumed that a stimulus person filled out with a personality would create higher press on the subject. The primary dependent measure was the Hass letter-drawing procedure.

The data showed an interaction (see Table 22.1). There was a simple effect within the low-conflict condition, such that perspective taking increased with the extent of press. In addition, there was a tendency toward a difference within the high-conflict condition, in that perspective taking declined with the extent of press. The difference between the low-conflict/low-press and high-conflict/low-press conditions was also significant. The correlation between liking for the target person and perspective taking was −.01.

One of the unexpected features of the data was the relatively high mean among subjects who insulted the confederate, but who knew nothing about her background (low press). We can conjecture that having made an insult generated an urge to do something to compensate for the injury, and that this urge heightened subject's overall orientation to the person. Thus as long as press was low, there was a positive effect for the insult manipulation in the direction of subjects' taking the target's perspective. However, when the insult was combined with high press, the effect was a relative collapse of perspective taking—a result that follows from our theoretical model.

The experiment thus shows that under certain conditions of conflict with another, there is less drawing upon cues in order to infer another's psy-

TABLE 22.1. Interaction between Press and Conflict in Perspective Taking

	Low conflict		High conflict	
	Low press	High press	Low press	High press
Correctness (all three trials)				
M	0.80	1.90	2.30	1.40
SD	1.03	1.28	0.95	1.17
Latency[a] (all three trials)				
M	1049	1226	1101	1005
SD	174	408	397	233

Note. $n = 10$ for each cell. Data from Steins and Wicklund (1993b).
[a]In hundredths of seconds.

chological state. In this case we had a condition in which the male subjects would have liked very much to influence the target, in the sense of explaining that the insult should not count; conflict was created by the fact that the subjects could not proceed with this clearing up of the situation. Given this preoccupation with dealing effectively with the other, and especially when the multifaceted character of the woman was salient, the subjects tended strongly to neglect the cue (the fact of the other's sitting at 180 degrees to each subject), and instead to make an egocentric judgment in writing the three letters for the other. In short, among subjects with guilt or inequity feelings vis-à-vis a target person with numerous personal qualities, the inference process failed.

PERSON PERCEPTION: MOTIVES AND ORIENTATIONS IN A CULTURAL CONTEXT

It is instructive to follow a line of thinking proposed by Levine (1985), who draws a strong qualitative distinction between certain thinking patterns in Western or highly technological cultures and other patterns in Third World, agrarian cultures. His prototypes for the West are North America and Europe. As Levine describes it, the use of words in the "advanced," technological cultures is characterized by efficiency and technical precision. There is a constant striving forward—toward effecting movement, toward reaching goals, toward efficient and instant communication. It suits such an orientation when the words and phrases are reality-oriented, when there exists a one-to-one correspondence between word and thing. Ambiguity in words or in expressions is not relished: A word with multiple meanings; or a phrase that is not grounded strictly in empirical, tangible events, disturbs the efficient movement of humans toward their pressing goals and schedules.

The Ethiopian culture Levine depicts is very different, and so are the examples he offers from China, Native American cultures, and India. In Ethiopian culture, great pleasure is ostensibly taken in being indirect in the use of words—in employing a phrase or symbol to denote a contradictory state of affairs. The abstraction, the concept, the metaphor, the paradox, and all other non-empirical-reality-based forms of communication are valued, and, according to Levine, also have their functions.

This would imply in our context that the building of constructs, the imagining of another's thoughts, and perhaps perspective taking in general would be frequent in such cultures as Ethiopia. Levine's descriptions imply a people open to nonphysicalistic events, to pure concepts. In North America (or, for that matter, in any "modern" society), reduction to a pure or singular physical essence should predominate.

As arbitrary as an anthropological bifurcation may seem, we should take Levine's (1985) distinction and detailed observations as a stimulus to thinking about what might underlie these disparate cultures. One element that seems to separate them is the domination of everyday goals and also long-term goals in the Western cultures—a kind of impatience to accomplish some physically based end. Often these are cognitive tasks, such as computer work, library work, financial work, communication tasks, or other technical undertakings. Efficiency is a concept that accompanies these enterprises. This means that the underlying variable that happens to be much more present in Western societies, at least among people who are under duress to produce and communicate, is a certain multifaceted press. This element is relatively lacking in the so-called Third World.

If it is a fair statement that these multiple sources of subjectively felt press constitute the critical element differentiating the "abstract thinking" societies from the "concrete, unambiguous thinking" societies, then we can apply the notion of press *within* a society as well. For example, if we move right to our issue of the perception of other people, it is not hard to locate a dimension of press within a Western society. It is easy to find individuals who interact with many strangers in an unintegrated, ill-defined manner, so that conflicts can easily ensue. In particular, if it is one's job to identify or evaluate others—for instance, as a personnel tester, as an evaluation psychologist, or possibly even as a psychologist whose *job* it is to explain complex human events, including person perception—then the conflict–control sequence can easily go into gear. If a salesperson has to predict how a customer will react, or if a psychologist has to be sure that a person will be highly predictable based on a given test, then the personal goal is just that: to be sure that the other person is highly predictable and consistent across time. As a result, this control will lead to reducing the other to a tangible, certain essence—to a batch of reliable behavioral tendencies, or to a set of reliable (unchanging) physical characteristics such as gender, race, age.

This is, then, one of the overriding messages of this chapter. Insofar as others are "important" in the sense of our having to make sense of them, "understand" them, or direct them, in order that we may arrive at some further goal efficiently, then person perception, in the sense of building a construct, collapses. Others are transformed, in a highly motivated society or group, into a physical essence that contains little besides one's own conflict or concern with moving toward the goal efficiently.

One of the difficulties throughout this analysis has been the problem of capturing adequately the character of the *open* side of person perception. It is easy to postulate that humans generally "tend to be open" insofar as no forces such as conflict are operating to close their thinking or perceiving of others (Easterbrook, 1959). However, are there not some systematic factors or chains of events that lead a person to build constructs, to move into that uncertain realm of the "other as phantom"? We have, for example, the waxing and waning need for cognition (as a function of deprivation; Cohen et al., 1955). Whether need for cognition leads to our construct-building variety of person perception is another question. Alternatively, we can begin with stimulus conditions such as moderate departures from expectation that engage curiosity (Harlow, 1950). Does curiosity mean entering the "phantom" realm of building constructs? Then we have the Levine's (1985) "functions"—that is, the conceivable purposes that are served by ambiguity in language and communication. These factors all constitute a start in the direction of telling us when and why a person comes to perceive another in terms of an open construct. To be sure, they are more difficult to pin down than is an analysis of "Why closure?" But they need to be understood in order for person perception as inference of mental states to be comprehended as a product of psychological conditions or events.

Probably the suggestion of Levine (1985) comes closest, in that he refers to the "understanding" function of ambiguity. Ultimately, one could postulate a set of principles—possibly a kind of deprivation principle—that talks about the relief of being able to transcend physical reality, to get away from it. In the fourth century B.C., Plato, in *The Republic* (1937), was intent on proving that the particulars (the tangible) are unreal, and that the only satisfying reality is the eternal or abstract. Akin to such statements would be a notion of escaping from boredom, moving toward fantasy, and possibly moving toward perceiving or maintaining something private to which no one else has access.

This latter "motive" could also be a reaction against being controlled. As long as we conduct all commerce on the plane of physical reality, we have a heavyweight common denominator with others. They know what we see and what we talk about, and the common control function is substantial. In a modern, technical society, those who stray too often from this plane are labeled as crazy and are excluded (i.e., they are uncontrollable within the technical environment).

A further hint would be the following. In postulating (inferring) a construct, the perceiver is responding to what *must* be there, in order that certain patterns of behaviors take place in the context of given perceivable cues. Those who are impatient with the plane of the construct are denying that there is a psychological reality. This denial can of course be regarded as the product of the conflict–control process and what has been described above.

The mystery is that this orientation toward construct building entails responding to what *must* be there, inside, independent of the perceiver's control needs. Therefore, such orientations have heretofore been analyzed as purely perceptual (i.e., curiosity phenomena). And perhaps this more perceptual, less behavioral level is the answer to our theoretical issue. Just as Gestalt mechanisms drive attention to the foreground (e.g., to the smaller figure), so can a set of cues drive one's attention to the inner state, to the explanation, insofar as the person perceiver does not reduce the other because of control issues.

ACKNOWLEDGMENTS

We are grateful to the Deutsche Forschungsgemeinschaft (Grant No. IIA4-Wi795/4-1) for support of the research reported here. A special note of thanks is due to Guido H. E. Gendolla, John A. Bargh, and Peter M. Gollwitzer for their invaluable suggestions for improvement in the manuscript.

REFERENCES

Adams, J. S. (1965). Inequity in social exchange. In L. Berkowitz (Ed.), *Advances in experimental social psychology* (Vol. 2, pp. 267–299). New York: Academic Press.

Adams, J. S., & Freedman, S. (1976). Equity theory revisited: Comments and annotated bibliography. In L. Berkowitz & E. Walster (Eds.), *Advances in experimental social psychology* (Vol. 9, pp. 43–90). New York: Academic Press.

Benenson, J. F., & Dweck, C. S. (1986). The development of trait explanations and self-evaluations in the academic and social domains. *Child Development, 57,* 1179–1187.

Berlyne, D. E. (1960). *Conflict, arousal and curiosity.* New York: McGraw Hill.

Buss, D. M., & Craik, K. H. (1983). The act frequency approach to personality. *Psychological Review, 90,* 105–126.

Campbell, D. T., & Fiske, D. W. (1959). Convergent and discriminant validation by the multitrait–multimethod matrix. *Psychological Bulletin, 56,* 81–105.

Cronbach, L. J., & Meehl, P. E. (1955). Construct validity in psychological tests. *Psychological Bulletin, 52,* 281–302.

Cofer, C. N., & Appley, M. H. (1964). *Motivation: Theory and research.* New York: Wiley.

Cohen, A. R., Stotland, E., & Wolfe, D. M. (1955). An experimental investigation of need for cognition. *Journal of Abnormal and Social Psychology, 51,* 291–294.

Cunningham, M. R. (1986). Measuring the physical in physical attractiveness: Quasi-experiments on the sociobiology of female face beauty. *Journal of Personality and Social Psychology, 50,* 925–935.

Dion, K., Berscheid, E., & Walster, E. (1972). What is beautiful is good. *Journal of Personality and Social Psychology, 24,* 285–290.

Easterbrook, J. A. (1959). The effect of emotion on cue utilization and the organization of behavior. *Psychological Review, 66,* 183–201.

Engel, R. (1928). Experimentelle Untersuchungen über die Abhängigkeit der Lust und Unlust von der Reizstärke beim Geschmackssinn. *Archiv für die gesamte Psychologie, 64,* 1–36.
Feigl, H. (1958). The mental and the physical. In H. Feigl, M. Scriven, & G. Maxwell (Eds.), *Minnesota studies in the philosophy of science: Vol. 2. Concepts, theories and the mind-body problem.* Minneapolis: University of Minnesota Press.
Flavell, J. H., Botkin, P. T., Fry, C. L., Wright, J. W., & Jarvis, P. E. (1968). *The development of role-taking and communication skills in children.* New York: Wiley.
Garner, W. R., Hake, H. W., & Eriksen, C. W. (1956). Operationism and the concept of perception. *Psychological Review, 63,* 149–159.
Hamilton, D. L. (1979). A cognitive attributional analysis of stereotyping. In L. Berkowitz (Ed.), *Advances in experimental social psychology* (Vol. 12, pp. 53–84). New York: Academic Press.
Harlow, H. F. (1950). Learning and satiation of response in intrinsically motivated complex puzzle performance by monkeys. *Journal of Comparative and Physiological Psychology, 43,* 289–294.
Hass, R. G. (1979). *A test of the bidirectional focus of attention assumption of the theory of objective self-awareness.* Paper presented at the annual meeting of the Eastern Psychological Association, Philadelphia.
Hass, R. G. (1984). Perspective-taking and self-awareness: Drawing an E on your forehead. *Journal of Personality and Social Psychology, 46,* 788–798.
Hebb, D. O. (1949). *The organization of behavior.* New York: Wiley.
Heider, F. (1958). *The psychology of interpersonal relations.* New York: Wiley.
Helson, H. (1964). *Adaptation-level theory.* New York: Harper & Row.
Katz, D., & Braly, K. W. (1933). Racial stereotypes of one hundred college students. *Journal of Abnormal and Social Psychology, 28,* 280–290.
Levine, D. N. (1985). *The flight from ambiguity.* Chicago: University of Chicago Press.
McArthur, L. Z., & Post, D. L. (1977). Figural emphasis and person perception. *Journal of Experimental Social Psychology, 13,* 520–535.
McClelland, D. C. (1961). *The achieving society.* Princeton, NJ: Van Nostrand.
McClelland, D. C., Atkinson, J. W., Clark, R. A., & Lowell, E. L. (1953). *The achievement motive.* New York: Appleton-Century-Crofts.
Mehrabian, A., & Epstein, N. (1972). A measure of emotional empathy. *Journal of Personality, 40,* 525–543.
Montgomery, K. C. (1954). The role of exploratory drive in learning. *Journal of Comparative and Physiological Psychology, 47,* 60–64.
Murray, H. A. (1938). *Explorations in personality.* New York: Oxford University Press.
Peak, H. (1955). Attitude and motivation. In M. R. Jones (Ed.), *Nebraska Symposium on Motivation* (Vol. 3, pp. 149–189). Lincoln: University of Nebraska Press.
Piaget, J. (1966). *Judgment and reasoning in the child.* Totowa, NJ: Littlefield, Adams. (Original work published 1924)
Piaget, J., & Inhelder, B. (1947). *La représentation de l'espace chez l'enfant.* Paris: Presses Universitaires de France.
Plato. (1937). The republic. In B. Jowett (Trans.), *The dialogues of Plato* (3rd ed., Vol. 1, pp. 591–870). New York: Random House. (Original work composed ca. 370–360 B.C.)
Steins, G., & Wicklund, R. A. (1992). *The pleasing person's paradox: The need to please others and collapse of perspective-taking.* Unpublished manuscript, Universität Bielefeld.

Steins, G., & Wicklund, R. A. (1993a). Zum Konzept der Perspektivenübernahme: Ein kritischer Überblick. *Psychologische Rundschau, 44,* 226–239.

Steins, G., & Wicklund, R. A. (1993b). *Perspective-taking, conflict and interaction intensity.* Unpublished manuscript, Universität Bielefeld.

Steins, G., & Wicklund, R. A. (in press). Perspective-taking, conflict, and press: Drawing an E on your forehead. *Basic and Applied Social Psychology.*

Taylor, J. A. (1952). A personality scale of manifest anxiety. *Journal of Abnormal and Social Psychology, 48,* 285–290.

Thibaut, J. W., & Kelley, H. H. (1959). *The social psychology of groups.* New York: Wiley.

Walster, E., Berscheid, E., & Walster, G. W. (1976). New directions in equity research. In L. Berkowitz & E. Walster (Eds.), *Advances in experimental social psychology* (Vol. 9, pp. 1–42). New York: Academic Press.

White, P. A., & Younger, D. P. (1988). Differences in the ascription of transient internal states to self and other. *Journal of Experimental Social Psychology, 24,* 292–309.

CHAPTER 23

Expectancy Influences in Social Interaction

The Moderating Role of Social Goals

Steven L. Neuberg

The first day of kindergarten. A first date. The birth of a first child. These are happy occasions, events to be celebrated. Why, then, are these moments so anxiety-laden? I think the answer lies in the inherent unpredictability of novel circumstances: "What if no one plays with me?" the child asks the parent. "What are we going to talk about at dinner?" frets the teenager. "What if the child is ill?" worries the parent-to-be. Uncertainty can be stressful; we want to know what to expect.

Because so many of our waking hours are spent with others, social expectations—expectations of what others will be like—become quite important. Indeed, the inclination to create for ourselves such expectations virtually guarantees that no social interaction begins free of them. Minimally, social expectations provide us with perceptions of control; such perceptions, it is well known, are fundamental to healthy psychological functioning (e.g., Seligman, 1975; Thompson, 1981). Moreover, social expectations suggest practical ways of behaving toward others, of interpreting their actions, and so forth. They enable us to take advantage of previous experience, saving us the difficult and time-consuming task of treating each new event as if it were novel. As such, social expectations are indispensable to the cognitive "toolbox"; we would be lost without them.

The problem with such a useful tool is that we may be tempted to rely on it indiscriminately. Unfortunately, most tools possess a range of usefulness, beyond which they become decreasingly effective. A microwave oven is a good example. It is great for warming leftovers and baking potatoes, but fails miserably at cooking steaks; its strength (heating food rapidly) becomes a liability as taste and appearance are sacrificed. Similarly, social expectations, when *accurate*—that is, when they represent their target well—are wonderful. Their use increases the likelihood that we will correctly interpret others' ambiguous behaviors, and helps us act appropriately toward them. Like the microwave, however, expectations can be used unwisely. When they are *in*accurate—as when they are based on misguided social stereotypes, unsubstantiated third-party hearsay, and previous self-produced errors of judgment—their benefits, too, become liabilities.

First, just as accurate expectations provide us with appropriate contexts for thinking about others' behaviors, inaccurate expectations furnish us with inappropriate cognitive contexts. To believe mistakenly that a student has little academic potential can bias a teacher's views of that student's subsequent performance, as the teacher emphasizes the few mistakes, attributes the frequent successes to the help received from others, and so on. Similarly, to believe mistakenly that a student has great promise can also produce a bias, this time in the favorable direction, as the teacher focuses instead on those rare flashes of insight, attributes infrequent successes to natural brilliance, and attributes repeated failures to external events outside the student's control. We often see what we expect to see, even when our expectations are inaccurate (Fiske & Neuberg, 1990; Fiske & Taylor, 1991; Hamilton, Sherman, & Ruvulo, 1990; Higgins & Bargh, 1987; Nisbett & Ross, 1980).

Second, we often *create* what we expect. Again, this is no problem when expectations are correct, as the reality we impose is the reality that already exists. When expectations are inaccurate, however, they can be transforming, creating "self-fulfilling prophecies" (Merton, 1948): Within the social realm, our actions can cause others to behave in ways consistent with our expectations, even if such behaviors are typically unrepresentative of them. Indeed, such demonstrations are plentiful (for reviews, see Brophy, 1983; Darley & Fazio, 1980; Jussim, 1986; Miller & Turnbull, 1986; Rosenthal, 1974; Snyder, 1984). For example, teachers can lead students whom they inappropriately expect to be promising to actually perform better than students who do not have the benefit of such expectations (e.g., Meichenbaum, Bowers, & Ross, 1969; Rosenthal & Jacobson, 1968); the expectations of therapists can lead to the anticipated symptomatology (e.g., Sibicky & Dovidio, 1986; Vrugt, 1990); job applicants expected to perform poorly are indeed more likely to do so (e.g., Christensen & Rosenthal, 1982; Neuberg, 1989; Word, Zanna, & Cooper, 1974; see Dipboye, 1982); and, closer to our everyday lives, expectations can lead people to shape the behaviors of others even in casual social encounters (e.g., Ickes, Patterson, Rajecki, & Tanford, 1982). Moreover, although not all expectations can lead to self-fulfilling prophecies (e.g., it is unlikely that anyone's expectation that I will become a world-class pole vaulter will ever be realized; see Jones, 1986, for a discussion), they can be produced by a wide range of expectations based on personality traits, abilities, and prejudices.

As a consequence of these cognitive and behavioral biases, we may exit encounters with others believing the others to be something they are not. And such mistaken impressions can have considerable implications. When inaccurate expectations are negative (e.g., when they are based on unflattering stereotypes), both the holders of the expectations and their targets incur costs of opportunity. For example, perceivers may make poor hiring decisions, lose potential friends and allies, and so forth; the targets of such expectations may lose employment, housing, and educational opportunities, and, perhaps more important, may encounter higher hurdles than others in their attempts to reach full potential. When expectations are inappropriately positive, perceivers again may make poor decisions, and targets may find themselves in situations for which they are unprepared (although the possibility of having their capabilities "developed" by others' favorable expectations may mitigate this cost to some degree). But in all cases, expectancy-biased processes support and maintain the culprit expectations, enabling their inappropriate influence to survive to affect subsequent encounters.

We see, then, that in a social world characterized by ambiguity, expectations are a necessary and functional part of everyday social life. We also see, however, that to use them inappropriately has its costs. It is thus important to understand better the nature of the expectancy confirmation process. In particular, I explore here the conditions that regulate this process—that both encourage and discourage the likelihood of expectancy confirmation. I begin by explicating briefly the cognitive and behavioral mechanisms by which we confirm our expectations. Then, because it is quite clear that expectancy confirmation is far from inevitable, I present a framework that better enables us to understand when we confirm expectations and when we do not. To anticipate the discussion to follow, I argue that the active social motivations of the interactants (Are we motivated to form accurate impressions of the person? Do we want the other person to like us? Are we motivated to be deferential?) regulate the mechanisms that underlie expectancy confirmation, in this way moderating the likelihood of its occurrence. Finally, relevant research is presented, including several studies from my own laboratory that address these issues directly.

A GENERAL MODEL OF EXPECTANCY CONFIRMATION

Psychologists have investigated for many years the interpersonal and intrapersonal processes creating expectancy confirmation. In the next several pages, I briefly summarize this work. This summary is far from exhaustive; my purpose is merely to outline the fundamentals of expectancy confirmation as they exist in everyday social encounters.

Setting the Stage

A social expectation is a belief that another individual is likely to be in a particular state, to possess a certain trait or ability, or to act in a particular manner at some point in the future. We expect people to be nervous before their weddings, librarians to be shy, and students to learn the assigned course material. The interpersonal process of expectancy confirmation thus requires at least two individuals; following convention, I designate the holder of the expectation as the "perceiver" and the individual who is the focus of the expectancy as the "target."

In the simplest scenario, the perceiver merely observes the target (who is unaware that he or she is being observed); in this case, the role of perceiver expectations is limited to their cognitive impact (e.g., their biasing effects on interpretation processes). This chapter focuses, however, on the more complex cases, in which the perceiver and target interact with each other, thus allowing expectations to influence not only perceiver cognitive processes but also, via the perceiver's actions, target behaviors.[1]

Perceiver Behaviors

How do expectations influence perceiver behaviors toward the target? First, they may determine whether or not a social encounter takes place. For example, if I expect the woman down the street to be a snob, I am likely to avoid her. As a consequence, I never discover that she is actually quite nice, and my unflattering expectation is maintained. In contrast, if I expect her to be friendly, I may look for occasions to interact with her. Such an approach tendency provides not only an opportunity to confirm my favorable expectation, but, importantly, also an opportunity to disconfirm it if it is indeed untrue. Thus, inaccurate negative expectancies often remain negative and strong, because our inclination is to avoid such people; in contrast, inaccurate positive expectations have a less stable future, as we are more likely to subject such expectations to a test (albeit often a weak one) against reality.

Second, when perceivers do interact with targets, expectations can create self-fulfilling prophecies, by biasing (1) the manner in which the perceivers gather information about their targets and (2) the manner in which the perceivers express themselves to their targets.

First, expectations, even when inaccurate, can influence perceivers' information-gathering behavior. People often ask questions of others that are "leading," in that they make it easier for targets to provide expectancy-consistent than expectancy-inconsistent information (e.g., Snyder, Campbell, & Preston, 1982; Snyder & Gangestad, 1981; Snyder & Swann, 1978; Swann & Ely, 1984). For example, an interviewer who expects a man applying for a job to get along famously with others may ask him to describe previous instances in which he has cooperated effectively with his coworkers. Even if the applicant typically has difficulty relating to others, he can probably discuss an instance or two where collaborative efforts went smoothly (indeed, almost anyone can do this). Thus, the interviewer's question elicits expectancy-consistent information. If the interviewer subsequently neglects to ask about instances where the applicant had problems with coworkers, the sample of cooperation-related information will be biased, and the interviewer will come to believe erroneously that the applicant is indeed predisposed toward interpersonal cooperation and collegiality. Note that an outsider, listening to the interview but unaware of the interviewer's expectations, will also believe the applicant to be cooperative, based on the information available.

There are other ways in which information gathering can be biased. For example, when perceivers hold unfavorable expectations, they tend to ask questions that are negatively tinged (Neuberg, 1989), to ask fewer questions (Harris & Rosenthal, 1985), and to spend less time with their targets (Word, Zanna, & Cooper, 1974). Such perceiver behaviors increase the likelihood that targets will present themselves in an undesirable manner, to the extent that targets accept the common rules of conversational discourse (Grice, 1975) and decline to "challenge" the perceiver (Jones, 1986; for more on this, see below). Thus, the manner in which a person gathers information from a target can create a self-fulfilling prophecy, leading the perceiver to exit his or her encounter with inaccurate expectations confirmed.

Perceivers' expressive behaviors can also mediate the impact of expectations on target actions. People holding expectations for others often express them—sometimes intentionally (e.g., "You're the friendliest person I've met in a long time"), but more often via unintended "leakage." For example, people often behave toward the targets of negative expectations with reduced warmth and sociability (Babad, Inbar, & Rosenthal, 1982; Harris & Rosenthal, 1985; Snyder, Tanke, & Berscheid, 1977), greater interpersonal distance (Word et al., 1974), fewer expressions of positive regard (Ickes et al., 1982), and more speech errors (Word et al., 1974). To the extent that such behaviors reveal perceivers' underlying unfavorable feelings, and "rules" of social engagement lead targets to respond to others with behaviors of a similar type (Goffman, 1959), these perceiver expressions are likely to lead targets to reciprocate in kind, in this way fulfilling the initial expectation. Thus, the expressive behaviors of perceivers also play an important mediating role in the expectancy confirmation process.

Target Responses to Perceiver Behaviors

There is no reason, however, why targets must respond to biased perceiver questions with unrepresentative responses, or to perceiver expressions with behaviors of a similar affective tone. The fact that an interviewer wants me to discuss my negative characteristics does not prohibit me from talking also about my strengths; the fact that a person is nasty to me does not constrain me from responding with extreme kindness. Indeed, even though the common conventions of conversation and social interaction encourage the acceptance of others' interactional scripts—we should "go with the flow" and avoid violating the "face-saving" contract implicit to social interaction (see Goffman, 1959; Grice, 1975; Jones, 1986)—we can instead decide to press our own agendas, to present ourselves as we wish to be seen. To some extent, then, the creation of a self-fulfilling prophecy requires the target's cooperation: He or she must accommodate the perceiver's interactional script, allowing the perceiver's information-gathering and expressive behaviors to constrain his or her responses. Such target deference need not be carefully considered and strategic, although at times it may indeed be; more often than not, accommodation may merely reflect social habit, engaged in for no better reason than to avoid creating an uncomfortable scene.

Some research implies the importance of targets' deference decisions to the self-fulfilling prophecy process. For example, women are particularly likely to succumb to self-fulfilling prophecies (Christensen & Rosenthal, 1982), as are individuals who reveal themselves to have "influenceable" personalities (Cooper & Hazelrigg, 1988; Harris & Rosenthal, 1986). To the extent that women and influenceable individuals are dispositionally more accommodating—for reasons of differential socialization, for example—these data fit well with the proposed importance of target deference. Moreover, targets believing themselves to be in low-power or low-status situations are more likely to behaviorally confirm the expectations of others (e.g., Copeland, 1994; Virdin & Neuberg, 1990). Given that deference is an adaptive strategy for low-power individuals, this too supports the proposed role of target accommodation in the self-fulfilling prophecy. Finally, a recent study by Snyder and Haugen (1995), reviewed later, further bolsters this view.

Perceiver Cognitive Processes

To this point, I have addressed the behavioral avenue toward expectancy confirmation—the creation of the self-fulfilling prophecy, in which the perceiver brings about target behaviors that are objectively consistent with expectations. As stated earlier, there also exists a cognitive avenue whereby expectations bias the way the perceiver thinks about target behaviors. Particularly when target actions are ambiguous, as social behaviors tend to be (e.g., consider that eye contact can be interpreted in many ways—as friendliness, interest, a sexual come-on, a means of intimidation, etc.), perceiver expectations play a central role in determining the apparent meaning of those actions. For example, in several studies within the stereotyping domain, behaviors performed by white children were looked upon more favorably by white perceivers than were the identical behaviors performed by black children (Duncan, 1976; Sagar & Schofield, 1980). Apparently, the perceivers' stereotypical expectations led the behaviors to be viewed as "assertive" when targets were white and "inappropriately aggressive" when targets were black, in line with the initial expectations. Other findings demonstrate comparable effects of stereotypical expectations (for reviews, see Brigham, 1971; Farina, 1982; Ruble & Ruble, 1982; Tavris & Offir, 1977).

In a similar vein, expectations influence what perceivers pay attention to: Perceivers often seek information that is expectancy-consistent, and these attentional biases mediate the development of expectancy-consistent impressions (e.g., Erber & Fiske, 1984; Fiske, Neuberg, Beattie, & Milberg, 1987;

Kruglanski & Freund, 1983; Neuberg & Fiske, 1987; Omoto & Borgida, 1988; see Fiske & Neuberg, 1990, for a review). More generally, the power of such cognitive biases can be so strong that targets may be viewed as confirming expectations even when their behavior is objectively *in*consistent with them (e.g., Farina & Ring, 1965; Ickes et al., 1982; Major, Cozzarelli, Testa, & McFarlin, 1988; Swann & Snyder, 1980).

Summary

In short, one can characterize the expectancy-confirming interaction in the following way: (1) A perceiver holds an expectation for a target; (2) this expectation biases the way the perceiver gathers information from the target and/or is revealed via the perceiver's expressive behaviors; (3) the target, either intentionally or not, allows himself or herself to be constrained by the "script" created by the perceiver, thus behaviorally confirming the perceiver's expectations; and (4) when the target's behaviors are ambiguous with respect to the expectation (and sometimes even when they are inconsistent with it), the perceiver—utilizing expectancy-biased attentional and interpretational processes—cognitively assesses the target's behaviors as being consistent with the initial expectation.

SOCIAL GOALS AS MODERATORS OF EXPECTANCY CONFIRMATION

People do not, however, always confirm their expectations for others. Perceivers do not invariably create self-fulfilling prophecies, nor do they always exhibit expectancy-consistent biases in their thinking about others (e.g., Andersen & Bem, 1981; Babad et al., 1982; Darley, Fleming, Hilton, & Swann, 1988; Hilton & Darley, 1985; Neuberg, 1989; Neuberg & Fiske, 1987; Swann & Ely, 1984; for reviews, see Brophy, 1983; Fiske & Neuberg, 1990; Higgins & Bargh, 1987; Hilton & Darley, 1991; Hilton, Darley, & Fleming, 1989; Jussim, 1986, 1991; Snyder, 1992). Indeed, some authors argue that expectancy biases are infrequent, and of only small magnitude when they do exist (e.g., Brophy, 1983; Brophy & Good, 1974; Cooper, 1979; Jussim, 1991; West & Anderson, 1976; but see Rosenthal & Rubin, 1978). How do we reconcile the adaptive nature of expectations, and the many demonstrations of their influences, with the literature documenting a lack of such influences? Is one of the literatures just wrong? This is not likely. Rather, the existence of apparently incongruent findings suggests the need for an integrative model—one that articulates the conditions under which expectancy confirmation does and does not occur. This is the present task: What factors moderate the expectancy confirmation effect, and why?

Two general assumptions characterize my approach. The first is simple and straightforward, grounded in the logic of mediation and moderation: To moderate any effect, one must first know how the effect came to be. That is, one must identify the mediational processes underlying the effect. Once mediators are recognized, the task is simplified, as moderators (factors that alter an effect) are merely those factors that change the mediation process. Within the specific context of expectancy confirmation, the implications are clear, as the processes mediating the influence of expectations on final impressions have already been identified. Thus, factors that (1) increase the likelihood that perceivers will gather information in an expectancy-biased manner, leak their expectancies in their expressive behaviors, and exhibit expectancy-biased attentional and interpretational processes, while (2) increasing the likelihood that targets will decide to accommodate perceivers' behavioral scripts, should boost the probability of expectancy confirmation. Factors that decrease the probability of such mediating thoughts and behaviors, perhaps by creating incompatible ones, should attenuate the likelihood of expectancy confirmation.

We need, then, to uncover factors with these properties. Unfortunately, there exists an infinite number of such moderator variables, because any condition that influences a mediator immediately qualifies as a moderator. The task is thus one of limiting the search to potentially *important* moderators. "Important" can be defined in terms of influence on effect size, ecological validity, ease of measurement, ease of manipulation in the laboratory, and so forth. It can also be defined in terms of compatibility with a favored metatheoretical perspective. This is my preference, bringing me to my second assumption: *The motivational system is the hub of human functioning*. Motives and goals direct relevant cognitive and behavioral processes to do their bidding; such thoughts and actions are merely the means (i.e., the mediators) by which people move toward their desires. Thus, we need to identify those motivational states that evoke (or inhibit) the four critical mediational processes documented above.

In the following pages, I begin to articulate the specific implications of this perspective (a more comprehensive presentation is found in Neuberg, 1996). In particular, I propose strong regulatory roles for perceiver impression formation and self-presentational goals, and for target self-presentational goals. Moreover, I suggest that these regulatory roles are typically constrained by the need for cognitive and behavioral resources, thus leading to a situation where strategies compatible with expectancy confirmation gain default status.

The Role of Perceiver Impression Formation Goals

Impression formation goals, simply enough, are social motives aimed at creating specified outcomes of the impression formation process. Sometimes we want to form accurate impressions of others; this may be particularly important, for instance, when target others control "resources" important to us (e.g., our jobs). Sometimes we desire to form impressions consistent with an existing expectation; such a desire may be especially strong for expectations linked to broad value systems of personal importance, as stereotypes and prejudices often are. And sometimes we want to form impressions rapidly; when we are under time pressure, for example, any impression may suffice.

Success in attaining these goals depends on the nature of available information. Accurate impressions require unbiased, representative target information, sampled broadly; confirming impressions require target information consistent with expectations; and rapid impressions require easily available information possessing little interpretational ambiguity. Information is the currency of impression formation, and distinct impression formation goals require specific types of information.

Impression formation goals use behavioral and cognitive information-gathering and interpretational processes as the means, the tools, for acquiring the desired information. Because such tools are highly relevant to expectancy confirmation, as reviewed above, the potential moderating role of perceiver impression formation goals comes into focus. When impression formation goals elicit processes compatible with expectancy confirmation—the gathering of expectancy-consistent information; the biased direction of attention toward expectancy-consistent behaviors and away from expectancy-incompatible behaviors; and the interpretation of ambiguous behaviors as being expectancy-consistent—perceivers are increasingly likely to confirm their expectations. When impression formation goals discourage these processes, expectancy confirmation should be less likely.

Perceivers motivated to form accurate impressions should thus be less likely to confirm their erroneous expectations, as their strategy should include (1) gathering a large amount of target information, sampling across different trait and behavioral "domains"; and (2) attempting to minimize cognitive biases when interpreting that information. Because these information-processing tactics are incompatible with those underlying expectancy confirmation, accuracy-motivated perceivers should be relatively unlikely to form inappropriate expectancy-consistent impressions.

In contrast, perceivers motivated either to confirm their expectations or to form a rapid impression should be particularly likely to confirm erroneous expectations, as they will presumably focus on gathering expectancy-consistent target information, attend primarily to expectancy-consistent target behaviors, and interpret ambiguous target behaviors as being expectancy-consistent—all of which encourage the formation of expectancy-consistent impressions. The confirmation-motivated perceivers should utilize this strategy for the straightforward reason that it provides them with the information needed to believe what they wish to believe. Perceivers desiring a rapid impression should adopt this strategy because expectancy-consistent processing is more cognitively efficient than expectancy-inconsistent processing (see Fiske & Neuberg, 1990).

Thus, because different impression formation goals regulate information-gathering and cognitive processes, and because the various strategies within these "classes" of processes have differential likelihoods of enabling expectancy confirmation, impression formation goals should play an important role in determining whether perceivers confirm their expectations. This indeed seems to be the case.

First, there exists abundant evidence supporting the notion that impression formation goals moderate the cognitive process of expectancy confirmation (for more comprehensive reviews, see Fiske & Neuberg, 1990; Hilton & Darley, 1991; Neuberg, 1996). Fiske and colleagues have documented accuracy-driven attenuations of expectancy confirmation when an accuracy motive is elicited by either a cooperative (Neuberg & Fiske, 1987) or a competitive (Ruscher & Fiske, 1990) outcome dependency situation, or by direct manipulation (Neuberg & Fiske, 1987). Tetlock and Kim (1987) demonstrated that perceivers' judgments of others are less biased by expectancy information when the perceivers believe that objective standards of judgmental accuracy exist. And Freund, Kruglanski, and Shpitzajzen (1985) found reduced influence of expectancy information when perceivers were aware that their judgments would have important implications for their targets (ostensibly activating in the perceivers an accuracy set). Importantly, these moderating effects of accuracy motivation are apparently mediated by reductions in expectancy-biased attentional and interpretational processes (Fiske & Neuberg, 1990).

Second, evidence from the behavioral domain also suggests an important moderating role for impression formation goals. When perceivers are motivated to be accurate—either by explicit accuracy instructions (Fein, von Hipple, & Hilton, 1989; Neuberg, 1989), by the belief that their expectations are particularly weak (Swann & Ely, 1984), or by the prospect of important future interactions with the target (Darley et al., 1988)—they are less likely to form expectancy-consistent impressions. And again, such moderating effects occur because of accuracy-driven changes in perceiver information-gathering behaviors. Indeed, an experiment from my own lab (Neuberg, 1989) traced the moderating impact of perceiver motives through a social encounter—from perceiver behavior to target behavior to perceiver impressions after the interaction.

Within a study presumably investigating phone interviewing techniques, interviewer subjects were led to believe that one of their two applicants was probably unqualified for the job (negative-expectancy condition), based on previously acquired personality assessment scores; such personality information was ostensibly unavailable for the other applicant (no-expectancy condition) because of a computer scoring error. Moreover, half of the interviewers were motivated to be particularly accurate, while the remaining interviewers were given no explicit goal beyond the basic interviewing instructions all interviewers received. Interviewers generated their own questions and were allowed to conduct the interviews as they wished. Applicants were told to impress their interviewers, and were additionally encouraged to perform well by the prospect that highly successful applicants would receive $50 prizes. When each interview was completed to the interviewer's satisfaction, both participants completed questionnaires assessing their impressions of each other. Finally, the interviews were unobtrusively audiorecorded; this provided independent information about interviewer behaviors and applicant performances.

Results strongly supported predictions. Whereas the no-goal interviewers tended to gather less favorable information from their negative-expectancy applicants than from their no-expectancy applicants (e.g., via the use of negatively tinged questions, fewer encouragements, and shorter interviews), the accuracy-motivated interviewers exhibited no such bias, indeed bending over backward to provide their negative-expectancy applicants with special opportunities to present themselves well. As a consequence, these applicants did not exhibit the performance deficit displayed by the negative-expectancy applicants with the no-goal interviewers. Finally, these performance differences translated into differences in the interviewers' final impressions: Whereas the no-goal interviewers evaluated their negative-expectancy applicants much less favorably than their no-expectancy applicants (i.e., the basic expectancy confirmation effect), the accuracy-motivated interviewers showed no such impression bias.

Finally, two recent studies suggest that explicitly activating the goal of confirming expectations leads to self-fulfilling prophecies, as one would predict. In an experiment by Snyder and Haugen (1994), some perceivers were led to focus particularly on their initial impressions of the target, manipulated via randomly assigned photographs of obese versus normal-weight college students. These perceivers created conversations in which the obese targets behaved less positively than the normal-weight targets. Not surprisingly, this self-fulfilling prophecy translated into an expectancy-confirming bias in perceivers' final impressions. We (Judice & Neuberg, 1994) have reported conceptually similar results, and our data also documented the predicted mediating role of biased perceiver information-gathering behaviors.

On the whole, then, there exists strong support for the idea that perceiver impression formation goals play an important role in moderating the expectancy confirmation process. Moreover, they appear do so via the proposed mechanisms—by regulating the impact of expectations on both behavioral information-gathering processes and attentional and interpretational processes.

The Role of Perceiver Self-Presentational Goals

We are frequently motivated to manage the impressions others form of us. We may want others to view us as likable, smart, competent, intimidating, and so forth (see Jones & Pittman, 1982), and we have at our disposal certain strategies for creating such images. For example, if I want someone to like me, I may make an effort to smile, maintain an appropriate level of eye contact, make flattering statements, exhibit "warm" body language, and avoid potentially uncomfortable topics. In contrast, if I want someone to fear me, my behaviors are likely to be quite different: I may frown, glare, make nasty statements, and introduce uncomfortable or unflattering issues. In each case, the strategy for creating the desired impression includes the tactical use of expressive and information-gathering behaviors—those classes of behavior discussed above as being so important to the expectancy confirmation process.

Furthermore, our self-presentational concerns may have implications for how we think about others. For instance, a personnel officer who wants the boss to view him or her as a good judge of character may adopt the goal of impression accuracy, leading him or her to pay special attention to individuating characteristics and reduce interpretive biases. Thus, self-presentational concerns may additionally influence the cognitive expectancy confirmation process by activating particular impression formation goals and their attendant expectancy-relevant strategies.

To the extent, then, that perceiver self-presentational goals regulate expressive and information-gathering behaviors, as well as attentional and interpretation processes, they should moderate expectancy confirmation.

Much less work has investigated the role of perceiver self- presentational goals. Nonetheless, the existing research does lend support to this hypothesis. Within the cognitive realm, self-presentational concerns can reduce the impact of stereotypical expectations. For example, judgments become less stereotypical when perceivers know they will have to justify their judgments to unknown others (Kruglanski & Freund, 1983) and when they fear that others may view them as being prejudiced (Snyder et al., 1982). Within the behavioral realm, Baumeister, Hutton, and Tice (1989) demonstrated that people's self-presentational concerns can elicit similar motives in others with whom they interact (e.g., a self-promoting perceiver can create a self-promoting target), although the implications of this for the expectancy confirmation process was not addressed.

A recent experiment from my lab, however, directly investigated the self-presentation hypothesis (Neuberg, Judice, Virdin, & Carrillo, 1993). The study employed the interview paradigm described above (Neuberg, 1989), in which interviewers were given negative expectations for one applicant and no expectations for the other. Moreover, half of the interviewers were motivated to get their applicants to like them, while the remaining interviewers received no explicit motivational instructions. As before, the interviewers conducted the interviews as they deemed fit, and we collected data on postinteraction impressions, interviewer behavior, and applicant performance.

We hypothesized that interviewers in the ingratiation-motivated conditions would perform behaviors incompatible with negative-expectancy confirmation. That is, instead of expressing unfavorable reactions to their negative-expectancy applicants and asking them uncomfortable, negatively tinged questions, they should instead strategically strive to display warmer, more favorable behaviors; ask easy, positively tinged questions; and so forth—all so their applicants would like them. Because such favorable expressive and information-gathering behaviors are incompatible with a negative self-fulfilling prophecy, we anticipated no performance deficit by these negative-expectancy applicants and a corresponding lack of postinteraction impression bias by these interviewers.

This was indeed the pattern observed. Moreover, these findings are corroborated by Snyder and Haugen's (1994) finding that perceivers motivated to create smooth, comfortable interactions were also less likely to create a self-fulfilling prophecy. In sum, perceiver self-presentational goals seem to regulate the presence or absence of expectancy-biased cognitive and behavioral processes, in this way moderating the likelihood of expectancy confirmation.

The Role of Target Self-Presentational Goals

Targets also have self-presentational concerns. Importantly, these concerns have direct implications for a target's willingness to accommodate his or her behavior to a perceiver's interactional script. Because accommodation decisions are central to the self-fulfilling prophecy, target self-presentational goals should also help moderate expectancy confirmation: When a target's self-presentation goal encourages a deferential stance toward the perceiver, self-fulfilling prophecies should be more likely; when a target's self-presentational goal discourages deference, summoning instead an expectancy-incompatible agenda, self-fulfilling prophecies should be less likely.

The following circumstances should thus be especially conducive to self-fulfilling prophecies. First, when targets wish to avoid awkward, potentially stressful social interactions (e.g., when the encounters are unimportant), they should be more likely to accommodate the perceivers' behavioral scripts, thus unwittingly confirming the perceivers' expectations. Recent data from Snyder and Haugen (1995), in which targets were encouraged to adjust their behaviors to those of the perceivers, support this notion. Second, if a target wants to be liked by a perceiver, behavioral accommodation may also be a tactic of choice. Third, a target who desires to be viewed as weak or vulnerable may also adopt a deferential behavioral posture. Indeed, several studies found that women were particularly likely to behaviorally confirm a male chauvinist's stereotypical expectations—by acting in a more sex-role-traditional manner (Zanna & Pack, 1975) or dressing more "femininely" (von Baeyer, Sherk, & Zanna, 1981)—but only when the male perceiver was attractive, implicating the motivational component. Fourth, when expectancy-consistent behavior is perceived to be associated with positive public perceptions, it should also become more likely. In one study, subjects underperformed relative to their potential when they were publicly expected to do so and when poor performance was ostensibly linked to a positive personality characteristic (Baumeister, Cooper, & Skib, 1979). Finally, under some circumstances, costs may be associated with challenging the behavioral script of a perceiver; thus, two recent studies indicating that self-fulfilling prophecies become more likely when targets are of apparent low status (Virdin & Neuberg, 1990) or low power (Copeland, 1994) are also compatible with the view that target goals encouraging deference are particularly likely to elicit expectancy confirmation.

Whereas the self-presentational goals described above may make target deference more likely, other self-presentational concerns should evoke strategies of nonaccommodation, thus reducing the likelihood of expectancy confirmation. For example, Hilton and Darley (1985) demonstrated that targets aware of a perceiver's unflattering expectations were particularly likely to disconfirm these expectations; one suspects that the knowledge of another's unfavorable views might evoke a motivated attempt to disabuse the person of the misconception. Similarly, Swann and Ely (1984) demonstrated that targets highly certain of their personality characteristics were particularly unlikely to behaviorally confirm their perceivers' expectations; this too fits with the present conceptualization if one reasonably assumes that self-certain individuals are especially likely to have self-presentational agendas of their own—agendas that may not conform to the scripts created by their perceivers.

On the whole, then, existing data support the hypothesis that a target's self-presentational goals, because of their implications for the target's deference decision, are important moderators of the expectancy confirmation process. Note, however, that few studies have directly tested this notion; current efforts in my own lab are investigating this hypothesis more fully.

When Perceiver and Target Goals Meet

To this point, I have addressed in isolation the social goals of perceivers and targets. A few thoughts on what happens when such goals meet head-to-head seem warranted. If we agree that the focal outcome of an expectancy-tinged interaction is the perceiver's final impression, then the "power" would seem to rest with the perceiver.

Let's consider first the case where a perceiver is strongly motivated to confirm his or her expectations. Regardless of target motives, the perceiver is likely to be successful. If the target decides for whatever reason to be accommodating, the perceiver exits the encounter with expectations confirmed. Even if the target decides to challenge the perceiver's constraining script, and even if he or she is able to do so effectively, the perceiver still holds the trump card—the ability to warp attentional and interpretational processes toward his or her desired outcome. A perceiver committed to expectancy confirmation is thus likely to be successful.

Or consider the case where the perceiver is motivated to be accurate. Because the perceiver's strategies are minimally constraining, and indeed encouraging of target disclosure, target decisions to accommodate mean little. Whether the target desires to defer to the perceiver or to follow a self-presentational agenda, he or she is likely to provide the perceiver with wide-ranging, self-determined information. Thus, although the target's behaviors constrain the particular impression formed by the accuracy-driven perceiver, this is because the perceiver wants it that way.

Let's contemplate one last case—that in which the perceiver is motivated to ingratiate the target. As a consequence, he or she exhibits favorable information-gathering and expressive behaviors. Again, this is a circumstance devoid of serious constraints; thus, although the target provides the expectancy-disconfirming information, he or she essentially does so at the invitation of the perceiver.

These three cases illustrate the perceiver's ability to control an interaction. In particular, because final impressions are ultimately created in the perceiver's mind, target control is limited to (1) presenting self-determined information when given the opportunity and (2) attempting to change the perceiver's goal. Of course, we should not underestimate this latter influence. It is only the highly dogmatic perceiver who maintains a confirmatory stance in the face of relentlessly disconfirmatory evidence. And by injecting a degree of personal relevance into the interaction, a target may be able to shift a perceiver toward accuracy and ingratiation concerns. Nonetheless, perceivers are in the driver's seat; their impressions are shaped by targets to the extent that they allow them to be.

The simultaneous consideration of perceiver and target highlights an additional issue. The present framework is one in which numerous variables are viewed as operating simultaneously in a dynamic, ongoing manner. (Indeed, space constraints have prohibited me from discussing other highly relevant factors, all of which have a place in the developing model—for example, the "compatibility" between perceiver expectation and goal, relative strengths of perceiver expectation and target self-concept, "distance" between the perceiver's expectation and the target's actual self, and so on.). The conventional manner of thinking in terms of simple two- and three-way interactions is thus inadequate, as are simple box-and-arrow visual presentations (although I present such a model below, to summarize my fundamental motivational hypotheses). My colleagues and I are presently using the more dynamic tools of connectionist modeling, hoping that they will better enable us to "work through" the conceptual complexities of such social-interactive processes.

The Role of Limited Resources

Any discussion of motivational influences requires a consideration of the availability of cognitive and behavioral resources, as the conscious pursuit of motivated strategies depends on them. What are the implications of resource unavailability for the expectancy confirmation process? I propose that there exists a set of default strategies—requiring little in the way of resources—that drive the critical mediators when they are not under the conscious control of one's presently active motives.

When resources are scarce, perceivers' information gathering should be limited and focused on the search for expectancy-consistent information, as such information requires fewer resources to process than does expectancy-inconsistent information (Fiske & Neuberg, 1990). This logic can also be applied to the cognitive domain: Perceivers should be particularly likely to focus their attention on expectancy-consistent information and to interpret ambiguous information as being expectancy-consistent. Third, perceivers' expressive behaviors should be more likely to "leak," revealing their underlying expectations, when resources are tight; it is typically more difficult to mask underlying feelings than it is to express them. Finally, because it is usually easier to accommodate another's script than it is to impose upon another a script of one's own, we might expect the unavailability of resources to increase target deference.[2]

Note that the proposed defaults all encourage expectancy confirmation. Existing data are compatible with this notion. For example, circumstances that reduce the availability of cognitive resources—time pressure, physiological arousal, circadian variations—increase the likelihood of stereotype-based judgments (e.g., Bechtold, Naccarato, & Zanna, 1986; Bodenhausen, 1990; Kim & Baron, 1988; Kruglanski & Freund, 1983; Wilder & Shapiro, 1989). Moreover, when resources are expended in one domain (e.g., concern with expressive behaviors), simplifying default processes are particularly likely to occur in neglected domains (e.g., Baumeister et al., 1989; Gilbert, Krull, & Pelham, 1988; Lord & Saenz, 1985; Saenz & Lord, 1989). Although no research has directly assessed the implications of scarce resources within the expectancy confirmation context, data from the Neuberg (1989) study indicated that the increased information-gathering efforts of accuracy-motivated interviewers made it difficult for them to minimize expectancy biases in their cognitive appraisal of the gathered information.

Ongoing research in my lab is focusing more directly on the issue of resource availability. The evidence that does exist, however, is compatible with the hypothesis: Limits in resource availability constrain the ability of social motives to regulate the expectancy confirmation process.

Summary: A Revised Model

The motivational framework, as addressed here, can be summarized by the following four working hypotheses:

1. Perceiver impression formation goals regulate information-gathering behaviors and attentional and interpretational processes, thus moderating the expectancy confirmation effect.
2. Perceiver self-presentational goals regulate information-gathering behaviors, expressive behaviors, and attentional and interpretational processes, thus moderating the expectancy confirmation effect.
3. Target self-presentational goals regulate the decision to accommo-

date the perceiver's behavioral script, thus moderating the expectancy confirmation effect.

4. A decreased availability of cognitive and behavioral resources reduces the ability of goals to regulate their attendant processes. As a consequence, when such resources are scarce low-effort default processes are likely to occur, increasing the likelihood of expectancy confirmation.

Evidence supporting the first two hypotheses seems solid; evidence for the third and fourth hypotheses is less direct, however, and we are currently exploring those issues.

Figure 23.1 presents a visual representation of the first three hypotheses (clarity of presentation prohibits the visual integration of the resource availability hypothesis). The expectancy-tinged social interaction process is conceived as a dynamic process, with both perceiver's and target's motivations leading to behaviors that influence the other's responses and, ultimately, the perceiver's postinteraction impressions. The interested reader should note that the proposed framework shares some similarities with the contributions of Hilton and Darley (1991) and Snyder (1992). Most important, all three frameworks stress the importance of the social-motivational context. The models differ in important ways, however, primarily in their intended scopes and levels of analysis. Elsewhere (Neuberg, 1996), I provide a more thorough comparison of the three models.

SOME FINAL COMMENTS

I have begun this chapter by proposing the necessity of expectation-based thought and action. Indeed, an analysis of resource constraints suggests that the use of expectations to guide cognitive and behavioral processes is the default state—the first option. Inherent in the motivational position, however, is the belief that expectations exist merely to serve active needs. So although expectations do provide people with quick judgments and an easy sense of understanding and control, we must recognize that the needs for quick judgments and superficial perceptions of control are not always predominant. Other goals prevail at times, and possess their own repertoire of strategies—strategies that may be incompatible with expectancy-based cognition and behavior: For example, when motivated to be accurate, people become somewhat suspicious of their expectations, and seem to test them in a reasonably rigorous way; when they are motivated to be ingratiating, there often is not much opportunity for negative expectancy-tinged interpersonal expressions to emerge. Thus, the functionality of expectations does not imply their dominance across all circumstances. Other strategies are equally adaptive, given the goals they serve (Neuberg, 1992), and are themselves dominant

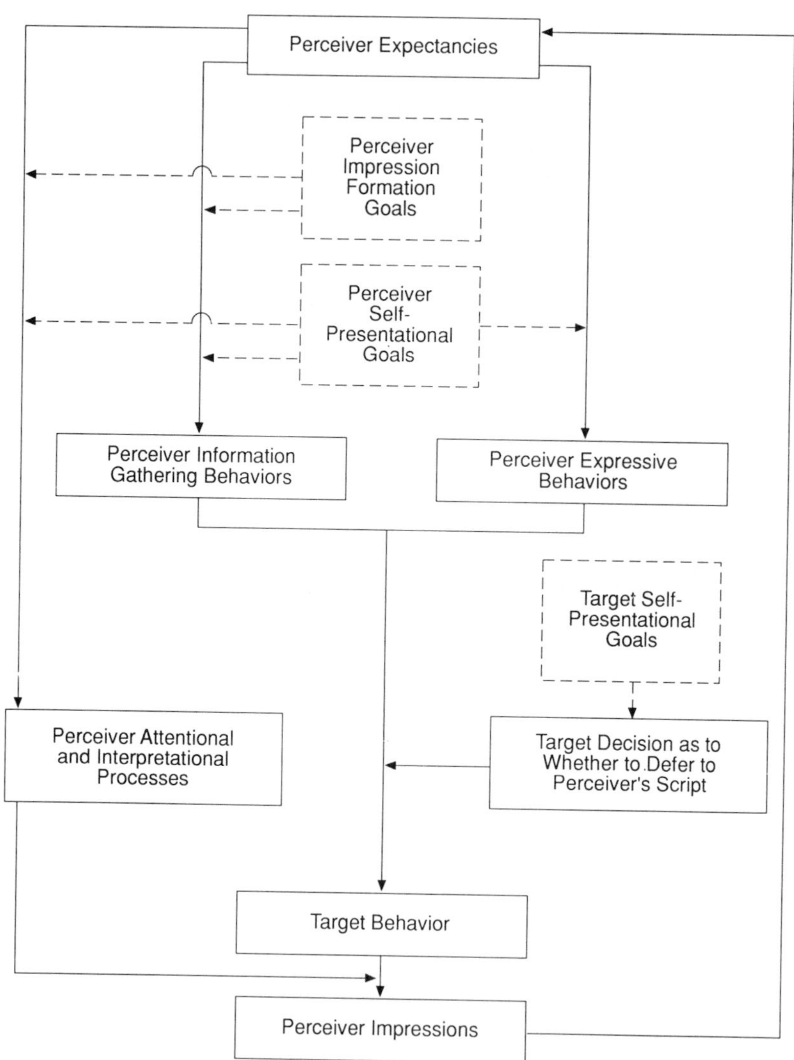

FIGURE 23.1. The proposed role of social motives in expectancy-tinged social encounters. The moderating influences of perceiver and target goals are represented by dotted arrows. For clarity's sake, the constraining impact of resource availability is not represented. From Neuberg (1994). Copyright 1994 by Lawrence Erlbaum Associates. Reprinted by permission.

when called upon. Thus, the apparently incompatible findings cited earlier—some implicating the existence of expectancy confirmation, some suggesting its nonexistence—are far from incompatible. Instead, expectancy confirmation occurs within some motivational contexts and not within others, and does so predictably.

Because the present framework helps explain when expectancy confirmation occurs and when it does not, we are in a better position to address the issue of what to do about the inappropriate confirmation of inaccurate expectations (see Neuberg, 1994, for a more comprehensive discussion of this issue within the context of stereotyping and prejudice). In general, the present analysis makes clear that (1) the holders of inaccurate expectations need to be more concerned with accuracy and/or the formation of positive social relationships; (2) the targets of such expectations need to be willing and able to pursue their own self-presentational agendas; and (3) the interactional contexts need to make available the behavioral and cognitive resources required for the execution of such goals. Because it is often easier to alter people's goals than it is to change their existing beliefs, the present approach may be particularly well suited to deal with this problem. Indeed, given the everyday impact of inaccurate expectations, it is my hope that the theoretical contributions of the present framework can be translated into tools of effective intervention.

ACKNOWLEDGMENTS

Some of the research reported here was supported by National Institute of Mental Health Grant No. MH45719. I appreciate the editors' helpful comments.

NOTES

1. Note that the designations of "perceiver" and "target" are arbitrary, as both individuals typically play both roles. I continue to follow the existing labeling practice, however, for two reasons. First, to do so reduces immeasurably the complexities of exposition. Second, because existing research has typically either focused on those situations in which clear perceiver–target asymmetries naturally exist (e.g., teacher–student and interviewer–applicant interactions) or created such asymmetries via experimental manipulation, the simplified perceiver–target distinction remains useful. Readers should recognize, however, that a full understanding of the expectancy-tinged social interaction process awaits a more complete analysis—one that embraces dual roles for each participant.

2. I do not claim that these proposed defaults are ubiquitous. For example, with frequent use, strategies can become automatized, thus requiring few resources (e.g., Bargh, 1990). For a salesperson well practiced at the art of ingratiation, smiles and compliments may be the default state; this person should thus be able to mask the expression of negative expectations with ease, even under conditions of severe resource constraint. Similarly, for experienced interviewers, comprehensive and un-

biased questioning strategies may be automatized, enabling them to minimize expectancy biases in information gathering when resources are scarce. Nonetheless, I believe that the posited default states hold for most people under most circumstances.

REFERENCES

Andersen, S. M., & Bem, S. L. (1981). Sex typing and androgeny in dyadic interaction: Individual differences in responsiveness to physical attractiveness. *Journal of Personality and Social Psychology, 41,* 74–6.

Babad, E. Y., Inbar, J., & Rosenthal, R. (1982). Pygmalion, Galatea, and Golem: Investigations of biased and unbiased teachers. *Journal of Educational Psychology, 74,* 459–474.

Bargh, J. A. (1990). Auto-motives: Preconscious determinants of social interaction. In E. T. Higgins & R. M. Sorrentino (Eds.), *Handbook of motivation and cognition: Foundations of social behavior* (Vol. 2, pp. 93–130). New York: Guilford Press.

Baumeister, R. F., Cooper, J., & Skib, B. A. (1979). Inferior performance as a selective response to expectancy: Taking a dive to make a point. *Journal of Personality and Social Psychology, 37,* 424–432.

Baumeister, R. F., Hutton, D. G., & Tice, D. M. (1989). Cognitive processes during deliberate self-presentation: How self-presenters alter and misinterpret the behavior of their interaction partners. *Journal of Experimental Social Psychology, 25,* 59–78.

Bechtold, A., Naccarato, M. E., & Zanna, M. P. (1986). *Need for structure and the prejudice–discrimination link.* Paper presented at the annual meeting of the Canadian Psychological Association, Toronto.

Bodenhausen, G. V. (1990). Stereotypes as judgmental heuristics: Evidence of circadian variations in discrimination. *Psychological Science, 1,* 319–322.

Brigham, J. C. (1971). Ethnic stereotypes. *Psychological Bulletin, 76,* 15–38.

Brophy, J. E. (1983). Research on the self-fulfilling prophecy and teacher expectations. *Journal of Educational Psychology, 75,* 631–661.

Brophy, J. E., & Good, T. (1974). *Teacher–student relationships: Causes and consequences.* New York: Holt, Rinehart & Winston.

Christensen, D., & Rosenthal, R. (1982). Gender and nonverbal decoding skill as determinants of interpersonal expectancy effects. *Journal of Personality and Social Psychology, 42,* 75–87.

Cooper, H. (1979). Pygmalion grows up: A model for teacher expectation communication and performance influence. *Review of Educational Research, 49,* 389–410.

Cooper, H., & Hazelrigg, P. (1988). Personality moderators of interpersonal expectancy effects: An integrative research review. *Journal of Personality and Social Psychology, 55,* 937–949.

Copeland, J. T. (1994). Prophecies of power: Motivational implications of social power for behavioral confirmation. *Journal of Personality and Social Psychology, 67,* 264–277.

Darley, J. M., & Fazio, R. H. (1980). Expectancy confirmation processes arising in the social interaction sequence. *American Psychologist, 35,* 867–881.

Darley, J. M., Fleming, J. H., Hilton, J. L., & Swann, W. B., Jr. (1988). Dispelling negative expectancies: The impact of interaction goals and target characteristics on the expectancy confirmation process. *Journal of Experimental Social Psychology, 24,* 19–36.

Dipboye, R. L. (1982). Self-fulfilling prophecies in the selection-recruitment interview. *Academy of Management Review, 7*, 579–586.

Duncan, S. L. (1976). Differential social perception and attribution of intergroup violence: Testing the lower limits of stereotyping of blacks. *Journal of Personality and Social Psychology, 34*, 590–598.

Erber, R., & Fiske, S. T. (1984). Outcome dependency and attention to inconsistent information. *Journal of Personality and Social Psychology, 47*, 709–726.

Farina, A. (1982). The stigma of mental disorders. In A. G. Miller (Ed.), *In the eye of the beholder: Contemporary issues in stereotyping* (pp. 305–363). New York: Praeger.

Farina, A., & Ring, K. (1965). The influence of perceived mental illness on interpersonal relations. *Journal of Applied Social Psychology, 70*, 47–51.

Fein, S., von Hipple, W., & Hilton, J. L. (1989, August). *The impact of interaction goals on expectancy confirmation.* Paper presented at the annual meeting of the American Psychological Association, New Orleans.

Fiske, S. T., & Neuberg, S. L. (1990). A continuum of impression formation, from category-based to individuating processes: Influences of information and motivation on attention and interpretation. In M. P. Zanna (Ed.), *Advances in experimental social psychology* (Vol. 23, pp. 1–74). New York: Academic Press.

Fiske, S. T., Neuberg, S. L., Beattie, A. E., & Milberg, S. J. (1987). Category-based and attribute-based reactions to others: Some informational conditions of stereotyping and individuating processes. *Journal of Experimental Social Psychology, 23*, 399–427.

Fiske, S. T., & Taylor, S. E. (1991). *Social cognition* (2nd ed.). New York: McGraw-Hill.

Freund, T., Kruglanski, A. W., & Shpitzajzen, A. (1985). The freezing and unfreezing of impression primacy: Effects of the need for structure and the fear of invalidity. *Personality and Social Psychology Bulletin, 11*, 479–487.

Gilbert, D. T., Krull, D. S., & Pelham, B. W. (1988). Of thoughts unspoken: Social inference and the self-regulation of behavior. *Journal of Personality and Social Psychology, 55*, 685–694.

Goffman, E. (1959). *The presentation of self in everyday life.* Garden City, NY: Doubleday.

Grice, H. P. (1975). Logic in conversation. In P. Cole & J. L. Morgan (Eds.), *Syntax and semantics* (Vol. 3, pp. 41–58). New York: Academic Press.

Hamilton, D. L., Sherman, S. J., & Ruvulo, C. M. (1990). Stereotype-based expectancies: Effects on information processing and social behavior. *Journal of Social Issues, 46*, 35–60.

Harris, M. J., & Rosenthal, R. (1985). Mediation of interpersonal expectancy effects: 31 meta-analyses. *Psychological Bulletin, 97*, 363–386.

Harris, M. J., & Rosenthal, R. (1986). Counselor and client personality as determinants of counselor expectancy effects. *Journal of Personality and Social Psychology, 50*, 362–369.

Higgins, E.T., & Bargh, J.A. (1987). Social cognition and social perception. *Annual Review of Psychology, 38*, 369–425.

Hilton, J. L., & Darley, J. M. (1985). Constructing other persons: A limit on the effect. *Journal of Experimental Social Psychology, 21*, 1–18.

Hilton, J. L., & Darley, J. M. (1991). The effects of interaction goals on person perception. In M. P. Zanna (Ed.), *Advances in experimental social psychology* (Vol. 24, pp. 235–267). San Diego, CA: Academic Press.

Hilton, J. L., Darley, J. M., & Fleming, J. H. (1989). Self- fulfilling prophecies and self-defeating behaviors. In R. C. Curtis (Ed.), *Self-defeating behaviors: Experimental* research, clinical impressions, and practical implications (pp. 41–65). New York: Plenum Press.

Ickes, W., Patterson, M. L., Rajecki, D. W., & Tanford, S. (1982). Behavioral and cognitive consequences of reciprocal versus compensatory responses to preinteraction expectancies. *Social Cognition, 1,* 160–190.

Jones, E. E. (1986). Interpreting interpersonal behavior: The effects of expectancies. *Science, 234,* 41–46.

Jones, E. E., & Pittman, T. S. (1982). Toward a general theory of strategic self-presentation. In J. Suls (Ed.), *Psychological perspectives on the self* (Vol. 1, pp. 231–262). Hillsdale, NJ: Erlbaum.

Judice, T. N., & Neuberg, S. L. (1994). *When perceivers desire to confirm their negative expectancies: Self-fulfilling prophecies and target misperceptions of their own performance.* Manuscript submitted for publication.

Jussim, L. (1986). Self-fulfilling prophecies: A theoretical and integrative review. *Psychological Review, 93,* 429–445.

Jussim, L. (1991). Social perception and social reality: A reflection-construction model. *Psychological Review, 98,* 54–73.

Kim, H.-S., & Baron, R. S. (1988). Exercise and the illusory correlation: Does arousal heighten stereotypic processing? *Journal of Experimental Psychology, 24,* 366–380.

Kruglanski, A. W., & Freund, T. (1983). The freezing and unfreezing of lay-inferences: Effects of impressional primacy, ethnic stereotyping, and numerical anchoring. *Journal of Experimental Social Psychology, 19,* 448–468.

Lord, C. G., & Saenz, D. S. (1985). Memory deficits and memory surfeits: Differential cognitive consequences of tokenism for tokens and observers. *Journal of Personality and Social Psychology, 49,* 918–926.

Major, B., Cozzarelli, C., Testa, M., & McFarlin, D. B. (1988). Self-verification versus expectancy confirmation in social interaction: The impact of self-focus. *Personality and Social Psychology Bulletin, 14,* 346–359.

Meichenbaum, D. H., Bowers, K. S., & Ross, R. R. (1969). A behavioral analysis of teacher expectancy effects. *Journal of Personality and Social Psychology, 13,* 306–313.

Merton, R. K. (1948). The self-fulfilling prophecy. *Antioch Review, 8,* 193–210.

Miller, D. T., & Turnbull, W. (1986). Expectancies and interpersonal processes. *Annual Review of Psychology, 37,* 233–256.

Neuberg, S. L. (1989). The goal of forming accurate impressions during social interactions: Attenuating the impact of negative expectancies. *Journal of Personality and Social Psychology, 56,* 374–386.

Neuberg, S. L. (1992). Evolution and individuation: The adaptiveness of nonstereotypical thought. *Psychological Inquiry, 3,* 178–180.

Neuberg, S. L. (1994). Expectancy-confirmation processes in stereotype-tinged social encounters: The moderating role of social goals. In M. P. Zanna & J. M. Olson (Eds.), *The psychology of prejudice: The Ontario Symposium* (Vol. 7, pp. 103–130). Hillsdale, NJ: Erlbaum.

Neuberg, S. L. (1996). Social motives and expectancy-tinged social interactions. In R. M. Sorrentino & E. T. Higgins (Eds.), *Handbook of motivation and cognition: Vol. 3. The interpersonal context* (pp. 225–261). New York: Guilford Press.

Neuberg, S. L., & Fiske, S. T. (1987). Motivational influences on impression formation: Outcome dependency, accuracy-driven attention, and individuating processes. *Journal of Personality and Social Psychology, 53,* 431–444.

Neuberg, S. L., Judice, T. N., Virdin, L. M., & Carrillo, M. A. (1993). Perceiver self-presentational goals as moderators of expectancy influences: Ingratiation and the disconfirmation of negative expectancies. *Journal of Personality and Social Psychology, 64,* 409–420.

Nisbett, R. E., & Ross, L. (1980). *Human inference: Strategies and shortcomings of social judgment.* Englewood Cliffs, NJ: Prentice-Hall.

Omoto, A. M., & Borgida, E. (1988). Guess who might be coming to dinner?: Personal involvement and racial stereotypes. *Journal of Experimental Social Psychology, 24,* 571–593.

Rosenthal, R. (1974). *On the social psychology of the self-fulfilling prophecy: Further evidence for Pygmalion effects and their mediating mechanisms* (Module No 53.). New York: MSS Modular.

Rosenthal, R., & Jacobson, L. F. (1968). *Pygmalion in the classroom.* New York: Holt, Rinehart & Winston.

Rosenthal, R., & Rubin, D. B. (1978). Interpersonal expectancy effects: The first 345 studies. *Behavioral and Brain Sciences, 3,* 377–386.

Ruble, D. N., & Ruble, T. L. (1982). Sex stereotypes. In A. G. Miller (Ed.), *In the eye of the beholder: Contemporary issues in stereotyping* (pp. 188–252). New York: Praeger.

Ruscher, J. B., & Fiske, S. T. (1990). Interpersonal competition can cause individuating impression formation. *Journal of Personality and Social Psychology, 58,* 832–842.

Saenz, D. S., & Lord, C. G. (1989). Reversing roles: A cognitive strategy for undoing memory deficits associated with token status. *Journal of Personality and Social Psychology, 56,* 698–708.

Sagar, H. A., & Schofield, J. W. (1980). Racial and behavioral cues in black and white children's perceptions of ambiguously aggressive acts. *Journal of Personality and Social Psychology, 39,* 590–598.

Seligman, M. E. P. (1975). *Helplessness: On depression, development, and death.* San Francisco: W. H. Freeman.

Sibicky, M., & Dovidio, J. F. (1986). Stigma of psychological therapy: Stereotypes, interpersonal reactions, and the self-fulfilling prophecy. *Journal of Counseling Psychology, 33, 148*–154.

Snyder, M. (1984). When belief creates reality. In L. Berkowitz (Ed.), *Advances in experimental social psychology* (Vol. 18, pp. 248–306)). New York: Academic Press.

Snyder, M. (1992). Motivational foundations of behavioral confirmation. In M. P. Zanna (Ed.), *Advances in experimental social psychology* (Vol. 25, pp. 67–114). San Diego, CA: Academic Press.

Snyder, M., Campbell, B. H., & Preston, E. (1982). Testing hypotheses about human nature: Assessing the accuracy of social stereotypes. *Social Cognition, 1,* 256–272.

Snyder, M., & Gangestad, S. (1981). Hypothesis-testing processes. In J. H. Harvey, W. Ickes, & R. F. Kidd (Eds.), *New directions in attribution research* (Vol. 3, pp. 171–196). Hillsdale, NJ: Erlbaum.

Snyder, M., & Haugen, J. A. (1994). Why does behavioral confirmation occur? A functional perspective on the role of the perceiver. *Journal of Experimental Social Psychology, 30,* 218–246.

Snyder, M., & Haugen, J. A. (1995). Why does behavioral confirmation occur? A functional perspective on the role of the target. *Personality and Social Psychology Bulletin, 21,* 963–974.

Snyder, M., & Swann, W. B., Jr. (1978). Hypothesis-testing processes in social interaction. *Journal of Personality and Social Psychology, 36,* 1202–1212.

Snyder, M., Tanke, E. D., & Berscheid, E. (1977). Social perception and interpersonal behavior: On the self-fulfilling nature of social stereotypes. *Journal of Personality and Social Psychology, 35,* 656–666.

Swann, W. B., Jr., & Ely, R. J. (1984). A battle of wills: Self- verification versus behavioral confirmation. *Journal of Personality and Social Psychology, 46,* 1287–1302.

Swann, W. B., Jr., & Snyder, M. (1980). On translating beliefs into action: Theories of ability and their applications in an instructional setting. *Journal of Personality and Social Psychology, 38,* 879–888.

Tavris, C., & Offir, C. (1977). *The longest war: Sex differences in perspective.* New York: Harcourt Brace Jovanovich.

Tetlock, P. E., & Kim, J. I. (1987). Accountability and judgment processes in a personality prediction task. *Journal of Personality and Social Psychology, 52,* 700–709.

Thompson, S. C. (1981). Will it hurt less if I can control it? A complex answer to a simple question. *Psychological Bulletin, 90,* 89–101.

Virdin, L. M., & Neuberg, S. L. (1990, August). *Is perceived status a moderator of expectancy confirmation?* Paper presented at the annual meeting of the American Psychological Association, Boston.

von Baeyer, C. L., Sherk, D. L., & Zanna, M. P. (1981). Impression management in the job interview: When the female applicant meets the male (chauvinist) interviewer. *Personality and Social Psychology Bulletin, 7,* 45–51.

Vrugt, A. (1990). Negative attitudes, nonverbal behavior and self-fulfilling prophecy in simulated therapy interviews. *Journal of Nonverbal Behavior, 14,* 77–86.

West, C., & Anderson, T. (1976). The question of preponderant causation in teacher expectancy research. *Review of Educational Research, 46,* 613–630.

Wilder, D. A., & Shapiro, P. (1989). The role of competition- induced anxiety in limiting the beneficial impact of positive behavior by an outgroup member. *Journal of Personality and Social Psychology, 56,* 60–69.

Word, C. O., Zanna, M. P., & Cooper, J. (1974). The nonverbal mediation of self-fulfilling prophecies in inter-racial interaction. *Journal of Experimental Social Psychology, 10,* 109–120.

Zanna, M. P., & Pack, S. J. (1975). On the self-fulfilling nature of apparent sex differences in behavior. *Journal of Experimental Social Psychology, 11,* 583–591.

CHAPTER 24

Beyond Accuracy

Defense and Impression Motives in Heuristic and Systematic Information Processing

Shelly Chaiken
Roger Giner-Sorolla
Serena Chen

Social psychologists have long realized that people process information in more than one way, and for more than one reason. By now, the literature is rich with multiple-process models that, in taxonomizing the "hows" of information processing, draw a distinction between more and less thoughtful ways of thinking (e.g., Chaiken, Liberman, & Eagly, 1989; Fiske & Neuberg, 1990; Gilbert, 1989; Petty & Cacioppo, 1986; Tetlock, 1985). Renewed attention has also been given to the "whys," or motivational underpinnings, of information processing (e.g., Chaiken & Stangor, 1987; Herek, 1986; Johnson & Eagly, 1989; Kunda, 1990; Snyder, 1992), often with explicit reference to pioneering taxonomies of attitude functions (Katz, 1960; Smith, Bruner, & White, 1956). Yet little effort has been made to explore the interaction of multiple processing modes on the one hand and multiple motivations on the other.

In this chapter, we consider the motivations governing information processing within the framework of the heuristic–systematic model (Chaiken, 1980, 1987; Chaiken et al., 1989). This model proposes two concurrent modes by which people process information and reach judgments: a relatively effortless *heuristic* mode, characterized by the application of simple decision rules (e.g., "Experts can be trusted"), and a more effortful and analytic *systematic* mode, in which particularistic or individuating information about objects of judgment is used. Which mode predominates in any situation depends on the individual's current motivation and capacity to engage in detailed processing.

The model's motivational predictions are based on the *sufficiency principle* (Figure 24.1), which embodies the tradeoff between minimizing effort and reaching an adequate level of confidence in one's judgment. The sufficiency principle proposes a continuum of judgmental confidence for any particular decision. On this continuum there exist two points of interest: the level of *actual* confidence in one's judgment, and the level of *desired* confidence, or *sufficiency threshold.* With adequate capacity to process information, a person will engage in processing until the level of actual confidence is raised to the level of desired confidence, thereby closing the gap between the two.

Although the systematic mode requires greater processing capacity, it is generally more effective in increasing subjective confidence than heuristic processing is. Consequently, systematic processing will occur when heuristic processing cannot completely close the gap between actual and desired confidence. Systematic processing, then, can be encouraged by increasing this gap, either by raising the sufficiency threshold (Figure 24.1B—e.g., by increasing the relevance or importance of information at hand) or by lowering the amount of actual confidence (Figure 24.1C—e.g., by introducing information that contradicts a previously presented heuristic cue) (Maheswaran & Chaiken, 1991). It should be noted, however, that systematic processing can only take placed if there is adequate *capacity* to process information effortfully.

The heuristic–systematic model originally assumed that perceivers were motivated to hold accurate attitudes and beliefs (Chaiken, 1980, 1987). While high levels of *accuracy motivation* tend to foster systematic processing, even heuristic processing was assumed to be motivated by accuracy concerns, albeit less pressing ones. However, in many situations, other motivations coexist with or supplant the desire to be objectively correct (Kruglanski, 1990; Swann, 1990; Taylor, 1991; Tesser, 1988; Trope, 1986). The heuristic–systematic model presently acknowledges two broad motives other than accuracy (Chaiken et al., 1989). *Defense motivation* is an orientation toward reinforcing important self-related beliefs, and *impression motivation* is an orientation toward holding and expressing beliefs dictated by the current interpersonal situation.[1] In the same way that both heuristic and systematic processing have been shown to serve accuracy concerns, both modes of processing can serve defense and impression concerns.

The heuristic–systematic model was also originally developed to apply to persuasion settings, and indeed most research inspired by this model has examined attitude formation and change (see Eagly & Chaiken, 1993, Ch. 7). However, we have argued that the concepts of heuristic and systematic processing are also applicable to information processing in other settings, such as person perception and the evaluation of evidence (Chaiken et al., 1989). In fact, several new studies reported here extend the model's concepts and predictions to information processing in the absence of an explicit attempt to persuade.

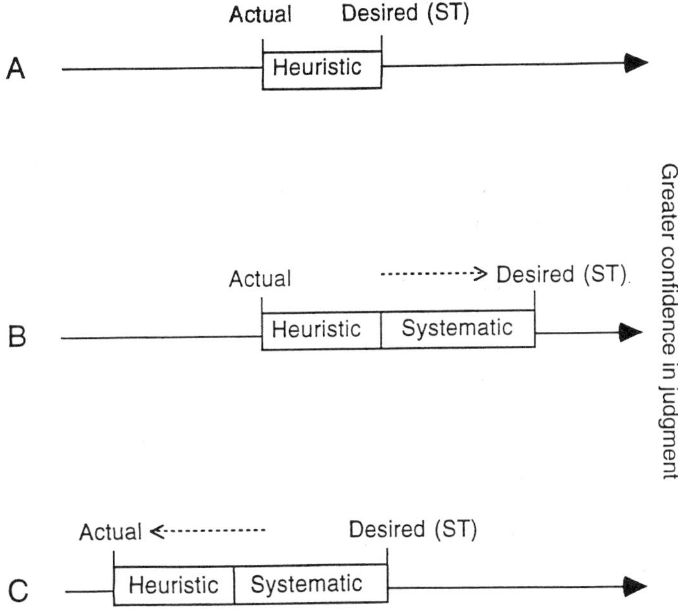

FIGURE 24.1. Illustration of the accuracy-motivated sufficiency principle in three different types of situations. (A) Small gap between actual and desired confidence; only heuristic processing is used. (B) Systematic processing promoted by increasing level of desired confidence. (C) Systematic processing promoted by lowering level of actual confidence. *Note.* "Actual" refers to the actual level of confidence; "Desired (ST)" refers to the desired level of confidence or sufficiency threshold.

NO MOTIVATION

We are about to consider the ways in which our three proposed motivations may create, sustain, or change attitudes and beliefs about the world. But what happens in the absence of any particular motivation? Like an unmotivated mass in the physical world, the unmotivated individual remains inert, maintaining existing attitudes and beliefs. Although information does impinge on the unmotivated person, it is processed in a superficial way, leaving knowledge structures essentially unchanged.

As Allport (1935) noted, attitudes serve a schematic function, organizing the world in a convenient way. When there is no motivation to change existing attitudes, they will persist. Cognitive conservatism in the absence of motivation, however, should not be confused with more motivationally based resistance to change, such as that which arises from defense motivation. This distinction is explored at more length when we discuss defense motivation.

ACCURACY MOTIVATION

Accuracy motivation is the desire to hold attitudes and beliefs that are objectively valid. Not only the heuristic–systematic model, but other influential theories of attitude formation and change (e.g., Petty & Cacioppo, 1986; Anderson, 1971) and of social information processing (e.g., Fiske & Neuberg, 1990) have explicitly or implicitly assumed that people are motivated to have an objectively true representation of the world. Accuracy motivation is also well represented among attitude theories that acknowledge multiple possible motives in persuasion. In particular, various typologies of attitude function have asserted that attitudes can serve the goal of realistic assessment, whether this function is labeled as "knowledge" (Katz, 1960) or as "object appraisal" (Smith et al., 1956). Accuracy motivation is also conceptually related to Chaiken and Stangor's (1987) discussion of issue involvement, as well as to Gollwitzer's (1990) discussion of the deliberative mind-set corresponding to the predecisional action phase, which is characterized by "an orientation toward accurate and impartial processing" (p. 65).

Although systematic processing does not necessarily lead to an objectively accurate judgment, in many cases it is the mode better suited to achieving accuracy goals. Careful scrutiny is needed to distinguish between valid and specious information (Petty & Cacioppo, 1986), and can attenuate the effects of such fallible heuristics as "Likeable people are correct" (Chaiken & Eagly, 1983). Thus, systematic processing is promoted in situations that induce high accuracy motivation, such as those in which the issue at hand will personally affect the subject (Petty & Cacioppo, 1979). However, it is crucial that the *capacity* to process systematically also be present. For example, the person must know enough about the issue to be able to process arguments about it (Wood, Kallgren, & Priesler, 1985), and must have enough time to be able to concentrate on the message (Chaiken & Lutz, 1993; Ratneshwar & Chaiken, 1991).

Heuristic processing also serves the goal of accuracy motivation, because heuristics tend to reduce uncertainty. When systematic processing is difficult or impossible, an accuracy-motivated person may have no choice but to base a decision on the best rule of thumb available; and when accuracy motivation is present but relatively low, heuristics provide a cognitively inexpensive way to gain a limited degree of confidence in the accuracy of one's judgment.

According to the sufficiency principle, the preferred processing mode is that which best closes the gap between actual and desired confidence, given adequate capacity to process. When the prevailing motive is accuracy, as we have noted, extensive systematic processing increases actual confidence to a greater level than does heuristic processing alone, which in turn increases actual confidence more effectively than no processing at all. However, the nature of information, and not just the way in which it is processed, can affect its ability to satisfy accuracy concerns. For example, a heuristic-based inference that is later called into doubt by contradictory information will be seen as an unsatisfactory basis for judgment even when accuracy motivation is low (Maheswaran & Chaiken, 1991). Similarly, one might predict that a message that comes from an obviously biased or self-interested source may not satisfy the accuracy-motivated person's need for reliable information, even if it is processed systematically.

Finally, even though a person may be driven to seek accuracy, the actual result of processing may fall short of this goal. Most persuasion heuristics are of limited diagnostic value: Not all experts can be trusted; not all majorities are right. Even when motivation is high, expectancies derived from these heuristics can bias systematic processing; for example, an expert's arguments may be evaluated more favorably than a nonexpert's (Chaiken & Maheswaran, 1994). Bias in prior knowledge can also affect the accuracy of systematic processing. For example, if the arguments on one side of an issue rest mainly on biological evidence, while those on the other side rest on sociological evidence, a person who is knowledgeable about potential fallacies in biological research but knows little about sociology may criticize the biological evidence especially harshly (see also Biek, Wood, Chaiken, & Nations, in press).

DEFENSE MOTIVATION

Defense motivation is the desire to hold attitudes and beliefs that are congruent with existing self-definitional attitudes and beliefs. By "self-definitional" we mean those attitudes and beliefs that are closely tied to the self, including terminal values (Rokeach, 1968); social identities such as one's gender, ethnicity, religion, or profession; attitudes supporting one's material vested interests; and beliefs about personal attributes such as intelligence, social sensitivity, and healthfulness.[2] The defense-motivated person's main goal, consciously or unconsciously, is not to have an accurate representation of the world, but to preserve the self-concept and associated world views. Therefore, the hallmark of defense motivation is a self-serving *bias* in processing.

Processing bias arising from defense motivation should be distinguished from other sources of bias that are more purely cognitive, such as the impact of prior knowledge or heuristic information on accuracy-motivated systematic processing (Biek et al., in press; Chaiken & Maheswaran, 1994). Defense motivation leads to a *directional* bias that is consistently in line with existing self-beliefs, whereas a bias arising only from cognitive sources can either favor or contradict existing self-beliefs.[3]

Our concept of defense motivation is similar to Chaiken and Stangor's (1987) discussion of position involvement, Tesser's (1988) discussion of self-evaluation maintenance, Johnson and Eagly's (1989) discussion of value-relevant involvement, and Kunda's (1990) discussion of motivated reasoning—all of which are described as motivations to defend pre-existing ideas.[4] Within the functional theories of attitude, defense motivation is closely linked to Katz's (1960) *ego-defensive* function, under which attitudes are formed, held, and changed to preserve existing beliefs about the self. Less obviously, we also see our concept of defense motivation as related to Katz's *value-expressive* function, under which attitudes are formed, held, and changed with the aim of reflecting core values and beliefs about the world.[5]

Defense-Motivated Heuristic and Systematic Processing

Under defense motivation, the overriding processing principle is *selectivity*. That is, people will selectively process information in the way that best meets their defensive needs. The sufficiency principle can still be applied under defense motivation. However, defensive sufficiency is determined not by whether information processing yields a judgment that is likely to be accurate, but by whether information processing yields a judgment that reinforces self-definitional attitudes and beliefs.

Motivational factors that raise a person's defensive sufficiency threshold for an issue include the perceived *relevance* of the issue to existing self-concepts, and the *centrality* of these concepts. Issues that obviously touch on core attitudes, beliefs, and identities are more likely to arouse defense motivation than issues that are only weakly linked to central concerns, or that are linked to more peripheral concerns. Threats to the self-concept can also increase defense motivation and raise the defensive sufficiency threshold. These threats may affect an area similar to (e.g., symbolic self-completion; Wicklund & Gollwitzer, 1982) or different from (e.g., self-affirmation; Steele, 1988) the aspect of the self currently under consideration. In addition, self-views about which a person is relatively certain are more likely to evoke defense motivation when threatened (Swann, 1990). In our terms, an initially high level of certainty creates a high standard of desired confidence that people are motivated to restore.

The defensive sufficiency threshold may be reached using either heuristic or systematic processing, or both modes. We propose that defense motivation leads to a congenial bias in the processing of information *within* the systematic and heuristic modes, so that the desired judgment will more easily be reached. Moreover, defensive concerns may determine whether heuristic *or* systematic processing is used, according to the strength of defense motivation and the nature of available information.

Within the systematic mode, selective processing involves the biased evaluation of evidence and arguments. Material that is congruent with existing self-relevant beliefs, such as research supporting one's position on capital punishment, will be judged as more valid and accurate than incongruent material (Lord, Ross, & Lepper, 1979; Pyszczynski, Greenberg, & Holt, 1985; Pyszczynski & Greenberg, 1987). We believe that this judgment bias pervades the defense-motivated individual's systematic processing, and that its strength varies mainly according to how much defense motivation is present.

Heuristics, too, can be applied in a biased way, and their implications may be accepted or rejected according to whether or not they support the individual's central beliefs and attitudes. The *reliability* of a particular piece of noncongenial heuristic information may be disparaged, as when a survey's sample size or sampling method is called into question (Hazlewood & Chaiken, 1990). Following the principle of selectivity, people will be especially likely to question the survey if its implications go against their beliefs. In addition, attitudes may be defended by disparaging the *validity* of a noncongenial heuristic; one may endorse the general rule "The majority is right" when public opinion supports one's own opinions, but dismiss it when the polls offer contrary findings.

As these examples indicate, we believe that defense-motivated people can and do use the same heuristics that accuracy-motivated people use, although in a biased way. It is also possible that defensive concerns may manifest themselves in heuristics that are *not* used by accuracy-motivated people. These heuristics, although determined idiosyncratically by the individual's core beliefs, would take the general form "If information supports belief *X*, it must be true," or the converse, "If information contradicts belief *X*, it must be false." Such defensive heuristics may provide quick and easy ways to reinforce important attitudes and beliefs, while dismissing threats to them.

Selectivity in the amount of processing given to information can manifest itself in two ways. First, a person may give more systematic scrutiny to hostile material in order to find flaws in it or generate counterarguments. When this process is driven by defense motivation, it may be labeled "defensive counterarguing." Conversely, hostile material may be ignored outright, or attended to less carefully than congenial material; we label this process "defensive inattention." Although associated with psychoanalytic perspectives on repression (e.g., Freud, 1933/1965), defensive inattention has also been acknowledged in social psychology by Janis and Feshbach's (1953) theoretical perspective on avoidance of fear-arousing stimuli; by Festinger's (1957, 1964) selective exposure hypothesis; and by Baumeister and Cairns's (1992) concept of self-deception, which they define as "the systematic, motivated avoidance of threatening or unpleasant information about the self" (p. 851).

Extensive study has not been given to the question of which conditions lead to the use of counterarguing versus inattention. But, as with accuracy motivation, we can predict that the individual's motivation and ability to process selectively will determine which type of selective processing is used. When defensive sufficiency thresholds are high (e.g., the issue is highly self-definitional) and actual defensive confidence is low (e.g., the material effectively threatens the person's self-image), selective counterarguing will be preferred, given the ability to do so. Such an active strategy is more likely to effectively reinforce existing self-relevant attitudes and beliefs. However, when defensive thresholds are low, when actual defensive confidence has been bolstered, or when ability to counterargue is not present, the less demanding inattention strategy will predominate (see also Eagly & Chaiken, 1993, Ch. 12).

The mode of processing favored by the defense-motivated person may also depend on the congeniality of existing information. For example, a message may be accompanied by hostile heuristic information, such as a poll showing that most people reject a political position that the individual is motivated to support. Because the poll undermines the individual's actual defensive confidence, biased systematic processing will be used to close the widened defensive sufficiency gap. Assuming that ability is present, then, a hostile cue can be expected to lead to greater levels of systematic processing, albeit biased. A congenial cue, on the other hand, can be expected to boost actual defensive confidence, narrowing the confidence gap so that biased systematic processing of the message is reduced.

Empirical Evidence

Although many empirical studies have shown defensively motivated selectivity in the evaluation of information (e.g., Lord et al., 1979; Pyszczynski et al., 1985), the processing mediation of these effects has not been fully examined within a dual-process framework. Nonetheless, several recent studies have found that evidence contradictory to such vital self-beliefs as "I am healthy" and "I am socially sensitive" may be subject to increased scrutiny or counterargument, rather than to defensive inattention. Wyer and Frey (1983) found that students who received negative feedback on an intelligence test, relative to neutral observers or to students who received positive feedback, recalled more pro-intelligence-test information from a message presenting information both for and against the test. However, negative-feedback subjects also judged intelligence tests more negatively, suggesting that pro-intelligence-test arguments were given special attention in order to be refuted.

Liberman and Chaiken (1992) gave women who either did or did not drink coffee a detailed message that either supported or disconfirmed a purported link between coffee drinking and fibrocystic disease, but presented studies on both sides of the issue. Coffee-drinking and non-coffee-drinking subject groups were matched on prior belief in the link, so that any biases found would clearly proceed from self-interest motivation rather than from cognitive factors. In addition to finding biased judgment of the message, Liberman and Chaiken found tendencies for coffee drinkers to expend more effort on the message and to find more weaknesses in pro-link than in anti-link information, suggesting the use of a defensive counterarguing strategy.

Finally, Ditto and Lopez (1992) present a particularly vivid illustration of the tendency to engage in greater scrutiny of threatening evidence. Subjects were told that a self-administered saliva test indicated either the presence or absence of an unfavorable medical condition. Those who were diagnosed as having the unfavorable condition not only were more likely to rate the test as less accurate and the condition as generally less serious, but were more likely to spontaneously give themselves the test again, subjecting the unwelcome information to a more intensive analysis.

Evidence for defensive inattention has been mixed. Research in the "fear appeals" tradition, in which subjects are typically exposed to fear-arousing persuasive communications, has generally failed to establish that the reduced persuasive effect of threatening information is mediated by reduced attention to information (Eagly & Chaiken, 1993). But in a related literature, Frey (1986) concluded that people who experience cognitive dissonance after a decision, when given a selection of information to peruse, tend to avoid decision-incongruent information and to seek out decision-congruent information. In line with our ability predictions, the tendency to select congruent material appears to be eliminated if the incongruent material is seen as easily refutable (Frey & Stahlberg, 1986).[6] Pyszczynski and Greenberg (1987) also report a line of research in which nondepressed subjects, given a selection of information after receiving self-relevant performance feedback, tend to request congenial material.

The general finding of defensive inattention when subjects are given a selection of information stands in contrast to the general findings of defensive counterarguing or unbiased attention when all subjects are actually exposed to mixed or hostile information, as in the fear appeal and health message literatures referred to above. This contrast has not yet been tested explicitly. However, it stands to reason, in line with our hypotheses, that actually presenting people with hostile material will lead to a greater drop in actual defensive confidence, and a greater reliance on biased systematic counterarguing, than merely giving people the option to select hostile material.

Apart from the above-described findings, there has been little work devoted to specifying the conditions under which defense-motivated perceivers employ inattention versus counterarguing. A recent study (see Chaiken, Pomerantz, & Giner-Sorolla, 1995) provides some evidence that the extent to which one's beliefs on an issue support one's attitudes, as measured by evaluative–cognitive consistency, affects which defensive style is used in processing a mixed message. Low-consistency subjects, who presumably lacked the cognitive resources with which to counterargue, remembered fewer hostile than congenial arguments on the issue of capital punishment, which suggests that they may have focused mainly on congenial arguments in an attempt to bolster their attitudes. High-consistency subjects showed the opposite bias, remembering more hostile arguments and judging them negatively, which suggests a greater tendency to counterargue.

Another recent experiment (Giner-Sorolla & Chaiken, 1995) examined the selective use of defensive processing modes in response to heuristic cues that either did or did not support defensive concerns. Subjects were classified according to their vested interest in the issue of making essay exams mandatory—that is, whether they said they generally did better in essay exams (vested interest pro), did better in multiple-choice exams (vested interest anti), or had no preference (vested interest neutral). In the laboratory, subjects were told that they were participating in an evaluation of a university proposal requiring that upper-level classes use only essay exams. Some subjects were exposed to a heuristic consensus cue in the form of poll results stating that the majority of students opposed (cue anti) or favored (cue pro) the proposal; others were not shown the poll results (no cue). All subjects then read a mixed message composed of equal numbers of arguments for the merits of essay and multiple-choice exams.

Consistent with earlier research, the experiment found evidence for biased processing of both the cue and the message. Subjects with a vested interest rated the poll as significantly more reliable, and criticized it significantly less in an open-ended thought listing, if its results supported their vested interest. Subjects also showed a significant congenial bias in evaluating the message, rating the arguments supporting their vested interest as stronger than the arguments against it.

Our main prediction was that a hostile heuristic cue would confer less judgmental confidence than a congenial cue, consequently increasing the gap between actual and desired confidence, and inducing higher levels of systematic processing to close the gap. We carried out a regression analysis in which attitude change was to be simultaneously predicted from cue valence weighted by perceived cue validity, which represented heuristic influences, and from the valence of subjects' listed specific thoughts about the issue (i.e., arguments for or against either type of exam), which represented the influence of systematic processing. In the two "noncongenial-cue" conditions (vested interest of opposite valence to cue), the valence of subjects' specific issue thoughts predicted attitude change, whereas cue valence had no effect on attitude change, suggesting that biased systematic processing mediated attitude change in these conditions. Conversely, in the two "congenial-cue" conditions (vested interest of same valence as cue), valence of specific issue thoughts was not a consequential predictor of attitude change.

Another index of systematic processing was the degree to which subjects' open-ended thought listings reflected specific thoughts about substantive aspects of the issue, rather than general statements of attitude, thoughts about the cue, or other thoughts. Here, the interaction of vested interest × cue significantly affected the proportion of specific issue-relevant thoughts listed, such that subjects who received a cue hostile to their vested interest listed more specific thoughts than did subjects who received a congenial cue. Taken together, these results tentatively indicate that when a cue fails to fulfill a person's defensive needs, biased systematic processing is more likely to be used.

The recent emphasis on motivated bias in information processing has at least partially answered Sears's (1986) critique of contemporary researchers' emphasis on cognitive and rational processes as a result of relying on student populations and laboratory settings. Although laboratory researchers have not literally taken up Sears's challenge to account for the strong motivations of people "such as Palestinian guerrillas, southern Italian peasants, . . . Archie Bunker, Ma Joad, Clarence Darrow or Martin Luther King" (p. 527), various issues—mainly academic and health-related—have been found to activate the defensive motives of the undergraduate subjects caricatured by Sears as "lone, bland, compliant wimps who specialize in paper-and-pencil tests" (p. 527). Our framework for examining defensively motivated processing, which encompasses both relatively thoughtful and thoughtless ways of rejecting threatening information, stands as a potentially useful guide to future research on the passions and biases of many different populations in many different settings.

IMPRESSION MOTIVATION

Thus far, we have seen that whereas accuracy-motivated perceivers search for judgments that reflect objective reality, defense-motivated perceivers desire judgments that are congruent with their existing self-defining attitudes and beliefs. In comparison, impression-motivated individuals express judgments that are called for by the social situations in which they find themselves.

Impression motivation involves the desire to express attitudes and beliefs that will address the specific interpersonal goals arising within different social contexts. Therefore, impression-motivated perceivers are primarily focused on the *interpersonal consequences* associated with expressing a given judgment in a particular social situation. In terms of its processing implications, impression motivation, like defense motivation, invokes processing that is guided by the principle of selectivity. Impression-motivated selectivity, however, promotes perceivers' current social goals rather than their existing self-views.

In considering the social context, impression-motivated perceivers may take into account the views of others who are actually present in the immediate social setting, as well as those of imagined others (Chaiken et al., 1989). For example, a political candidate anticipating that a particular audience will be viewing a televised debate may engage in impression-motivated processing and express judgments that are tailored to fit the audience (e.g., Cialdini, Levy, Herman, Kozlowski, & Petty, 1976; Tetlock, 1983). However, it is important to note that when real and imagined others comprise important self-defining reference groups, defense motivation is likely to be paramount.

In past research on various forms of impression motivation, when the views of anticipated audiences were known, impression-motivated subjects expressed judgments that mirrored these views; when the views of anticipated audiences were unknown, impression-motivated subjects formed moderate judgments (e.g., Cialdini, Levy, Herman, & Evenbeck, 1973; McFarland,

Ross, & Conway, 1984; Tetlock, 1983). In our broader conception of impression motivation, it is also recognized that certain interpersonal goals (e.g., the desire to end an unsatisfying relationship) may be facilitated by expressing judgments *opposite* to those of one's audience. Moreover, the pursuit of impression-motivated goals may often extend beyond merely expressing directional judgments; that is, the amounts and kinds of beliefs that impression-motivated individuals search for and process vary with the social setting and its concomitant interpersonal goals. For example, one's desire to appear particularly well informed in front of a group of peers may result in expressing judgments that are backed by an extensive array of supportive beliefs.

Past theoretical perspectives have proposed numerous constructs similar to impression motivation. Theories of impression management (e.g., Schlenker, 1980; Tetlock & Manstead, 1985) and self-presentation (e.g., Jones, 1990; Tedeschi & Riess, 1981) examine impression motivation primarily in the form of a concern with public appearances. For example, several of these theorists posit that people may be motivated to act in ways that will enhance "desired social identity images," or images that individuals wish to project in particular social contexts (Schlenker, 1980; Mori, Chaiken, & Pliner, 1987). Another closely aligned construct is Johnson and Eagly's (1989, 1990) impression-relevant involvement, or the form of involvement that induces a concern with the social acceptability of opinions. Zimbardo (1960) and others (e.g., Leippe & Elkin, 1987) have considered impression motivation in terms of response involvement, or the form of involvement that leads individuals to desire attitudes that can "successfully undergo public evaluation" (Leippe & Elkin, 1987, p. 270).

In terms of Deutsch and Gerard's (1955) distinction between "normative" and "informational" influence, impression motivation can be viewed as having a normative impact in that others' "expectations of appropriate conduct" are implicated (Eagly & Chaiken, 1993, p. 630). From a functional perspective, impression-motivated judgments may reflect the social adjustment function of attitudes (Smith et al., 1956; Snyder & DeBono, 1987); attitudes serving this particular function are formed on the basis of their implications for one's social relationships.[7] For example, individuals may express opinions congruent with those of their employers, with whom they wish to establish and maintain smooth interactions and relationships.

Of the various theoretical distinctions drawn between the different aspects of the self, impression motivation is most closely aligned with the "public" self. Impression motivation is likely to implicate, in Scheier and Carver's (1983) terms, the public or "socially apparent" self versus the inwardly focused "private" self. Similarly, impression-motivated individuals are most closely attuned to the public facets of themselves (Breckler & Greenwald, 1986), as evidenced in their sensitivity to others' evaluations and in their search, oftentimes, for the approval of others.[8]

Finally, several constructs have been proposed to measure individual differences in impression motivation. For instance, research has shown that high versus low *self-monitors* exhibit greater attitude change when persuasive messages are designed to heighten concern with public approval or appearances—concerns closely linked to impression motivation (e.g., Snyder & DeBono, 1985; DeBono, 1987; DeBono & Edmonds, 1989, Experiment 2). Fenigstein (1979) found that people high versus low in *public self-consciousness* were more sensitive to and reacted more negatively to social rejection. Given a social setting in which impression motivation may be aroused, we would expect higher levels of public self-consciousness to correspond to pronounced degrees of impression motivation.

Levels of impression motivation may depend not only on individual-difference factors such as self-monitoring status, but also on varying situational factors. For example, impression motivation may be enhanced to the degree that the attitudinal preferences of real or imagined others are salient, social norms are obvious, or social relationships are important (Chaiken et al., 1989). More generally, to the extent that individuals perceive the social implications of expressing particular judgments to be consequential or far-reaching, impression motivation is heightened. To illustrate, impression motivation is likely to be enhanced to the extent that the significance of a social relationship increases one's perception that expressing certain judgments will have large consequences for the maintenance of the relationship.

Impression-Motivated Heuristic and Systematic Processing

Impression-motivated processing may invoke either the heuristic or systematic mode, independently or interactively. Importantly, as we have stated, this form of motivated processing is selective in direct response to the interpersonal goals relevant in the surrounding social environment. As with the other two broad motives, the sufficiency principle can be used to make predictions regarding the form and extent of impression-motivated processing. However, impression motivation sufficiency is determined by whether information processing produces a judgment that serves current social goals, rather than one's accuracy or self-defining goals.

Like accuracy- and defense-motivated systematic processing, impression-motivated systematic processing involves a relatively deep analysis of judgment-relevant information, given the requisite cognitive capacity. Impression-motivated systematic processing is selective in that it varies consistently with situation-specific social goals; the amount and type of information that the impression-motivated perceiver chooses to process extensively will reflect a motivational bias toward the fulfillment of these goals. For example, an impression-motivated individual whose goal is merely to obtain a positive evaluation may selectively attend to information that supports an evaluator's opinions. Impression-motivated perceivers who desire not only to secure a positive evaluation, but also to appear particularly knowledgeable in an upcoming interaction with an evaluator, may also prepare to counterargue information that opposes the evaluator's opinions. Finally, impression-motivated individuals may carefully scrutinize *all* of the available information if, for example, their primary interpersonal goal is to appear flexible and well informed to others in a future discussion.

Impression-motivated heuristic processing involves the use of simple decision rules to guide the selection of judgments that address individuals' current interpersonal goals. The likelihood that a given heuristic will be used depends on the particular social situation and its accompanying interpersonal goals. For example, impression-motivated individuals may invoke the heuristic "Moderate opinions minimize disagreement" if they merely desire a smooth social interaction with a person whose opinions are not known. Given a situation where others' views are known, the same individuals may choose instead to follow an "Agreement leads to liking" heuristic. In essence, we propose that impression-motivated perceivers may selectively invoke the *same* heuristics used under our other forms of motivation if these rules are perceived as serving their current social goals. To illustrate, the heuristic "Expert opinions are correct" can serve the accuracy-motivated goal of forming a valid opinion, or the impression-motivated goal of appearing knowledgeable to others by expressing correct opinions.

Predictions about the relative extent of our two modes of processing are guided by the sufficiency principle. The impression sufficiency threshold refers to that point of processing at which perceivers feel adequately confident that a particular judgment will facilitate their interpersonal goals (actual confidence reaches desired confidence). Heuristic processing should confer sufficient judgmental confidence in situations that elicit low levels of impression motivation; these situations involve relatively lower sufficiency thresholds, or, in other words, are ones in which the perceived social consequences of expressing certain judgments are minimal. However, if heuristics that are capable of serving one's impression-motivated goals are neither available nor applicable in a given social context (and hence impression motivation sufficiency has not been reached), the likelihood of impression-motivated systematic processing is enhanced. In short, impression-motivated systematic processing is likely to occur in social situations in which heuristic processing has failed to close the gap between one's desired and actual level of confidence that a particular judgment will fulfill one's current interpersonal goals.

To illustrate, suppose Bob is anticipating a job interview with a company whose views on certain issues are well known. To ensure a positive evaluation, Bob may simply invoke an agreement or "acceptability" heuristic by shifting his opinions to match those of his anticipated audience (Tetlock, Skitka, & Boettger, 1989). However, to the extent that Bob views the interview as particularly consequential (i.e., his sufficiency threshold is raised), he may engage in impression-motivated systematic processing. For example, Bob may research the issues, paying selectively close attention to information that supports the company's views.

Empirical Evidence

Explicit tests of our hypotheses about impression-motivated processing are few in number. Tetlock's (1983) accountability research lends support to our assertion that the nature of impression-motivated processing varies with the interpersonal context. Social context in this research was manipulated by making subjects either aware or unaware of the views of the person to whom they had to justify their opinions. To serve their accountability concerns, aware subjects merely invoked an acceptability heuristic and expressed attitudes directionally consistent with that of the person to whom they were accountable. The same heuristic could not be used by the unaware subjects, who not only indicated relatively moderate attitudinal positions, but also listed thoughts that were more integratively complex and evaluatively inconsistent than those of aware subjects. From our perspective, Tetlock's results suggest that unaware subjects were forced to engage in relatively more systematic forms of processing in order to achieve a level of impression motivation sufficiency (brought on by the accountability manipulation) comparable to that of the aware subjects.[9]

Leippe and Elkin's (1987) study of issue and response involvement bolsters our propositions concerning the selectivity of impression-motivated processing. In contrast to the impression-motivated concerns of the response-involved individual, issue-involved perceivers are motivated to "form an attitude . . . in a way that best fits their personal goals, standards, and values" (p. 270). Issue involvement was varied by manipulating the personal relevance of the experimental issue, and response involvement was varied by manipulating whether or not subjects were told that they would later discuss the issue with another person. Although Leippe and Elkin found that both high issue involvement and high response involvement led to relatively more extensive processing of message information, they suggested that cognitive elaboration in the service of these two forms of involvement differed qualitatively. Issue-involved subjects' processing was highly sensitive to variations in message argument quality; in contrast, response-involved subjects generated evaluatively balanced thoughts and engaged in "maintenance" processing, or processing aimed merely at obtaining and retaining attitudinally relevant information. Presumably, the selective nature of response-involved subjects' processing reflected their impression-motivated concerns both with appearing well informed and with not appearing extreme (i.e., seeming flexible) in their issue opinions.

Before presenting our own research, we need to clarify and expand on past "strategic" interpretations of impression motivation and related constructs. Several researchers have argued that attitudes expressed under impression motivation are often merely "elastic" responses to impression-motivated concerns elicited by the situation (e.g., Cialdini & Petty, 1981). For instance, McFarland et al. (1984, Experiment 3) found that once interpersonal pressures were removed, subjects' expressed opinions demonstrated a considerable degree of "snap-back" toward prior attitudes. Other researchers, however, provide evidence for the persistence of expressed judgments resulting from processing that was initially in the service of impression-motivated goals (e.g., Chen, Shechter, & Chaiken, 1995; Higgins & McCann, 1984; Higgins, 1992; Sedikides, 1990). For example, Higgins and McCann (1984) demonstrated not only that subjects processed judgment-relevant information in a manner that would facilitate their interpersonal goals, but also that this "strategic" processing had enduring effects on their subsequently assessed judgments.

A tentative resolution may lie within the principles of the heuristic–systematic model. Impression-motivated processing is "strategic" in the sense that it is, by definition, directed toward achieving situational social goals. However, we propose that to the extent that impression-motivated processing is *systematic,* resulting beliefs and judgments will tend to endure over time. Impression-motivated judgments resulting from systematic forms of processing persist because they are backed by an extensive and relatively more complex consideration and array of judgment-relevant information. In short, we speculate that impression-motivated systematic processing may lead perceivers to genuinely adopt the judgments that they once formed and expressed with primarily strategic or goal-directed intent.[10] Clearly, further research is needed to substantiate and discover the limits of our theoretical speculations. Below we present our own research bearing on several of the propositions we have made regarding impression-motivated processing.

In two separate studies, we led subjects to anticipate an upcoming discussion with a partner about their issue opinions—an interpersonal situation in which we believed impression motivation would be aroused. In our first study (Shechter, 1987), high and low self-monitors were recruited as subjects. On the basis of past research using the self-monitoring construct (e.g., DeBono & Harnish, 1988; Snyder & DeBono, 1987), we expected our experimental setting to arouse higher levels of impression motivation among high self-monitors and lower (or no) impression motivation among low self-monitors; we reasoned that expecting a discussion would lead high self-monitors to be relatively more concerned with getting along with their discussion partners and low self-monitors to be relatively more concerned with expressing accurate opinions. Subjects were led to believe that their alleged discussion partner held either a favorable, an unfavorable, or an unknown attitude on the issue. Subjects' attitudes and thoughts were assessed after exposure to a judgment-relevant message.

In the two partner-attitude-known conditions, although both high and low self-monitors aligned their immediate attitudes with those of their alleged partners, this effect was stronger among high self-monitors. To serve their impression-motivated goals of "getting along with others" or "having a smooth interaction," high self-monitors were especially likely to use their partners' attitudes as a heuristic to determine their own attitudes. High self-monitors in the partner-attitude-unknown condition expressed significantly less extreme attitudes on the issue than did their counterparts in the partner-attitude-known conditions; in contrast, the attitudes of low self-monitors in the unknown condition differed only from those of their counterparts in the favorable-partner-attitude condition. Presumably, particularly nonextreme opinions reflected high self-monitors' use of a "Moderation minimizes disagreement" heuristic in addressing their interpersonal objectives in a situation where a simple agreement heuristic was not applicable (i.e., their partners' attitudes were unknown).

For the two partner-attitude-known conditions, thought-listing analyses revealed that high and low self-monitors engaged in similar overall amounts of processing. However, on a valenced index of systematic processing (specific message-related thoughts), a significant partner attitude effect emerged only among high self-monitors, indicating that the valence of their systematic processing was directionally congruent with their partners' attitudes. In contrast, the valence of low self-monitors' thoughts was not significantly affected by our manipulation of partner attitude. Thus, it appears that high self-monitors selectively processed judgment-relevant information in a way that was appropriate for their upcoming discussion, not with the goal of forming an accurate judgment.

To extend our findings, we conducted a second study using a similar discussion situation (Chen et al., 1995). In this second study, however, we sought to directly compare impression and accuracy motivation by using a motivation-priming manipulation (see Bargh, 1990). In an ostensibly unrelated study, subjects were asked to read and respond to a set of three "imagination" scenarios specifically designed to prime either accuracy or impression motivation concerns. All subjects were then led to anticipate a discussion with a partner who they were told held either a favorable or an unfavorable opinion on the discussion issue. Subjects' laboratory-expressed attitudes, thoughts, and delayed attitudes were recorded after exposure to an essay containing arguments for both sides of the issue.

Analyses on laboratory-expressed attitudes revealed that only those subjects who were primed for impression motivation were affected by knowledge of their partners' attitude; impression-motivated subjects reliably aligned their attitudes with those of their partners. Moreover, in several regression analyses, we found that while both impression- and accuracy-motivated subjects' valenced thoughts predicted their laboratory-expressed attitudes, our partner attitude manipulation significantly predicted the valence of only impression-motivated subjects' thoughts. Once again, impression motivation led to biased systematic processing, or processing tailored to fit prevailing interpersonal goals. Finally, laboratory-expressed attitudes for all of our subjects were reliably correlated with delayed attitudes. These final results appear to bolster the notion that systematic processing in the service of strategic impression-motivated goals may subsequently lead to attitudinal persistence.

Taken together, our two studies have produced results that are consistent with our impression motivation propositions. We have shown that the nature of both impression-motivated heuristic and systematic processing differs qualitatively from that of relatively more accuracy-motivated processing. Impression-motivated individuals took as their primary referent the social situation; that is, they used the opinion of their anticipated partner as a cue in addressing their interpersonal agenda. Furthermore, we have presented evidence suggesting that impression-motivated systematic processing may result in judgments that persist over time.

CONCLUSION

We have described the motivated individual throughout this chapter as one who "strategically" processes information in accordance with certain motivational "goals." In spite of the connotations of these terms, we do not necessarily believe that the individual is always aware of motivational influences on information processing. Recent trends in social-psychological research are leading to an increased appreciation of the power of motives to guide thought and behavior without the motivated person's conscious knowledge (Bargh & Barndollar, Chapter 20, this volume). In this light, we can ask two questions about the motivational states we have heretofore described. Are people aware that their processing strategies are motivationally influenced? And are they aware even of the existence of the motivation?

Of the three motives we have described, accuracy motivation is the least reprehensible motive with which to deal with information in contemporary Western culture, especially in the context of young students brought into laboratory settings (see Sears, 1986). Pressures to hide the existence or influence of truth-seeking motives, either from others or from oneself, are virtually nonexistent. Although the accuracy-motivated individual may not be aware of habitual flaws in reasoning, or of the influence of certain heuristics on judgments, we are reasonably confident that accuracy-motivated people believe themselves and their processing strategies to be accuracy-motivated.

Defense motivation, on the other hand, has been associated with the unilluminated side of human consciousness ever since Freud proposed the notion of psychological defenses. Indeed, the *sine qua non* of an effective ego defense is its invisibility to full awareness. Similarly, the most effective world views rest on the acceptance of their central values and beliefs as the stuff of objective reality. Thus, whether or not the core concepts to be defended have emerged into awareness, we believe that people are generally unaware of biases originating in defensive concerns. Like Pyszczynski and Greenberg (1987), we suspect that defense-motivated individuals maintain an "illusion of objectivity"—a belief that their processing is guided by accuracy concerns.

Although research has not directly addressed this question, Lord, Lepper, and Preston (1984) found that instructions to "be objective" were ineffective in reducing biased processing, suggesting that subjects' defensive biases can coexist with a conscious accuracy goal. Research on the "hostile media" phenomenon (Vallone, Ross, & Lepper, 1985; Giner-Sorolla & Chaiken, 1994) also indicates that, far from recognizing their own biases, defense-motivated partisans see a hostile bias in balanced presentations, which they judge to be imperfect conveyors of the partisan "truth." Nevertheless, these findings are only suggestive, and we believe that future research should strive to empirically clarify the claim that defensively biased people are unaware of their own biases.

Similarly, our characterization of impression motivation as strategically directed toward fulfilling interpersonal goals by no means implies that people are always aware of these goals or of the influence that these goals may have on their processing and subsequently expressed judgments. For example, one can imagine that for some individuals (e.g., high self-monitors), certain frequently encountered interpersonal situations may unconsciously lead to impression-motivated processing. Tetlock and Manstead (1985) support this idea in suggesting that impression management, a form of impression motivation, may be the "product of highly overlearned scripts, the original functions of which people have long forgotten" (p. 62). Jones and his colleagues (Jones, 1990; Jones & Pittman, 1982) concur with this notion in their assertion that various self-presentational strategies (e.g., ingratiation) may become "semiautomatic reactions triggered by interpersonal threats and opportunities" (Jones & Pittman, 1982, p. 258).

Although it seems possible that individuals may not be consciously aware of their impression-motivated concerns, we consider it more likely that impression-motivated perceivers are aware of their particular social goals, but unaware of the ways in which these interpersonal goals color their information processing and judgments. For example, it is likely that individuals who are motivated to agree with an attractive date are aware that they are seeking the affections of this other person, yet unaware that this goal leads them to selectively process information that is favored by this person. These speculations, however, await future empirical testing.

Finally, in drawing distinctions among accuracy, defense, and impression motives, we do not wish to imply that only one motive is present in all or even most situations. When multiple motives are present, their effects on information processing may counteract or complement one another. For instance, the fact that people are not entirely free to reinterpret the world as they would like it has been interpreted in terms of a dialectic between accuracy and defense motives (Kunda, 1990; Pyszczynski & Greenberg, 1987), implying that many situations present a conflict between the biased processing demanded by defensive concerns and the more objective view demanded by accuracy concerns. Impression management concerns calling for greater scrutiny of information may also conflict with, and indeed override, defensive processing (Baumeister & Cairns, 1992).

Despite the existing literature's focus on conflicting motivations, we believe that under the right circumstances, motivations may have a complementary effect on processing outcomes. Sometimes, impression motives can actually reinforce the biases created by defense motives—as when a Republican is given the chance to discuss politics with his or her conservative idol, Rush Limbaugh. Accuracy motives, too, may work to reinforce defensive biases if the information to be scrutinized itself tends to favor the person's point of view—as when a Democrat peruses the liberal-leaning editorial page of *The New York Times.* Although the complexity of multiple-motive situations is great, we see them as especially fertile grounds for future inquiry.

ACKNOWLEDGMENTS

We thank Stacey Lutz, Eva Pomerantz, Rosalind Tordesillas, and Jonathan Zimmerman for their comments on an earlier version of this chapter.

NOTES

1. Although our taxonomy does not categorically rule out other motives, we believe that this set of three adequately represents the possible reference points of most epistemic motivations. Defense motivation takes the self as a reference point; impression motivation takes others as a reference point; and accuracy motivation refers to an objective reality independent of the personal perspective of either self or others.
2. As Solomon, Greenberg, and Pyszczynski (1991) assert, beliefs that serve to fend off thoughts of one's mortality can play an important role in the self-system. The idea that one's health is not in danger, which people are evidently motivated to defend (Ditto & Lopez, 1992; Kunda, 1990; Liberman & Chaiken, 1992), is a relatively self-evident example of such beliefs.
3. We side with Kunda (1990) and Pyszczynski and Greenberg (1987) in asserting that defensive biases in processing are ultimately motivational, and not merely cognitive, in nature. Although we have defined defense motivation as a tendency to protect certain self-definitional cognitions, we also recognize that motivational factors determine which cognitions are protected—namely, those closest to the self-concept.
4. Although Kruglanski's (1990) need for specific closure encompasses defense motives, it can also describe impression motivation (see our later discussion) when a desired conclusion is dictated by interpersonal concerns.
5. By including the value-expressive function under defensive rather than accuracy motivation, we assume that values function primarily as ends in themselves, rather than as guides to the nature of objective reality.
6. It should be noted that some of the studies reviewed by Frey (1986) may not have involved defense motivation as we have defined it. For example, Frey and Rosch (1984) asked subjects to choose whether or not to prolong a manager's contract—a decision apparently with little consequence for self-relevant attitudes or beliefs. Moreover, high levels of cognitive dissonance may produce results more akin to accuracy motivation, as the individual seeks to change his or her beliefs to fit reality.

Frey (1982) has in fact found a curvilinear relation between intensity of dissonance and selective information seeking.

7. Smith et al.'s (1956) social adjustment function can be used to refer to attitudes that are strategically expressed to achieve current interpersonal goals, or to those attitudes that are expressed to affirm one's valued group identities (see Eagly & Chaiken, 1993). Impression motivation is more closely aligned with a strategic interpretation of the social adjustment function, whereas one's valued group identities may invoke defense-motivated processes.

8. The obvious connection drawn between the public self and impression motivation is not meant to rule out the possibility that other motives may also implicate the public self. For instance, Gollwitzer's (e.g., 1986) theory of symbolic self-completion proposes that identity goals, conceptually related to defense motives, are best served in the public domain; that is, "people feel that they need to make self-symbolizing public in order to move toward attainment of their identity goals" (p. 148).

9. Tetlock (e.g., Tetlock et al., 1989) has proposed that accountability concerns may lead to the use of the low-effort acceptability heuristic; to multidimensional, flexible processing; *or* to defensive forms of processing. The accountability strategy that people choose to employ depends on whether the views of an anticipated audience are known and on the attitudinal constraints of past commitments. We propose that accountability is appropriately characterized as an impression motivation manipulation in cases where the views of an audience are either known or unknown, *and* past attitudinal commitments are minimal. When past commitments are high, accountability is likely to lead to defense-motivated processing.

10. The idea that attitudes once expressed for primarily strategic reasons may nevertheless persist is consistent with the notion of "sleeper effects" in attitude research. That is, over time the initial strategic or goal-directed intent of impression-motivated processing becomes disassociated with expressed judgments, thereby leading to the delayed impact of judgment-relevant information on later assessed judgments (Eagly & Chaiken, 1993). The sleeper effect interpretation is also consistent with research on the "communication game" (e.g., Higgins, 1992), which has repeatedly demonstrated that communication and judgments that are initially tailored to fit one's audience may act back on the communicator's own attitude over time.

REFERENCES

Allport, G. W. (1935). Attitudes. In C. Murchison (Ed.), *Handbook of social psychology* (pp. 798–844). Worcester, MA: Clark University Press.

Anderson, N. H. (1971). Integration theory and attitude change. *Psychological Review, 78,* 171–206.

Bargh. J. A. (1990). Auto-motives: Preconscious determinants of thought and behavior. In E. T. Higgins & R. M. Sorrentino (Eds.), *Handbook of motivation and cognition: Foundations of social behavior* (Vol. 2, pp. 93–130). New York: Guilford Press.

Baumeister, R. F., & Cairns, K. J. (1992). Repression and self-presentation: When audiences interfere with self-deceptive strategies. *Journal of Personality and Social Psychology, 62,* 851–862.

Biek, M., Wood, W., Chaiken, S., & Nations, C. (in press). Working knowledge, cognitive processing, and attitudes: On the inevitability of bias. *Personality and Social Psychology Bulletin.*

Breckler, S. J., & Greenwald, A. G. (1986). Motivational facets of the self. In R. M. Sorrentino & E. T. Higgins (Eds.), *Handbook of motivation and cognition: Foundations of social behavior* (Vol. 1, pp. 145–164). New York: Guilford Press.

Chaiken, S. (1980). Heuristic versus systematic information processing and the use of source versus message cues in persuasion. *Journal of Personality and Social Psychology, 39,* 752–766.

Chaiken, S. (1987). The heuristic model of persuasion. In M. P. Zanna, J. M. Olson, & C. P. Herman (Eds.), *Social influence: The Ontario Symposium* (Vol. 5, pp. 3–39). Hillsdale, NJ: Erlbaum.

Chaiken, S., & Eagly, A. H. (1983). Communication modality as a determinant of persuasion: The role of communicator salience. *Journal of Personality and Social Psychology, 45,* 241–256.

Chaiken, S., Liberman, A., & Eagly, A.H. (1989). Heuristic and systematic processing within and beyond the persuasion context. In J. S. Uleman & J. A. Bargh (Eds.), *Unintended thought* (pp. 212–252). New York: Guilford Press.

Chaiken, S., & Lutz, S. (1993, October). *Time pressure and social judgment.* Paper presented at the meeting of the Society of Experimental Social Psychology, Santa Barbara, CA.

Chaiken, S., & Maheswaran, D. (1994). Heuristic processing can bias systematic processing: Effects of source credibility, argument ambiguity, and task importance on attitude judgment. *Journal of Personality and Social Psychology, 66,* 460–473.

Chaiken, S., Pomerantz, E., & Giner-Sorolla, R. (1995). Structural consistency and attitude strength. In R. E. Petty & J. A. Krosnick (Eds.), *Attitude strength: Antecedents and consequences* (pp. 387–412). Hillsdale, NJ: Erlbaum.

Chaiken, S., & Stangor, C. (1987). Attitudes and attitude change. *Annual Review of Psychology, 38,* 575–630.

Chen, S., Shechter, D., & Chaiken, S. (1995). *Getting at the truth or getting along: Accuracy- and impression-motivated heuristic and systematic processing.* Manuscript submitted for publication.

Cialdini, R. B., Levy, A., Herman, C. P., & Evenbeck, S. (1973). Attitudinal politics: The strategy of moderation. *Journal of Personality and Social Psychology, 25,* 100–108.

Cialdini, R. B., Levy, A., Herman, C. P., Kozlowski, L. T., & Petty, R. E. (1976). Elastic shifts of opinion: Determinants of direction and durability. *Journal of Personality and Social Psychology, 34,* 663–672.

Cialdini, R. B., & Petty, R. E. (1981). Anticipatory opinion effects. In R. E. Petty, T. M. Ostrom, & T. C. Brock (Eds.), *Cognitive responses in persuasion* (pp. 217–235). Hillsdale, NJ: Erlbaum.

DeBono, K. G. (1987). Investigating the social-adjustive and value-expressive functions of attitudes: Implications for persuasion processes. *Journal of Personality and Social Psychology, 52,* 279–287.

DeBono, K. G., & Edmonds, A. E. (1989). Cognitive dissonance and self-monitoring: A matter of context? *Motivation and Emotion, 13,* 259–270.

DeBono, K. G., & Harnish, R. J. (1988). Source expertise, source attractiveness, and the processing of persuasive information: A functional approach. *Journal of Personality and Social Psychology, 55,* 541–546.

Deutsch, M., & Gerard, H. B. (1955). A study of normative and informational social influences upon individual judgment. *Journal of Abnormal and Social Psychology, 51,* 629–636.

Ditto, P. H., & Lopez, D. F. (1992). Motivated skepticism: Use of differential decision criteria for preferred and nonpreferred conclusions. *Journal of Personality and Social Psychology, 63,* 568–584.

Eagly, A. H., & Chaiken, S. (1993). *The psychology of attitudes.* Fort Worth, TX: Harcourt Brace Jovanovich.

Fenigstein, A. (1979). Self-consciousness, self-attention, and social interaction. *Journal of Personality and Social Psychology, 37,* 75–86.

Festinger, L. (1957). *A theory of cognitive dissonance.* Evanston, IL: Row, Peterson.

Festinger, L. (1964). *Conflict, decision, and dissonance.* Stanford, CA: Stanford University Press.

Fiske, S. T., & Neuberg, S. L. (1990). A continuum of impression formation, from category-based to individuating processes: Influences of information and motivation on attention and interpretation. In M. P. Zanna (Ed.), *Advances in experimental social psychology* (Vol. 23, pp. 1–74). New York: Academic Press.

Freud, S. (1965). *New introductory lectures on psychoanalysis.* (J. Strachey, Ed. and Trans.). New York: Norton. (Original work published 1933)

Frey, D. (1982). Different levels of cognitive dissonance, information seeking, and information avoidance. *Journal of Personality and Social Psychology, 43,* 1175–1183.

Frey, D. (1986). Recent research on selective exposure to information. In L. Berkowitz (Ed.), *Advances in experimental social psychology* (Vol. 19, pp. 41–80). New York: Academic Press.

Frey, D., & Stahlberg, D. (1986). Selection of information after receiving more or less reliable self-threatening information. *Personality and Social Psychology Bulletin, 12,* 434–441.

Frey, D. & Rosch, M. (1984). Information seeking after decisions: The roles of novelty of information and decision reversibility. *Personality and Social Psychology Bulletin, 10,* 91–98.

Gilbert, D. T. (1989). Thinking lightly about others: Automatic components of the social inference process. In J. S. Uleman & J. A. Bargh (Eds.), *Unintended thought* (pp. 189–211). New York: Guilford Press.

Giner-Sorolla, R., & Chaiken, S. (1994). The causes of the hostile media effect. *Journal of Experimental Social Psychology, 30,* 165–180.

Giner-Sorolla, R., & Chaiken, S. (1995). *Selective use of heuristic and systematic processing under defense motivation.* Manuscript submitted for publication.

Gollwitzer, P. M. (1986). Striving for specific identities: The social reality of self-symbolizing. In R. F. Baumeister (Ed.), *Public self and private self* (pp. 143–159). New York: Springer-Verlag.

Gollwitzer, P. M. (1990). Action phases and mind-sets. In E. T. Higgins & R. M. Sorrentino (Eds.), *Handbook of motivation and cognition: Foundations of social behavior* (Vol. 2, pp. 53–92). New York: Guilford Press.

Hazlewood, J. D., & Chaiken, S. (1990, August). *Personal relevance, majority influence, and the law of large numbers.* Paper presented at the 98th annual meeting of the American Psychological Association, Boston.

Herek, G. M. (1986). The instrumentality of attitudes: Toward a neofunctional theory. *Journal of Social Issues, 42*(2), 99–114.

Higgins, E. T. (1992). Achieving 'shared reality' in the communication game: A social action that creates meaning. *Journal of Language and Social Psychology, 11,* 107–131.

Higgins, E. T., & McCann, C. D. (1984). Social encoding and subsequent attitudes, impressions, and memory: "Context-driven" and motivational aspects of processing. *Journal of Personality and Social Psychology, 47,* 26–39.

Janis, I. L., & Feshbach, S. (1953). Effects of fear-arousing communications. *Journal of Abnormal and Social Psychology, 48,* 78–92.

Johnson, B. T., & Eagly, A. H. (1989). The effects of involvement on persuasion: A meta-analysis. *Psychological Bulletin, 106,* 290–314.

Johnson, B. T., & Eagly, A. H. (1990). Involvement and persuasion: Types, traditions, and the evidence. *Psychological Bulletin, 107,* 375–384.

Jones, E. E. (1990). *Interpersonal perception.* New York: Freeman.

Jones, E. E., & Pittman, T. S. (1982). Toward a general theory of strategic self-presentation. In J. Suls (Ed.), *Psychological perspectives on the self* (Vol. 1, pp. 231–262). Hillsdale, NJ: Erlbaum.

Katz, I. (1960). The functional approach to the study of attitudes. *Public Opinion Quarterly, 24,* 163–204.

Kruglanski, A. W. (1990). Motivations for judging and knowing: Implications for causal attribution. In E. T. Higgins & R. M. Sorrentino (Eds.), *Handbook of motivation and cognition: Foundations of social behavior* (Vol. 2, pp. 333–368). New York: Guilford Press.

Kunda, Z. (1990). The case for motivated reasoning. *Psychological Bulletin, 108,* 480–498.

Leippe, M. R., & Elkin, R. A. (1987). When motives clash: Issue involvement and response involvement as determinants of persuasion. *Journal of Personality and Social Psychology, 52,* 269–278.

Liberman, A., & Chaiken, S. (1992). Defensive processing of personally relevant health messages. *Personality and Social Psychology Bulletin, 18,* 669–679.

Lord, C. G., Lepper, M. R., & Preston, E. (1984). Considering the opposite: A corrective strategy for social judgment. *Journal of Personality and Social Psychology, 47,* 1231–1243.

Lord, C. G., Ross, L., & Lepper, M. R. (1979). Biased assimilation and attitude polarization: The effects of prior theories on subsequently considered evidence. *Journal of Personality and Social Psychology, 37,* 2098–2109.

Maheswaran, D., & Chaiken, S. (1991). Promoting systematic processing in low-motivation settings: Effect of incongruent information on processing and judgment. *Journal of Personality and Social Psychology, 61,* 13–25.

McFarland, C., Ross, M., & Conway, M. (1984). Self-persuasion and self-presentation as mediators of anticipatory attitude change. *Journal of Personality and Social Psychology, 46,* 529–540.

Mori, D., Chaiken, S., & Pliner, P. (1987). "Eating lightly" and the self-presentation of femininity. *Journal of Personality and Social Psychology, 53,* 693–702.

Petty, R. E., & Cacioppo, J. T. (1979). Issue involvement can increase or decrease persuasion by enhancing message-relevant cognitive responses. *Journal of Personality and Social Psychology, 37,* 1915–1926.

Petty, R. E., & Cacioppo, J. T. (1986). *Communication and persuasion: Central and peripheral routes to attitude change.* New York: Springer-Verlag.

Pyszczynski, T., & Greenberg, J. (1987). Toward an integration of cognitive and motivational perspectives on social inference: A biased hypothesis-testing model. In L. Berkowitz (Ed.), *Advances in experimental social psychology* (Vol. 20, pp. 297–340). New York: Academic Press.

Pyszczynski, T., Greenberg, J., & Holt, K. (1985). Maintaining consistency between self-serving beliefs and available data: A bias in information evaluation following success and failure. *Personality and Social Psychology Bulletin, 11,* 179–190.

Ratneshwar, S., & Chaiken, S. (1991). Comprehension's role in persuasion: The case of its moderating effect on the persuasive impact of source cues. *Journal of Consumer Research, 18,* 52–62.

Rokeach, M. (1968). *Beliefs, attitudes, and values: A theory of organization and change.* San Francisco: Jossey-Bass.

Scheier, M. F., & Carver, C. S. (1983). Two sides of the self: One for you and one for me. In J. Suls & A. E. Greenwald (Eds.), *Psychological perspectives on the self* (Vol. 2, pp. 123–157). Hillsdale, NJ: Erlbaum.

Schlenker, B. R. (1980). *Impression management: The self-concept, social identity, and interpersonal relations.* Monterey, CA: Brooks/Cole.

Sears, D. O. (1986). College students in the laboratory: Influences of a narrow data base on social psychology's view of human nature. *Journal of Personality and Social Psychology, 51,* 515–530.

Sedikides, C. (1990). Effects of fortuitously activated constructs versus activated communication goals on person impressions. *Journal of Personality and Social Psychology, 58,* 397–408.

Shechter, D. (1987). *Relational and integrity involvement as determinants of persuasion: The self-monitoring of attitudes.* Unpublished doctoral dissertation, New York University.

Smith, M. B., Bruner, J. S., & White, R. W. (1956). *Opinions and personality.* New York: Wiley.

Snyder, M. (1987). *Public appearances/private realities: The psychology of self-monitoring.* New York: Freeman.

Snyder, M. (1992). Motivational foundations of behavioral confirmation. In M. P. Zanna (Ed.), *Advances in experimental social psychology* (Vol. 25, pp. 67–114). New York: Academic Press.

Snyder, M. & DeBono, K. G. (1985). Appeals to images and claims about quality: Understanding the psychology of advertising. *Journal of Personality and Social Psychology, 49,* 586–597.

Snyder, M., & DeBono, K. G. (1987). A functional approach to attitudes and persuasion. In M. P. Zanna, J. M. Olson, & C. P. Herman (Eds.), *Social influence: The Ontario Symposium* (Vol. 5, pp. 107–125). Hillsdale, NJ: Erlbaum.

Solomon, S., Greenberg, J., & Pyszczynski, T. (1991). A terror management theory of social behavior: The psychological functions of self-esteem and cultural world views. In M. P. Zanna (Ed.), *Advances in experimental social psychology* (Vol. 24, pp. 93–159). New York: Academic Press.

Steele, C. M. (1988). The psychology of self-affirmation: Sustaining the integrity of the self. In L. Berkowitz (Ed.), *Advances in experimental social psychology* (Vol. 21, pp. 261–302). New York: Academic Press.

Swann, W. B., Jr. (1990). To be adored or to be known?: The interplay of self-enhancement and self-verification. In E. T. Higgins & R. M. Sorrentino (Eds.), *Handbook of motivation and cognition: Foundations of social behavior* (Vol. 2, pp. 408–448). New York: Guilford Press.

Taylor, S. E. (1991). Asymmetrical effects of positive and negative events: The mobilization–minimization hypothesis. *Psychological Bulletin, 110,* 67–85.

Tedeschi, J. T., & Riess, M. (1981). Identities, the phenomenal self, and laboratory research. In J. T. Tedeschi (Ed.), *Impression management theory and social psychological research* (pp. 3–22). New York: Academic Press.

Tesser, A. (1988). Toward a self-evaluation maintenance model of social behavior. In L. Berkowitz (Ed.), *Advances in experimental social psychology* (Vol. 21, pp. 181–227). New York: Academic Press.

Tetlock, P. E. (1983). Accountability and complexity of thought. *Journal of Personality and Social Psychology, 45,* 74–83.

Tetlock, P. E. (1985). Accountability: The neglected social context of judgment and choice. In L. L. Cummings & B. M. Staw (Eds.), *Research in organizational behavior* (Vol. 7, pp. 297–332). Greenwich, CT: JAI Press.

Tetlock, P. E., & Manstead, A. S. R. (1985). Impression management versus intrapsychic explanations in social psychology: A useful dichotomy? *Psychological Review, 92,* 59–77.

Tetlock, P. E., Skitka, L., & Boettger, R. (1989). Social and cognitive strategies for coping with accountability: Conformity, complexity, and bolstering. *Journal of Personality and Social Psychology, 57,* 632–640.

Trope, Y. (1986). Self-assessment and self-enhancement in achievement motivation. In R. M. Sorrentino & E. T. Higgins (Eds.), *Handbook of motivation and cognition: Foundations of social behavior* (Vol. 1, pp. 350–378). New York: Guilford Press.

Vallone, R. P., Ross, L., & Lepper, M. R. (1985). The hostile media phenomenon: Biased perception and perceptions of bias in television coverage of the Beirut massacre. *Journal of Personality and Social Psychology, 49,* 577–585.

Wicklund, R. A., & Gollwitzer, P. M. (1982). *Symbolic self-completion.* Hillsdale, NJ: Erlbaum.

Wood, W., Kallgren, C. A., & Priesler, R. M. (1985). Access to attitude-relevant information in memory as a determinant of persuasion: The role of message attributes. *Journal of Experimental Social Psychology, 21,* 73–85.

Wyer, R. S., Jr., & Frey, D. (1983). The effects of feedback about self and others on the recall and judgment of feedback-relevant information. *Journal of Experimental Social Psychology, 19,* 540–559.

Zimbardo, P.G. (1960). Involvement and communication discrepancy as determinants of opinion conformity. *Journal of Abnormal and Social Psychology, 60,* 86–94.

CHAPTER 25

Awareness of Influence as a Precondition for Implementing Correctional Goals

Fritz Strack
Bettina Hannover

As occasional writers of prose (scientific or literary), we sometimes catch ourselves repeatedly using a rather uncommon word. Such repetitions, of course, are not the elements of good style, and we may therefore correct our previous productions when we edit the manuscript. Note that such corrections do not occur at the time we are using the incriminated word for the second or third time; at the time we fall prey to this repetitive tendency, we are unaware that it is operating. Thus, in a sense, we are "under the influence" but cannot do anything about it—until we later become aware of what has happened.

Although this chapter is about social judgment, the example just described is the prototype of situations to be addressed. More generally, the chapter deals with circumstances under which our psychological processes are affected by some external determinant of which we are not aware at the time, and the circumstances under which we engage in a correction when our attention is directed toward the influence (for a more complete account, see Strack, 1992; see also Bargh, 1992; Martin & Achee, 1992; Schwarz & Bless, 1992; Wilson & Brekke, 1994).

MOTIVATIONAL DETERMINANTS OF CORRECTION

A crucial precondition for the kinds of corrections we are addressing in this chapter is that people are motivated to correct. In our initial example, the corrective action depends on people's desire to write well. Whether people will employ corrective procedures in judgment tasks depends on their epistemic goals. One person, for example, may want to generate a judgment that is as accurate as possible, whereas another may be interested in arriving at the judgment in a minimal amount of time (e.g., Kruglanski, 1990). The first judge, of course, will be more likely to correct his or her judgment than the second (e.g., Martin, Seta, & Crelia, 1990).

The correctness of judgments, however, is not solely defined by people's own standards; societal forces are influenced by norms dictating the opinions that are appropriate to hold or express, and, more importantly, by norms dictating the opinions or attitudes that are inappropriate. These influences are particularly apparent in the case of prejudice. Members of a tolerant society are not supposed to be prejudiced against members of minority groups, and the public expression of prejudice tends to be met with social censure. More recently, norms of "political correctness" have been disseminated to proscribe the use (and avoidance) of certain concepts or labels descriptive of certain minority groups.

Usually, such proscriptions are justified according to criteria of both validity and social desirability. The expression of prejudice, for example, is often viewed as both factually incorrect and socially undesirable (for a review of definitions, see Brigham, 1971). Corrective attempts may therefore be motivated by concerns for both accuracy or validity and social desirability. However, conflicts between the two goals (i.e., being right and obeying social norms) are conceivable. For example, jurors who are instructed to disregard a piece of inadmissible but relevant evidence may experience a conflict between two incompatible goals: Should they correct their judgments in accordance with judicial instructions, or should they strive for a valid assessment of the defendant's guilt by refraining from such a correction (e.g., Sue, Smith, & Coldwell, 1973)? Of course, in other cases of conflict, social norms may induce judges to correct their overt responses without modifying their private judgments (e.g., Strack, Schwarz, Chassein, & Kern, 1990).

PRIMING AND REMEMBERING

Let us return to the initial writing example. The tendency to repeat uncommon words can be understood as a priming situation in which the first task has a facilitative effect on the subsequent performance of the same or similar task (see Tulving, 1983). In our example, the prior use of a word increases the likelihood that the same word will be used again. In other priming situations, the prior use of a specific concept will increase the likelihood that this concept will be employed again, even in a different context. In social psychology, person judgments have been studied as a function of priming. In the first studies addressing this phenomenon (Higgins, Rholes, & Jones, 1977; Srull & Wyer, 1979, 1980), participants who had been induced to use a particular concept were later asked to interpret an ambiguous stimulus that could potentially be subsumed under the critical category. Results consistently demonstrated that the activated information was used to interpret an ambiguous stimulus. As a consequence, subsequent judgments were assimilated toward the content of the activated information.

As in the writing example, priming should be most effective when participants are unaware that they were primed. Indeed, most studies on categorical priming have used rather subtle induction procedures that have proved effective even when the priming occurred subliminally (e.g., Bargh & Pietromonaco, 1982). Under such conditions, it is difficult to correct for unwanted influences. If judges in a priming situation are unaware of being primed in the direction of the implication of the primed information, or if they do not remember the primed information at the time they make their judgments, it is reasonable to expect assimilation effects to be particularly pronounced.

Indeed, available research findings clearly suggest that this is the case: Judges who are unaware of a prime, or who do not remember a prime, are likely to manifest assimilation effects in their subsequent judgments (for a recent review of the literature, see Higgins, in press). In contrast, judges who remember a priming episode should be less likely to manifest assimilation effects and may even manifest contrast effects in their judgments. Studies by Lombardi, Higgins, and Bargh (1987) and by Newman and Uleman (1990) confirmed this prediction. Their evidence, however, was correlational, and precluded the unequivocal conclusion that remembering the priming episode did in fact cause the contrast effect. Consider, for example, the following alternative explanation: Judgmental contrast may require more extensive processing of the relevant information, and may thus increase the information's memorability. Therefore, to test whether the memory for the priming episode has a causal effect, Strack, Schwarz, Bless, Kübler, and Wänke (1993) conducted an experiment in which some participants were actively reminded of the priming episode.

Participants expected to complete a series of perceptual and cognitive tasks. In one task, tones were associated with auditorily presented prime words, and participants had to classify the tones and write down filler words (i.e., unrelated words not paired with a tone). After a distractor task, participants heard an ambiguous story and rated the protagonist. The ambiguous story was an episode adapted from a study conducted by Carlston (1980). Specifically, a male target person behaved in a morally questionable manner. In his capacity as research assistant, he had access to faculty offices and desks, and he provided a friend who had previously failed an exam with the forthcoming exam questions. Of course, this behavior can be interpreted as both helpful and dishonest, and is thus evaluatively ambiguous.

The prime words were semantically related to the two concepts, and it was expected that ratings of the target person made by participants who were not reminded of the priming episode would be assimilated toward the content of the primes. For unreminded participants, this was the case on three measures: (1) The protagonist was rated as more or less likeable, depending on the primed words; (2) ascriptions of specific traits ("honest" vs. "friendly/helpful") were consistent with prime words; and (3) free-response descriptions of the target were evaluatively consistent with the primes.

So far, both procedures and results resembled those of the typical priming experiment. Recall that in addition, however, half of the participants were reminded of the priming event. This was done by having participants (1) rate how well they could discriminate the tones, (2) estimate the proportion of adjectives and nouns, and (3) rate how well they were able to remember specific associations of words and tones. Thus, reminding was indirect, so that participants were not instructed to recall the specific content of the priming words.

The results clearly indicated that participants primed with words semantically related to "friendly/helpful" actually rated the target as more likeable than did participants exposed to "dishonest" words. These findings replicate those of previous priming studies (e.g., Higgins et al., 1977; Srull & Wyer, 1979, 1980). This assimilation effect was not found, however, for participants who were reminded of the priming episode. In this condition, participants initially exposed to words of positive valence expressed less liking for the target person than did participants exposed to negatively valenced words. The same was true for the specific trait ratings. For the open characterizations, reminding leveled out the priming effect, but no contrast effect occurred.

These findings are consistent with previous results (Lombardi et al., 1987; Newman & Uleman, 1990). Moreover, they provide clear evidence for a causal relation between awareness of the priming episode and the attenuation of assimilation effects (or even judgmental contrast).

A JUDGMENTAL EXPLANATION

Why is this the case? That is, why would participants who were made aware of a priming episode fail to manifest assimilation effects in subsequent judgments? We believe (for alternative accounts, see Martin & Achee, 1992; Petty & Wegener, 1993; Schwarz & Bless, 1992) that awareness of a contextual influence facilitates cognitive operations, and that these operations modify the impact of that awareness on the judgment process. Such modification may be invoked if, for any reason, the situational influence is not representative for the judgment. In the course of judgment formation, people may engage in a representativeness check (Strack, 1992). Specifically, people may check (1) whether the activated information is itself a relevant basis for the judgment ("content representativeness"), and (2) whether the determinant that activated the information is relevant for the judgment ("process representativeness"). For example, a person who has retrieved information about life events from memory to generate a judgment of his or her present subjective well-being (e.g., Schwarz & Strack, 1991) may become aware that the sampled information describes events that occurred in the distant past. Such information, however, may not be representative as an informational basis for the present judgment of well-being. As a consequence, the person may engage in correction by forgoing use of the information, or by using it as a standard of comparison (e.g., Strack, Schwarz, & Gschneidinger, 1985). Alternatively, he or she may consider using current feelings as a basis for the well-being judgment, may become aware that these current feelings were elicited by a determinant that is completely irrelevant for the judgment (e.g., Schwarz & Clore, 1983), and may then attempt to correct for that irrelevant determinant.

One way to delimit the conditions under which a representativeness check will occur is to ask ourselves when such a check is least likely to occur. The most general answer is that it is least likely under any kind of suboptimal judgment conditions. Time pressure is an example of such a suboptimal condition. When judges must reach a conclusion in the face of an imminent deadline, or when they feel rushed while working on a task, they are less likely to reconsider their tentative judgments and less likely to engage in corrective attempts. In fact, to reach their goal in a timely fashion, judges may use simplifying strategies that preclude an effortful representativeness check. To test this notion, Strack, Erber, and Wicklund (1982) conducted a study in which participants were provided with biographical sketches implying that a target person was either active or passive. To increase target salience for some participants, we showed them a photo of the target person. All participants were then asked to assess how active or passive the target person was. During this assessment task, however, half of the participants were put under time pressure. This was achieved by having the experimenter act rushed while waiting for the participant to answer the questions. The experimenter's alleged agitation was elicited by a phone call informing him that his car was preventing another motorist from leaving the parking garage. In the presence of the harried experimenter, participants under time pressure judged the salient target person in a more extreme fashion than participants who were not forming their assessment under time constraints. That is, participants who were rushed in making their judgments described the target as more passive if passivity was implied in the original description; similarly, these hurried participants described the target person as more active if activity was suggested in the biographical sketch. These results suggest that participants generated judgments consistent with their original impressions and attributed more of the characteristic in question to the target when the target was salient and when there was no opportunity to correct for the influence of participants' initial impressions.

Martin (1986) was the first to recognize that judges must be aware of priming for that priming to intervene actively in judges' subsequent processing of information. He showed that context stimuli produce either assimilation or contrast effects, depending on whether priming occurs in a subtle or blatant manner. To account for these findings, Martin proposed a "set–reset" model (for a recent summary, see Martin & Achee, 1992), which predicts that judges who become aware of the priming episode will suppress this influence and "reset" their judgmental procedure. Such "partialing out" of priming influences reduces assimilation effects and may even result in contrast effects. Conditions that reduce awareness of priming prevent resetting. In addition, participants must be able and motivated to expend the cognitive effort associated with the described intervention. Several priming studies (e.g., Martin et al., 1990) illustrate the phenomenon.

Supportive evidence was also provided by Gilbert and his associates (e.g., Gilbert, Pelham, & Krull, 1988; Gilbert & Hixon, 1991). These authors investigated the conditions under which explanations of observed behavior fell prey to the "correspondence bias" (Gilbert & Jones, 1986); that is, they explored the determinants of participants' tendency to engage in correspondent inferences even when there existed relevant situational determinants of the target behavior to be explained (see also Ross, 1977). The authors proposed that such a bias would be particularly strong under suboptimal judgment conditions. In a series of studies, Gilbert and his collaborators reduced attributors' awareness of situational influences by keeping them busy with irrelevant tasks that prevented them from noticing situational influences and from correcting their judgment. As their studies consistently showed, lowering attributors' cognitive capacity increased the likelihood of correspondent inferences. From our perspective, these results were obtained because participants were prevented from checking the representativeness of a preliminary judgment and from correcting for the influence of that preliminary judgment.

Whereas Gilbert and colleagues' studies directed participants' attention away from relevant influences, the priming experiment by Strack et al. (1993) used the converse procedure. Here, participants' attention was directed toward a critical determinant, which increased the likelihood of a representativeness check. The general paradigm of this procedure dates back to Schachter and Singer's (1962) seminal work on the attribution of arousal. In Schachter and Singer's original study, participants' attention was directed to one of two possible determinants of their previously induced arousal; this directed attention subsequently affected participants' self-reports of their internal states. More recently, Zillmann and his colleagues (e.g., Zillmann & Bryant, 1974) used a similar procedure to explain the transfer of autonomic arousal from a nonemotional situation to an emotional situation and from one emotion to another. In their basic paradigm, Zillmann and colleagues (for a review, see Zillmann, 1983) elicited autonomic arousal through an emotionally irrelevant task (e.g., physical exercise), and influenced the direction of participants' attention toward the source of the arousal by varying the time that elapsed between the induction episode and subsequent assessment of emotions. Specifically, it was found that the initial exercise task intensified various emotional responses to the extent that the time interval between the induction of arousal and later emotional assessments was at once short enough to ensure that arousal was still present and long enough that the cause of the arousal was no longer the focus of participants' attention. In other words, the transfer of excitation was found to be effective if the nonrepresentative cause of that excitation went unnoticed.

Damrad-Frye and Laird (1989) extended this idea to explain the dynamics of boredom. They argued that people may interpret distraction from the execution of a certain task as a sign of boredom. However, if people's attention is directed toward a situational cause of the distraction, an alternative explanation becomes salient, and they should report feeling less bored. This was in fact the case in an experiment in which participants who listened to a passage of text were distracted by a noise that was either very loud or just audible. In a control group, participants were not distracted. As predicted, most boredom was reported under moderate distraction; in this condition, participants were sufficiently distracted but failed to attribute their diminished attention to the external factor. As a consequence, they attributed their diminished attention to the text passage to their own feeling of boredom.

In describing the machinations of a judge who must decide on the relevance of his or her current feelings to a judgment task, we have earlier alluded to a study by Schwarz and Clore (1983). In fact, in their study, Schwarz and Clore (1983) directed participants' attention toward an extraneous cause of their current mood (e.g., the prevailing weather conditions), and found that subsequent judgments of well-being were corrected when participants took the influence of the weather into account.

Finally, Jacoby, Kelley, Brown, and Jasechko (1989) directed participants' attention toward an episode of prior exposure to a particular name; consequently, participants refrained from using their feelings of familiarity to attribute fame to that name.

Taken together, the results of these studies suggest that increasing judges' awareness of the determinants of their own psychological states or of the outcomes of mental operations is a crucial precondition for various judgmental modifications, corrections for nonrepresentativeness being one. As previously noted, and according to the same logic, a reduction of such awareness should prevent modifications of judgments. Several phenomena from the area of persuasive communication and social influence seem relevant here. A prominent example is the ubiquitous "sleeper effect" (Hovland, Lumsdaine, & Sheffield, 1949), which explains why the persuasive effect of a message increases over time, as recipients forget aspects of the message (e.g., a noncredible communicator) that would otherwise lead them to resist the persuasive appeal. On the basis of our previous reasoning, we would assume that reminding the recipient of the original circumstances of exposure to the message would initiate a corrective endeavor. Indeed, Kelman and Hovland (1953) conducted a study in which for some participants, the communicator was reinstated at the time of the delayed attitude assessment. Whereas communicator effects dissipated for participants in the control condition, a (non)credibility effect was restored for participants re-exposed to the original communicator.

Other persuasion research findings suggest that when message recipients are able and motivated to draw a conclusion themselves, persuasive attempts are more successful if the desired conclusion is not explicitly provided by the persuader, but rather is actively generated by the recipients themselves (Fine, 1957; Kardes, 1988; Thistlethwaite & Kamenetzky, 1955; for a discussion of this issue, see McGuire, 1985). Our present analysis suggests that this more effective persuasion may arise at least in part from the recipient's decreased awareness of the persuader's influence. Consequently, final evaluations appear representative of recipients' own opinions.

Yet another example comes from Cialdini's work on subtle influence attempts. Reviewing the evidence, Cialdini (1993) concluded that, on the one hand, influence attempts are most successful when interventions are subtle and agents' true intentions are well disguised. On the other hand, targets of persuasion attempts can best defend themselves against influence if they can correctly identify the influence.

As a final example, Freud's distinction between (neurotic) anxiety and (objective) fear is worthy of mention (Freud, 1926/1963; see also Spielberger, 1985). Freud conceptualized anxiety as a free-floating emotional experience, the cause of which is repressed and therefore unconscious, whereas he conceptualized fear as an emotion whose presumable cause is apparent to the experiencer. To identify repressed causes of anxiety and to bring them into consciousness are integral to psychoanalytic therapy.

Taken together, the results of a large body of research on social cognition and persuasion (and even the tenets of psychoanalytic theory) suggest the pervasiveness of a mechanism whereby people's awareness of the determinants of their own psychological processes often serves as an impetus to engaging in corrective actions. Judges made aware of primes are less likely to fall prey to their assimilative effects in making subsequent judgments; targets of persuasion who are made aware of subtle influence attempts are less likely to become victims of persuasion; judges made aware of possible influences on their judgments or evaluations (whether these influences are recollections of past emotions, current feelings induced by the weather, or distraction caused by an audible noise) are likely to correct for these "irrelevancies" in making subsequent judgments or evaluations. And judges for whom such awareness is made impossible—via distracting tasks, time pressures, or the appropriate passage of time—fail to engage in judgmental corrections when asked to assess other persons or their own emotional experience. Of course, the consequences of these psychological mechanisms extend beyond the confines of the social-psychological laboratory; there are important intra- and interpersonal consequences of social judgments, including those judgments based on stereotypes.

CORRECTING STEREOTYPES

In the priming study previously described (Strack et al., 1993), judges may have been concerned about the factual correctness of their assessments when the eliciting situation was entirely unrelated to the required judgment. Similarly, people may be concerned about being "politically correct" in the expression of their opinions. Regardless of whether this corrective concern arises from the motivation to be right (validity) or to be liked (social desirability), it should be relevant when it comes to rectifying prejudices and stereotypes.

Support for this contention comes from a study conducted by Darley and Gross (1983), who showed that observers were less likely to base judgments of a target on stereotypes when the observers' attention was directed toward those features of the target that were related to the stereotype. In contrast, more stereotype-based judgments were found when observers focused on target features that were unrelated to the stereotype. From the present perspective, this lesser impact of a stereotype on a judgment appears to be the result of a corrective process. Specifically, if judges' attention is directed to a stereotypic feature and they become "alerted" that their assessments of another person may be inordinately influenced by the stereotype, judges may initiate attempts to correct for the presumed influence of stereotypic information. If, in contrast, judges' attention is directed to specific individuating information about the target person, they may remain unaware of the extent to which stereotypes color their interpretation of the specific information (e.g., Devine, 1989), and judges may be less likely to correct for the influence of those stereotypes.

This interpretation of Darley and Gross's (1983) findings was tested in an independent study conducted in the spring of 1992, using students at the Technical University of Berlin (Hannover, 1994) as participants. Since the reunification of Germany, students from both the former West Germany ("Wessis") and the former East Germany ("Ossis") have attended the universities of Berlin. Results of representative sample opinion surveys (Spiegel-Spezial, 1991) have revealed that decidedly different stereotypes are associated with members of these two groups. Wessis are considered to be more active, competent, arrogant, know-it-all types, whereas Ossis are held to be more passive, credulous, submissive, warm-hearted, and helpful. Although there are some differences between the stereotypes endorsed by Wessis about Wessis (and by Ossis about Ossis) compared to the stereotypes endorsed by members of the other group, the Wessi stereotype is generally more positive than the Ossi one, and this is true for both autostereotypes (i.e., about one's own group) and heterostereotypes (i.e., about the other group).

It was hypothesized that if stereotypes serve as primes, then thinking about themselves as "typical Ossis" or "typical Wessis" should activate participants' self-descriptive information, the content of relevant group stereotypes, and/or denotatively and connotatively related characteristics, some or all of which should be used by participants for self-descriptions. Given that in general Wessi stereotypes are more positive than Ossi stereotypes, West German students should describe themselves more positively than should East German students.

To test this notion, psychology students from both East and West Germany were recruited for an experiment in which they were asked to describe typical members of different groups. They did this by writing down as many appropriate adjectives as they were able to generate within 1 minute. To avoid possible interference, all participants were asked to count backward for 30 seconds after each description. To familiarize themselves with the task, participants started out by listing adjectives characteristic of the typical artist. Subsequent tasks defined the three experimental conditions to which participants were randomly assigned. In the first condition, participants described themselves after an unobtrusive and subtle priming procedure. This interpolated priming task consisted of having participants describe both a typical member of their own group and a typical member of the other group (the order of presentation was varied) before describing themselves. The purpose of this interpolated task was to activate relevant information contained in the stereotype. It was predicted that only the applicable information from the stereotype of participants' own group would be used for subsequent self-descriptions (see Higgins et al., 1977; Banaji, Hardin, & Rothman, 1993).

To determine whether participants whose attention was directed toward the potential influence of the stereotype prime would engage in judgmental correction, a second condition was introduced. In this condition, a direct connection was made between participants' self-descriptions and the stereotypes associated with their own group. Specifically, participants in this second group were instructed to think about Ossis and Wessis and to describe themselves using typical characteristics of their own group. Finally, a third group of participants generated self-descriptions before listing stereotypic adjectives characteristic of the two groups. The adjectives used by all participants for the self-descriptions were classified as positive, negative, or neutral by raters unaware of the experimental conditions.

Under all three conditions, participants used more positive than negative adjectives to describe themselves, particularly when they were not induced to think about their group stereotype. When no stereotype was activated, West German students described themselves more positively than did their East German counterparts. This difference was greatly increased when group stereotypes were activated; when participants were unobtrusively reminded about the stereotypes associated with their groups, the self-descriptions of the East Germans turned dramatically more negative, whereas the valence of West Germans' self-descriptions remained largely unchanged. This pattern, however, was reversed when participants were alerted to the potential influence of the stereotype. That is, when the potential self-relevance of stereotypes was called to participants' attention by making the priming episode salient, East German students generated more positive self-descriptions than West German students, who in turn described themselves more negatively than in any other condition.

These findings suggest that the information contained in Wessi–Ossi stereotypes exacerbated original differences in self-descriptions and resulted in an assimilation effect, the direction of which depended on participants' own group membership. When participants were merely induced to generate stereotypic characteristics, they used the activated information about the stereotype of their own group when they were asked to describe themselves. However, when participants' attention was focused on the relation between their own characteristics and those of the group stereotype, their self-descriptions did not reflect the content of the accessible stereotypic information. Rather, participants seemed to correct for the influence of the stereotype. The West German students in particular described themselves in terms that were evaluatively inconsistent with the information activated in the stereotype generation task; in a sense, they were less presumptuous in their self-descriptions, and overcorrected for the positivity of self-relevant stereotypes.

Why do people engage in this type of correction? First, stereotypes and their potential influence are considered to be threats to the validity of a judgment. In public opinion, stereotypes are often considered to be false (Brigham, 1971). Their use may therefore distort a judgment, and attempts to forgo the use of stereotypes may arise from an epistemic motivation to strive for veridical judgments (Kruglanski, 1990). At the same time, the use of stereotypes is often socially undesirable. Therefore, it is increasingly difficult to demonstrate effects of prejudices and stereotypes when people are aware that they are using stereotypic information (e.g., Devine, 1989). Thus, refraining from the use of stereotypes as a basis for judgment may be motivated by people's attempt to create a positive impression, or at least to avoid creating a negative one. Of course, it is difficult to disentangle concerns for validity from concerns for social desirability when one has no further information about the specific conditions leading to corrective attempts.

There are, however, a few clues. A corrected judgmental outcome that reflects more negatively on the respondent than an uncorrected judgment would may be one indication of a validity-driven correction. However, findings also show that under certain conditions, social desirability concerns may lead participants to manifest negative evaluations (e.g., Strack et al., 1990). In addition to the valence of a response, the circumstances of its delivery may serve as indicators of social desirability. As findings from survey research suggest (e.g., Smith, 1979), public responding may be more likely than private responding to elicit concerns of social desirability (see also Schlenker, 1980).

CORRECTIVE STRATEGIES

The studies described in this chapter demonstrate that when people are aware of undesired influences on their judgments, they may modify those judgments. Such corrections may occur in the pursuit of different epistemic and social goals: to increase the validity of a judgment or to obey social rules. Conditions under which different judgmental goals are activated have been extensively discussed by Kruglanski (1990). Whatever the motivation, people made aware of irrelevant influences on their judgments or assessments will—given the ability and incentive—correct their judgments accordingly, and the question then arises as to how people implement their goals.

First, perhaps people recompute (correct by recomputation) their judgments (Strack, 1992; Wyer & Srull, 1989). Ideally, judges should disregard inappropriate information. Such a correction by recomputation is only feasible if the corrected judgment can be based on alternative information that is not "contaminated" (see also Wilson & Brekke, 1994). For example, a juror who has been instructed to disregard an inadmissible piece of evidence may focus on other aspects of testimony. Of course, the original inadmissible evidence may elicit expectations and beliefs that distort the interpretation of new (admissible) information, so that no "contaminating" influence can be completely negated (e.g., Fischhoff, 1977); in principle, however, people may select information that seems to be unaffected by the inappropriate influence. Of course, how people go about separating the wheat from the chaff—selecting uncontaminated information over contaminated information—is another question. Possibly one may identify uncontaminated information by its incongruence with either the factual content or the valence of the inappropriate contaminated information. If this endeavor is successful, a recomputation of the judgment should diminish the original influence of the contaminated information. Of course, "overcorrections" (compared to a no-influence control group) may occur and manifest themselves as contrast effects, yielding what may be another form of inaccurate judgment. It is important to note that corrections by recomputation merely require an awareness of the influence of irrelevant or contaminate information. It is not necessary that judges have any notion about the direction or magnitude of the unwanted influence.

The second type of correction, however, presupposes not only that judges are aware of unwanted influence, but also that they have a conception of its direction and its strength. Specifically, attempts at decontamination may also be made by adjusting one's response. This type of correction by adjustment does not require a recomputation of the judgment per se; it merely involves a modification of the response. This sounds deceptively simple; in reality, to compensate for an influence through adjustment, one must know more about the nature of the effect for which one is controlling. For example, a person who holds a hand in ice-cold water and is then asked to estimate the actual temperature of some lukewarm water may want to correct the judgment by adjusting his or her assessment. To do that, the person must possess some intuitive knowledge about the probable impact of exposure to the ice-cold water on his or her subsequent temperature sensations. In this example, the person may be an intuitive adaptation theorist who believes that sensations of a moderate temperature will "feel" warmer after exposure to an extremely cold stimulus. As a consequence, the corrected temperature judgment will be adjusted toward the value of the contaminating influence: The person will report that the lukewarm water is actually cooler than it "feels."

This example shows that corrective adjustments may manifest themselves as assimilation effects if an intuitive theory about a primary influence predicts contrast (for experimental demonstrations, see Petty & Wegener, 1993). Conversely, corrective adjustments will produce a contrast effect if the intuitive theory of influence predicts assimilation. This has been demonstrated in the studies described in this chapter. In priming studies, judges may adopt intuitive theories about the effect of the valence of the prime, and may compensate for its undesirable influence by adjusting their responses in the evaluatively opposite direction. Interestingly, the studies described here revealed an asymmetry, such that the correction was stronger when the priming stimuli were negative than when they were positive. Similar results were obtained in a series of experiments conducted by Hatvany and Strack (1980) and by Wyer and his associates (Wyer & Budesheim, 1987; Wyer & Unverzagt, 1985). Wyer and his associates assume that the stronger correction under negative-prime conditions can be attributed to judges' intuitive belief that people are more likely in general to have positive characteristics. Alternatively, an incorrect negative evaluation may be considered more costly than an incorrect positive evaluation. A heuristic based on these differential costs may also produce such an asymmetry.

In the arena of stereotype research, positive corrections have often been observed. An example is a courtroom study by Shaffer and Case (1982), in which some participants were presented with information subtly implying that the defendant was homosexual. The results revealed that the group of participants who were assumed to be most motivated to reach a fair verdict (i.e., those low in dogmatism) provided the most positive judgments when the potentially biasing characteristic was introduced. Specifically, participants who were low in dogmatism rated the defendant more leniently when he was subtly portrayed as homosexual than when he was portrayed as heterosexual. In contrast, highly dogmatic participants were not influenced by the defendant's sexual orientation.

However, just how individuals go about correcting for prejudice or stereotypes remains an open question. The present data suggest that in the case of self-ratings, corrections may result in judgments that may be either more positive or more negative. Given the prevalence and consequences of stereotypes, specific correctional mechanisms are worthy of continued exploration.

Several possible correctional mechanisms exist. First, people may moderate their judgments on those specific dimensions that are included in the stereotype. As a consequence, the valence of an overall assessment depends on the valence and the composition of the stereotype's salientic dimensions. For example, if judges want to avoid the influence of a specific ethnic stereotype, a salient component of which is aggression, they may judge a target to whom the stereotype may apply to be less aggressive. Second, people may simply use the overall valence of the stereotype and adjust the corrected judgment in the opposite direction. As most prejudices include negative evaluations, corrections based on the latter strategy tend to result in more positive evaluations. In the present example, a person identified as a member of the stereotyped group will receive a more positive evaluation that is independent of judges' corrections on a more specific level.

SUMMARY AND CONCLUSIONS

It has been our intent in the present chapter to shed some light on preconditions of judgmental corrections and to discuss possible means by which such corrections may be executed. It has become apparent that preconditions for corrections may be both motivational and factual in nature. On the motivational side, judges may enlist a correction in an attempt to compensate for contaminating influences that would otherwise threaten the validity of a conclusion or produce a socially inacceptable outcome. On the factual side, judges must be aware of a particular influence. This may be achieved by directing judges' attention to the source of the effect. Attempts to counteract such influences may take at least two routes. Judges may execute corrections by recomputing a judgment using different information; alternatively, judges may adjust their responses for the presumed influence. The first strategy merely requires judges' awareness of the contaminating influence; the second strategy requires additional knowledge about the likely direction and strength of the undesirable influence.

Cognitive preconditions of and strategies that bring about judgmental correction are deserving of increasing attention in future research. Although research has focused on motivational antecedents of cognitive functioning (e.g., Kruglanski, 1990; Tetlock, 1992; Thompson, Roman, Moskowitz, Chaiken, & Bargh, 1994) and on specific correctional mechanisms in the context of attribution research (e.g., Gilbert et al., 1988; Trope, Cohen, & Maoz, 1988), judgmental correction has only recently been discussed as a psychological phenomenon in its own right (e.g., Martin & Achee, 1992; Strack, 1992; Wilson & Brekke, 1994; see also Baumeister & Newman, 1994).

We suggest that correctional processes constitute an integral part of most judgment formation. If our assertion is correct, it is not sufficient simply to identify the motivational states that bring about such cognitive consequences. To understand the correctional dynamics of human judgment, it is equally important to explore both the cognitive conditions that elicit such motives, and the cognitive operations that effect judgmental consequences.

REFERENCES

Banaji, M. R., Hardin, C., & Rothman, A. J. (1993). Implicit stereotyping in person judgment. *Journal of Personality and Social Psychology, 65,* 272–281.

Bargh, J. A. (1992). Does subliminality matter to social psychology? Awareness of the stimulus versus awareness of its influence. In R. F. Bornstein & T. S. Pittman (Eds.), *Perception without awareness* (pp. 236–255). New York: Guilford Press.

Bargh, J. A., & Pietromonaco, P. (1982). Automatic information processing and social perception: The influence of trait information presented outside of conscious awareness on impression formation. *Journal of Personality and Social Psychology, 43,* 437–449.

Baumeister, R. F., & Newman, L. S. (1994). Self-regulation of cognitive inference and decision-processes. *Personality and Social Psychology Bulletin, 20,* 3–19.

Brigham, J. C. (1971). Ethnic stereotypes. *Psychological Bulletin, 76,* 15–33.

Carlston, D. E. (1980). The recall and use of traits and events in social inference processes. *Journal of Experimental Social Psychology, 16,* 303–328.

Cialdini, R. B. (1993). *Influence: Science and practice* (3rd ed.). New York: HarperCollins.

Damrad-Frye, R., & Laird, J. D. (1989). The experience of boredom: The role of self-perception of attention. *Journal of Personality and Social Psychology, 57,* 315–320.

Darley, J. M., & Gross, P. H. (1983). A hypothesis-confirming bias in labeling effects. *Journal of Personality and Social Psychology, 44,* 20–33.

Devine, P. G. (1989). Stereotypes and prejudice: Their automatic and controlled components. *Journal of Personality and Social Psychology, 56,* 5–18.

Fine, B. J. (1957). Conclusion-drawing, communicator credibility, and anxiety as factors in opinion change. *Journal of Abnormal and Social Psychology, 54,* 369–374.

Fischhoff, B. (1977). Perceived informativeness of facts. *Journal of Experimental Psychology: Human Perception and Performance, 3,* 349–358.

Freud, S. (1963). *The problem of anxiety* (Henry Alden Benkes, Trans.). New York: The Psychoanalytic Quarterly/Norton. (Original work published 1926)

Gilbert, D. T., & Hixon, J. G. (1991). The trouble of thinking: Activation and application of stereotypic beliefs. *Journal of Personality and Social Psychology, 60,* 509–517.

Gilbert, D. T., & Jones, E. E. (1986). Perceiver-induced constraint: Interpretations of self-generated reality. *Journal of Personality and Social Psychology, 50,* 269–280.

Gilbert, D. T., Pelham, B. W., & Krull, D. S. (1988). On cognitive busyness: When person perceivers meet persons perceived. *Journal of Personality and Social Psychology, 54,* 733–740.

Hannover, B. (1994). *Activating and correcting auto-stereotypes: The case of Ossis and Wessis.* Unpublished manuscript, Technical University of Berlin.

Hatvany, N., & Strack, F. (1980). The impact of a discredited key witness. *Journal of Applied Social Psychology, 10,* 490–509.

Higgins, E. T. (in press). Knowledge activation: Accessibility, applicability, and salience. In E. T. Higgins & A. W. Kruglanski (Eds.), *Social psychology: Handbook of basic principles.* New York: Guilford Press.

Higgins, E. T., Rholes, W. S., & Jones, C. R. (1977). Category accessibility and impression formation. *Journal of Experimental Social Psychology, 13,* 141–154.

Hovland, C. I., Lumsdaine, A. A., & Sheffield, F. D. (1949). *Experiments on mass communication.* Princeton, NJ: Princeton University Press.

Jacoby, L. L., Kelley, C., Brown, J., & Jasechko, J. (1989). Becoming famous overnight: Limits on the ability to avoid unconscious influences of the past. *Journal of Personality and Social Psychology, 56,* 326–338.

Kardes, F. R. (1988). Spontaneous inference processes in advertising: The effects of conclusion omission and involvement in persuasion. *Journal of Consumer Research, 15,* 225–233.

Kelman, H. C., & Hovland, C. I. (1953). "Reinstatement" of the communicator in delayed measurement of opinion change. *Journal of Abnormal and Social Psychology, 48,* 327–335.

Kruglanski, A. W. (1990). Motivations for judging and knowing: Implications for causal attribution. In E. T. Higgins & R. M. Sorrentino (Eds.), *Handbook of motivation and cognition: Foundations of social behavior* (Vol. 2, pp. 333–368). New York: Guilford Press.

Lombardi, W. J., Higgins, E. T., & Bargh, J. A. (1987). The role of consciousness in priming effects on categorization: Assimilation versus contrast as a function of awareness of the priming task. *Personality and Social Psychology Bulletin, 13,* 411–429.

Martin, L. L. (1986). Set/reset: The use and disuse of concepts in impression formation. *Journal of Personality and Social Psychology, 51,* 493–504.

Martin, L. L., & Achee, J. W. (1992). Beyond accessibility: The role of processing objectives in judgment. In L. L. Martin & A. Tesser (Eds.), *The construction of social judgments* (pp. 195–216). Hillsdale, NJ: Erlbaum.

Martin, L. L., Seta, J. J., & Crelia, R. (1990). Assimilation and contrast as a function of people's willingness and ability to expend effort in forming an impression. *Journal of Personality and Social Psychology, 59,* 27–37.

McGuire, W. J. (1985). Attitudes and attitude change. In G. Lindzey & E. Aronson (Ed.), *Handbook of social psychology* (3rd ed., Vol. 2, pp. 233–346). New York: Random House.

Newman, L. S., & Uleman, J. S. (1990). Assimilation and contrast effects in spontaneous trait inference. *Personality and Social Psychology Bulletin, 16,* 224–240.

Petty, R. E., & Wegener, D. T. (1993). Flexible correction processes in social judgment: Correcting for context-induced contrast. *Journal of Experimental Social Psychology, 29,* 137–165.

Ross, L. (1977). The intuitive psychologist and his shortcomings. In L. Berkowitz (Ed.), *Advances in experimental social psychology* (Vol. 10, pp. 173–220). New York: Academic Press.

Schachter, S., & Singer, J. E. (1962). Cognitive, social, and physiological determinants of emotional state. *Psychological Review, 69,* 379–399.

Schlenker, B. R. (1980). *Impression management. The self-concept, social identity, and interpersonal relations.* Monterey, CA: Brooks/Cole.

Schwarz, N., & Bless, H. (1992). Constructing reality and its alternatives: An inclusion/exclusion model of assimilation and contrast effects in social judgment. In L. L. Martin & A. Tesser (Eds.), *The construction of social judgments* (pp. 217–245). Hillsdale, NJ: Erlbaum.

Schwarz, N., & Clore, G. L. (1983). Mood, misattribution, and judgments of well-being: Informative and directive functions of affective states. *Journal of Personality and Social Psychology, 45,* 513–523.

Schwarz, N., & Strack, F. (1991). Evaluating one's life: A judgment model of subjective well-being. In F. Strack, M. Argyle, & N. Schwarz (Eds.), *Subjective well-being* (pp. 27–47). Oxford: Pergamon Press.

Shaffer, D. R., & Case, T. (1982). On the decision to testify in one's own behalf: Effects of withheld evidence, defendant's sexual preferences, and juror dogmatism on juridic decisions. *Journal of Personality and Social Psychology, 42,* 335–346.

Smith, T. W. (1979). Happiness: Time trends, seasonal variations, inter-survey differences, and other mysteries. *Social Psychology Quarterly, 42,* 18–30.

Spiegel-Spezial. (1991, January). *Das Profil der Deutschen* [Special issue]. Hamburg: Spiegel-Verlag.

Spielberger, C. D. (1985). Anxiety, cognition and affect: A state–trait perspective. In A. H. Tuma & J. Maser (Eds.), *Anxiety and the anxiety disorders* (pp. 171–182). Hillsdale, NJ: Erlbaum.

Srull, T. K., & Wyer, R. S. (1979). The role of category accessibility in the interpretation of information about persons: Some determinants and implications. *Journal of Personality and Social Psychology, 37,* 1660–1672.

Srull, T. K., & Wyer, R. S. (1980). Category accessibility and social perception: Some implications for the study of person memory and interpersonal judgments. *Journal of Personality and Social Psychology, 38,* 841–856.

Strack, F. (1992). The different routes to social judgments: Experiential vs. informational strategies. In L. L. Martin & A. Tesser (Eds.), *The construction of social judgment* (pp. 249–275). Hillsdale, NJ: Erlbaum.

Strack, F., Erber, R., & Wicklund, R. (1982). Effects of salience and time pressure on ratings of social causality. *Journal of Experimental Social Psychology, 18,* 581–594.

Strack, F., Schwarz, N., Bless, H., Kübler, A., & Wänke, M. (1993). Awareness of the influence as a determinant of assimilation vs. contrast. *European Journal of Experimental Social Psychology, 23,* 53–62.

Strack, F., Schwarz, N., Chassein, B., & Kern, D. (1990). The salience of comparison standards and the activation of social norms: Consequences for judgments of subjective well-being. *British Journal of Social Psychology, 29,* 203–314.

Strack, F., Schwarz, N., & Gschneidinger, E. (1985). Happiness and reminiscing: The role of time perspective, affect, and mode of thinking. *Journal of Personality and Social Psychology, 49,* 1460–1469.

Sue, S., Smith, R.E., & Coldwell, C. (1973). Effects of inadmissible evidence on the decisions of simulated jurors: A moral dilemma. *Journal of Applied Social Psychology, 3,* 345–353.

Tetlock, P. E. (1992). The impact of accountability on judgment and choice: Toward a social contingency model. In M. P. Zanna (Ed.), *Advances in experimental social psychology* (Vol. 25, pp. 331–376). San Diego, CA: Academic Press.

Thistlethwaite, D. L., & Kamenetzky, J. (1955). Attitude change through refutation and elaboration of audience counterarguments. *Journal of Abnormal and Social Psychology, 51,* 3–9.

Thompson, E. P., Roman, R. J., Moskowitz, G. B., Chaiken, S., & Bargh, J. A. (1994). Accuracy motivation attenuates covert priming: The systematic reprocessing of social information. *Journal of Personality and Social Psychology, 66,* 474–489.

Trope, Y., Cohen, O., & Maoz, Y. (1988). The perceptual and inferential effects of situational inducements on dispositional attributions. *Journal of Personality and Social Psychology, 55,* 165–177.

Tulving, E. (1983). *Elements of episodic memory.* London: Oxford University Press.

Wilson, T. D., & Brekke, N. (1994). Mental contamination and mental correction:

Unwanted influences on judgments and evaluations. *Psychological Bulletin, 116,* 117–142.

Wyer, R. S., & Budesheim, T. L. (1987). Person memory and judgments: The impact of information that one is told to disregard. *Journal of Personality and Social Psychology, 53,* 14–29.

Wyer, R. S., & Srull, T. K. (1989). *Memory and cognition in its social context.* Hillsdale, NJ: Erlbaum.

Wyer, R. S., & Unverzagt, W. H. (1985). The effects of instructions to disregard information on its subsequent recall and use in making judgments. *Journal of Personality and Social Psychology, 48,* 533–549.

Zillmann, D. (1983). Transfer of excitation in emotional behavior. In J. T. Cacioppo & R. E. Petty (Eds.), *Social psychophysiology: A sourcebook* (pp. 215–240). New York: Guilford Press.

Zillmann, D., & Bryant, J. (1974). Effect of residual excitation on the emotional response to provocation and delayed aggressive behavior. *Journal of Personality and Social Psychology, 30,* 782–791.

PART VII

Discussions

In the closing chapters, Kruglanski (Chapter 26), Sorrentino (Chapter 27), and Carver (Chapter 28) provide syntheses of important themes that flow through most chapters in this book. Each of them is a scholar well known for a long-standing concern with motivational phenomena, and especially with the links among motivation, cognition, and action. We asked them to provide discussions of the themes and points they felt should be highlighted, from the vantage point of their own perspectives on the field.

Kruglanski provides a conceptualization of goals as cognitive knowledge structures, and draws from this premise several hypotheses about the source, structure, and malleability of goals over time. Important questions that he raises and discusses are these: Where do goals come from? How are they selected? How do other epistemic needs and motives of the person influence which goals are selected for pursuit? How does success or failure in achieving the goal feed back on goal selection in the future? How do goals linked in memory to other knowledge structures, such as plans and strategies, result in goal-directed action? Kruglanski's formulation of goals as mental representations should prove very valuable in future research on the interface between motivation and cognition.

Sorrentino focuses on the role and functionality of conscious thought in producing action. He notes that many of the contributing authors take a stand, at least implicitly, as to how intentional and consciously determined the effects they describe are. Using Atkinson and Birch's framework of the three possible causal roles consciousness may play—epiphenomenal, amplifying of unconscious impulses, or serving as the sole causal influence—Sorrentino classifies several authors' positions on this central issue. Like Wicklund and Steins, Neuberg, and Chaiken et al., he highlights the importance of uncertainty feelings as a motivator of information processing, and describes his program of research on chronic uncertainty motivation to illustrate his points about the role of conscious thought.

In a thoughtful and introspective analysis of the themes inherent in several other chapters in the volume, Carver is concerned primarily with how goals vary in important ways from one another. For one thing, goals are related to one another hierarchically: Some goals are more abstract, whereas others are more concrete and serve to satisfy the higher-order concerns. That higher-order goals can be satisfied by the completion of several lower-order goals is also a theme of the Tesser et al. chapter in the present volume, and, as Carver notes, is the basis of Wicklund and Gollwitzer's earlier self-completion theory as well. Carver points to other critical dimensions on which goals seem to vary, as themes in the chapters by Dweck, Ajzen, Ryan et al., Emmons, Vallacher and Kaufman, and Higgins: whether the goal is dynamic or static in nature, and whether the motivation satisfies intrinsic or extrinsic needs. Finally, Carver relates his own cybernetic framework for understanding motivated progress toward a goal to the self-discrepancy model of Higgins and the dynamic model of Vallacher and Kaufman. All of these models underscore the importance of the discrepancy between where the individual is now and where he or she wants to be as a motivational factor in its own right. Like Vallacher and Kaufman, and also Cantor and Blanton, Carver leaves us with perhaps the most important question for future research: how people juggle the many purposes and goals they are trying to achieve at the same time.

CHAPTER 26

Goals as Knowledge Structures

Arie W. Kruglanski

Much human activity revolves around the pursuit of goals. Goals energize our behavior and guide our choices; they occupy our thoughts and dominate our reveries. Failure to attain them causes pain and suffering, whereas their successful attainment may bring about pleasure and satisfaction. Goals lend meaning and direction to our existence; a purposeless life, devoid of significant goals, is often decried as inferior and empty.

It is not surprising, therefore, that the goal concept has received mention in major psychological theories from psychoanalysis (Freud, 1923/1961) to notions of artificial intelligence (Ortony, Clore, & Collins, 1988). Yet there exists a relative paucity of explicit theorizing about goals, and they typically occupy the "ground" rather than the "figure" of various motivational anlyses. Clearly, however, there exist many important questions directly pertaining to goals: Why do individuals need them, and do all individuals need them to the same degree? How are they formed, and what role do they play in the self-regulatory process? What are the psychological consequences of their attainment and nonattainment? A general theory of goals should provide answers to such questions. In the pages that follow, I attempt a preliminary outline of such a theory. It is cast from a cognitive perspective, and is intended as a framework for organizing past research and suggesting directions for future work.

A THREE-LEVEL ANALYSIS OF GOALS

The basic premise of my analysis is that goals belong in a unique category of knowledge characterized by its own generic meaning. From this perspective, variability in goal-related phenomena may be explained on three levels of analysis. The most abstract or general level is that of knowledge structures per se. Thus, the same principles that govern the acquisition, change, or activation of all knowledge structures should also apply to goals. The second level pertains to the unique properties of goals as a category. A goal is a particular class of knowledge characterized by its own meaning, which appropriately constrains its psychological properties and functions. Finally, the third level of analysis is that of specific goals, or goal types. All goals are not created equal (Ryan, Sheldon, Kasser, & Deci, Chapter 1, this volume); therefore, to understand specific goal-driven action and affect, it is essential to comprehend the specific goal contents in which these are embedded.

THE KNOWLEDGE STRUCTURE LEVEL OF ANALYSIS

What then is a goal? In an important sense, it is a knowledge category whose generic definition is "a desirable future state of affairs one intends to attain through action." Thus, to state that one's goal is *X*—say, to write a novel or become a nuclear physicist—is to profess subjective knowledge that *X* represents such an intended state of affairs.

Evidence for "Goal-Worthiness"

A particularly important property of any knowledge is its acceptance by the individual as true or valid. Such validation presupposes a process of *proof* via relevant evidence. How then does one "prove" to oneself, or come to believe, that *X* is worthy to be adopted as a goal? Two major categories of evidence seem relevant here: (1) that *X* is desirable, at least more so than its alternatives; and (2) that *X* is attainable, given one's resources. The notions of "attainability" and "desirability" resemble the familiar motivational concepts of "expectancy" and "value," respectively (Atkinson, 1958). In the present analysis, they are treated as evidential categories considered by the individual in forming a goal. This framing has various implications, discussed later, that do not follow from the traditional expectancy × value approach.

Effects of Motivation and Construct Accessibility on Goal Setting

Thinking of goals as a knowledge category affords several insights. Consider goal setting, or the formation of goal intentions (Gollwitzer, 1990). According to the present proposal, this is accomplished via a normal judgmental process that is affected by activation of constructs in memory and by motivation. For instance, individuals with a heightened need for cognitive closure (Kruglanski, 1989, 1990a, 1990b) may process relatively little evidence before adjudging some state of affairs as goal-worthy. In this motivational condition, individuals may quickly "freeze" on whatever relevant evidence (for goal-worthiness) is accessible in memory, rather than extensively seeking out further relevant evidence and choosing among several potential goal options. It also follows that individuals with a heightened need for closure may be positively biased toward evidence that a given object is (rather than is not) goal-worthy. This is because a positive judgment on such an issue furnishes closure (as to what one's goal should be), whereas a negative judgment prolongs a state of ambiguity.

Individuals stably characterized by a high need for closure should be more likely to have well-formed goals than their counterparts with a low need for closure. Because goals furnish closure on pervasively important questions concerning the direction or "meaning" of people's lives, they are more likely to be formed and crystallized by persons with a strong preference for cognitive clarity and a distaste for ambiguity. At the same time, individuals with a high need for closure may "succumb" more to temptation—that is, form situational goals on the basis of contextually primed notions. In terms of the "synapse" model of accessibility effects (Higgins, Bargh, & Lombardi, 1985), persons with a high (vs. low) need for closure should both succumb more to momentary temptations (i.e., exhibit stronger effects of *recent* primes) and abandon them more quickly in favor of their long-term objectives (i.e., exhibit stronger effects of *frequent* primes). Because they tend to base judgments on accessible constructs (Ford & Kruglanski, 1994; Thompson, Roman, Moscowitz, Chaiken, & Bargh, 1994), individuals with a high (vs. low) need for closure may exhibit greater inclination to shift from chronically accessible to recently primed goals, which are temporarily more accessible, and back again to chronic goals when their accessibility dominance re-emerges. Those tendencies may cause considerable goal conflict for such individuals.

It also seems plausible that the formation of goal intentions is not always "objective" or impartial, but is occasionally biased by individuals' "needs for specific closure" (Kruglanski, 1989, 1990a, 1990b). These are related to *contents* of specific intentions, yet may not be consciously recognized by individuals as reasons for their choice. For example, an individual may decide to acquire a slick sports car that promises to lend him or her a "sexy," carefree image, without admitting (even to himself or herself) to such "frivolous" motives. The person may feel instead that ease of parking and fuel economy are the true reasons for the choice.

Influence of Unconscious Motivations on Goal Setting

In other words, just as other judgments can be shaped by factors outside individuals' awareness (e.g., Nisbett & Wilson, 1977; Higgins, Chapter 5, this volume), so can judgments related to goals. Furthermore, some out-of-consciousness factors affecting goal formation may themselves be motivational (i.e., may represent other goals). For example, possible need-for-closure effects on extent of information processing in forming a goal are probably unconscious, and do not "officially" figure as reasons for one's choice. It is more likely that such effects operate "behind the scenes" of cognition, or constitute a "power behind the throne" of judgment (Bargh, 1989).

Knowledge Utilization Processes

The knowledge structure level of analysis pertains also to the way previously formed goals may function. Specifically, the principles of knowledge activation (Higgins, in press) should also be applicable to the activation of goals. For example, any construct or knowledge structure can be activated by priming; the same should be true of goals. Meeting a friend with a specific goal orientation (e.g., a materialistic or an idealistic one) may prime one's own goals in those domains and may trigger discrepancy-related thoughts (Higgins, 1987) that were largely absent prior to the priming event (e.g., "I should save more and invest more wisely," "I should do more volunteer work for the homeless"). Similarly, some persons may have chronically accessible goals of "looking good," "being fit," or "being productive." Many of these persons' actions and feelings may relate to those particular goals.

Recent research by Bargh and Gollwitzer (1994) demonstrates how knowledge activation principles are relevant to the operation of goals. For instance, Bargh, Barndollar, and Gollwitzer (1994, Experiment 1) placed subjects in a conflict between the goals of affiliation and achievement, after priming one or the other in an allegedly unrelated context. Subjects primed with the achievement goal behaved in the conflict situation in a more achievement-related manner (i.e., they performed significantly better when paired with an "inept" confederate on a team task) than subjects primed with the affiliation goal. Further studies by Bargh et al. (1994, Experiments 2 and 4) also created an affiliation–achievement conflict after one or the other goal was primed. Again, subjects tended to resolve the conflict in the direction of the primed goal construct. Those for whom the achievement goal was primed exhibited more achievement-related and less affiliative behaviors than those for whom the affiliation goal was primed. Furthermore, consistent with the "synapse" model of construct accessibility (Higgins et al., 1985; Lombardi, Higgins, & Bargh, 1987), effects of the recently primed goals were manifested only on early trials or after no delay, and were overridden by chronically accessible (achievement or affiliation) goals on later trials or after a 5-minute delay. Finally, Bargh et al. (1994, Experiment 3) demonstrated that priming an achievement goal led subjects to persist significantly longer at an achievement task, compared to subjects in a neutral-prime condition.

Summary

Thus, just like other knowledge structures, goals too appear to be derived from relevant evidence during a process in which construct accessibility and motivational factors play an important role. Furthermore, semantic priming may appropriately affect goal activation and utilization. Those examples highlight how the knowledge structure level of analysis may illuminate significant motivational phenomena.

GOALS AS A SPECIFIC KNOWLEDGE CATEGORY

Useful though it may be, the knowledge-structure level of analysis is unlikely to explain all of the variance in goal-driven phenomena. Consider the research by Bargh et al. (1994), described above. The major dependent variables in much of this research—that is, activity choice or task persistence (related to achievement or affiliation goals)—derive not from a theory of knowledge structures per se, but rather from generic properties of goals as a category (e.g., their capacity to guide choices and affect persistence). It seems useful at this point to consider what such properties of the goal construct are. Many of those derive from the generic meaning of the goal concept as a "desirable state of affairs intended to be attained through action." Such meaning identifies issues relevant to (1) goal setting; (2) goal striving or implementation; and (3) reactions to goal-related outcomes, primarily nonattainment and attainment.

Goal Setting

Desirability Evidence

As already noted, in deciding that a given entity (object, activity, or event) is worthy of being adopted as a goal, the individual may consider two categories of evidence: its "desirability" and "attainability." Evidence for desirability may vary in accordance with higher values or standards in terms of which the specific goal is rationalized. For instance, one may adopt the goal of loosing weight for beauty or health reasons, and succeeding at an exam for achievement reasons.

Though no evidence appears to exist on this point, it seems likely that a goal will appear particularly desirable if it is seen to represent a standard from which the individual feels discrepant, particularly if the discrepancy is highly accessible to awareness (Higgins, 1987). For instance, a person with an accessible discrepancy between the "actual" self and the "ideal" self may find a goal particularly desirable if its positive attributes are couched in terms of this person's ideal self. A person whose accessible actual–ideal discrepancy consists of feeling unattractive may be readily convinced by arguments extolling the virtues of products (e.g., cosmetics), or treatments promising to reduce the discrepancy, and may readily adopt goals (make purchases, pursue treatments) implied by those arguments. By comparison, individuals lacking this particular actual–ideal discrepancy may be less convinced by the same arguments and may be more responsive to arguments corresponding to a discrepancy they do possess (e.g., a discrepancy between the actual self and the "ought" self) (Higgins, 1987).

Furthermore, individuals may be particularly responsive to desirability arguments promising to remove the *specific negative affect* associated with those persons' unique self-discrepancies. For instance, an individual with an accessible actual–ideal discrepancy may suffer from feelings of dejection (Strauman & Higgins, 1987), and thus may accept as goals activities or objects depicted as happiness-inducing (e.g., an exciting trip or a gourmet meal). By contrast, individuals with an actual–ought discrepancy may suffer from agitation, and thus may more readily view an activity (e.g., jogging, physical exercise, or a tranquil vacation) worthy of adopting as a goal if it is portrayed as relaxing or tension-reducing. These issues could be profitably investigated in the future.

Attainability Evidence

Beyond desirability, a major category of evidence for goal-worthiness concerns the attainability of a state of affairs. Most people seem at least subjectively realistic in their goal setting and are unlikely to adopt goals they themselves believe to be unattainable. This does not necessarily imply objective realism. In fact, major approaches to cognitive therapy, such as those of Albert Ellis (e.g., 1962) or Aaron Beck (1982), view it as a major task to uproot patients' "dysfunctional" goals (e.g., "succeeding at every single task," "being liked by every single person") on the grounds of their lack of realism—that is, their (perennially frustrating) unattainability.

The dysfunctional aspects of exaggerated attainability beliefs are illustrated by the research of Baumeister, Heatherton, and Tice (1993) on individuals with high self-esteem, whose excessive optimism about goal attainment led to failure under some conditions. Specifically, whereas in the absence of ego threat high-self-esteem individuals set appropriate goals and performed effectively, under ego threat (e.g., the mention of choking under pressure) these subjects set for themselves inappropriately risky goals that were beyond their performance capabilities; consequently, they ended up with smaller rewards than low-self-esteem subjects.

Of course, unrealistically low attainability beliefs may be equally harmful in preventing individuals from realizing their potential. Bandura's work on self-efficacy emphasizes the adaptive value of the tenacity and resolve characterizing high-self-efficacy persons. Presumably because of their strong beliefs about goal attainability, such individuals may adopt high-level goals and may be undaunted by initial setbacks and difficulties. As Bandura (1989) put it, "a striking common characteristic of people who eventually achieved eminence in their respective fields was an inextinguishable sense of self-efficacy that enabled them to override innumerable rejections of their early work" (p. 40).

Attainability beliefs may have important social consequences in affecting the degree to which an individual develops a dependence on others. For instance, persons who underestimate their ability to attain a goal may act dependently, even when objectively they possess the potential to succeed on their own. A colleague and I (Ellis & Kruglanski, 1992) investigated this phenomenon in reference to people's ability to benefit from experiential learning. Specifically, we assessed individuals' "self-ascribed epistemic authority" in mathematics—that is, their beliefs in their ability to grasp mathematical notions and principles readily. Subjects classified as high or low in self-ascribed authority were exposed either to experiential learning of several mathematical principles through performing the relevant examples, or to "frontal instruction" in those same principles by an external authority (a math teacher). It turned out that in the experiential learning condition, subjects with low self-ascribed "epistemic authority" in mathematics did appreciably more poorly than those with high self-ascribed authority. This difference held even when actual mathematical ability was statistically controlled for, and it disappeared in the "frontal instruction" condition. Apparently the low-authority subjects did not have faith in their ability to learn mathematics on their own (i.e., they did not consider this goal as attainable). As a consequence, they may not have tried sufficiently hard, and thus failed to realize their learning potential.

The issue of attainability is relevant to Dweck's and Leggett's (1988) discussion of "performance" and "learning" goals. Essentially, a performance goal involves the *manifestation* of one's positive qualities (e.g., intelligence), whereas a learning goal involves the *enhancement* of one's potential. Dweck and Leggett have reported that children who tend to adopt learning goals tend to subscribe to the "incremental" theory of intelligence, in which intelligence is a malleable rather than a fixed quantity. By contrast, children with performance goals tend more to subscribe to the "entity" theory of intelligence, in which intelligence is a fixed property of the individual. In terms of the present analysis, incremental theorists believe that improvement of intelligence via learning is attainable, and hence they adopt it as a goal. Similarly, entity theorists believe that manifesting one's "true" (i.e., fixed) intelligence through performance is attainable, and hence they adopt this as a goal.

Often it may be functional for individuals to modify their attainability beliefs. I have already mentioned cases in which persons' goals seem objectively unattainable. Reducing their subjective (or perceived) attainability may help to reduce the suffering that prolonged nonattainment may induce (Ellis, 1962; Beck, 1982). In other cases—for instance, where attainment of certain goals (academic, professional, social) is expected by society, and nonattainment may invite adverse social consequences—increasing the goals' perceived attainability may boost an individual's flagging enthusiasm and prevent him or her from relinquishing these objectives.

Cantor's (1994) work on people's strategies of coping with different life tasks illustrates possible ways in which individuals may manipulate their own environments to appropriately affect attainability beliefs. For instance, one group of women oriented toward academic outcomes used their friends as "encouragers"; that is, they induced their friends to boost their self-esteem after setbacks on important tests, thus increasing their perceived likelihood of attaining their eventual academic goals. Another group of Cantor's subjects employed a different strategy, consisting of having a "good time" before important academic trials. Possibly, the mood enhancement such lighthearted socializing induced may have increased these individuals' general optimism, and generalized to greater perceived attainability of the academic goals. Finally, a subgroup of Cantor's subjects, characterized by a high actual–ideal self-discrepancy (Higgins, 1987), pursued the strategy of studying with successful people. Among other things, identification with such individuals, or "upward" social comparison (Waymont & Taylor, 1992), may have increased these subjects' perceived goal attainability and consequently enhanced their tendency to commit themselves unequivocally to the goal and strive forcefully to attain it.

Heuristic Goal Setting

Though the categories of desirability and attainability may be essential to the concept of goal-worthiness, there may be instances in which they are not considered particularly carefully before a goal is adopted. Specifically, the knowledge structure level of analysis considered earlier suggests that depending on the accessibility of evidence in the desirability and attainability categories, and on the individual's motivational state, such evidence may be processed more or less extensively. For instance, an individual with a high need for cognitive closure may process goal-relevant information briefly and give weight to the more accessible evidence (concerning desirability *or* accessibility), paying less attention to subsequent relevant information. Note that the notion of such differences in processing information relevant to goal setting is unique to the present analysis and is not implied by traditional expectancy–value approaches, which assume that individuals have definite beliefs about both these motivational parameters.

In yet other instances, rather than collecting goal-worthiness information "systematically" on basis of desirability and attainability considerations, individuals may render the relevant judgments "heuristically" (Chaiken, Liberman, & Eagly, 1989; Chaiken, Giner-Sorolla, & Chen, Chapter 24, this volume). In this vein, Locke and colleagues (Locke & Kristof, Chapter 16, this volume; Locke, Latham, & Erez, 1988) have discussed "passive choosing"—that is, selecting goals because everyone else seems to be choosing them, or choosing what others in authority (e.g., one's parents, boss, or military commander) have instructed one to choose.

As already indicated, the present framework affords the possibility of asking several empirical questions about goals. How do individuals' cognitive (e.g., their world knowledge and personal theories) and motivational (e.g., self-discrepancy) characteristics affect the kind of evidence for goal-worthiness they find compelling? When might an individual be convinced more by desirability versus attainability evidence? When might he or she adopt goals on the basis of systematic (desirability and attainability) versus heuristic evidence? And so on.

Goal Execution (Implementation)

Planning

Once a goal has been set, it needs to be implemented through appropriate action. After all, attainment via action is precisely what the goal construct implies. The exact mode of implementation needs to be planned. In turn, planning may depend on the individual's specific notions or theories or "narratives" as to what means may serve what ends.

Social-psychological theory and research related to goal implementation has essentially addressed two separate cases. In the first of these, the goal's mental representation is well developed and contains a fairly routinized set of procedures for goal attainment. For instance, the goal of having one's hair cut may be associated with a fairly specific activity script, including setting the appointment, driving to a specific hair salon, sitting in the hairdresser's chair, and paying for his or her services. Wyer and Srull (1986) discuss the case of such well-developed goal structures, in which the strategies and tactics of goal attainment are immediately evoked by activation of the goal itself. Presumably, implementation of those goals requires relatively little planning.

The second case is that in which the mental representation of goals is relatively undeveloped and the individual initially lacks specific ideas about implementation. For instance, goals of "becoming a millionaire," "being a good parent," or "learning to speak Italian" may evoke few specific ideas as to their accomplishment. In such a case, effective goal pursuit will require considerable planning.

To be sure, at least some planning is required in the case of well-evolved goals of the first type discussed above. Action occurs in time; therefore, even in the case of highly developed and routinized goal structures, it is necessary to decide on the specific time and place at which goal implementation will occur. Research by Gollwitzer (Chapter 13, this volume), and Taylor and Pham (Chapter 10, this volume) suggests that making specific implementation decisions is critically important in determining individuals' success in attaining their adopted goals.

Energetics of Goal Implementation

Beyond planning, or forming an implementation-intention, the implementation process itself raises several interesting issues for inquiry. One of its essential aspects is allocation of energy to a given goal system in accordance with apparent requirements. The energy-related aspects of self-regulation have been relatively neglected in past research. Kurt Lewin (1951) had an interest in these issues; he conceived of goals as tension systems, drained of their charge by goal attainment. The Zeigarnik (1927) effect of greater recall of uncompleted versus completed tasks provides some support for this conception, if it is assumed that systems in tension maintain the related cognitions in a state of activation (Higgins, in press) that facilitates recall. However, several questions remain. For instance, will the energy stay in the unattained-goal system even after a new goal is adopted? If energy resources at an organism's disposal are finite, it seems plausible that investing energies in a new goal should reduce the magnitude of energies tied to the old goal. This should reduce the magnitude of the Zeigarnik effect. A somewhat similar implication follows from cognitive capacity considerations discussed by Wyer and Srull (1986). They assume that goals reside in a capacity-limited "goal specification box," Therefore, as additional objectives and procedures for attaining them enter the unit, others are displaced and consequently cease to affect any current information-processing activity. This seems to suggest that the Zeigarnik effect should disappear following the adoption of a new goal. Martin and Tesser's (1989) work on rumination provides evidence consistent with this notion.

Finally, a goal may be abandoned without its being replaced by a new goal. Thus, if compelling evidence against desirability or attainability exists. an individual may be persuaded to give up a goal. Consistent with this notion, Wright (Chapter 19, this volume) finds that when the task appears too demanding (implying that a success is unattainable) and/or the individual's self-ascribed ability appears low, energy investment in the task declines—indicating that the individual may have relinquished the goal.

Means–Ends Relations: Equifinality, Contingency, and Substitutability

Equifinality. An important notion related to the goal concept is that of "equifinality" (McDougal, 1923; Heider, 1958). Specifically, the "desirable state of affairs" that a goal category represents may be often attained via multiple possible actions, that is, multiple means. In motivated social cognition, the equifinality concept has been investigated in two distinct connections: (1) that of the "contingency principle," whereby the choice of proper means may depend on situational circumstance; and (2) that of the "substitutability principle," whereby the affective, cognitive, or behavioral consequences of blocking a path to a goal may be removed if an alternative means to the same goal is adopted.

Contingency. Activation of a goal may activate the set of means, or attainment strategies, associated with that goal (e.g., Wyer & Srull, 1986). A subset of these means may be further activated by situations to which they are applicable (see Higgins, in press). Thus, choice of means may be contingent upon the situation. For example, research by Tetlock (1992) suggests that social accountability motivation may prompt different cognitive activities, depending upon the circumstances. When individuals can tell what opinions are acceptable to those to whom they feel accountable, they tend to adopt those particular opinions (Tetlock, 1983a; Tetlock, Skitka, & Boettger, 1989).

In the absence of such knowledge, however, accountable (vs. less accountable) individuals will engage more in flexible, multidimensional information processing in search of the most defensible judgment (Tetlock, 1983b; Tetlock & Kim, 1987). Finally, when irrevocably committed to a course of action, accountable individuals will expend cognitive effort aimed at generating reasons "why they are right and potential critics wrong" (Tetlock, 1992, p. 340; see also Festinger, 1964; Kiesler, 1971; Tetlock et al., 1989).

Stated broadly, the contingency principle suggests that people will pursue an activity affording the "best" or most effective satisfaction of the underlying motivation. According to Tetlock (1992), an essential ingredient of the accountability motivation is the need for approval and status. Thus, knowing what significant others find acceptable may suggest that the best way of securing status and approval is adopting their opinion. Not knowing what these others find acceptable, however, may suggest that the best path to status and esteem is having a well-thought-out, thoroughly considered viewpoint. Finally, having made an irrevocable commitment may, suggest that the best path to accountability is defensive bolstering of one's position.

The contingency principle also seems implicated in a study (Kruglanski, Webster, & Klem, 1993) where subjects with high (vs. low) dispositional need for closure, or subjects whose need for closure was situationally elevated via environmental noise, tended to resist persuasion when they possessed a firm initial opinion on an issue, and tended to be readily persuaded when lacking such an opinion. Presumably for subjects with an initial opinion, the motivation for closure was best satisfied by "freezing" upon it and refraining from reopening the issue in the light of new arguments. By contrast, for subjects without an initial opinion, the same motivation may have been best gratified by adopting the persuader's view.

Substitutability. A different implication of the equifinality notion is that different paths to the same goal are substitutable for each other, or functionally equivalent. Thus, if a given path to a goal is blocked, it may be possible to attain the same goal via alternate means. Several recent research programs in motivated social cognition bear on this possibility. For instance, Steele and his colleagues (Steele & Liu, 1983; Liu & Steele, 1986; Steele, 1988) have demonstrated that making salient to oneself an important personal value (thereby self-affirming one's worth) can turn off or reduce the extent of attitude change under dissonance-producing circumstances.

Tesser and Cornell (1991; Cornell & Tesser, 1994) showed in a series of studies that (1) providing subjects with a self-affirmation opportunity (responding to a subjectively important Study of Values subscale) lowered their tendency to engage in self-esteem maintenance behaviors (by choosing a difficult task for a friend); (2) making salient a positive self-esteem maintenance context (writing an essay about having outperformed a close other on a highly relevant dimension) lowered subjects' tendency to engage in dissonance reduction; and (3) making salient a negative self-esteem maintenance context (writing an essay about having been outperformed by a close other on a highly relevant dimension) increased subjects' tendency to self-affirm (see also Martin & Tesser, 1989).

These findings support the notion that different processes related to self-evaluation constitute diverse paths to the same superordinate goal of self-esteem maintenance, and are therefore functionally equivalent or mutually substitutable. Attaining positive self-esteem via one means may reduce the tendency to pursue a different means of self-esteem enhancement (see Cornell & Tesser, 1994). Similarly, when one's attempts to elevate self-esteem via a given means are thwarted, this may strengthen one's attempts to do so via alternative means.

Though the confluence of modes whereby self-esteem may be maintained integrates several heretofore separate notions in social cognition (dissonance reduction and self-affirmation, among others), an even broader integration may be possible. Thus, a non-esteem-related positive experience (e.g., having a gourmet meal, taking a walk on the beach, winning a lottery)—that is, *any* mood-repairing event—may serve as an adequate substitute for failure at an esteem-related activity. Equally general in scope is anxiety avoidance. Solomon, Greenberg, and Pyszczynski (1991) proposed in this connection that the motivation to maintain positive self-esteem is itself subordinate to the goal of buffering mortality anxiety. Research reported by Solomon et al. (1991) suggests specifically that once the buffering is undermined (via making one's mortality salient), there exist two alternate routes whereby it may be restored: self-esteem enhancement, or reaffirmation of one's world view and values (i.e., the system from which esteem-lending outcomes derive their meaning). For example, in one experiment Greenberg et al. (1991, Study 1) found that death scenes led to an elevation in self-reported anxiety for subjects previously given neutral personality feedback, but not for those given positive feedback. In other research, Rosenblatt, Greenberg, Solomon, Pyszczynski, and Lyon (1989) found that increasing mortality salience led to recommendations of a more severe punishment for a moral transgression (prostitution) and of a greater reward for courageously upholding cultural values (turning in a criminal).

Outcomes of Goal Strivings

Nonattainment

Because a goal represents a desirable state of affairs, its nonattainment in the expected time should be experienced as undesirable, giving rise to negative affect. In addition to means substitution, or as a strategy when the set of substitutable means has been exhausted, it is possible to cope with such negative affect via goal substitution, or execution of a "goal shift" (Kruglanski & Jaffe, 1988). Research on cognitive complexity (Linville, 1985, 1987; Showers, 1992) is relevant here. It suggests that depending on the degree of differentiation among the individual's goal systems, failure with respect to one goal may be experienced as more or less devastating. Individuals characterized by low cognitive complexity have most of their "eggs" in relatively few motivational "baskets" or goal systems. The failure-engendered negative affect may be difficult to escape in these circumstances. By contrast, individuals with high cognitive complexity have numerous goal systems, which may "buffer" them from the consequences of failure in one system. The tradeoff, however, seems to involve relatively muted positive affect when success is experienced. Presumably, the amount of affective investment such a person is capable of is limited. An individual who spreads such investment across numerous goals may therefore invest less in any one goal (and hence may react less intensely to attainment as well as nonattainment) than an individual who invests the same amount of affect in fewer goals.

It is also of interest to ask how nonattainment of a goal affects the choice of a subsequent goal. Early research on levels of aspiration (Festinger, 1942; Lewin, Dembo, Festinger, & Sears, 1944) found that following a failure to attain a task at a given difficulty level, subjects exhibited shifts to easier tasks. Presumably, because the previous task seemed unattainable, subjects were willing to lower the desirability level of their goal (assuming that in an achievement domain desirability was positively related to task difficulty) to assure the attainability of at least some objective.

But the question is whether such lowering of aspiration levels is a general phenomenon, or whether it occurs only in restricted circumstances. For instance, one might ask whether, rather than lowering the desirability level of their goals, people might not prefer to switch to a different activity domain where highly desirable goals are still attainable. For instance, rather than "realistically" switching to a lower-level task, an individual may abandon the activity altogether and attempt to attain an equally desirable goal in a different domain. A person who failed an academic task may switch to athletics, go shopping, or engage in social interaction with friends (Cantor & Blanton, Chapter 15, this volume).

Whether or not an individual exhibits such compensatory switching may depend on a number of factors—for instance, the availability of equally desirable alternative dimensions. As noted earlier, highly self-differentiated individuals (Linville, 1985, 1987) may have numerous alternative dimensions available, whereas individuals with relatively low degrees of self-differentiation may have fewer such alternatives. Furthermore, it may matter whether the individuals perceive the desirability reduction as temporary or permanent. For example, entity theorists (Dweck, Chapter 4, this volume), who believe intelligence is a fixed quantity, may believe that the desirability reduction is permanent. Therefore, they may be more inclined to abandon the activity if provided with a desirable alternative. By contrast, instrumental theorists, who believe intelligence to be a malleable attribute, may regard the desirability reduction as temporary and may thus be more inclined to persist at the activity (Dweck & Leggett, 1988).

Attainment

Whereas responses to goal nonattainment have received a considerable amount of research attention (e.g., in clinical and personality psychology), goal attainment has been relatively neglected in research. Yet several aspects of goal attainment seem rather poorly understood. Research has consistently shown that goal attainment is not highly correlated with happiness (Andrews & Withey, 1976); this is intriguing in light of the popular view that happiness does follow goal attainment. I am aware of no systematic research on this issue, but it is possible to consider some speculative possibilities. For instance, the presence of tension in the goal system (prompting, e.g., physiological arousal) may magnify the perceived attractiveness of the goal object and lead to the belief that attainment will be highly desirable, which may induce an expectation of happiness. Upon attainment, however, tension may be drained from the system; thus the perceived desirability of the goal may wane, and the degree of satisfaction may be reduced.

Furthermore, goal attainment may create an "epistemic vacuum" or ambiguity concerning what to do next. For some individuals—those high in the need for cognitive closure (Webster & Kruglanski, 1994), for example—such ambiguity may be aversive and may detract from the positive affect engendered by goal attainment as such. It is also likely that such individuals are likely to proceed to form their next goal rather quickly, rather than "resting on their laurels" for too long. If it is further assumed (1) that indiviudals high in the need for closure may make a particularly strong commitment to their yet-to-be-attained goals because those lend much-wanted structure to their activities, and (2) that such commitment may make those goals appear all the more desirable, it follows that these individuals' goal-related affect may be rather inconsistent and labile: Their *anticipated* pleasure of goal attainment may be higher than that of low-need-for-closure individuals, whereas their *actual* pleasure may be less.

As in the case of nonattainment, it is of interest to ask how a new goal is chosen following attainment. Among others, this may depend on what has made the new goal desirable in the first place, or what evidence for its desirability has been activated in the postattainment period. Thus, it is possible that the new goal will resemble the old one on dimensions represented by the activated desirability evidence. Consider a just-attained goal *X* (graduation from college) whose desirability was originally based on two separate arguments: *A* (pleasing one's parents) and *B* (gratifying one's intellectual interests). If argument *A* is more accessible during the postattainment period (e.g., is activated by one's parents' presence during the graduation ceremony), the new goal *Y* may resemble *X* on the *A* dimension (e.g., one may accept a nonstimulating job because of its closeness to the parents' home). By contrast, if argument *B* is more accessible, the new goal *Y* may resemble *X* on the *B* dimension (e.g., one may accept a stimulating job even if its location is far from the parents' home).

Furthermore, the tendency for the new goal to resemble the old one on *any* dimension may decline as a function of time passage following attainment. As noted earlier, energy tied to the goal system may dissipate with the passage of time, reducing the goal's perceived appeal. One may no longer feel as "excited" about the goal, and any argument for its desirability may seem less compelling; hence it may be less likely to form the basis for the adoption of other goals.

Summary

In summary, consideration of goals as a unique category of knowledge affords ways of thinking about a wide range of goal-related phenomena, including goal setting, goal implementation, and reactions to goal-relevant outcomes (i.e., nonattainment and attainment). Most of the understanding at this level of analysis derives from the generic understanding of the goal concept as a "desirable future state of affairs one intends to attain through action." If we assume that this understanding of goals is widely shared, it is possible to use it as a basis for theoretical developments and empirical research into goal-related thought, affect, and action.

SPECIFIC GOAL SYSTEMS

Beyond insights from properties goals share with other knowledge structures, and those they share in common with other goals, a significant understanding of goal-related phenomena depends upon an understanding of properties on which goals *differ* from other goals. Identification of such properties seems essential if one is to affect the formation or modification of goals, or understand individuals' reactions to events whose subjective meaning derives from the representational contents of specific goal systems.

Though the variety of such specific goal systems can be considerable, it is restricted somewhat by the fact that most goals are culturally defined, and hence are shared to a large extent by members of a culture. In fact, clinical, social, and personality psychologists have conducted extensive research on specific, culturally shared goal systems chosen for their significance for broad domains of human functioning. Detailed discussion of such goal systems exceeds the scope of the present chapter, but a few examples may be helpful.

Consider, for instance, the lists of "irrational beliefs" compiled by cognitive therapists like Beck (1982) and Ellis (1962). These lists consist of goals regarded as largely unattainable (e.g., "to succeed on every single task I attempt" or "to be liked by every single person I meet"); yet such goals are held by some individuals and cause them perennial frustration and suffering. The potential utility of these lists is that they provide a basis for developing generally compelling counterarguments whereby clients may be persuaded to abandon the dysfunctional goals.

A different example of work pertinent to specific goal systems is Higgins's (1987) research on self-discrepancies from "ideal" and "ought" standards, mentioned earlier in this chapter. An ideal standard involves goals one would like to have attained, and an ought standard involves goals one feels one should have attained. An important aspect of this work relates to qualitative differences in negative affect as a consequence of failure to attain an ideal or an ought goal. Higgins and his colleagues (e.g., Strauman & Higgins, 1987) find that in the former case the typical affect is dejection, whereas in the latter it is agitation.

Also as described earlier, Dweck and Leggett, (1988; see also Dweck, Chapter 4, this volume) have distinguished in the domain of intellectual achievement between learning goals, "in which individuals are concerned with increasing their competence" (1988, p. 256), and performance goals, "in which individuals are concerned with gaining favorable judgments of their competence" (1988, p. 256). The importance of this distinction lies, among others, in its implications for individuals' ability to cope with failure—an inseparable counterpart of any learning.

Finally, Mischel (Chapter 9, this volume; Mischel, Shoda, & Rodriguez, 1989) has discussed children's ability to pursue long-term (vs. short-term) goals—that is, their capacity for the delay of gratification. One focus of this work is on cognitive strategies individuals use to delay gratification. This has important applied implications, as the ability to pursue long-term goals is surely essential to any significant achievement.

CONCLUDING COMMENT

In this chapter, I have argued that the understanding of goal-driven thought, affect, and action may be approached at three levels of analysis: that of knowledge structures per se, that of the goal construct as a unique knowledge category, and that of specific goal contents of broad significance. Though these analytic levels are conceptually separate, we may gain predictive power by combining them in the explanation of particular phenomena. For instance, consider the notions (derived from the knowledge structure level of analysis) that there may exist stable individual differences in the chronic accessibility of different goals, and that goal accessibility may play a more important part in goal setting under high (vs. low) need for cognitive closure (Ford & Kruglanski, 1994; Thompson et al., 1994). Given specific goal contents, these notions may interact with the situational appropriateness of goals an individual may adopt. For instance, a person whose chronically accessible goals are based on what Higgins (1987) calls an "ought" standard may, under heightened need for closure, adopt such goals inappropriately even in a situation that calls for "ideal" (i.e., hedonistic) goals (e.g., at a party or during a vacation). In the same context, heightened need for closure may, if anything, increase the situational appropriateness of adopted goals for individuals with chronically accessible goals derived from the "ideal" standard.

Or consider combining the second and third levesl of analysis (the goal category and specific goals). Thus, in attempting to get a child to adopt a given socially desirable goal—for example, a learning goal (Dweck, Chapter 4, this volume) or a long-term goal (Mischel, Chapter 9, this volume)—it may be useful to consider whether the evidence the child would find most compelling would concern the goal's desirability (relative to alternatives) or its attainability. Such possibilities highlight the potential advantages of the present three-level framework for understanding goal-related phenomena.

REFERENCES

Andrews, F. M., & Withey, S. B. (1976). *Social indicators of well-being.* New York: Plenum.

Atkinson, J. W. (1958). *Motives in fantasy, action and society.* Princeton, NJ: Van Nostrand.

Bandura, A. (1989). Self-regulation of motivation and action through internal standards and goal systems. In L. A. Pervin (Ed.), *Goal concepts in personality and social psychology* (pp. 55–85). Hillsdale, NJ: Erlbaum.

Bargh, J. A. (1989). Conditional automaticity: Varieties of automatic influence in social perception and cognition. In J. S. Uleman & J. A. Bargh (Eds.), *Unintended thought: Limits of awareness, intention, and control* (pp. 3–51). New York: Guilford Press.

Bargh, J. A., Barndollar, K., & Gollwitzer, P. M. (1994). *Environmental control of behavior.* Manuscript in preparation, New York University.

Bargh, J. A., & Gollwitzer, P. M. (1994). Environmental control of goal-directed action: Automatic and strategic contingencies between situations and behavior. In W. D. Spaulding (Ed.), *Nebraska Symposium on Motivation: Vol. 41. Integrative views of motivation, cognition, and emotion* (pp. 71–124). Lincoln; University of Nebraska Press.

Baumeister, R. F., Heatherton, T. F., & Tice, D. M. (1993). When ego-threats lead to self-regulation failure: Negative consequences of high self-esteem. *Journal of Personality and Social Psychology, 64,* 141–156.

Beck, A. T. (1982). *Depression: Clinical, experimental and theoretical aspects.* New York: Raven Press.

Cantor, N. (1994). Life task problem solving: Situational affordances and personal needs. *Personality and Social Psychology Bulletin, 20*(3), 235–243.

Chaiken, S., Liberman, A., & Eagly, A. H. (1989). Heuristic and systematic information processing within and beyond the persuasion context. In J. S. Uleman & J. A. Bargh (Eds.), *Unintended thought: Limits of awareness, intention, and control* (pp. 212–252). New York: Guilford Press.

Cornell, D. P., & Tesser, A. (1994). *On the confluence of self-processes: II. SEM affects self-affirmation.* Unpublished manuscript, University of Georgia.

Dweck, C. S., & Leggett, E. L. (1988). A social-cognitive approach to personality and motivation. *Psychological Review, 95,* 256–273.

Ellis, A. (1962). *Reason and emotion in psychotherapy.* Secaucus, NJ: Lyle Stuart.

Ellis, S., & Kruglanski, A. W. (1992). Self as epistemic authority: Effects on experiential and instructional learning. *Social Cognition, 10,* 357–375.

Festinger, L. (1942). A theoretical interpretation of shifts in level of aspiration. *Psychological Review, 49,* 235–250.

Festinger, L. (Ed.). (1964). *Conflict, decision and dissonance.* Stanford, CA: Stanford University Press.

Ford, T. E., & Kruglanski, A. W. (1994). *Effects of epistemic motivations on the use of accessible constructs in social judgment.* Unpublished manuscript, Kalamazoo College.

Freud, S. (1961). The ego and the id. In J. Strachey (Ed. and Trans.), *The standard edition of the complete psychological works of Sigmund Freud* (Vol. 19, pp. 3–66). London: Hogarth Press. (Original work publishe 1923)

Gollwitzer, P. M. (1990). Action phases and mind-sets. In E. T. Higgins & R. M. Sorrentino (Eds.), *Handbook of motivation and cognition: Foundations of social behavior* (Vol. 2, pp. 53–92). New York: Guilford Press.

Greenberg, J., Solomon, S., Burling, J., Rosenblatt, A., Pysczynski, T., Simon, L., & Lyon, D. (1991). *The effects of raising self-esteem on physiological and affective responses to subsequent threat.* Unpublished manuscript, University of Arizona.

Heider, F. (1958). *The psychology of interpersonal relations.* New York: Wiley.

Higgins, E. T. (1987). Self-discrepancy: A theory of relating self and affect. *Psychological Review, 94,* 319–340.

Higgins, E. T. (in press). Knowledge activation: accessibility, applicability, and salience. In E. T. Higgins & A. W. Kruglanski (Eds.), *Social psychology: handbook of basic principles.* New York: Guilford Press.

Higgins, E. T., Bargh, J. A., & Lombardi, W. (1985). The nature of priming effects on categorization. *Journal of Experimental Psychology: Learning, Memory, and Cognition, 11,* 59–69.

Kiesler, A. C. (1971). *The psychology of commitment.* New York: Academic Press.

Kruglanski, A. W. (1989). *Lay epistemics and human knowledge: Cognitive and motivational bases.* New York: Plenum.

Kruglanski, A. W. (1990). Motivations for judging and knowing: Implications for causal attribution. In E. T. Higgins & R. M. Sorrentino (Eds.), *Handbook of motivation and cognition: Foundation of social behavior* (Vol. 2, pp. 333–368). New York: Guilford Press.

Kruglanski, A. W. (1990b). Lay epistemic theory in social cognitive psychology. *Psychological Inquiry, 1,* 181–197.

Kruglanski, A. W., & Jaffe, Y. (1988). Curing by knowing: The epistemic approach to cognitive therapy. In L. Abramson (Ed.), *Social cognition and clinical psychology* (pp. 254–291). New York: Guilford Press.

Kruglanski, A. W., Webster, D. M., & Klem, A. (1993). Motivated resistance and openness to persuasion in the presence or absence of prior information. *Journal of Personality and Social Psychology, 64,* 861–876.

Lewin, K. (1951). *Field theory in social science: Selected theoretical papers.* New York: Harper & Row.

Lewin, K., Dembo, T., Festinger, L., & Sears, P. S. (1944). Level of aspiration. In J. M. Hunt (Ed.), *Personality and the behavior disorders* (pp. 333–378). New York: Roland Press.

Linville, P. W. (1985). Self-complexity and affective extremity: Don't put all of your eggs in one cognitive basket. *Social Cognition, 3,* 94–120.

Linville, P. W. (1987). Self-complexity as a cognitive buffer against stress-related illness and depression. *Journal of Personality and Social Psychology, 52,* 663–676.

Liu, T. J., & Steele, C. M. (1986). Attributional analysis as self-affirmation. *Journal of Personality and Social Psychology, 51,* 531–540.

Locke, E., Latham, G. P., & Erez, M. (1988). The determinants of goal-commitment. *Academy of Management Review, 13,* 21–29.

Lombardi, W. J., Higgins, E. T., & Bargh, J. A. (1987). The role of consciousness in priming effects on categorization. *Personality and Social Psychology Bulletin, 13,* 411–429.

Martin, L. L., & Tesser, A. (1989). Toward a motivational and structural theory of ruminative thought. In J. S. Uleman & J. A. Bargh (Eds.), *Unintended thought: Limits of awareness, intention, and control* (pp. 306–326). New York: Guilford Press.

McDougal, W. (1923). *Outline of psychology.* New York: Scribner's.

Mischel, W., Shoda, Y., & Rodriguez, M. I. (1989). Delay of gratification in children. *Science, 244,* 933–938.

Nisbett, R. E., & Wilson, T .D. (1977). Telling more than we can know: Verbal reports on mental processes. *Psychological Review, 84,* 231–259.

Ortony, A., Clore, G. L., & Collins, A. (1988). *The cognitive structure of emotions.* Cambridge, England: Cambridge University Press.

Rosenblatt, A., Greenberg, J., Solomon, S., Pyszczynski, T., & Lyon, D. (1989). Evidence for terror management theory: I. The effects of mortality salience on reactions to those who violate or uphold cultural values. *Journal of Personality and Social Psychology, 57,* 681–690.

Showers, C. (1992). Compartmentalization of positive and negative self-knowledge: Keeping bad apples out of the bunch. *Journal of Personality and Social Psychology, 62,* 1036–1049.

Solomon, S., Greenberg, J., & Pyszczynski, T. (1991). A terror management theory of social behavior: The psychological functions of self-esteem and cultural worldviews. In M. P. Zanna (Ed.), *Advances in experimental social psychology* (Vol. 24, pp. 93–159). New York: Academic Press.

Steele, C. M. (1988). The psychology of self-affirmation: Sustaining the integrity of the self. In L. Berkowitz (Ed.), *Advances in experimental social psychology* (Vol. 21, pp. 261–302). New York: Academic Press.

Steele, C. M., & Liu, T. J. (1983). Dissonance processes as self-affirmation. *Journal of Personality and Social Psychology, 45,* 5–19.

Strauman, T. J., & Higgins, E. T. (1987). Automatic activation of self-discrepancies and emotional syndromes: When cognitive structures influence affect. *Journal of Personality and Social Psychology, 53,* 1004–1014.

Tetlock, P. E. (1983a). Accountability and the complexity of thought. *Journal of Personality and Social Psychology, 45,* 74–83.

Tetlock, P. E. (1983b). Accountability and the perseverance of first impressions. *Social Psychology Quarterly, 46,* 285–292.

Tetlock, P. E. (1992). The impact of accountability on judgment and choice: Toward a social contingency model. In M. P. Zanna (Ed.), *Advances in experimental social psychology* (Vol. 25, pp. 331–376). New York: Academic Press.

Tetlock, P. E., & Kim, J. (1987). Accountability and overconfidence in a personality prediction task. *Journal of Personality and Social Psychology, 52,* 700–709.

Tetlock, P. E., Skitka, L., & Boettger, R. (1989). Social and cognitive strategies of coping with accountability: Conformity, complexity, and bolstering. *Journal of Personality and Social Psychology, 57,* 632–641.

Tesser, A., & Cornell, D. P. (1991). On the confluence of self-processes. *Journal of Experimental Social Psychology, 27,* 501–526.

Thompson, E. P., Roman, R. J., Moscowitz, G. B., Chaiken, S., & Bargh, J. A. (1994). Accuracy motivation attenuates covert primary: The systematic reprocessing of social information. *Journal of Personality and Social Psychology, 66,* 474–489.

Waymont, H. A., & Taylor, S. E. (1933). Paper presented at the meeting of the American Psychological Association, Toronto.

Webster, D. W., & Kruglanski, A. W. (1994). Individual differences in need for cognitive closure. *Journal of Personality and Social Psychology, 67,* 1049–1062.

Wyer, R. S., & Srull, T. K. (1986). Human cognition in its social context. *Psychological Review, 93,* 322–359.

Zeigarnik, B. (1927). Das Behalten erledigter und unerledigter Handlugen. *Psychologische Forschung, 9,* 1–85.

ˈhe Role of Conscious ..ought in a Theory of Motivation and Cognition

The Uncertainty Orientation Paradigm

Richard M. Sorrentino

I have been thinking about the problem of the role of conscious thought in a theory of motivation and action for a long time. In my course on motivation and cognition, my students insist that conscious thought has some role; if it does not, then they have no free will. "How can you have free will if conscious thought is not important?" they ask. In two volumes of our *Handbook of Motivation and Cognition* (Higgins & Sorrentino, 1990; Sorrentino & Higgins, 1986), we see a large array of theorists, none of whom deal directly with this issue. Often, however, they appear to contradict or to be at odds with one another. For example, Cantor, Markus, Niedenthal, and Nurius (1986) postulate that all motivated behavior stems from people's decisions about what they want to be or would like to become. After imagining a number of possible selves, they pick the most desired and pursue it. Motivation, then, stems from conscious decision making, and nonconscious motives or cognitions have little relevance. On the other hand, the second volume includes a chapter by John Bargh (1990) on unintended thought, and one by Jacoby and Kelley (1990) on episodic memory. Both of these chapters would indicate that nonconscious memories and unintended thought play major roles in determining much of human behavior. Many of the other contributors fall somewhere in between. There are those accepting nonconscious forces, but only to a point—basically implying that when things become really important, and/or individuals are aware of nonconscious forces, then the individuals can control them by using conscious thought (cf. Fazio,

1986; Kuhl, 1986; Weiner, 1986). Interestingly, there are others such as Polivy (1990) who argue that it is unwise to try to interfere with people's biological or natural tendencies.

In addition to our own *Handbook,* I (Sorrentino, 1993) recently had an opportunity to contribute a review chapter to an edited book on control motivation and social cognition (Weary, Gleicher, & Marsh, 1993). Here too, I discovered that consciousness is seen to play an important role in restoration of control. Whether a person is simply trying to regain control over a specific situation, or faces more general problems such as depression, ill health, or even terminal illness, he or she will strive to regain understanding over his or her environment, and will only engage in activities that permit such an understanding. So who is right? Who is wrong? How do we reconcile these differences?

OVERVIEW

As a consequence of my concerns, I have chosen the role of conscious thought as the theme of this chapter. In pursuing this theme, I have begun to realize that much of my deliberation has a lot to do with my own research. Also, many of the other chapters in the present volume touch upon this problem in one way or another. In what follows, I present a brief history of this problem; next, I attempt to show how I believe my own research speaks to the issue (albeit indirectly); and then I attempt to show how some of the other contributors to this volume aid in our understanding of the dynamics behind this issue. I think I understand the role of conscious thought a little better now, and I hope to share this understanding with my readers at the conclusion of this chapter.

HISTORY

In seeking answers to the questions above, I sought opinions of others who had gone before me. Much to my surprise and delight, just as I was getting this chapter underway, I came upon a plaster cast of a very famous sculpture at the Museum D'Orsay in Paris. It was a copy of Rodin's "The Gates of Hell." I was so struck by its implications that I ran over to the Rodin Museum to see the original. And there it was in all its glory—a sculpture of people plunging through the gates of Hell for eternity. And what is the cause of this eternal damnation? Well, at the very top of the sculpture is a replica of Rodin's most famous statue, "The Thinker." It seems clear to me what role Rodin had in mind for the functional significance of conscious thought: It is a precursor to all that is evil about human beings, and it ultimately leads to their demise.

Although I will not know for a while (I hope) whether Rodin is correct, there are others who consider conscious thought a relatively recent occurrence in human history. For example, there is the work of Julian Jaynes (1976), who sees the origin of consciousness in the breakdown of the bicameral mind.[1] He asserts that human beings got along quite well without cons

ness until ab

to e

> We have been brought to the conclusion that consciousness is not what we generally think it is. It is not to be confused with reactivity. It is not involved in hosts of perceptual phenomena. It is not involved in the performance of skills and often hinders their execution. It need not be involved in speaking, writing, listening, or reading. It does not copy down experience, as most people think. Consciousness is not at all involved in signal learning, and need not be involved in the learning of skills or solutions, which can go on without any consciousness whatever. It is not necessary for making judgments or in simple thinking. It is not the seat of reason, and indeed some of the most difficult instances of creative reasoning go on without any attending consciousness. And it has no location except an imaginary one!

From these two sources, one might conclude that consciousness is both evil and quite unnecessary. A little closer to home (or at least my scholarly abode) is the work by John W. Atkinson. In coming up with his tour de force, *The Dynamics of Action* (Atkinson & Birch, 1970), Atkinson constantly battled those who embraced extreme points of view. As can be seen in Figure 27.1, he and David Birch laid out three possible alternatives or models for the significance of conscious thought or *r* (covert activity) for a theory of motivation and action or *R* (overt activity).

Model A: Conscious Thought May Correlate with Action but Does Not Influence Action

The first alternative, Model A, sees conscious thought as merely a concomitant or correlate of overt behavior, as both overt and covert activity are determined by nonconscious forces. Conscious thought, then, has no role in directly determining overt behavior or action. This model is best represented by Freud and psychoanalysis (Freud, 1943). That is, conscious thought is manifested by correlates of unconscious motivation, and although one can get at the latent content of thought by analysis of conscious thought, it has no predictive power by itself for behavior. I think also that other noncognitive views of behavior such as Skinner's (1953) behaviorism, Hull's (1943) drive habit theory, Baron and Byrne's (Byrne, 1971) reinforcement–affect theory, and Zajonc's (1965) social facilitation theory, can all be placed in this camp. None of them assume consciousness has any role in the behavior they specify.

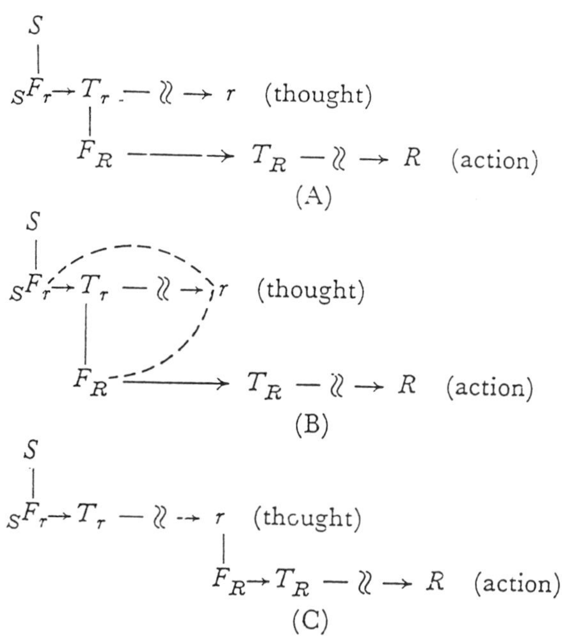

FIGURE 27.1. The graphic representation of three possible relationships between conscious thought (r) and action (R), treated as covert and overt activity in the text. In A, instigation to action is mediated by the perceptual–imaginal tendency (T_r), which, when dominant, is expressed in thought. The content of though and action are correlated, and so the content analysis of thought is diagnostic of action. In B, conscious though is considered an additional source of instigating force for both covert and overt activity. It thus functions to *amplify* trends that are already implicit in the unconscious process. In C, all instigation and resistance to over action are mediated by conscious though. The unconscious perceptual–imaginal tendency (T_r) does not mediate instigation or resistance to overt action. S, stimulus force, F, instigating force, for the activity that is occuring. From Atkinson and Birch (1970). Copyright 1970 by John W. Atkinson. Reprinted by permission of John Wiley & Sons.

Model B: Conscious Thought May Amplify a Process Already Implicit in the Conditions of the Moment

The second alternative stresses the importance of underlying or nonconscious sources of motivation. Behavior can occur without reference to conscious thought; however, conscious thought can serve to accentuate these dispositions by instigating or inhibiting action. It does not do this independently, however. So for example, if people perceive that a situation is of moderate difficulty, this can increase or decrease their tendency to undertake activity in this situation, depending upon the strength of their underlying motivation to succeed. To the extent that the underlying motive is strong and positive (i.e., people are success-oriented), then they will jump at the chance to engage in this activity and probably perform well. If the motive is strong and negative (i.e., people are failure-threatened), then they will avoid this activity or perform poorly if forced to engage in the activity.[2] In short, conscious thought may be part of an instigating force or resisting force, and it combines multiplicatively with underlying sources of motivation.

This model covers the work of many of my heroes in social psychology, including Lewin (1938) with his field theory, Tolman (1932) with his purposive behavior in animals and humans, Atkinson and Raynor (1974) with their general theory of achievement motivation, and of course Atkinson and Birch (1970) with *The Dynamics of Action* itself. All these theories assume that behavior is purposive and that it is directed toward some goal as a function of personality and situational determinants. Furthermore, they assume that nonconscious determinants of action are propelled by nonconscious or conscious perceptions of the environment. These thinkers are, in fact, expectancy–value theorists. They believe that the organism undertakes an activity if and only if it has some expectancy regarding the outcome and it values that outcome.

Model C: All Instigation to Action and Resistance to Action Must be Mediated by Conscious Thought

Atkinson first discussed the third model in speaking of "common-sense" approaches to motivation and action (see Atkinson, 1964). Originally it was meant to represent the theorizing of William James, but then Atkinson used it to represent challenges to his theory by various self-assessment theories of achievement motivation (e.g., Trope, 1975) or attribution theories (e.g., Weiner, 1972; see Atkinson & Birch, 1978). All of these theories assume that whenever the environment can tell individuals something new about themselves or the world around them, they will be motivated to act in order to achieve this understanding. These theories argue, then, that all motivated action is preceded by conscious thought. Atkinson (1964) believed that to the extent that a theory postulates that any important overt activity must be screened by covert action, the theory is akin to that of William James, and to a rational or "common-sense" approach to psychological investigation as described above. Thus when Weiner (1972), and later Trope (1975), offered deep cognitive challenges to his theory, Atkinson responded accordingly (Atkinson & Birch, 1978, p. 359):

> What is essential for any cognitive theory of motivation . . . is that it contain explicit statements of how action is determined by cognition and that these statements be used to derive expected characteristics of the measurable stream of behavior. . . . The rebirth of interest in cognitive approaches to motivation must not lead to theories which . . . leave the individual lost in thought (Birch and others, 1974).

Other Options

Since the publication of the original *The Dynamics of Action* (Atkinson & Birch, 1970), two other streams of theories relating covert activity to motivation and cognition have become rather prominent in social psychology. Following from the work of Posner and Snyder (1975), Shallice (1972), and Logan (1980), these theories argue that both nonconscious (automatic) and conscious processes are operating simultaneously, and that both can influence behavior just as they influence thought, emotion, perception, and so on (J. A. Bargh & P. M. Gollwitzer, personal communication, 1994).[3] Shallice (1972), for example, suggests an information-processing model for cognitive processes, which has as a main characteristic that only one action system can be maximally activated at any time. For Shallice, the selector input to the dominant action system corresponds to what is meant by consciousness. That is, the selector input has the functions of selecting which action system is dominant and of setting its goal (Shallice, 1972).

Much work has been done demonstrating that conscious thought in the form of intentions or current concerns (see Klinger, Barta, & Maxeiner, 1981) can override unconscious or automatic tendencies (Bargh, 1984; Logan, 1980; Posner & Snyder, 1975). However, one must ask, "Where do these conscious thoughts come from?" and "Where does the desire to override automatic or nonconscious thoughts come from?" I have little doubt that Atkinson would say, "Why, of course, they come from other action tendencies." I say this because the major premise of *The Dynamics of Action* is that there are many competing tendencies going on at once. Although people are motivated to do many things at any particular point in time, they can only do one. For Atkinson and Birch (1970), that one thing is determined by which tendency is strongest at that point. So if some thought enters consciousness either through cues from the environment or from internal forces, or both, it will override other conscious or nonconscious forces only if its motivational strength is greater. In short, automatic or other nonconscious forces can be overridden simply by the combined strength of some other action tendency.

To the extent, then, that conscious thought selects actional systems in conjunction with underlying motivational forces, this model is no different from Model B.[4] If this selection is not initiated from nonconscious forces, then, as Atkinson and Birch (1970) have said, the model must contain explicit statements of how action is determined by cognition, and these statements must be used to derive expected characteristics of the measurable stream of behavior. I have more to say about this later.

The second cognitive variant has emerged from Schneider and Shiffrin's (1977; Shiffrin & Schneider, 1977) distinction between automatic and controlled information processing. Recent "motivated-tactician" models (see Fiske & Taylor, 1991) are included in this classification. These models assume that more or less automatic or nonconscious processing of information occurs, unless the issue is important. To the extent that the issue or message is personally relevant, controlled or systematic forms of information processing emerge (see Fazio, 1986; Petty & Cacioppo, 1984; Weary et al., 1993). In a sense, this distinction is much like William James's (1890) notion that involuntary control or habit takes precedence unless the individual consciously (voluntarily) seeks control over the situation. Thus, there is automatic or heuristic processing going on when things are not very important, but personal relevance increases voluntary control or systematic processing of information.

Although this model acknowledges nonconscious or automatic forms of information processing, I do not see it as a significant departure from Model C. The organism is simply more efficient, reserving its conscious control over behavior for important matters. More on this variant follows as well. Having examined a few instances in the past, I now turn to my own research to see what answers it provides.

UNCERTAINTY ORIENTATION

My colleagues and I have been working for some time now on what we consider a major domain-nonspecific individual-difference variable, uncertainty orientation (see Sorrentino & Short, 1986; Sorrentino, Raynor, Zubek, & Short, 1990). Briefly, we conceive of people as ranging along a continuum from the "uncertainty-oriented personality" to the "certainty-oriented personality." Those we call "uncertainty-oriented" have a need to know and find out new things about themselves and the world around them. Any time there is uncertainty with regard to just about anything, they are motivated to resolve this uncertainty. These we call "certainty-oriented," by contrast, believe it is not good to find out new things. They are motivated by situations where there is nothing new to find out about themselves or the world around them. They like clarity and avoid or ignore confusion.

The construct of uncertainty orientation was developed by drawing on the work of Kagan (1972), and Rokeach (1960). Kagan (1972) argued that uncertainty reduction is a primary motive, with other motives (e.g., achievement, affiliation), in its service. He noted that "incompatibility between cognitive structures, between cognitive structures and experience, or between cognitive structures and behavior" (p. 54) leaves a person in a state of uncertainty about the self and the environment. In his work on the "open" versus "closed" mind, Rokeach (1960) distinguishes between people who do not appear to be afraid of uncertainty and are capable of resolving it, and people who find new beliefs or inconsistent information threatening.

Clearly, in a broader sense, the concept of uncertainty is seen as a major force to be reckoned with. Fiddle (1980, p. 3) writes:

> The twentieth century has been colored by the principle of uncertainty, taken both in its original Heisenberg meaning of 1927, to refer to a fundamental incommensurability, and in its broadest sense, as a general characteristic of the life of modern man since Einstein's miracle year of 1905 and the killing of the archduke in 1914. Along with relativity, uncertainty is a sort of charismatic concept, exciting those who filter conventional concepts and data through its perspectives.

Our concept of uncertainty orientation can also be seen as part of two of the major dimensions Hofstede (1991) uses to distinguish one culture from another: "avoidance of uncertainty," and "individualism" (vs. "collectivism"). High avoidance of uncertainty would be associated with the certainty-oriented person, and individualism (i.e., self-orientation) would be a feature of the uncertainty-oriented person (see Sorrentino & Short, 1986). Interestingly, much as we speculate for uncertainty-oriented persons (see Sorrentino et al., 1990), Hofstede finds Western cultures highest in individualism and lowest in uncertainty avoidance; Eastern cultures are more likely collectivistic and high in uncertainty avoidance, much as we speculate for certainty-oriented persons (Sorrentino et al., 1990).

Finally, it is important to note that we do get the within-culture differences we expect. We (Sorrentino et al., 1990) have found that university populations are indeed higher in uncertainty orientation than lay populations (e.g., factory workers), and these findings have been replicated (Sorrentino, Holmes, Hanna, & Sharp, 1995). This is important, because we believe that many theories in social psychology mistakenly assume that *all* people are like our uncertainty-oriented people, when in fact *most* people outside of academia are probably certainty-oriented. As we shall see, this fact has considerable bearing on our discussion of conscious thought and action. But now let us look at the research. Much of our research can be split into two parts: The first deals with motivation to process information, whereas the second deals with motivation and action or performance. We have developed a model for each.

Uncertainty Orientation and Information Processing

Figure 27.2 represents our model for information processing. As the figure indicates, we distinguish between more or less automatic forms of information processing (A) and controlled or systematic forms of information processing (C). The crucial situational dimension is the extent to which concerns with uncertainty or certainty are activated. Situations where information about the self, the outcome of the activity, or the environment is uncertain activate concerns about uncertainty. Situations where information about the self, the outcome of the activity, or the environment is certain activate concerns about certainty.[5] The third dimension in Figure 27.2 is, of course, uncertainty orientation. Uncertainty-oriented persons are motivated to process information in situations where uncertainty concerns are activated. Certainty-oriented persons are motivated to process information in situations where concerns about certainty are activated.

Using this information processing model, we can see in Figure 27.2 that an uncertainty-oriented person follows the behavior of what is typically meant by the "motivated tactician" (Fiske & Taylor, 1991). When uncertainty concerns are activated—that is, when the situation contains uncertainty about the self—the uncertainty-oriented person increases his or her controlled

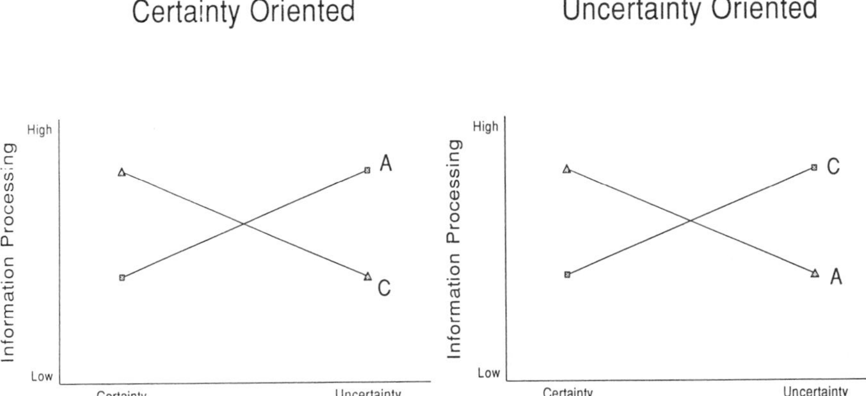

FIGURE 27.2. Strength of controlled (C) versus automatic (A) information processing as a function of certainty and uncertainty activation and of uncertainty orientation.

processing of information, and decreases utilization of more automatic forms. For example, the more personally relevant an issue is—that is, the more it will provide an opportunity to find out new information about the self—the more a person will systematically process the message, such as by attending to the strength of the arguments. Also, the more personally relevant the issue is, the less the person will rely on heuristics, such as source expertise.

The certainty-oriented person, however, behaves in just the opposite fashion. For this person, it is when certainty is activated that he or she will engage in controlled rather than automatic forms of information processing. Hence, as personal relevance increases, controlled processing of information will actually decrease, and automatic forms of information processing will actually increase. This person, in fact, will be more likely to rely on the heuristic of source expertise and less likely to rely on a systematic evaluation of the arguments when an issue is really important.

This specific example refers to one of our studies on attitudes and persuasion (Sorrentino, Bobocel, Gitta, Olson, & Hewitt, 1988, Study 2), where we found exactly what we predicted. Table 27.1, summarizes this study and some of our other research in support of this model. At the top of Table 27.1 are our two dimensions of uncertainty orientation as well as whether the situations studied were likely to activate concerns with uncertainty or certainty. For each study, the table gives the differences between levels of a situational variable on a dependent measure that gives us an idea of the type of information processing being engaged. So for example, we see that the difference in persuasibility as a function of strong versus weak arguments (Sorrentino et al., 1988, Study 2a), indicative of controlled processing, was higher (i.e., 1.55) for the uncertainty-oriented subjects when personal relevance was high (uncertainty activation), and lower (i.e., 0.68) when personal relevance was low (certainty activation). Conversely, for the certainty-oriented subject, the difference in persuasibility as a function of strong versus weak arguments was higher (i.e., 1.52) when personal relevance was low, and lower (i.e., 0.77) when personal relevance was high. So it seems that both uncertainty-oriented and certainty-oriented persons use systematic processing, depending upon the situational relevance of uncertainty or certainty to their underlying personality. Similarly, we see that automatic processing, as judged by an expert source versus a nonexpert source, decreased for the uncertainty-oriented subjects (in fact, there was no difference, 0.00) when personal relevance was high as opposed to low (0.70); yet it increased for the certainty-oriented subjects (from −0.71 to 0.48) when personal relevance was high.[6]

So far, all of our research on information processing has been consistent with this model. This began with our study on self-assessment (Sorrentino & Hewitt, 1984), shown in Table 27.1. Here we demonstrated that Trope's (1979) hypothesis that people will seek information to reduce uncertainty about their ability (i.e., whether they are good or bad at something) applied only to uncertainty-oriented subjects, who choose to take a test with items diagnostic as opposed to nondiagnostic of a new and potentially important ability. Certainty-oriented people did not seek such information, choosing to take a test with more nondiagnostic as opposed to diagnostic items. This was done regardless of whether they believed the potential outcome was likely to be bad or good (not shown in Table 27.1). More recently, we (Brouwers & Sorrentino, 1993) have extended this model to a test of protection motivation theory (Rogers, 1984; Maddux & Rogers, 1983). According to this theory, the motivation to undertake health compliance behavior or preventive action depends upon how threatening the situation is and how efficacious the action will be in preventing the threat from occurring. From our point of view, only uncertainty-oriented persons should be motivated to find out potentially threatening information about the self; hence we thought this would also be a good test of our model.

Here, subjects were invited to seek out additional information concerning a new disease, or in fact to sign up for a kit where they could test for themselves whether or not they had the disease. As can be seen in Table 27.1, compliance with these requests, or the opportunity to find out more about the disease, depended upon threat and efficacy in a manner similar to that in the persuasion study. That is, if we subtract the compliance scores in the low-efficacy condition from those in the high-efficacy condition, we get exactly what the model predicts if we assume that high threat is equivalent to high personal relevance. Uncertainty-oriented subjects were more persuaded by high efficacy under high threat, whereas certainty-oriented subjects were more persuaded by high efficacy under low threat. Certainty-oriented persons' desire to ignore personally relevant information, then, carries over even into life-threatening situations.

Another example shown in Table 27.1 is our research on mind-set the-

TABLE 27.1. Information Processing as a Function of Certainty and Uncertainty Activation and of Individual Differences in Uncertainty Orientation

	Certainty-oriented		Uncertainty-oriented	
Study	Certainty activation	Uncertainty activation	Certainty activation	Uncertainty activation
Brouwers & Sorrentino (1993)				
Mean compliance scores as a function of threat and efficacy (E)				
	Low threat	High threat	Low threat	High threat
(High E − low E)	0.97	−0.15	0.14	0.53
Sorrentino, Bobocel, Gitta, Olson, & Hewitt (1988)				
Study 1. Mean persuasion scores as a function of personal relevance (PR) and one- vs. two-sided communication				
	Low PR	High PR	Low PR	High PR
(Two-sided − one-sided)	−0.25	−1.10	−1.32	−0.60
Study 2a. Mean persuasion scores as a function of personal relevance (PR) and strength of arguments				
	Low PR	High PR	Low PR	High PR
(Strong − weak)	1.52	0.77	0.68	1.55
Study 2b. Mean persuasion scores as a function of personal relevance (PR) and source expertise				
	Low PR	High PR	Low PR	High PR
(Expert − nonexpert)	−0.71	0.48	0.70	0.00
Hanna, Sorrentino, & Gollwitzer (1995)				
Mean number of deliberate thoughts as a function of task diagnosticity (D)				
	Low D	High D	Low D	High D
	2.33	2.03	2.50	3.19
Sorrentino & Hewitt (1984)				
Mean number of items chosen as a function of diagnosticity (D)				
	Low D	High D	Low D	High D
	9.80	8.35	8.63	10.75
Sorrentino, Hewitt, & Raso-Knott (1992)				
Study 1. Mean percentage of ring tosses as a function of risk (R)—skilled				
	Low R	High R	Low R	High R
	38.15	23.57	23.93	50.86
Study 2. Mean percentage of choices as a function of risk (R)—chance				
	Low R	High R	Low R	High R
	54.25	41.50	42.00	67.00
Study 3. Mean percentage of choices as a function of risk (R)—chance				
	Low R	High R	Low R	High R
	44.75	62.00	41.75	68.25
Sorrentino, Holmes, Hanna, & Sharp (1995)				
Mean frequency of partners in close relationships as a function of trust (T) and uncertainty orientation				
	Low or high T	Mod T	Low or high T	Mod T
	20.50	11.00	14.00	25.00

ory (Hanna, Sorrentino, & Gollwitzer, 1995). Using the deliberative phase of Peter Gollwitzer's (1990) mind-set analysis of motivation, we found in the Hanna et al. (1994) study that when a task was perceived as highly diagnostic of a new and important ability (High D), uncertainty-oriented subjects were more likely to engage in deliberative thinking than when the task was perceived as low in diagnosticity (Low D). Again, a reversal was seen for certainty-oriented subjects: They engaged in deliberative thought more when the task was seen as being of low diagnosticity than of high diagnosticity.

Table 27.1 also shows our three studies on risk taking in games of chance and skill (Sorrentino, Hewitt, & Raso-Knott, 1992). Here we found that regardless of whether the uncertainty was about subjects' own skill (Study 1) or simply about chance (Studies 2 and 3), uncertainty-oriented subjects most preferred, and certainty-oriented subjects most avoided, moderate risk, for this was the point of highest uncertainty; high risk and low risk had more certain outcomes of failure or success, respectively. In any skilled situation, moderate risk also enables one to find out most about one's ability (see Trope, 1975; Weiner, 1972).

Finally, we have expanded the model shown in Figure 27.2 to research on close relationships (Sorrentino et al. 1995). Since uncertainty-oriented persons should systematically process information in personally relevant situations, whereas certainty-oriented persons should not, we predicted that uncertainty-oriented partners would have only moderate trust for their partners, as they would always be testing their relationship. We felt that certainty-oriented persons, however, would avoid testing their relationship and would be at more extreme levels of trust. This hypothesis was supported, as shown in Table 27.1. In various self-report measures, diary data, and memory recall of important events, this study also found a definite pattern of discomfort (and indeed psychopathological disturbances) for certainty-oriented persons when they had moderate trust for their partners; this was in fact greater than when they had low trust for their partners. Uncertainty-oriented persons, however, were as much or more satisfied with their relationships in many ways when they had moderate as opposed to high trust for their partners (see Sorrentino et al., 1995)

At present, we are considering the implications of this model for cognitive dissonance, consensus utilization, "groupthink," control motivation and cognition, depression and information processing, and self-disclosure therapy. In all of these, we predict that where these theories predict systematic processing of information, this will only be true for uncertainty-oriented persons when, the information is personally relevant, and for certainty-oriented persons when it is not.

Uncertainty Orientation and Action

When we move to overt activity or performance, a paradigm that is conceptually similar to the information-processing paradigm is observed, as shown in Figure 27.3. Here, instead of automatic versus controlled processing, we have inserted performance differences as a function of achievement-related motives. If we extend our notion that motivation should increase under uncertainty activation for uncertainty-oriented persons, and under certainty activation for certainty-oriented persons, we get the following. For the uncertainty-oriented group, uncertainty activation leads to an increase in performance for "success-oriented" persons, or those who value pride in accomplishment and have little shame over failure, and to a decrease in performance for "failure-threatened" persons, or those who fear failure more than they pride accomplishment. Exactly the reverse occurs for certainty-oriented individuals: They appear to be more motivated and to perform better or worse (depending upon the underlying achievement-related motives) under certainty activation than under uncertainty activation. It is important to note that uncertainty activation does not simply lead to better performance for the uncertainty-oriented persons, nor does certainty activation simply lead to better performance for the certainty-oriented persons. Rather, the outcome depends upon relevant underlying sources of motivation. If these persons are also success-oriented, then everything is fine and certainty or uncertainty activation leads to high performance. However, if persons are also failure-threatened, they become even more anxious and perform more poorly in situations that motivate them to act.

Table 27.2 demonstrates the persistent robustness of this finding. Beginning with the Sorrentino, Short, and Raynor (1984) studies, we see differences in performance between success-oriented and failure-threatened subjects as our model predicts (i.e., across uncertainty orientation and acti-

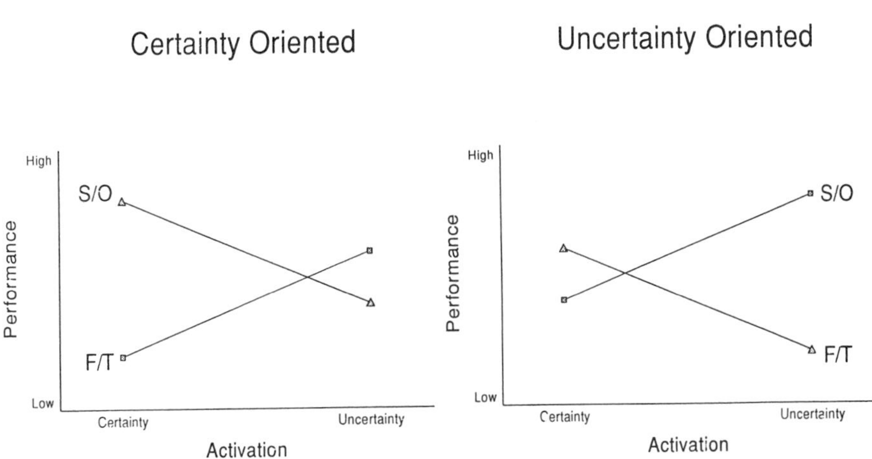

FIGURE 27.3. Performance as a function of certainty and uncertainty activation, uncertainty orientation, and achievement-related motives (S/O success-oriented; F/T, failure-threatened).

TABLE 27.2. Performance Due to Achievement-Related Motives (Success-Oriented vs. Failure-Threatened) as a Function of Certainty and Uncertainty Activation and of Individual Differences in Uncertainty Orientation

	Certainty-oriented		Uncertainty-oriented	
Study	Certainty activation	Uncertainty activation	Certainty activation	Uncertainty activation
Roney & Sorrentino (in press)				
Study 1. Mean differences in complex arithmetic ability as a function of self-discrepancy (SD)				
	Low SD	High SD	Low SD	High SD
	1.93	−1.27	−2.12	2.29
Study 2. Mean differences in midterm (and final) course examinations as a function of ought–other self-discrepancy (SD)				
	Low SD	High SD	Low SD	High SD
	5.30	−3.70	1.67	7.86
Sorrentino, Brouwers, Hanna, & Roney (1995)				
Mean differences in verbal IQ scores as a function of task diagnosticity				
	Non-diagnostic	Diagnostic	Non-diagnostic	Diagnostic
	9.38	5.57	−0.87	7.33
Hanna, Sorrentino, & Gollwitzer (1995)				
Mean differences in complex arithmetic ability during the actional phase of mind-set as a function of task diagnosticity				
	Non-diagnostic	Diagnostic	Non-diagnostic	Diagnostic
	1.02	−3.65	−0.79	2.75
Sorrentino & Roney (1986)				
Mean differences in complex arithmetic ability as a function of task diagnosticity				
	Non-diagnostic	Diagnostic	Non-diagnostic	Diagnostic
	2.23	−2.50	−0.63	3.18
Sorrentino, Short, & Raynor (1984)				
Study 1. Mean difference in complex arithmetic ability scores as a function of uncertain vs. certain outcomes				
	Certain	Uncertain	Certain	Uncertain
	3.10	−1.05	1.70	7.70
Study 2. Mean difference in complex arithmetic ability scores as a function of contingency of outcome to future goals				
	Non-contingent	Contingent	Non-contingent	Contingent
	1.23	−1.20	−0.17	4.00
Study 3. Mean differences in course grades as a function of instrumentality of course to future goals				
	Noninstrumental	Instrumental	Noninstrumental	Instrumental
	8.38	2.24	−1.55	5.48

vation). This is seen where we manipulated the uncertainty of the outcome (Study 1), where we made subjects think future success was contingent or noncontingent on performance at the immediate activity (Study 2), or where subjects perceived their course as instrumental or noninstrumental to future goals (Study 3). We can also see this pattern of results when the task was perceived as diagnostic or nondiagnostic of an important ability (Sorrentino & Roney, 1986), or whem there was a high or low self-discrepancy (Roney & Sorrentino, 1995) in cases where self-discrepancies (see Higgins, Strauman, & Klein, 1986) were varied on a test of arithmetic ability (Study 1) or on final course examinations (Study 2). The latter occurred 7 months following establishment of the discrepancy.

In a very recent study (Sorrentino, Brouwers, Hanna, & Roney, in press), we have extended our research to IQ testing situations. On Jackson's (1984) measure of verbal IQ, which correlates very highly with the total IQ of the Wechsler Adult Intelligence Scale—Revised (Wechsler, 1981), performance varied as a function of whether we introduced the IQ test as diagnostic of subjects' ability (i.e., we told them that it was an IQ test) or nondiagnostic (we told them we did not really know what the test measured and we were just collecting norms). As can be seen in Table 27.2, the pattern of interaction for IQ test performance as a function of uncertainty orientation × achievement-related motives × diagnosticity is the same as those for complex arithmetic ability or course grades, shown in the other studies in Table 27.2. We are particularly proud of this study because it challenges many views regarding supposed trait, genetic, racial, or ethnic differences inintelligence. Atkinson (1974) was right all along: IQ tests are no less the domain of motivation and situational determinants than they are of ability.

Finally, Table 27.2 shows the performance part of the study we completed in collaboration with Peter Gollwitzer (Hanna et al., 1995).[7] Recall that only uncertainty orientation made a difference with regard to thought processing, but here performance interacted with achievement-related motives in support of our model. Interestingly, then, when it comes to overt behavior instead of thought, achievement-related motives "kick in" to increase or decrease performance.

FUNCTIONAL SIGNIFICANCE OF CONSCIOUS THOUGHT

So what does all this have to do with the functional significance of conscious thought? In short, I believe that our data can only be understood in terms of Model B (i.e., conscious thought can amplify a process already implicit in the conditions of the moment). As can be gleaned from Tables 27.1 and 27.2, the behavior of certainty-oriented persons appears to be rather peculiar, indeed almost alien, to those who feel that the need for understanding the self and the world is a universal trait. In our information-processing model, for example, we see that certainty-oriented persons appear to be more likely to use systematic or controlled processing of information when certainty is activated—that is, when the task is of low personal relevance and/or the outcome is fairly predictable. When the task activates uncertainty, they are more likely to use heuristics than to attend to the actual information. As I have mentioned earlier, certainty-oriented persons, though they may appear abnormal or peculiar, are not a small part of society, but in fact may constitute the largest segment of society (see Sorrentino et al., 1990).

If we use Model B, then we can better understand the behavior of both uncertainty-oriented and certainty-oriented persons. On the basis of *The Dynamics of Action* (Atkinson & Birch, 1970), we can think of automatic and controlled processing of information as two competing tendencies, one effortful and the other noneffortful. When uncertainty-oriented persons perceive uncertainty in a situation, this perception feeds back to the unconscious tendency to systematically process information, and propels this tendency into action. For certainty-oriented persons, perceptions of uncertainty serve as an inhibitory force or negaction tendency, preventing the tendency to systematically process information from being expressed in action. In this case, the noneffortful tendency—that is, automatic processing—is expressed in action.

Similar processes takes place when certainty is activated. Here, uncertainty-oriented people lose interest; more precisely, their tendency to process information is blocked, leading to heuristic processing. However, this is precisely where certainty-oriented people express their tendency to systematically process information.

Now, using our performance model, we can see the same instigating and inhibitory forces in operation, but these interact with the additional nonconscious forces surrounding achievement-related motives. Again, conscious perceptions of uncertainty or certainty feed back to nonconscious tendencies, leading uncertainty-oriented and certainty-oriented persons to increase or decrease effort in the situation. However, in achievement-oriented situations, additional tendencies to succeed or avoid failure are "kicked in," leading to increases in instigating or inhibiting forces affecting action.

A good example of this is our work with Peter Gollwitzer on mind-set theory (Hanna et al., 1995). Note in Table 27.1 that when it came to simply thinking about which situation to choose, deliberative thinking increased for uncertainty-oriented subjects when they perceived the task as diagnostic of their abilities, whereas it increased for certainty-oriented subjects when they perceived the task as nondiagnostic. But when it came to actual performance, Table 27.2 shows that achievement-related motives were also affected, leading to greater increases or decreases in performance, depending upon their perceptions of the situation and subjects' uncertainty orientation.

Although this is complex, I think it should be clear that the other two models cannot account for these data. Model A says that conscious thought is irrelevant to actual behavior, but it is clear that conscious attention to the uncertainty or certainty inherent in a situation can accentuate nonconscious tendencies, leading to greater expression or inhibition of action. This is true for both information processing and actual performance. Model C says that all behavior must be mediated by conscious thought, but I think our data clearly show that this is only true to the extent that conscious thought can feed back to tendencies already implicit in the situation. Furthermore, it would be difficult if not impossible to use Model C to explain the behaviors included in these tables. This is particularly true for certainty-oriented persons in general, and for uncertainty-oriented persons when we consider their behavior in conjunction with achievement-related motives.

All of this again would seem to indicate that we have an incomplete picture of what determines information processing and performance if we do not look at both conscious and nonconscious forces as they interact with each other. Conscious thoughts help us to define the situation, but then motivation takes over. My research is only part of the picture, however. I now turn to some of the other contributors in this volume whose work I believe helps support this view and/or suggests possible avenues for future research on the functional significance of conscious thought.[8]

OTHER CONTRIBUTIONS

John Bargh's "auto-motive" model of goal-directed behavior posits three stages through which features of the social environment direct one's behavior automatically. First, mental representations of one's chronic goals or motives within frequently experienced situations come to be automatically linked with representations of those situations. Second, the goal or motive so activated then operates to cause goal-directed behavior, without the need for the individual to consciously choose those behavioral responses with the choice stage bypassed by the automatic link. Third, the individual is not aware of the source of the goal-directed action, making possible misunderstandings and misattributions as to the reasons for the behavior.

Evidence in support of Bargh's model in this volume (see Bargh & Barndollar, Chapter 20) and earlier (see Bargh, 1990) leaves little room for those who believe that all behavior must be preceded by conscious thought, or Model C. Clearly, much behavior can occur without knowledge of the reasons for that behavior. For those of us embracing Model B, Bargh's work presents a particular challenge. For example, one could argue that all the research I have just presented on uncertainty orientation, with or without achievement-related motives, can comfortably fit within his model. That is, uncertainty orientation and achievement-related motives are individual differences in chronically accessible goals, and the situation simply propels or inhibits those goals into or away from action. Although I would argue (or would like to think) that conscious thought in many instances is unnecessary for much behavior, I would agree with Atkinson that conscious thought can accentuate the tendencies implicit in the situation. This can happen in two ways: The motivation of the individual can evoke a thought into consciousness, or the environment can evoke the thought into consciousness. Once the thought is evoked, then it can serve as an additional force, and the strength of the behavior may be increased or decreased. So the thought "I would really like to get an A in this course," occurring from the underlying motivation from within the individual, or from some cue from the environment, may increase performance if the person is high in achievement motivation (it may also decrease performance if the person is failure-threatened). Hence, the thought itself may be a cue, pulling motivational forces. This is an empirical question, and I think it would be an interesting direction for future research.

It seems to me that Daniel Wegner's work (see Ansfield & Wegner, Chapter 21, this volume) shows the wonderful interplay between conscious and nonconscious forces. Here we see that attempts to control the mind result in two processes. There is an operating process that promotes the intended change by searching for mental contents consistent with the intended state. Also, there is a monitoring process that tests whether the operating process is needed by searching for mental content inconsistent with the intended state. Many of us can indeed relate to Ansfield and Wegner's example of how the monitoring of attempts to sleep can in fact keep a person awake. This is an excellent example of how one conscious thought leads to one or more other conscious thoughts that work in opposition to the intended thought.

Atkinson would probably see this as conscious thought serving as an additional instigating force for a number of action tendencies that are inconsistent with the intended thought. For example, when I can't sleep, I may think that it has something to do with my work, and my underlying achievement-related motives and uncertainty orientation bring these thoughts into consciousness. Eventually, the monitoring force kicks in, leading to still other reasons with their competing forces. Cognitive load should by definition bring to mind other competing action tendencies (e.g., causes of stress, reasons for drinking, or depression). Wegner's work clearly indicates that nonconscious forces rule the day, but only in connection with conscious thought; hence Model B would seem most compatible with this approach as well.

Norbert Schwarz's work on motivational implications of feelings and phenomenal experiences (see Schwarz & Bohner, Chapter 6, this volume) endorses an evolutionary, biological approach to the study of emotion and cognitive processing. Although different situations yield distinct affective reactions, resulting in different types of information processing, this is all part of human biological makeup. Schwarz states that emotions exist for the sake of signaling states of the world that have to be responded to, or that no longer need response and action. He also places his work within the framework of evolutionary cognitive psychology (e.g., Cosmides & Tooby, 1989), arguing for a greater range of moods than the happy–sad dichotomy. He notes that evolutionary psychology has maintained that human reasoning is probably *not* characterized by the application of a few general-purpose tools. Rather, humans seem to use a large variety of specialized tools appropriate for different tasks.

For this reason, then, Schwarz's model would appear to embrace Model A. That is, people are biologically predisposed to react to a range of different situations with specific emotions that steer their information processing in a biologically functional direction. I think this is very interesting work and again shows the importance of nonconscious forces governing the systematic processing of information in some instances, and the absence of information processing in others. As far as it goes, it does seem to fit Model A better than the others. However, similar to his feelings-as-information work (see Schwarz, 1990), in which drawing attention to nonconscious sources of mood eliminates feelings as a source of information, it seems likely that conscious thought can also play a role in increasing or decreasing a particular emotional state.

Schwarz's work makes it very clear that those of us interested in the motivation–cognition interface must examine the role emotion plays along with motivation and cognition. Similarly, it would seem that motivation and cognition can interact with many of the predictions made by the evolutionary cognitive approach. For example, I notice that whereas the research reviewed by Schwarz is very successful in predicting information processing and related "cognitive" constructs such as attitudes and persuasion, he points out that it has not been very successful in predicting performance. I think this would be a good place to start looking at the role of other sources of motivation combining with emotional responses in predicting behavior. For example, recall that in our own research testing Peter Gollwitzer's mind-set theory (Hanna et al., 1995), when it came to information processing, uncertainty orientation predicted the amount of deliberative processing as a function of the uncertainty of the situation; when it came to performance, however achievement motivation kicked in, subsuming this lower-order interaction.

Shelly Chaiken was once a Model C person, but has changed her theoretical orientation to be more in line with Model B. Earlier, she followed the motivated-tactician model by arguing that heuristic processing occurs unless the situation is personally relevant; then deliberative or systematic processing of information ensues, and people make a more or less rational decision based on the available evidence (see Chaiken, 1980). Now I think the reader can see from both of our research paradigms that systematic processing of information does not necessarily follow from perceptions of relevance or importance, but may be an orthogonal dimension. I am also excited to see that Chaiken's new work (see Chaiken, Giner-Sorolla, & Chen, Chapter 24, this volume) stresses the importance of personality and underlying sources of motivation as crucial in predicting the type of information processing that will occur as a function of their interaction with situational determinants. All of this clearly indicates that information processing is dependent not only on the information's personal relevance to an individual, but to nonconscious forces governing that person's type of information processing in response to personal relevance.

Eric Klinger's work (see Klinger, Chapter 8, this volume) shows the almost incredible power nonconscious forces can have on our conscious behavior throughout the day and night. Expanding on his classic work on current concerns (Klinger et al., 1981), Klinger develops strong evidence to show that unconscious forces are repeatedly pulled into play by environmental cues, leading to distraction or alternative courses of behavior. Clearly distractor stimuli, or those that evoke an emotional response, are competing tendencies that at least temporarily interfere with ongoing conscious processing of information. This work is highly reminiscent of Freud's (1943) notion that a wish persists until satisfied, or Lewin's (1938) notion that a tension in the life space persists until the goal is reached (i.e., the Zeigarnik effect; Zeigarnik, 1927). It is also a wonderful example of a competing action tendency, much like Wegner's monitoring process (discussed above). I elaborate more on this in the final section.

One issue I wish Klinger had addressed is that of whether conscious thought has any influence on subsequent behavior. So far, the research paradigm appears to consider only nonconscious forces at work. However, it is not unreasonable to assume that conscious thought can have similar effects. Insofar as conscious thought, like nonconscious thought, may serve as a feedback mechanism to emotional arousal, I feel comfortable with the placement of Klinger's theory in Model B.

Fritz Strack (see Strack & Hannover, Chapter 25, this volume) presents an impressive array of research showing that calling attention to the activated nonconscious information can override nonconscious influences. This inevitably results in an overreaction to the nonconscious influence, producing a contrast effect. Although this suggests that conscious thought can override nonconscious impulses, I believe that Strack's future research should and will address the question of what creating awareness of nonconscious influences does to the individual. One could reasonably argue that the person consciously and rationally rules out the role of unconscious forces, thus wielding control over these nasty irrational impulses. On the other hand, Strack's contrast effects are very interesting, in that his subjects appeared to "go out of their way" or "bend over backward" to prove that this did not affect their judgment. This would seem to indicate in and of itself that "reminding" serves as an instigating force to bring other actional tendencies (of which the individual is unaware), such as impression formation or self-evaluation, into action.

Gifford Weary (see Weary & Gannon, Chapter 7, this volume) presents a very important analysis of depression, control motivation, and the processing of information about others. Her work fits in very nicely with Model B. That is, when there is a congruence between depressed and nondepressed perceivers' dispositional goals (control and self-esteem enhancement, respectively) and situational affordances, perceivers will be more motivated to understand the social situation, and as a result will attend more to goal-relevant information. Hence, we see a nice interplay between motivation to process information in order to regain control, and perceptions of the situation in terms of whether it is congruent with these goals.

I am also pleased to see that Weary is moving in the direction of considering whether underlying sources of motivation enhance or decrease the tendency to process information. I have commented on Weary's work before (see Sorrentino, 1993), and there is a striking similarity between Weary's work with moderately depressed people and ours with uncertainty orientation (i.e., the primary goal of moderately depressed people is to reduce uncertainty, and they are most likely to do this when the situation is highly likely to provide information). This raises the question of whether in fact moderately depressed people tend to be uncertainty-oriented, or whether Weary's samples of moderately depressed people are primarily uncertainty-oriented.

The additional question of the behavior of certainty-oriented persons is also raised. I would guess that if they are moderately depressed, they may be more inclined to use heuristic rather than systematic processing of information, relying on experts or others to help them restore control. Much as in Chaiken's views, then, it is quite possible that heuristic versus systematic processing of information is orthogonal to goals of controllability, and depends upon its relevance to the individual.

NEW DIRECTIONS

From mulling over Atkinson and Birch's (1970) *The Dynamics of Action*, our own research on uncertainty orientation, and the issues raised by the authors mentioned above and other contributors to this volume, I believe now that conscious thought is far more important than I originally supposed. Up to this point I have talked about my own research as well as those of the other theorists in terms of the three models listed by Atkinson and Birch in *The Dynamics of Action*. The other theorists, however, have led me to realize that I was overlooking the most important part of that theory—a part I have alluded to earlier.

Recall that by "dynamics," Atkinson and Birch (1970) meant just that. The organism is not static, addressing one goal or action tendency at a time, but is filled with a number of action tendencies competing for expression or overt action. Hence, as I sit here writing, I am not only motivated to write (possibly to gain pride in accomplishment, avoid shame over failure, gain approval from others, avoid fear of social rejection, influence others, etc.); I am simultaneously tempted to listen to the news (I have CNN on in the background), have lunch, watch a movie, go for a walk, have a martini, study my German, and so on and so forth. All of these tendencies (albeit some are stronger than others) are in competition with my current tendency being expressed in action. Thus, although fatigue, consummation of the current action tendency, and/or increases in other action tendencies (e.g., hunger, thirst) may lead me to change what I am currently doing at the nonconscious level, conscious thought can serve to help me choose among action tendencies. Thoughts about the world may turn my attention to watching the news for a moment. Perceiving my stomach growling may lead me to look at my watch, or indeed to get up and go to lunch. On the other hand, thoughts about the deadline I have to finish this chapter may sustain my activity a little longer. In other words, there are numerous forces acting upon me. Any single thought not only may accentuate the ongoing tendency being expressed in action, but may change my behavior, or keep my behavior from changing.

This, then, is the functional significance of conscious thought for a theory of motivation and action. It may not only strengthen or weaken a particular action tendency being expressed in action, but change (or sustain) behavior by strengthening or weakening other action tendencies at any given point in time.

We can see this behavior in the work of some of the theorists discussed above. Clearly Wegner's monitoring process leads to a chain of thoughts, leading to a string of other thoughts, as does cognitive load, preventing us from falling asleep. With Klinger's work, it is clear that current concerns are more or less just "sitting there" waiting to be evoked. When they are, people cannot sustain or at least fully attend to their current action. Strack's awareness manipulations in fact change the nature of action tendencies already implicit in conditions of the moment, leading to other action tendencies (i.e., contrast effects). And although biological processes (Schwarz), control deprivation (Weary), and personal relevance (Chaiken) may lead to particular forms of information processing (depending upon personality and/or biological factors), success or failure of this type of information processing may result in a strengthening or weakening of the current tendency being expressed in action vis-à-vis other tendencies (see Atkinson & Birch, 1970).

Thus, although nonconscious behavior does indeed occur, conscious thought can also strengthen, weaken, or change the very nature of the behavior. With that said, let me state clearly that conscious thought does not occur in a vacuum; it is often the product of nonconscious forces. It can also occur by association or by environmental cues. So I would not go so far as to say that I am speaking of free will in this sense. People's choices are probably the products of past intentions, and it remains for us to show how all of these are products of conscious and nonconscious forces. On the other hand, it is comforting to know that conscious thought is good (or bad) for something.

ACKNOWLEDGMENTS

The research reported here was supported by various Social Sciences and Humanities Research Council of Canada research grants to me as principal investigator. My thanks to John Bargh and Peter Gollwitzer, as well as Steve Hanna, Gordon Hodson, Günter Huber, and Joel Raynor, for their helpful comments during various drafts of this chapter.

NOTES

1. My thanks to Abe Tesser for pointing this work out to me.

2. This example is only for a one-step contingent path (see Atkinson & Raynor, 1974). When the task is *perceived* as relevant to future goals, then circumstances change, depending upon how many steps are in the path (see Atkinson & Raynor, 1974). Again, however, conscious perceptions can amplify tendencies implicit in the conditions of the moment.

3. My thanks to Peter Gollwitzer and John Bargh for pointing this out.

4. It is interesting to note that Shallice's (1972) information-processing model has motivation systems as a key part of the selector input.

5. My thanks to Tory Higgins for suggesting the term "activation" here.

6. Study 1 of this series, shown in Table 27.1, examined the hypothesis that uncertainty- oriented persons would be less persuaded by a one-sided message and more persuaded by a two-sided message as personal relevance increased, whereas the reverse would occur for certainty-oriented persons. Although a significant main effect was found for a one-sided message's being more effective than a two-sided message (accounting for the minus signs in Table 27.1), the predicted pattern of interaction was significant ($p < .001$).

7. This study is not without its problems, but is presented here because it is highly suggestive of ways we can compare information processing with overt behavior or performance.

8. My apologies to the many important contributors I left out of this segment. I would have liked to include them all, but space is restricted.

REFERENCES

Atkinson, J. W. (1964). *An introduction to motivation.* Princeton, NJ: Van Nostrand.

Atkinson, J. W., & Birch, D. (1970). *The dynamics of action.* New York: Wiley.

Atkinson, J. W. (1974). Motivational determinants of intellectual performance and cumulative achievement. In J. W. Atkinson & J. O. Raynor (Eds.), *Motivation and achievement* (pp. 389–410). New York: Holt, Rinehart, & Winston.

Atkinson, J. W., & Birch, D. (1978). *The dynamics of achievement-oriented activity.* New York: Van Nostrand.

Atkinson, J. W., & Raynor, J. O. (1974). *Motivation and achievement.* Washington, DC: V. H. Winston.

Bargh, J. A. (1984). Automatic and conscious processing of social information. In R. W. Wyer, Jr., & T. K. Srull (Eds.), *Handbook of social cognition* (Vol. 3, pp. 1–44). Hillsdale, NJ: Erlbaum.

Bargh, J. A. (1990). Auto-motives: Preconscious determinants of social interaction. In E. T. Higgins & R. M. Sorrentino (Eds.), *Handbook of motivation and cognition: Foundations of social behavior* (Vol. 2, pp. 93–130). New York: Guilford Press.

Birch, D., Atkinson, J. W., & Bongort, K. (1974). Cognitive control of action. In B.

Weiner (Ed.), *Cognitive views of human motivation* (pp. 71–84). New York: Academic Press.

Brouwers, M. C., & Sorrentino, R. M. (1993). Uncertainty orientation and protection motivation theory: The role of individual differences in health compliance. *Journal of Personality and Social Psychology, 65,* 102–112.

Byrne, D. (1971). *The attraction paradigm.* New York: Academic Press.

Cantor, N., Markus, H., Niedenthal, P., & Nurius, P. (1986). On motivation and the self-concept. In R. M. Sorrentino & E. T. Higgins (Eds.), *Handbook of motivation and cognition: Foundations of social behavior* (Vol. 1, pp. 96–121). New York: Guilford Press.

Chaiken, S. (1980). Heuristic versus systematic information processing and the use of source versus message cues in persuasion. *Journal of Personality and Social Psychology, 39,* 752–756.

Cosmides, L., & Tooby, J. (1989). Evolutionary psychology and the generation of culture: II. Case study: A computational theory of social exchange. *Ethology and Sociobiology, 10,* 51–97.

Fazio, R. (1986). How do attitudes guide behavior? In R. M. Sorrentino & E. T. Higgins (Eds.), *Handbook of motivation and cognition: Foundations of social behavior* (Vol. 1, pp. 204–243). New York: Guilford Press.

Fiddle, S. (Ed.) (1980). *Uncertainty: Behavioral and social dimensions.* New York: Praeger.

Fiske, S. T., & Taylor, S. E. (1991). *Social cognition* (2nd ed.). New York: McGraw-Hill.

Freud, S. (1943). *A general introduction to psychoanalysis.* Garden City, NY: Doubleday.

Gollwitzer, P. M. (1990). Action phases and mind-sets. In E. T. Higgins & R. M. Sorrentino (Eds.), *Handbook of motivation and cognition: Foundations of social behavior* (Vol. 2, pp. 53–92). New York: Guilford Press.

Hanna, S. E., Sorrentino, R. M., & Gollwitzer, P. M. (1995). *Informational and affective influences on mind-sets during goal-oriented achievement behaviour.* Manuscript submitted for publication.

Higgins, E. T., & Sorrentino, R. M. (Eds.). (1990). *Handbook of motivation and cognition: Foundations of social behavior* (Vol. 2). New York: Guilford Press.

Higgins, E. T., Strauman, T., & Klein, R. (1986). Standards and the process of self-evaluation: Multiple affects from multiple stages. In R. M. Sorrentino & E. T. Higgins (Eds.), *Handbook of motivation and cognition: Foundations of social behavior* (Vol. 1, pp. 23–63). New York: Guilford Press.

Hofstede, G. (1991). Empirical models of cultural differences. In N. Bleichrodt & P. J. D. Drenth (Eds.), *Contemporary issues in cross-cultural psychology* (pp. 4–20). Amsterdam: Swets & Zeitlinger.

Hull, C. L. (1943). *Principles of behavior.* New York: Appleton-Century-Crofts.

Jackson, D. N. (1984). *MAB: Multidimension Aptitude Battery Manual.* Port Huron, MI: Research Psychologists Press.

Jacoby, L. L., & Kelley, C. M. (1990). An episodic view of motivation: Unconscious influences of memory. In E. T. Higgins & R. M. Sorrentino (Eds.), *Handbook of motivation and cognition: Foundations of social behavior* (Vol. 2, pp. 451–481). New York: Guilford Press.

James, W. (1890). *Principles of psychology* (2 vols.). New York: Henry Holt.

Jaynes, J. (1976). *The origin of consciousness in the breakdown of the bicameral mind.* Boston: Houghton Mifflin.

Kagan, J. (1972). Motives and development. *Journal of Personality and Social Psychology, 22,* 51–66.

Klinger, E., Barta, S. G., & Maxeiner, M. E. (1981). Current concerns: Assessing therapeutically relevant motivation. In P. C. Kendall & S. D. Hollon (Eds.), *Assessment and strategies for cognitive-behavioral interventions* (pp. 161–196). New York: Academic Press.

Kuhl, J. (1986). Motivation and information processing: A new look at decision making, dynamic change, and action control. In R. M. Sorrentino & E. T. Higgins (Eds.), *Handbook of motivation and cognition: Foundations of social behavior* (pp. 404–434). New York: Guilford Press.

Lewin, K. (1938). *The conceptual representation and the measurement of psychological forces.* Durham, NC: Duke University Press.

Logan, G. D. (1980). Atention and automaticity in Stroop and priming tasks: Theory and data. *Cognitive Psychology, 12,* 523–553.

Maddux, J. E., & Rogers, R. W. (1983). Protection motivation and self-efficacy: A revised theory of fear appeals and attitude change. *Journal of Experimental Social Psychology, 19,* 469–479.

Petty, R. E., & Cacioppo, J. T. (1984). The effects of involvement on reponses to argument quanity and quality: Central and peripheral routes to persuasion. *Journal of Personality and Social Psychology, 46,* 69–81.

Polivy, J. (1990). Inhibition of internally cued behavior. In E. T. Higgins & R. M. Sorrentino (Eds.), *Handbook of motivation and cognition: Foundations of social behavior* (Vol. 2, pp. 131–147). New York: Guilford Press.

Posner, M. I., & Snyder, C. R. R. (1975). Attention and cognitive control. In R. Solso (Ed.), *Information processing and cognition: The Loyola Symposium.* Hillsdale, NJ: Erlbaum.

Rogers, R. W. (1984). Changing health-related attitudes and behaviors: The role of preventative health psychology. In J. H. Harvey, J. E. Maddux, R. P. McGlynn, & C. D. Stoltenberg (Eds.), *Social perception in clinical and counselling psychology* (Vol. 2, pp. 91–112). Lubbock, TX: Texas Tech University Press.

Rokeach, M. (1960). *The open and closed mind: Investigations into the nature of belief systems and personality systems.* New York: Basic Books.

Roney, C. J. R., & Sorrentino, R. M. (1995). Reducing self-discrepancy or maintaining self-congruence: Uncertainty orientation, self-regulation, and performance. *Journal of Personality and Social Psychology, 68*(3), 485–487.

Schneider, W., & Shiffrin, R. M. (1977). Controlled and automatic human information processing: I. Detection, search, and attention. *Psychological Review, 84,* 1–66.

Schwarz, N. (1990). Feelings as information: Informational and motivational functions of affective states. In E. T. Higgins & R. M. Sorrentino (Eds.), *Handbook of motivation and cognition: Foundations of social behavior* (Vol. 2, pp. 527–561). New York: Guilford Press.

Shallice, T. (1972). Dual functions of consciousness. *Psychological Review, 79,* 383–393.

Shiffrin, R. M., & Schneider, W. (1977). Controlled and automatic human information processing: II. Perceptual, learning, automatic attending, and a genereral theory. *Psychological Review, 84,* 127–189.

Skinner, B. F. (1953). *Science and human behavior.* New York: Macmillan.

Sorrentino, R. M. (1993). The warm look in control motivation and social cognition. In G. Weary, F. Gleicher, & L. Marsh (Eds.), *Control motivation and social cognition* (pp. 291–322). New York: Springer-Verlag.

Sorrentino, R. M., Bobocel, C. R., Gitta, M. Z., Olson, J. M., & Hewitt, E. C. (1988). Uncertainty orientation and persuasion: Individual differences in the effects of personal relevance on social judgements. *Journal of Personality and Social Psychology, 55*(6), 357–371.

Sorrentino, R. M., Brouwers, M. C., Hanna, S. E., & Roney, C. J. R. (in press). The nature of the test taking situation: Informational and affective influences on test performance. *Learning and Individual Differences.*

Sorrentino, R. M., & Hewitt, E. C. (1984). The uncertainty reducing properties of achievement tasks revisted. *Journal of Personality and Social Psychology, 4,* 884–899.

Sorrentino, R. M., Hewitt, E. C., & Raso-Knott, P. A. (1992). Risk-taking in games of chance and skill: Individual differences in affective and information value. *Journal of Personality and Social Psychology, 62,* 522–533.

Sorrentino, R. M., & Higgins, E. T. (Eds.). (1986). *Handbook of motivation and cognition: Foundations of social behavior* (Vol. 1). New York: Guilford Press.

Sorrentino, R. M., Holmes, J. G., Hanna, S. E., & Sharp, A. (1995). Uncertainty orientation and trust: Individual differences in close relationships. *Journal of Personality and Social Psychology, 68*(2), 314–327.

Sorrentino, R. M., Raynor, J. O., Zubek, J. M., & Short, J. C. (1990). Personality functioning and change: Informational and affective influences on cognitive, moral, and social development. In E. T. Higgins & R. M. Sorrentino (Eds.), *Handbook of motivation and cognition: Foundations of social behavior* (Vol. 2, pp. 193–228). New York: Guilford Press.

Sorrentino, R. M., & Roney, C. J. R. (1986). Uncertainty orientation, achievement-related motivation, and task diagnosticity as determinants of task performances. *Social Cognition, 4,* 420–436.

Sorrentino, R. M., & Short, J. C. (1986). Uncertainty orientation, motivation and cognition. In R. M. Sorrentino & E. T. Higgins (Eds.), *Handbook of motivation and cognition: Foundations of social behaviour* (Vol. 1, pp. 379–403). New York: Guilford Press.

Sorrentino, R. M., Short, J. C., & Raynor, J. O. (1984). Uncertainty orientation: Implications for affective and cognitive views of achievement behaviour. *Journal of Personality and Social Psychology, 46,* 189–206.

Tolman, E. C. (1932). *Purposive behavior in animals and men.* New York: Appleton-Century.

Trope, Y. (1975). Seeking information about one's own ability as a determinant of choice among tasks. *Journal of Personality and Social Psychology, 32,* 1004–1013.

Trope, Y. (1979). Uncertainty-reducing properties of achievement tasks. *Journal of Personality and Social Psychology, 37,* 1505–1518.

Weary, G., Gleicher, F., & Marsh, K. L. (Eds.). (1993). *Control motivation and social cognition.* New York: Springer-Verlag.

Wechsler, D. (1981). *Manual for the Wechsler Adult Intelligence Scale—Revised.* New York: Psychological Corporation.

Weiner, B. (1972). *Theories of motivation: From mechanism to cognition.* Chicago: Rand McNally.

Weiner, B. (1986). Attribution, emotion, and action. In R. M. Sorrentino & E. T. Higgins (Eds.), *Handbook of motivation and cognition: Foundations of social behavior* (Vol. 1, pp. 281–312). New York: Guilford Press.

Zajonc, R. B. (1965). Social facilitation. *Science, 149,* 269–274

Zeigarnik, B. (1927). Das Behalten erledigter und unerledigter Handlugen. *Pscyholgische Forschung, 9,* 1–85.

CHAPTER 28

Some Ways in Which Goals Differ and Some Implications of Those Differences

Charles S. Carver

The contributions on which the editors of this volume have asked me to comment represent a diverse array of topics. The topics do, however, share a number of common threads, and in this chapter I point to some of them. I also point to a few places where I have questions, concerns, and observations. In many cases, the questions and concerns reduce to the wish that I knew more than I do about how something works, or a concern about whether a process will generalize past the setting in which it has been studied. In a few cases, I have something to add that I think goes beyond the points these authors have made themselves.

My reactions to these chapters have arisen within the framework of a particular view of behavior that I find familiar and congenial. Accordingly, I begin this commentary with a brief sketch of that viewpoint, to serve as background.

BACKGROUND: GOALS AND EXPECTANCIES

The concept that forms the backbone of this group of chapters—indeed, perhaps the entire book—is the goal concept. This is a concept that is fundamental to the way I view the world (e.g., Carver & Scheier, 1990a, 1990b, in press), though I haven't emphasized it as much as other ideas that go hand in hand with it (i.e., feedback processes). I see virtually all behavior as goal-directed, even though people often don't have a perfectly clear idea (either as observers or as actors) of what goal lies behind a particular action; even though the goals are not always planned or even held in consciousness while they are being pursued; and even though the goals are sometimes so small-scale and concrete that they are of interest to motor control researchers (e.g.,

Rosenbaum, 1991; Schmidt, 1988) rather than to personality and social psychologists.

As do many of the other authors represented in this volume, I see a person's goals and the nature of those goals as providing form and structure to the person's life. It is important to keep in mind, in this regard, that goals can be dynamic in quality as well as static. Goals aren't solely places that people are trying to get to as endpoints; goals often constitute entire paths of movement. For example, the goal to "having a holiday" is not to emerge relaxed at the other end of a blank 4-day period, but to experience whatever leisure activities the holiday comprises.

Another idea I've found useful as a heuristic for thought and discussion is the idea that a person's goals have a natural hierarchicality in their ordering. This, of course, is a more central idea in other people's theories—action identification being the most prominent among them (Vallacher & Wegner, 1985, 1987). People have abstract, high-level goals that they pursue by means of lower-level activities. An actor can view a given action at many levels and control it from many levels. Sometimes trying a new task is simply trying a new task. Sometimes, however, the person trying the new task isn't focused on trying a new task, but instead is trying to live up to his or her idealized self-image. This is an altogether different thing to be doing, even if the physical movements that take place are exactly the same. This view assumes that whichever level of abstraction the person is focused on while performing the behavior is the level that is functionally superordinate, with action qualities at lower levels of abstraction being subsumed and engaged automatically by that one (see Carver & Scheier, in press, for a broader discussion).

A final set of ideas I've found indispensable in trying to talk about behavior concerns the fact that people often find it difficult to do what they set out to do. What happens when people confront adversity on the way to their destinations? Along with many others, I've assumed that the answer depends in part on people's expectancies about the eventual outcomes of their efforts, given the situation they're in (Carver & Scheier, 1981, 1990a, in press). With favorable expectancies, people keep trying to move toward their goals. If expectancies are unfavorable enough, people quit trying. This issue of continued effort versus disengagement is a critical one in talking about goal pursuits (cf. Klinger, 1975).

These assumptions represent reference points for me in what I have to say in the remainder of my comments. With this in mind, then, let me turn to the chapters themselves.

COMMENTS ON THE CHAPTERS

Dweck: Implicit Theories as Organizers of Goals and Behavior

Carol Dweck's contribution to this volume (Chapter 4) represents an eloquent opening statement about goals—a statement that makes a number of important points. One of those points is really a first emphatic statement of a more general theme that stands behind several of of these chapters, and which I have assimilated into my own title: the idea that goals are not all alike. In the research reported here, it becomes very clear that goals are not all alike, even when the task is the same. Furthermore, it's clear that people's goals are related to their broader views of reality, their sense of the way the world is constructed—and, more particularly, to their sense of the way human beings function. I have several reactions to the way in which these ideas play themselves out.

Hierarchicality

I believe that there is a hierarchical organization implicit behind Dweck's view of the goals used by her subjects (Figure 28.1). Task performances represent a means by which they hold onto their self-esteem, or their general sense of fit between their present self and their desired or ideal self. The issue of self-esteem is particularly obvious in the behavior of the group Dweck has called "helpless" children—those with performance goals who are experiencing failure. These children's self-inflating verbalizations (e.g., talking about skills in other domains, boasting of wealth and possessions) clearly reflect a desire to regain threatened self-esteem in ways other than in the domain that's responsible for the current threat. This behavior suggests the themes of symbolic self-completion theory (Wicklund & Gollwitzer, 1982), with its assumption that people can fill in an experienced incompleteness in diverse ways.

This strong sense of a connection between performance goal and threatened self-esteem initially seduced me into thinking that the hierarchies of the two groups Dweck and her colleagues focus on differ in their degree of elaboration. My first inference was that performance goals are directly tied to broad sense of self-worth, and that learning goals are linked more indirectly, with an intermediate goal of acquiring greater skills. But this doesn't really capture what the research shows. Both of these orientations have an intermediate goal concerning ability. However, the learning-goal hierarchy (Figure 28.1A) is one where the intermediate goal is more dynamic in nature (*gain* task ability), compared to the more static goal in the performance hierarchy (*have* task ability). This difference in the dynamic versus static quality becomes more apparent as the goals themselves are linked to entity versus incremental views of what ability consists of. Upon further reflection, then, I see a hierarchicality in both groups (or both construals of reality), but the midlevel element in the hierarchy is more dynamic (focused on change rather than on absolute level) in the one case than in the other.

Let me step away from this point for a moment to say that one of the questions raised by the general theme that goals are not all alike is "What are the parameters on which goals differ?" What is the best way to think about *how* goals differ? One of the answers from Dweck's contribution to this volume

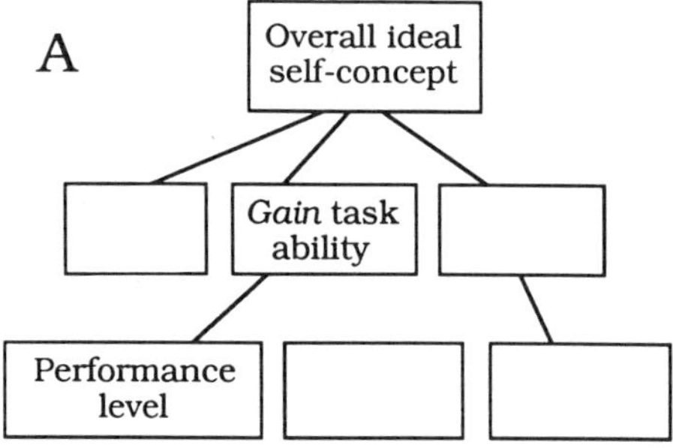

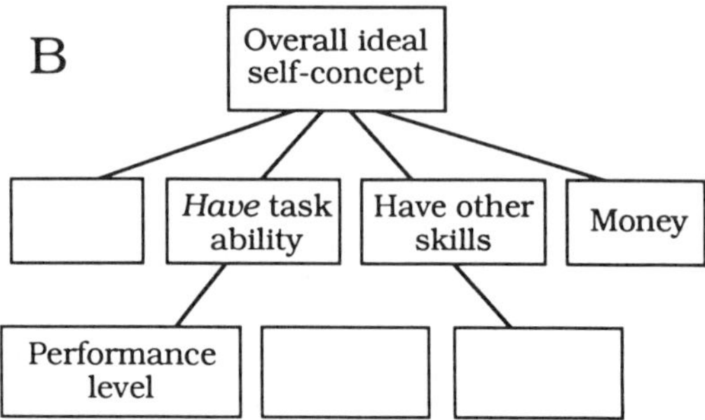

FIGURE 28.1. Three-level goal hierarchy (A) of a child who holds a learning goal and (B) of a child who holds a performance goal. For the child with the learning goal, performing well (eventually) provides evidence of gaining in the ability relevant to the task, which contributes to the overall sense of self-esteem. For the child with the performance goal, performing well creates the sense of having a high level of the ability, which contributes to the overall sense of self-esteem. (Other qualities, of course, also contribute to self-esteem in both cases. In the case of children with performance goals who were failing at the task, however, several other contributors were mentioned spontaneously.) From Carver and Scheier (in press).

is that goals vary in the extent to which they incorporate a dynamic quality. This, I think, represents a very important contribution in itself.

I find the analysis particularly intriguing—and compelling—with respect to social domains of application. I am someone who has tended to have performance goals concerning relationship issues and an entity orientation to the skills involved, and my behavior in the face of adversity is pretty much the same as that of the helpless children who confront rejection. The perspective taken by Dweck has a great deal to say about the problems that people develop in their social interactions, and potentially about the ways in which those problems can be diminished. I will be interested in further developments as Dweck and her collaborators think more about that sort of question—how to get people to shift their orientations toward the more dynamic, learning goals in social contexts.

Disengagement

Dweck's recent analysis of the nature of children's goals builds in part upon her earlier work, in which the two types of children responded differently to failure (Diener & Dweck, 1978). These two patterns of responses were labeled as "mastery-oriented" and "helpless." The patterns clearly reflect the same kinds of responses that have been postulated by many to follow from confidence and doubt about succeeding. The mastery-oriented group showed continued efforts, no deterioration in strategies, and positive, hopeful affect. The helpless group showed reduction in effort, off-task thinking, deterioration in strategy, negative affect, and performance deficit.

One thing the later work has added to this is the idea that the disengagement tendency that follows from failure and doubt can be circumvented by somehow instituting a learning orientation in place of a performance orientation (Dweck & Leggett, 1988). This would appear to be a very important point. It even begins to suggest that expectancies of success can be made to be unimportant. I want to be careful, though, about being carried away too quickly with this inference, because I suspect it is only partly correct.

What has been shown in this research is that if they are induced to take a learning orientation, even children who perceive their ability as being low fail to show deficits (Table 28.1, line 2). To put it differently, deficits can be circumvented even among those subjects who have doubts about the adequacy of their performances. What has not been addressed yet is whether having a different kind of doubt—doubt about being able to *increase one's ability*—will recreate the deficits.

It's important to keep in mind that having a learning orientation doesn't necessarily imply that the person will be successful in acquiring the new skill—only that the person has the belief that the skill is acquirable. The incremental view can be held as long as increments do occur periodically. But what happens in the face of extended failure? One failure doesn't mean inability to learn, but enough failure begins to carry that message. I have to suspect that extended failure will create the perception of doubt about reaching the desired goal—in this case, the goal of extending one's ability—and yield the deficits one would like to avoid (Table 28.1, line 3).

I also suspect that what Deci and Ryan (Chapter 1, this volume) call "optimally challenging" situations are likely to prove most effective for persons who hold learning goals. These are the situations where people don't succeed all the time, but they do succeed some of the time. Without success some of the time, even an incremental view of the skill involved is likely to become undermined.

In short, although it's clear that the shift to a learning orientation is facilitative of continued efforts, I don't think this shift gets us entirely around

TABLE 28.1. Under a Learning Goal, Relationships among Perceived Ability, Confidence about Performance, Confidence about Learning, and Performance Deficit

Ability	Confidence about performance	Confidence about increasing ability	Is there a deficit?
1. High	High	High	No
2. Low	Low	High	No
3. Low	Low	Low	?

Note. When subjects have a learning goal, their perceived level of ability has less impact on the display of deficits than in other circumstances (lines 1 and 2). Confidence about performing well seems to be no longer an issue, apparently because subjects of both ability levels have confidence about being able to increase their ability. But what happens if something about one's experience threatens that sense of confidence (line 3)?

the problems that result from doubts. Rather, it puts off the doubts somewhat, because they necessarily take longer to develop. This is an important step in itself, of course, but it doesn't entirely remove the problem.

Ryan, Sheldon, Kasser, and Deci: All Goals Are Not Created Equal

Let me turn now to the contribution by Ryan, Sheldon, Kasser, and Deci (Chapter 1), which has the theme of diversity among goals embedded in its very title (my own title being but a pale echo of theirs). Ryan et al. take a different approach to this issue than others of this group have taken. Their emphasis is on the origins of the intent to act, and on the forces that a person sees as influencing the creation of that intention. Some actions are undertaken out of interest in the activity or the belief that the activity is intrinsically valuable. These are called "self-determined" behaviors. Some actions are undertaken for extrinsic reasons—for example, to gain payment or to satisfy someone's pressures or demands. These are called "controlled" behaviors. Behaviors can be controlled even if the control occurs entirely inside one's own mind. Thus, people who engage in actions because they know they would feel guilty if they didn't do so are engaging in controlled behavior.

Although some of us are accustomed to thinking in terms of differences between intrinsically motivated and extrinsically motivated behaviors, this model distinguishes among extrinsically motivated actions on the basis of the extent to which the activities are integrated into the structure of the self. In most respects these latter distinctions are what matter most, rather than the distinction between intrinsic and extrinsic motivation. That is, in the findings reviewed by Ryan et al., there appears to be a functional split between what they call "introjected regulation" and "identified regulation."

In introjected regulation, the individual engages in the behavior for extrinsic and controlling reasons, although the regulation is happening intrapsychically (e.g., the behavior is done to avoid a sense of guilt). In identified regulation, the individual has accepted the behavior as personally important and meaningful. For all practical purposes, identified regulation appears to be equivalent to intrinsic motivation in its consequences. Identified regulation (and the even more advanced "integrated regulation") can be viewed as self-determined, even though the behavior is extrinsically motivated.

I want to draw two simple links between these ideas about these two classes of behaviors and ideas that appear in two other chapters (Table 28.2). One link is to the Higgins model of self-guides (see Chapter 5). In many ways it sounds as though self-determined behaviors reflect the operation of what Higgins calls "ideals," whereas controlled behaviors reflect the operation of "oughts." Ideals are self-guides one intrinsically aspires to. Oughts are duties or obligations—values to which one accedes in order to avoid criticism or disapproval (or self-criticism or disapproval). The other link is to Ajzen's discussion of intentions (see Chapter 17), which derive both from one's own personal desires and from implicit pressures that originate outside the self. Rather than emphasize the divergent effects of these two sources of influence, as both Ryan et al. and Higgins have done, Ajzen emphasizes that most intentions people develop incorporate elements of both of these sources of influence.

Despite these similarities, there are differences in psychological tone among these three theories. Ryan et al. have said that behavior initiated by either external or internal pressures lacks a sense of volition or choice, despite the fact that the behavior is intentional. In thinking about this assertion, I began to wonder whether the similarity stands up that well after all between the self-determined behaviors of Ryan et al. and either the attitude-based intentions of Ajzen or the ideal-based behavior of Higgins (though I have much less concern about the comparability of controlled behaviors and oughts).

Part of the problem for me here is that I find the concept of self-determination a very hard one to hold onto. I have the feeling that just as I have a handle on it, it slips away from me. Ryan et al. indicate that behavior is self-determined only when there is no sense of coercion. I find myself wondering about whether a person's ideals, no matter how pure, are noncoercive. If ideals do become coercive of an action, the behavior is controlled instead of self-determined. For example, if you are writing a book for pure-

TABLE 28.2. Parallels among Three Theories in Considering Two Classes of Behavior

	Ryan et al.	Higgins	Ajzen
Class 1	Self-determined	Ideal-based	Attitude-based
Class 2	Controlled	Ought-based	Subjective-norm-based

Note. See the theorists' respective chapter for greater detail on the distinctions they draw between the two classes.

ly self-determined reasons, but you force yourself to keep working through a weekend when you'd really rather be doing something else, the behavior of that weekend would seem to be controlled rather than self-determined. The critical element seems to be how a person is oriented to an experience when it occurs.

In thinking about this issue, I find myself thinking of the reactance phenomenon of self-induced threat to freedom, in which just having an initial preference for one of several options can come to constitute a perceived infringement on one's freedom of choice (Linder & Crane, 1970; Linder, Wortman, & Brehm, 1971). Can behavior that follows from having an initial preference be self-determined if one doesn't think about it and just does it, but controlled if one thinks about it hard enough to realize that having the preference limits one's options? In much the same vein, while working on a textbook chapter on Carl Rogers, I found myself asking the question of how to decide when one's desires for oneself are really self-imposed conditions of worth, as opposed to goals for self-actualization. It's perhaps unfair to treat self-determination as equivalent to self-actualization, but it's hard to think about the issues that Ryan et al. raise without gravitating to this broader question as well.

Perhaps a large part of the problem for me is knowing how to tell whether an activity has been incorporated into the self or only introjected (this may be a personal problem, since I also have trouble telling my ideals from my oughts). There must be criteria beyond simply whether the behavior feels as though it's being done spontaneously with no subjective sense of coercion. But that seems to be the clearest clue to whether an action should be viewed as self-determined or not. I find myself very uncomfortable with this idea for the reasons just outlined, but I don't know exactly what to do about it. This is one of those cases where I wish I understood better than I do how things work.

An important strength of the approach of Ryan et al. is its emphasis on an issue that goes beyond self-determination: the issue of how people's goals relate to organismic needs. They note that selfish greed and generativity would be equivalent in value if the only thing that mattered was efficacy in performing the behavior. They suggest that the critical question in evaluating the value of a behavior is whether it satisfies a need directly or is only a means to an end. In general, greed-driven behavior is a means to an end. (I am forced to ask, though, whether this is inevitably so; in principle, can't this desire be integrated into the self?)

The evidence indicates that psychological investment in intrinsic goals is associated with higher levels of vitality, whereas investment in financial and other extrinsic goals is associated with personal and social dysfunction. Thus, the intrinsic–extrinsic distinction appears to stand as an important one, as goals relate to psychological well-being (though I raise a question about the meaning of this pattern of findings a little farther along, in the context of the chapter by Emmons). The substance of this pattern is quite consistent with a theme that underlies this body of work as a whole: that the best of human experience is characterized by growth and self-actualization.

Ajzen: The Directive Influence of Attitudes on Behavior

Let me turn now to Ajzen's chapter (Chapter 17). In it he discusses the role of attitudes and subjective norms in the adoption of intentions toward actions. His focus is on the controlled and deliberate aspects of the decision-making process that often lies behind action. Goals are even more deeply embedded in this analysis than in most, though this may or may not be apparent at first glance. At first glance the most obvious application of the goal construct is in the intention itself; that is, the intention is a goal for the eventual behavior. In another sense, however, there are two other goals that always lie behind the intention and behind the behavior that results from it. One of these goals is provided by the person's attitude, the other by the subjective norm. Thus, in Ajzen's model any intention-based action reflects at least a two-level hierarchy of behavior. An additional goal may also lie behind the development of at least some intentions, if the individual's personal opinions and subjective norms both relate to the overall sense of desired self (Figure 28.2).

Ajzen tends to take the position that the determination of behavior is a rational process, in which attitudes, subjective norms, and perceptions of personal control in the domain to which the intention is relevant become influential to the extent that they are brought to consciousness during the decision process. An interesting question is the extent to which the intentions that result are self-determined. An intention based primarily on a subjective norm has a very different character in that respect than does an intention based primarily on an attitude. Subjective norms are the internal

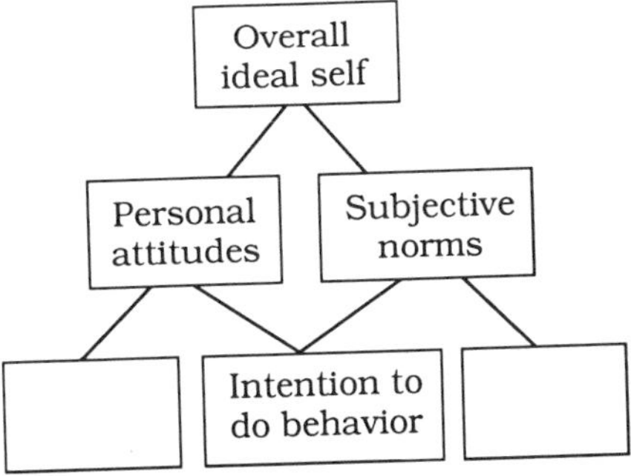

FIGURE 28.2. Ajzen's model of intentions implies a potential hierarchy of three further goals behind the development of a specific behavioral intention. Carrying out an intention thus may serve to enhance conformity to one's attitude, the internalized norms of one's comparison group, and even the overall idealized self.

representation of the wishes of others; behaviors based on these are controlled. Attitudes are personal; behaviors based on these are more self-determined (in Ryan et al.'s sense).

I find myself asking more questions about this contribution than about some of the others. Given the division of underlying goal values into attitudes and subjective norms, I find it curious that so little is known concerning possible differences between the intentions that result from these two sources of influence. Are intentions that are heavily weighted by attitudes different in any way from those that are heavily biased by subjective norms? If they differ in the extent to which they are self-determined, there may also be further consequences. Intentions based on attitudes may be associated with indicators of higher levels of vitality, compared to intentions based on subjective norms. This seems to me an interesting direction for future inquiry.

I would like to note briefly what I regard as the importance of a shift from the older theory of reasoned action to its successor, the theory of planned behavior (Ajzen, 1988). In the newer model, it is acknowledged that behaviors cannot always be assumed to be effective in moving toward desired ends. One might view this variable as controllability (as Ajzen does), or as efficacy (as Bandura does), or as expected success in attaining the outcome (as I do). What one calls the variable is less important to me at present than the fact that this issue is now explicitly recognized within this model as important. The evidence is clear that even at the level of forming intentions, people take into account their perceptions of whether the behavior will yield the desired outcome. People don't form intentions to do things they're sure won't work.

Wicklund and Steins: Person Perception under Pressure

The contribution of Wicklund and Steins (Chapter 22) diverges considerably from the others in this group of chapters. It addresses themes involved in the viewing and construing of other persons with whom an individual is interacting. The overriding message of this chapter is that person perception is always influenced by the perceiver's own goals regarding the other. Wicklund and Steins argue that accurate person perception involves more than the noticing of particular physical and behavioral characteristics of the other. If the perceiver is to make meaningful inferences about the other, the process must involve taking the other's perspective.

Taking the other's perspective may be a naturally occurring phenomenon in some circumstances, but there are forces that influence its likelihood of occurrence. Specifically, Wicklund and Steins argue that the processing of social situations changes as a result of the other person's motivational significance to the subject ("press") and the presence in the observer of some intrapsychic conflict. It is argued that press serves to exaggerate the potential impact of other forces. In the absence of any force that counters perspective taking, press enhances perspective taking. But if the element of

With respect to cultural diversity, Wicklund and Steins suggest that the ess of Western society induces a tendency to disregard others' perspec- es. I can readily agree with this opinion. I am less confident, however, about e other side of their assertion: that living in an undeveloped country is pecially conducive to perspective taking. Nevertheless, their overriding essage—that the attempt to determine what another person is like is un- rmined by having strong motivation-relevant connections to that person— an interesting and important one.

ttingen: Positive Fantasy and Motivation

very different question about goals was taken up by Oettingen (Chapter . The question concerns how expectancies and fantasies influence be- vior. Data from several studies indicate that positive expectations promote ter outcomes (compared to more negative expectations), but that posi- e fantasies often have the opposite effect. Positive fantasies seem to have potential to interfere with effort and consequent goal attainment.

Why is this so? The answer suggested by Oettingen is that positive fan- ies undermine effort by creating the sense that the outcome will be at- ned effortlessly. In this view, then, positive fantasies tend to move a person m a "try" mode of functioning into a mode in which the goal seems al- dy attained and trying is unnecessary. This view rests on the assumption t attaining most important goals in life entails dealing with hardship and iculty along the way. Only by exerting effort under adversity can people successful in reaching such goals. If positive fantasy undermines effort, nperils goal attainment. Support for the notion that fantasies have this ect comes from the finding that among subjects searching for jobs, posi- fantasy was related to sending out fewer job applications.

Oettingen goes on to argue that positive fantasy need not always have e bad effects. Positive fantasy can be mobilized to facilitate action (provid- hat one's expectancies are also positive). The trick is to juxtapose the itive fantasy with reflection on one's current reality. Given simultaneous sideration of these two images, the fantasy is apparently treated as a goal action (which it otherwise is not treated as being), and the current-reality ge makes it salient that the goal hasn't yet been attained. The result— n favorable expectations—is engagement in active goal-directed effort. h unfavorable expectations, on the other hand, the result is a clearer ten- cy to disengage effort.

Note that this induced juxtaposition between goal and present reality sentially the same comparison as that which occurs in a feedback loop ver & Scheier, 1981, 1990a, in press). The pattern thus seems to fit a ure in which feedback loops need to have all their elements in place for on to occur. The data also appear to indicate that when a person is ex- ning one of these mental representations in the absence of the other, eedback loop is incomplete. As a result, the engagement in action that conflict is present, press causes that conflict to have a stronger i it otherwise would.

One difficulty I have with this analysis concerns the role tha for conflict. Wicklund and Steins argue that conflict creates a wish to change the other to suit the needs of what the observer complish. To put it differently, the perceiver is no longer motiv the true character of the person perceived, but desires to see in a way that is temporarily expedient. Thus, there is no nee other's perspective. As press increases, the wish to transform comes more intense. The combination of high press and high imally disrupts perspective taking. So far, so good.

What's harder for me to understand in this analysis, thoug flict should not *uniformly* interfere with perspective taking. Tha and Steins speculate that if there is a near-total absence of may itself engage a tendency to take the other's perspective; speculation seems to me to be at odds with their conceptual ing drawn this conclusion, I began to wonder whether their holds up, or whether I understand it properly. The picture b ble one in which small amounts of information that link th the perceived (via either press or conflict regarding the per the perspective-taking tendency, but larger amounts (the comb and conflict) overwhelm it.

This interpretation would suggest that press and confl extent interchangeable. This inference appears to be compat certain aspects of the discussion by Wicklund and Steins. In use of an empathy scale to assess individual differences in one they describe this measure as assessing how sensitive people chic conflict with others. The measure is characterized as ta cy to transform others' thoughts into one's own problems, an attunement to problematic facets of other people and a come absorbed in those problematic facets. I agree that th individual difference in potential for intrapsychic conflict. L this same variable is discussed as a difference in press. T is not a typographical one; rather, the concepts of press an in this chapter) do overlap conceptually to a considerable ceiver has an intrapsychic conflict regarding the other, th ly has more motivational significance for the perceiver.

This interpretation changes somewhat the implication na observed. It would imply that there is nothing specifi a causal force in producing the pattern of effects. Rathe rely entirely on an accumulation of press (a possibility t and Steins also allude in their comments about cultura be that the study in which press (without conflict) led line spective taking simply failed to obtain a high enough leve ate the undermining effect.

follows from confidence fails to take place; so too does the disengagement that follows from having doubt about success.

Oettingen closes by arguing that something special happens when people actively confront both the fantasy and the present reality. She points out that discrepancies *exist* when only one of the two images is considered closely, but they aren't acted on in the same way as when both sides are focused on. Thus, rehearsing the discrepancy "in the mind's eye" causes the fantasy to become bound to real-life considerations in a way that otherwise is not the case. The fantasy ceases to be a hypothetical possibility and becomes a goal—perhaps because this rehearsal somehow creates an implemental mindset on the goal implied in the fantasy (Gollwitzer, 1990).

One of the interesting things about this research is also something about which Oettingen says very little in her chapter. Work on behavior change and performance enhancement often makes a good deal of use of imagery, treating it as a positive tool for productive change. Some of the imagery used in such work verges on fantasy. This raises a question: What's the difference between helpful imagery and counterproductive fantasy? Since the use of imagery for behavior change and performance enhancement does not especially rely on juxtaposing positive imagery with a representation of current conditions, the difference between good and bad fantasy must lie somewhere else. Presumably the difference is partly the difference between fantasizing about the successful negotiation of pathways (good) and fantasizing about endpoints (bad). I think that the continuum between these kinds of fantasy represents an interesting avenue for further investigation, and I hope this question will become part of the research agenda in this area.

Emmons: Striving and Feeling

I turn now to the chapter by Emmons (Chapter 14). This chapter has links to a number of themes that have already arisen in my discussion.

Hierarchicality

One comment I have on this chapter concerns high- versus low-level strivings, which closely resemble what Vallacher and Wegner (1985, 1987) call high- versus low-level action identifications. Emmons has found that people who are high-level strivers are vulnerable to higher levels of distress. There are two ways in which I find this easy to understand. Both are implicit in the logic of hierarchically organized feedback systems. First a higher-order system intrinsically has a longer lag time for discrepancies to be diminished. This greater time lag must be taken into account in evaluating the system's success at reducing the discrepancies, though people probably don't do this very well. From my point of view, negative affect results from perceptions of not moving toward one's goals fast enough (Carver & Scheier, 1990b). Thus, all other things being equal, longer lag times (thus, perceptions of minimal forward movement) make negative affect more likely.

Another (complementary) way of viewing this finding is that higher-level identifications are closer to the core sense of self. If you think about the majority of your day-to-day actions as having implications for your core self, and if you are struggling with any of them, it's no wonder you may feel distressed (cf. Carver & Ganellen, 1983). If you think about your behavior in ways that are more peripheral from the core self (ways that characterize lower-level strivers), the behaviors are less important; the reduced importance, in turn, means that there is less chance that negative affect will arise.

This general line of argument would seem to be compatible with the principles of Vallacher and Wegner's (1985, 1987) action identification theory. This theory holds that people tend to use lower-level identifications for their behavior when they can't successfully maintain higher-level ones. An attempt to hold onto an ineffective higher-level identification will generate distress, because of its ineffectiveness. By moving to a more concrete level, a person becomes more successful in self-regulating within that more limited domain and is consequently less distressed.

It should be noted that there are theoretical arguments to be made on either side of this question. It might be argued, for example, that people who are self-actualizing are less prone to distress than people who aren't self-actualizing (compare this with findings in the Ryan et al. chapter). One wonders, though, whether the issue of high- versus low-level striving really is the same as self-actualization versus its absence. How distress relates to levels of striving is obviously a complex question, and there are many angles from which it might be viewed. As such, this question would seem to be worthy of further attention.

Approach versus Avoidance

Emmons also discusses research examining differences between people who hold primarily approach goals and people with higher proportions of avoidance goals. The distinction between these two classes of goals has had a long history in theories of motivation (e.g., Atkinson, 1957; McClelland, Atkinson, Clark, & Lowell, 1953; Schneirla, 1959). Most obviously, the distinction between the motive to approach success and the motive to avoid failure has played an important role in theories of achievement behavior. More recently, the broad distinction between approach and avoidance goals has been echoed by Markus and Nurius (1986) in their concept of the "feared self," and also in the recent work of Higgins and his colleagues (to which I turn later on). In the language of Markus and Nurius, the avoidance strivers in the research discussed by Emmons are people whose lives are dominated by attempts to avoid feared possible selves.

The research Emmons discusses found that people with higher proportions of avoidance strivings tend to report higher levels of distress than do those more focused on approach strivings. It is certainly reasonable to expect people who are trying to escape from feared selves to be vulnerable to anxiety, to the extent that they see themselves as unsuccessful in avoiding those feared futures. Implicit in my interpretation of this finding is that it depends on the occurrence of a higher perceived rate of failure at goal attainment among the avoidance-motivated strivers than among the approach-motivated strivers. This is something that apparently can't be verified from the data collected. This inference is consistent, though, with the observation that there is an asymmetry in the amount of analytic reasoning required by approach and avoidance situations (Schwarz, 1990). People trying to avoid must block many possible paths by which the undesired event can occur; those trying to approach must find only one path to the desired goal. It may follow that with more things to worry about, there is a greater likelihood of perceiving that there is something amiss.

One might also argue, on the basis of the findings reviewed by Ryan et al., that subjects with primarily avoidance strivings are more extrinsically motivated (i.e., they engage in more controlled behavior) than subjects with primarily approach strivings. It's worth noting in this regard that Ryan et al.'s illustrations of introjected (controlled) regulation are both cases in which a behavior is being performed to *avoid some undesired outcome*. Thus, there is a potential link between the two sets of work. If being dominated by controlling motives (rather than self-determined motives) is tied to adverse psychological outcomes (which seems to be the import of the evidence reviewed in the Ryan et al. chapter), perhaps this is what underlies the finding reported by Emmons.

On the other hand, the emphasis on avoidance in Ryan et al.'s characterization of introjected regulation raises questions about their own work. That is, is it possible that their findings depend on a difference between approach and avoidance, rather than on a difference in terms of integration of behavior with the self? Are people who report being motivated by financial success trying to avoid an undesired state of affairs (e.g., being rejected and disapproved), rather than trying to approach a desired end (e.g., being liked)? If that were so, it would cast a different light on the meaning of their findings. I don't think the answer to this question is available in the data collected thus far, but I think this also represents an interesting avenue for further study.

One more brief comment here concerning approach and avoidance strivers: Consistent with discussion in the Emmons chapter, it wouldn't surprise me to find that avoidance strivers are characterized by sensitive behavioral inhibition systems, in the terms of Gray's (1985, 1987, 1990) analysis of motives. Someone who is especially attentive to punishment, by virtue of being biologically sensitive to it, may come to spend large amounts of time striving to avoid it (Fowles, 1980). An alternative possibility is that the biological sensitivity may interact with the extent of avoidance striving in a person's life, serving to amplify the adverse effects of such strivings when they occur. Yet another possibility (complementary to either of these) is that individual differences in the sensitivity of the behavioral activation system may also contribute to differences in striving patterns, as people with highly sensitive activation systems are more closely focused on approach striving than people with less sensitive activation systems.

Let me turn briefly now to the notion of conflict. It's no surprise that conflict between strivings is associated with negative affect. When actions pertain to more than one higher-order goal, it sometimes is the case that movement toward one goal means a lack of movement, or even a slipping backward, regarding another goal. In such a case, the result must be negative feeling. I find particularly congenial the way of thinking about this that Emmons employs, undoubtedly because it shares a good deal with my own way of thinking about it. His is a viewpoint that incorporates the sense of hierarchical organization—conflict as pulling apart the coherent sense of self—and also some of the same ways of viewing the sources of affect as I hold.

Vallacher and Kaufman: Time in Action

Another view that is explicitly hierarchical is presented in the chapter by Vallacher and Kaufman (Chapter 12), which deals with action identification processes from a newer angle than most of us have seen before. In thinking of action identification in terms of dynamic systems, Vallacher and Kaufman emphasize the concept of "self-organization," the tendency for an organization to emerge from disorder. They argue that people who are construing their actions in low-level terms are, in effect, in a condition of disorder. Their behavior is being guided by goals that are restricted in scope and brief and transitory in their application (indeed, Vallacher and Kaufman make the further assertion that lower-level identifications aren't goals at all—an assertion with which I disagree).

In trying to arrive at a higher-order understanding of their behavior (because of the natural tendency to gravitate to high-level identifications as long as they can be maintained), people use the unstable low-level information as raw material. This raw material can be packaged in many different ways (using portions of what's available in different mixes), each of which would represent a higher-order identification of the action. According to Vallacher and Kaufman, the many possible higher-order identifications come and go in brief bursts, until one identification emerges and takes hold in a person's mind. They refer to this process with the phrase "selected by the environment," in part to indicate that many cues from outside the person as well as processes inside the person contribute to the determination of the identification eventually reached.

In support of this line of argument, Vallacher and Kaufman describe a study in which subjects thought about a previous interaction with someone of the same sex in either high-level or low-level terms. They then indicated continuously for 2 minutes how they felt about their having behaved in the way they described. The assumption was that subjects with low-level construals would have a quickly shifting sense of the meaning of their behavior, until they selected some particular high-level identification. Since the various identifications would be associated with different self-evaluative reactions, subjects' feelings would not be stable until a high-level identification of the behavior had been arrived at. The data from the study were consistent with these assumptions.

These findings, and the interpretation that Vallacher and Kaufman apply to them, suggest that when people move upward to a higher-order identification of their behavior from a more primitive elemental one, there is a burst of chaotic switching among images, with one of them emerging as the adopted construal. This depiction raises a number of questions. For example, what happens when a person shifts from one higher-level action identification to another? Such a lateral shift can happen either when the person reconstrues the ongoing activity in a new light, or when the person stops one activity to take up another. Although Vallacher and Kaufman do not discuss either of these cases, it's tempting to infer that a similar burst of mental turbulence should arise between the one construal and the other.

This inference seems particularly appropriate for cases in which an ongoing activity is reconceptualized while it's taking place. After all, what is it that causes the shift in construal, except information at a low level that doesn't fit the picture of the current construal? Perhaps an accumulation of inconsistent low-level information causes the person to drop briefly to the lower level, mentally reshake the package of elements (now a package somewhat different from the one previously considered), and let the multiple possible higher-level identities flash chaotically past (like a random miniversion of *Wheel of Fortune*) until one identity fits the package well enough to emerge and become locked in.

The fit of this line of thought to the other case—ending one activity and starting another one—seems less intuitive but not entirely implausible. At the point where one action ends and another has not yet begun, the person probably is more readily distracted by cues signifying another action than at any other point in the behavioral stream. (All other things being equal, if your plan is to finish writing a letter and then go to the supermarket, you are more easily thrown off track at the moment you finish the letter than during either writing the letter or going to the store.) This relative distractibility may imply a return to the lower level to reshake the package of lower-level behavioral elements.

This portrayal of behavior is one in which periods of intentionality and identification of the goals of one's action are punctuated by brief bursts of what amounts to mental static. If so, these bursts of static must in many cases be quite brief, since people do sometimes shift quite abruptly from one activity to another. In other cases, the periods of static may not be so brief at all. I might also note that using words such as "static," "turbulence," or "chaos" to refer to these periods is evocative in one sense but is probably very misleading in another sense. Subjectively, these periods may not feel like "turbulence" at all, since their occurrence is quite familiar. The chaos may feel instead like "implicit decision making"—which it is, even though the form Vallacher and Kaufman assume for the decision process isn't much like traditional views of decision making.

I would like to make at least a brief further comment on the conceptual underpinnings of the Vallacher and Kaufman chapter (cf. Vallacher & Nowack, 1994). The shift from one identification of an action to another can be thought of as an illustration of a "phase transition" (a phrase that Vallacher and Kaufman refrain from using in their chapter, but one that is used elsewhere). Phase transitions are relatively abrupt changes, involving not a gradual emergence of a property but a reorganization of the Gestalt. In applying this idea to human experience, it is perhaps easiest to think about shifts in perceptions. The well-known "perceptual catastrophe" process (e.g., Stewart & Peregoy, 1983)—in which a given perception is held as the stimulus gradually changes in form, until suddenly the perception reorganizes—may be the clearest example of a phase transition (Figure 28.3). It illustrates the nonlinearity of the transition, as well as the tendency to hold onto a given perceptual organization as long as possible (reflected in the diverging perceptions of the most ambiguous stimuli, depending on which percept was held initially).

Although phase transitions in perception may be most familiar, we can also talk of phase transitions in a person's goals and in the person's constru-

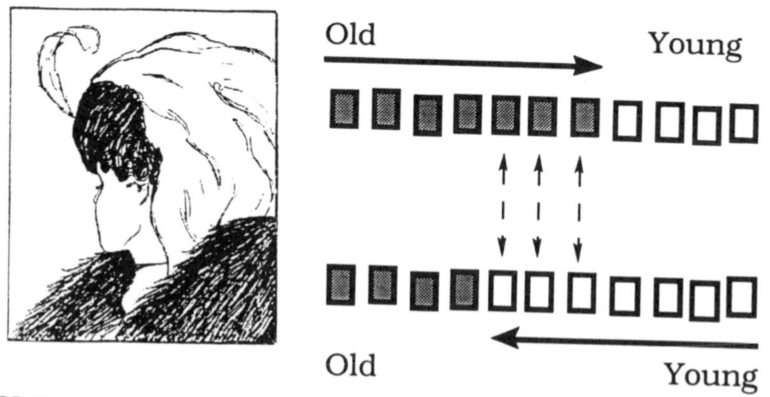

FIGURE 28.3. A perceptual catastrophe (see, e.g., Stewart & Peregoy, 1983). Images are created that vary gradually from a clear depiction of a young woman, through a highly ambiguous image (the image shown here at left, adapted from Boring, 1930), to a clear depiction of an old woman. Subjects view the series starting at one extreme or the other (where the image is clear and unambiguous). At some point in the series, the initial percept gives way and reorganizes abruptly into the other percept, illustrating the nonlinearity of some changes in perception. However, the most ambiguous of the images (those in the middle of the series) are usually perceived in terms of whichever was the initial percept (as indicated at right). This illustrates the tendency to hold onto a given perceptual organization as long as possible, until it can no longer be sustained. From Carver and Scheier (in press).

als of his or her action (discussions of action identification tend to emphasize the perception of the action, but the identification that occurs is also the identification of a goal for the action). As implied a little earlier, I think what Vallacher and Kaufman have described can be applied more widely than to shifting construals of a given act from lower to higher identifications. It also provides a perfectly reasonable way of thinking about what happens when people put one goal down, either permanently or for a while, to pursue another one instead. Whereas the process of doing this is all continuously dynamic (involving the simultaneous operation of many different forces that wax and wane but remain in place), its surface appearance is a set of abrupt shifts in one's activity, from one behavior to another and then to another.

Consider an analogy (sophisticated readers will recognize this as a dumbed-down version of the description of a chaotic attractor [see, e.g., Barton, 1994] but I trust they won't be offended by my analogizing in this way). Imagine a planetary system in which there are several large bodies, and you are following the orbit of a fast-moving smaller body among them (Figure 28.4). The small body is always attracted to all three of the larger bodies, of course, and is therefore influenced by all of them in a continuous, dynamic way. It orbits erratically around A for a while, then is pulled away to orbit C, as C's gravitational pull (along with that of B) joins with the small body's inertia on a particularly wide sweep to overcome the pull of A. The orbits are always erratic, and shifts occur periodically (and somewhat unpredictably) in which body is the center of the orbital motion. These transitions in orbit all represent phase transitions. If you plotted a time line of which body this object was orbiting, changing labels as soon as the break occurred from one orbit to another, you'd have a shifting series of discrete events, even though the entire flow reflects constant simultaneous pressure of forces from all the bodies in the system. You'd see a pattern of doing one thing, then something else, and then something else.

This extraction of linear meaning from the dynamic process closely resembles a point made a long time ago within the motive perspective on personality (Murray, 1938)—that the surface topography of behavior reflects an underlying dynamic of continually shifting motive strengths (see also Atkinson & Birch, 1970). Although the motives all rise and fall in intensity continuously, behavior tends to reflect one motive at a time, with behavior changing qualititatively from one time to another. Which motive is strongest at any given moment determines what behavior is performed then. As the motives shift in relative intensity, behavior changes its focus.

The similarity betwen a point made now in terms of dynamic system constructs and a point made long ago in terms of motives raises a question: What does the dynamic system view add that's new (at least in this respect)? There are two ways to look at this question, though. Maybe the question represents a challenge to the dynamic system perspective (by implying that it isn't saying anything new). But maybe the point is really that the motive

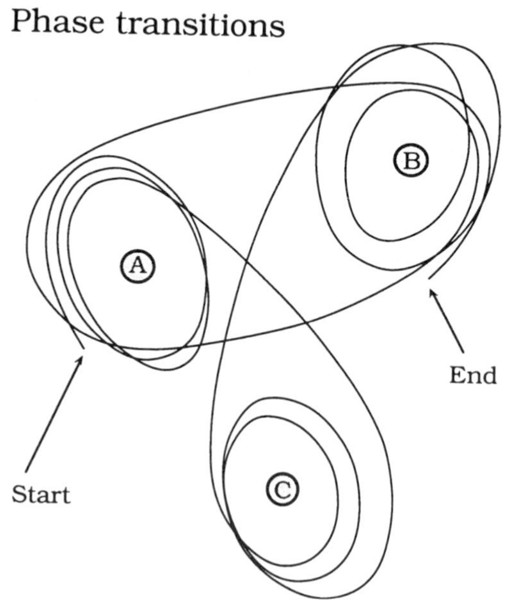

FIGURE 28.4. A moving body attracted to three larger bodies may orbit erratically around one, then another, and then another of the attractors; each shift in focus represents a phase transition. The focus of the orbits can be plotted across time (below), creating a picture of the topography of the "behavior" of the moving body. From Carver and Scheier (in press).

view is really more of a dynamic system perspective than has thus far been recognized.

Higgins: Ideals, Oughts, and Regulatory Outcome Focus

I turn finally to the chapter by Higgins (Chapter 5), whose work on the effects of various self-guides has mushroomed over the past several years. The work is both extensive and elaborated. I won't try to dissect the large body of work here, but I do want to make several points about this model in conjunction with conceptually related work done by myself and by others.

The Higgins theory connects with my own view of things at several points. In one case, the two of us have published somewhat contrasting ideas. Higgins holds that the extent of the discrepancy between the actual self and particular class of self-guides is responsible for negative affect (Higgins, 1987). Michael Scheier and I havve argued that what matters is not the size of the discrepancy, but the equally subjective sense of whether the discrepancy is being reduced at an acceptable rate or not (Carver & Scheier, 1990b, in press).

I think one consequence of this difference between theories is that it's a little easier for our model to address *positive* feelings than it is for the Higgins theory. In the Higgins theory, there is an implicit tendency to treat positive affect as what's left when all the negative affect has been whittled away; and I don't think that's an accurate view. Alternatively, one could argue that if there are many actual–ideal matches, there will be positive affect. But if one takes that approach, it's difficult to specify what circumstances produce an *absence* of affect.

Another consequence of this difference between models concerns fluctuation in affect from minute to minute or hour to hour. I think there are many times when people feel good even when they aren't matched to their ideals. Our model treats positive, negative, and neutral affective tones as determined by whether rates of discrepancy reduction are above some criterion, below it, or just at it. Thus, for any particular salient goal, it's relatively easy to see how any of these affective tones may exist, even if there is still a discrepancy with respect to the goal.

These differences are not what I want to focus on, though. What's special about the Higgins model is the idea that people use multiple guides for self-evaluation, which yield different affects. The idea that depressed (dejection related) affect follows from discrepancies with ideals, whereas anxious (and other agitation-related) affect follows from discrepancies with oughts, is interesting and important. It has many implications, some of which Higgins and his colleagues have pursued, and some of which they are still in the midst of pursuing.

I would like to examine more closely here the difference between the processes that create the two kinds of distress, with the goal of integrating elements of the Higgins model with other ideas. To do this, I must present some background on differences between positive and negative feedback loops (for more detail, see Carver & Scheier, in press). In a negative loop (so labeled because it is discrepancy-*negating*, or -reducing), the pressure is always to move *toward* some particular goal (Figure 28.5) that is positively valenced. (That negative feedback loops use positive reference values can be confusing at first, but the labeling here is correct.) In a positive loop (discrepancy-enlarging), the pressure is to move *away* from some negatively valenced goal value, but with no specification of where to go *to*. Away is away, no matter what direction the deviation.

For effective self-management, however, it's useful to have some value to move toward, at the same time as one is trying to move away from something else (Figure 28.6). Indeed, it has been argued that the effects of positive loops in living systems are typically overridden or bounded by effects of negative loops (McFarland, 1971). This seems to be what usually happens

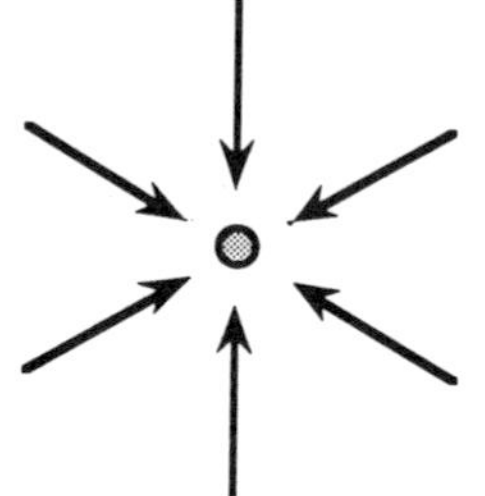

Negative
(discrepancy *reducing*)
feedback loop—
comparison value
as attractor

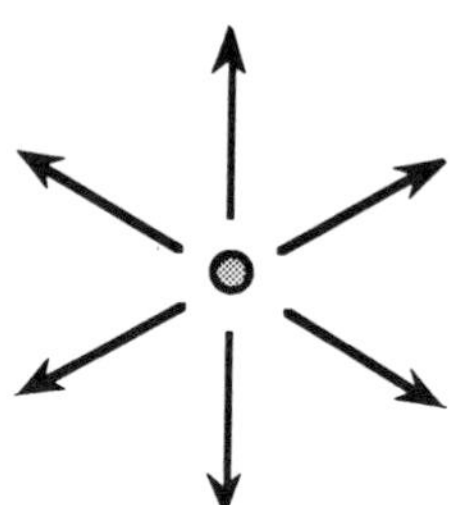

Positive
(discrepancy *enlarging*)
feedback loop—
comparison value
as repeller

FIGURE 28.5. Negative feedback loops cause sensed qualities to shift *toward* positively valenced reference points. Positive feedback loops cause sensed qualities to shift *away from* negatively valenced reference points. From Carver and Scheier (in press).

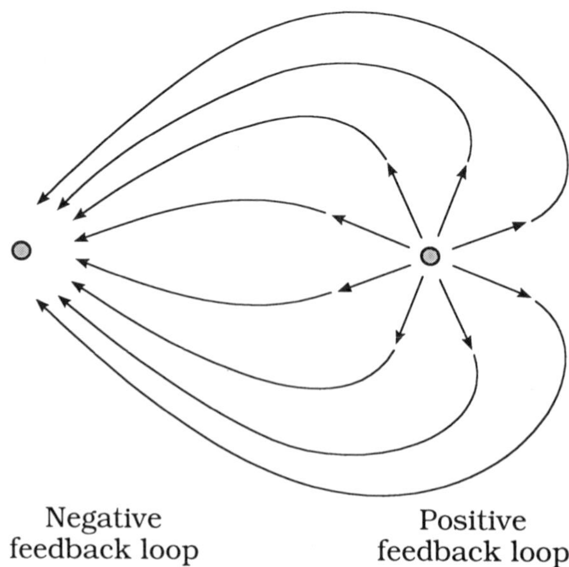

FIGURE 28.6. Positive feedback systems are often bounded or constrained by negative feedback systems—one often avoids some undesired condition by moving toward a desired condition. From Carver and Scheier (in press).

in cases where human behavior displays the characteristics of positive feedback processes.

As an example, consider the following. It appears to be a near-universal phenomenon of life in the United States that adolescents want to be different from their parents (thus they take parents as a negative reference group). There are, of course, innumerable ways to be unlike someone else. Although there is some degree of diversity within any group of adolescents in how they deviate from their parents, there is also a strong tendency for a positive reference group to emerge (i.e., other adolescents and their various role models). Through social comparison, this positive reference group evolves its norms, to which an adolescent adheres. Thus, the adolescent is a nonconformist with respect to the parent by being a conformist to a different value.

Now let's return to the Higgins model. There is an important difference in this model between the dynamics of the processes that create depression and those that create anxiety. Self-regulation with respect to ideals is straightforward: If you want to be something, you try to be that way, and that's it. This logical structure looks very much like a simple negative feedback system. Oughts are a more complicated case. Oughts are desired qualities, but they are desired principally because they keep you away from undesired punishing events. Oughts involve trying to be something and also trying to escape from something else. This suggests to me that ought-based self-regulation is another case of a positive loop's being overridden or bounded by a negative loop (Figure 28.7). First and most basic is the desire to escape and avoid the undesired value—a positive feedback process. What gives this effort form and coherence, however, is the desirable value of the ought, a value that the person can move toward—a negative feedback process.

In first developing our view of the source of affect (Carver & Scheier, 1990b), we attended primarily to discrepancy-reducing loops. We argued that such a loop can yield either positive or negative affect, depending on how well it's doing at what it's trying to do. But if we can talk about a discrepancy-*reducing* loop's doing well or poorly, why shouldn't the same idea be applicable to a discrepancy-*enlarging* loop? If it's doing well at what it's trying to do, the result should be a positive feeling; if it's doing poorly, the result should be a negative feeling. We have since made this argument more explicitly (Carver & Scheier, in press).

Since the two kinds of systems have different focuses, it's reasonable to expect the affects they yield to differ somewhat (see Figure 28.8). In characterizing the dimensions of affect that I believe are created by these two kinds of systems, I'm relying on the empirical findings of self-discrepancy theory as well as on other sources of information. I think that the dimensions could well be characterized as representing elation versus depression and anxiety versus relief/tranquility/contentment/serenity. One end of each dimension in Figure 28.8 is thus occupied by a feeling class postulated in self-discrepancy theory. The other end is occupied by a positive feeling relevant to successful approach and successful avoidance, respectively. Figure 28.8 thus

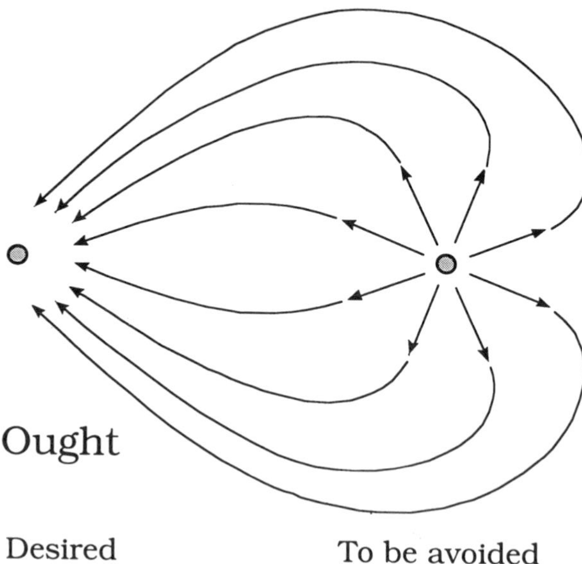

FIGURE 28.7. An "ought" self-guide can be seen as involving both an explicit desire to move toward a prescribed value and an implicit desire to move away from a proscribed value—in other words, a positive feedback loop whose effects are given form by those of a negative feedback loop. From Carver and Scheier (in press).

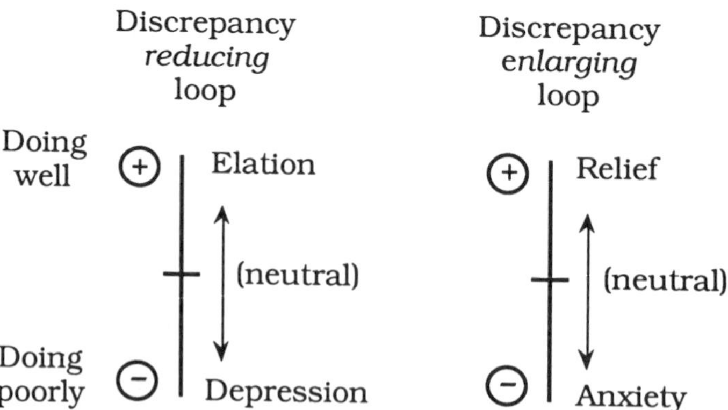

FIGURE 28.8. Two dimensions of affect created by two kinds of self-regulatory systems. For a discrepancy-reducing (approach) system, the negative feeling that can develop when self-regulation is going poorly is dysphoria. For a discrepancy-enlarging (avoidance) system, the negative feeling that can develop when self-regulation is going poorly is anxiety. Both kinds of system can also lead to positive affect, which also differs in tone from one system to the other. From Carver and Scheier (in press).

represents a partial integration of self-discrepancy theory with our feedback model of behavior.

Approach versus Avoidance as Basic

The line of thought shown in Figure 28.8 raises one more question however. Self-discrepancy theory holds that the discrepancy between the actual and the ought is what determines anxiety. Higgins and his colleagues have in their recent work begun to examine more closely the fact that self-regulation with regard to oughts involves more than trying to conform to oughts. The findings reviewed in the Higgins chapter seem to confirm that ought-based self-regulation involves trying to avoid something, as well as trying to approach the oughts. However, I am led to wonder whether the avoidance tendency is still being accorded too little importance. In a sense, the avoidance tendency has motivational primacy. It's the starting point (Figure 28.7), and thus the most fundamental part of the ought pattern. Perhaps, then, the trying to escape is more important in some ways than the trying to approach.

We have recently collected data bearing on this question (Carver, Lawrence, & Scheier, 1995). Subjects in this study rated how discrepant they were from their self-generated ought and ideal selves, and they also rated how discrepant they were from their self-generated *feared* selves. Of particular interest were findings from analyses in which the sample was divided into two sets: subjects who were relatively close to their feared selves and subjects who were relatively distant from their feared selves.

Among those who were close to their feared selves, actual-feared discrepancies, but no other discrepancies, related strongly to anxiety, guilt, and depression. Among subjects who were relatively removed from their feared selves, however, a very different picture emerged. Among these subjects, actual–ought discrepancies predicted agitation-related affects and actual–ideal discrepancies predicted dejection-related affects, just as suggested by self-discrepancy theory. Actual–feared discrepancies played a far smaller role in this subsample.

These findings appear to suggest that the move-away push inherent in the positive feedback process is a very important predictor of affect among people who are in relatively close proximity to their feared selves. Only when people have some degree of removal from that aversive reference point does the move-toward pull that's inherent in the negative feedback process begin to exert its influence. This pattern suggests further that there may be something about the "escape" process that is more demanding than the "attain" process. In this sense the pattern is consistent with the observation that people attend more to negative than positive events, and with the idea that evolution places a greater premium on escaping danger than on attaining desired ends (Pratto & John, 1991; Taylor, 1991).

Further Integration

In closing this discussion, let me point out that the dimensions of affect outlined in Figure 28.8 bear considerable resemblance to those identified by Zevon and Tellegen (1982) and Watson and Tellegen (1985), widely known as "positive affect" and "negative affect." Though these labels are in widespread use, I think they are somewhat misleading (see also Larsen & Diener, 1992, in this regard). Despite their labels, both dimensions have both positive and negative poles. To the extent that the data sets reviewed by Watson and Tellegen contained descriptors reflecting depression (and there were not many), they loaded on the *positive* affect factor. To the extent that descriptors reflecting relief were represented in the data sets (the closest were "calm," "carefree," and "satisfied"), they loaded on the *negative* affect factor. Indeed, Watson and Tellegen (1985) noted explicitly that both dimensions have markers that are both positive and negative, though I have seen no discussion concerning how this is to be reconciled with the position that the dimensions are unipolar.

I think that the two dimensions underlying the affective experiences labeled "positive affect" and "negative affect" are closely aligned with the two dimensions shown in Figure 28.8. The core of what is termed "positive affect" is the bipolar dimension from elation to depression. The core of what is termed "negative affect" is the bipolar dimension from anxiety to relief/serenity. Each of these dimensions is related to the actions of a behavioral self-regulatory system. One of these systems involves approach and the other involves avoidance (for reviews of neuropsychological data bearing on this viewpoint, see Davidson, 1992a, 1992b). This line of argument suggests that the affective dimensions discussed under the labels "positive affect" and "negative affect" have strong points of contact both with the Higgins (1987) self-discrepancy theory and with the Carver and Scheier (1990b, in press) model of action and affect. These points of contact, which have been little noted until now, would seem to deserve further exploration.

ACKNOWLEDGMENTS

Preparation of this chapter was supported in part by Grant No. BNS 90-11653 from the National Science Foundation and Grant No. PBR-56 from the American Cancer Society. The chapter was written while I was a visiting scholar at the University of California, Los Angeles.

REFERENCES

Ajzen, I. (1988). *Attitudes, personality, and behavior.* Chicago: Dorsey Press.

Atkinson, J. W. (1957). Motivational determinants of risk-taking behavior. *Psychological Review, 64,* 359–372.

Atkinson, J. W., & Birch, D. (1970). *The dynamics of action.* New York: Wiley.

Barton, S. (1994). Chaos, self-organization, and psychology. *American Psychologist, 49,* 5–14.

Boring, E. G. (1930). A new ambiguous figure. *American Journal of Psychology, 42,* 444–445.

Carver, C. S., & Ganellen, R. J. (1983). Depression and components of self-punitiveness: High standards, self-criticism, and overgeneralization. *Journal of Abnormal Psychology, 92,* 330–337.

Carver, C. S., Lawrence, J. W., & Scheier, M. F. (1995). *Self-discrepancies and affect: Incorporating the role of feared selves.* Manuscript under review.

Carver, C. S., & Scheier, M. F. (1981). *Attention and self-regulation: A control-theory approach to human behavior.* New York: Springer-Verlag.

Carver, C. S., & Scheier, M. F. (1990a). Principles of self-regulation: Action and emotion. In R. Sorrentino & E. T. Higgins (Eds.), *Handbook of motivation and cognition: Foundations of social behavior* (Vol. 2, pp. 3–52). New York: Guilford Press.

Carver, C. S., & Scheier, M. F. (1990b). Origins and functions of positive and negative affect: A control-process view. *Psychological Review, 97,* 19–35.

Carver, C. S., & Scheier, M. F. (in press). *On the self- regulation of behavior.* New York: Cambridge University Press.

Davidson, R. J. (1992a). Anterior cerebral asymmetry and the nature of emotion. *Brain and Cognition, 20,* 125–151.

Davidson, R. J. (1992b). Prolegomenon to the structure of emotion: Gleanings from neuropsychology. *Cognition and Emotion, 6,* 245–268.

Diener, C. I., & Dweck, C. S. (1978). An analysis of learned helplessness: Continuous changes in performance, strategy, and achievement cognitions following failure. *Journal of Personality and Social Psychology, 36,* 451–462.

Dweck, C. S., & Leggett, E. L. (1988). A social-cognitive approach to motivation and personality. *Psychological Review, 95,* 256–273.

Fowles, D. C. (1980). The three arousal model: Implications of Gray 's two-factor learning theory for heart rate, electrodermal activity, and psychopathy. *Psychophysiology, 17,* 87–104.

Gollwitzer, P. M. (1990). Action phases and mind-sets. In R. Sorrentino & E. T. Higgins (Eds.), *Handbook of motivation and cognition: Foundations of social behavior* (Vol. 2, pp. 53–92). New York: Guilford Press.

Gray, J. A. (1985). Issues in the neuropsychology of anxiety. In A. H. Tuma & J. D. Maser (Eds.), *Anxiety and the anxiety disorders* (pp. 5–25). Hillsdale, NJ: Erlbaum.

Gray, J. A. (1987). *The psychology of fear and stress.* Cambridge, England: Cambridge University Press.

Gray, J. A. (1990). Brain systems that mediate both emotion and cognition. *Cognition and Emotion, 4,* 269–288.

Higgins, E. T. (1987). Self-discrepancy: A theory relating self and affect. *Psychological Review, 94,* 319–340.

Klinger, E. (1975). Consequences of commitment to and disengagement from incentives. *Psychological Review, 82,* 1–25.

Larsen, R. J., & Diener, E. (1992). Promises and problems with the circumplex model of emotion. In M. S. Clark (Ed.), *Review of personality and social psychology* (Vol. 13, pp. 25–59). Newbury Park, CA: Sage.

Linder, D. E., & Crane, K. A. (1970). Reactance theory analysis of predecisional cognitive processes. *Journal of Personality and Social Psychology, 15,* 258–264.

Linder, D. E., Wortman, C. B., & Brehm, J. W. (1971). Temporal changes in predecision preferences among choice alternatives. *Journal of Personality and Social Psychology, 19,* 282–284.

Markus, H., & Nurius, P. (1986). Possible selves. *American Psychologist, 41,* 954–969.

McClelland, D. C., Atkinson, J. W., Clark, R. A., & Lowell, E. I. (1953). *The achievement motive.* New York: Appleton-Century-Crofts.

McFarland, D. J. (1971). *Feedback mechanisms in animal behavior.* New York: Academic Press.

Murray, H. A. (1938). *Explorations in personality.* New York: Oxford University Press.

Pratto, F., & John, O. P. (1991). Automatic vigilance: The attention-grabbing power of negative social information. *Journal of Personality and Social Psychology, 61,* 380–391.

Rosenbaum, D. A. (1991). *Human motor control.* San Diego: Academic Press.

Schwarz, N. (1990). Feelings as information: Informational and motivational functions of affective states. In R. Sorrentino & E. T. Higgins (Eds.), *Handbook of motivation and cognition: Foundations of social behavior* (Vol. 2, pp. 527–561). New York: Guilford Press.

Schmidt, R. A. (1988). *Motor control and learning: A behavioral emphasis* (2nd ed.). Champaign, IL: Human Kinetics Publishers.

Schneirla, T. C. (1959). An evolutionary and developmental theory of biphasic processes underlying approach and withdrawal. In M. R. Jones (Ed.), *Nebraska Symposium on Motivation* (Vol. 7, pp. 1–42). Lincoln: University of Nebraska Press.

Stewart, I. N., & Peregoy, P. L. (1983). Catastrophe theory modeling in psychology. *Psychological Bulletin, 94,* 336–362.

Taylor, S. E. (1991). Asymmetric effects of positive and negative events: The mobilization–minimization hypothesis. *Psychological Bulletin, 110,* 67–85.

Vallacher, R. R., & Nowack, A. (Eds.). (1994). *Dynamical systems in social psychology.* San Diego, CA: Academic Press.

Vallacher, R. R., & Wegner, D. M. (1985). *A theory of action identification.* Hillsdale, NJ: Erlbaum.

Vallacher, R. R., & Wegner, D. M. (1987). What do people think they're doing? Action identification and human behavior. *Psychological Review, 94,* 3–15.

Watson, D., & Tellegen, A. (1985). Toward a consensual structure of mood. *Psychological Bulletin, 98,* 219–235.

Wicklund, R. A., & Gollwitzer, P. M. (1982). *Symbolic self-completion.* Hillsdale, NJ: Erlbaum.

Zevon, M. A., & Tellegen, A. (1982). The structure of mood change: An idiographic/nomothetic analysis. *Journal of Personality and Social Psychology, 43,* 111–122.

Index

accuracy motivation, 554
  heuristic–systematic information processing, 556–557
action, 27–29
  mental simulation, 228–229
  phases, planning, 288–294
  sequence and moods, 126–138
  theory, 383
  uncertainty orientation, 630–633
action control models, 28
action identification, 660–664
  dynamics
    and action expression, 276–277
    mental dynamics state, 274–276
    and psychological process, 277–278
action understanding
  control, 261–264
    action levels, 261–263
    emergence process, 263–264
  dynamism
    assessment, 266–269
    and identification level, 269–272
  generalizability, 273–274
  instability and low-level understanding, 264–266
actional phase
  of action sequence, 129, 136–137
  of planning, 290
actual–ideal discrepancy, 93
actual–ought discrepancy, 93
acute illness recovery and positive fantasies, 241–242
affect as mediator in self-oriented processes, 62–64
Air Traffic Controller Task, 410–414
  effect of conditions on practice, 413–414
  goal setting effects, 411–413
ambivalence and goal conflict, goal parameters, 325–327
approach and avoidance goals, 322–324, 658–660
approach vs. avoidance, 669–670
  and regulatory focus, 98–108
association hypothesis vs. goal tension hypothesis, 52
attainability evidence, goal setting, 604–606
attainment, goal strivings, 612–613
attention
  and defensive responses, 30–33
  and depression, 175–176
attitude–behavior relation, 386–392
  automatic-process models, 391–392
  controlled-process model, 387–391
attitudes
  planned behavior theory, 393–396
attribution processes, 50, 87
automatic writing, 483
automaticity, 457–476
  auto-motive model, 461–464
  in feeling of doing, 492–493
  unconscious
    intelligence of, 464–465
    as routinized consciousness, 460–461
    as source of error, 458–460
  and unconscious intentions, 466–475
    cognitive processing goals, 467–469
    social behavior, 469–475
automatic-process models, 391–392
automatisms
  feeling of doing, 483–493
  and ironic processes, 499–502
auto-motive model, 461–464
  and conscious thought, 635–636
  avoidant defenses, 30–33
  avoiding threat, defensive response, 30–34

B

bad moods, 120–126
behavior
  and depression dispositional control motives, 159–161
  orientation in planning, 302–303
behavioral readiness in planning, 297–300
behavioral schema and unconscious intentions, 470–471
belief equivalence vs. mode congruence, 393
Brehm's motivation theory, 424–449
  difficulty effects, 430–434
  interactional influences, 435–441
  perceived ability role, 441–444

C

cardiovascular response and motivation theory, 424–449
causal uncertainty and helplessness–hopelessness model of depression, 149–152
character, implicit theories of, 75–87
Chevreul's pendulum illusion, 483
  feeling of doing, 483, 496–499
child–caretaker interactions, 92
children
  and delayed gratification, 199
  long-term implications of
    delayed gratification, 210–212
  and rewards, 200–202
  and self-control, 213
chronic illness recovery and positive fantasies, 240–241
cognitive dissonance theory, 56–57
  and affect hypothesis, 62–63
cognitive focus
  and willpower, 204–207
cognitive processing, 168–169
  and concern-related stimuli, 171–174
  and depression, 153–157
  goals and unconscious intentions, 467–469
  motivational influences on, 170–174
commitment in volitional theory, 375
concern-related stimuli and cognitive processing, 171–174
conflict
  and expressing emotion, 327–328
  and person perception, 516–517
  and volitional theory, 375–376
conflict motivation and person perception, 516–517
conscious thought, 619–640
  auto-motive model, 635–636
  functional significance, 633–635
  history, 620–625
  uncertainty orientation, 625–633
    and information processing, 626–630
constructs
  accessibility, 177–181
  accessibility and emotions, 177–181
  building, 515–516
    to egocentrism, 518
  person perception, 513–516, 518
content and mental health, 17–19
contextual information, providing, 78–79
contingencies
  goal execution, 608–609
  and goals, 38
  uncertainty, 150
continuum model of impression formation, 154
controlled-process model of attitude-behavior relation, 387–391
coping and mental simulation, 223–224
correctional goals, 579–592
  correcting stereotypes, 587–589
  corrective strategies, 590–592
  motivational determinants, 579–580
  priming and remembering, 580–582
cultural context in person perception, 523–525
current concerns and fantasies, 245

D

defense motivation, 554
  heuristic–systematic information processing, 557–563

defensive preoccupation, 32
defensive responses
  and attention, 30–33
  avoiding threat, 30–34
  and interpretive defenses, 34–36
  and self-regulation, 29–37
delay of gratification
  in children, 199
    long-term implications of, 210–212
  goal-directed, 199
  instrumental activity in, 207–209
  and willpower, 198
depression, 50, 146–163
  and attention, 175–176
  and cognitive processing, 153–157
  and negative affect, 161–162
  processing of social information, 154–155
  sensitivity to social information, 152–153
  social-cognitive consequences of, 147–152
desirability evidence, in goal setting, 603–604
diastolic blood pressure, 426
directive influence of attitudes on behavior, 385–400, 653–654
  models of attitude–behavior relation, 386–392
  reasoned vs. spontaneous processes, 396–400
disengagement
  and fantasy, 252–253
  and implicit theories, 649–650
dispositional control motives in depression
  and behavior, 159–161
  and social context, 157–159
disrupted goal pursuits, in planning, 306–307
dissociation hypothesis, in feeling of doing, 490–491
distinct processing sensitivities
  and ideals, 96–98
  and oughts, 96–98
distractions, in planning, 304–305
domain-specific implicit theories, 70–71
dowsing or divining, in feeling of doing, 485
dynamics
  of action, 621, 623, 624, 634, 639
  and action expression, 276–277
  and psychological process, 277–278
dynamism and identification level
  action understanding, 269–272
dynamism assessment
  action understanding, 266–269

E

effort expenditure, actional phase of action sequence, 136–137
effort experience, 353–355
  effortful or spontaneous, 353–355
effort mobilization, 303–304
effortful interventions, 342–343
effortful motivation, 340–345
  effortful interventions, 342–343
  effortful pursuit as patterned behavior, 343–345
effortful or spontaneous effort experience, 353–355
effortful pursuits
  locating effort in life task pursuit, 352–353
  negotiating multiple pursuits, 345–352
    life task interrelations and spillover, 349–352
    resource limitations and role strain, 347–349
  as patterned behavior, 343–345
ego threats, 29
  and self-management, 40–43
  and self-regulation, 27–44
egocentrism, person perception, 518
emotional faces, 76–77
emotions, 168–169
  and construct accessibility, 177–181
  implications for theories, 181–182
  influences on cognitive processing, 174–177
  and recall, 176–177
  regulation and mental simulation, 221
encoding information, implicit theories of personality and character, 81–83

engagement and disengagement, fantasy, 252–253
entity theory of intelligence, 70–75
  and learning goals, 72–73
  and performance goals, 72–73
equifinality, 53
  goal execution, 608
evoked potentials and protoemotional processes, 183–184
external regulation, 11
extrinsic focus, goals, 19–20
extrinsic motivation, 9–10

F

failure and frustration, volitional theory, 376
fantasies
  and current concerns, 245
  engagement and disengagement, 252–253
  fantasy–reality contrast, 253–254
  and stream of thought, 244–245
  Thematic Apperception Test fantasies, 243–244
feedback loops, 128
feeling and striving, 657–660
feeling of doing, 482–502
  automatic writing, 483
  automatic-habit hypothesis, 492–493
  automatisms, 483–493
  Chevreul's pendulum illusion, 483, 496–499
  dissociation hypothesis, 490–491
  dowsing or divining, 485
  facilitated communication, 485–486
  hypnosis, 486
  imagination hypothesis, 487–490
  ironic process theory, 493–496
  motor automatisms, 486–487
  Ouija board spelling, 484
  social pressure hypothesis, 491–492
  table turning, tilting, tapping, 484–485
  trance states, 486
feelings and motivational implications of moods, 119–141
focus, 367
focused attention disruption, 296–297
free will theory, 365–366

G

goal concept, 645–646
goal execution
  contingency, 608–609
  energetics of implementation, 607–608
  equifinality, 608
  means–ends relations, 608–610
  planning, 607
  substitutability, 609–610
goal orientation
  approach and avoidance goals, 322–324
  and goal specification, 319–322
  relative autonomy, 325
  and subjective well-being, 319–325
goal parameters, 325–331
  conflict over expressing emotion, 327–328
  goal conflict and ambivalence, 325–327
  goal differentiation, 331
goal setting
  attainability evidence, 604–606
  desirability evidence, 603–604
  in the Air Traffic Controller Task, 411–413
  goals as knowledge structures, 603–606
  heuristic, 606
  vs. goal striving, 129
goal specification
  and goal orientation, 319–322
  volitional theory, 373
goal strivings
  attainment, 612–613
  nonattainment, 610–611
  vs. goal setting, 129
goal systems, 613–614
goal tension systems, 49
  and self-protective mechanisms, 51–53
goal theories, 7
goal-directed delayed gratification, 199
goals, 650–653
  analysis, 599–600
  attainment, 132–133
  and behavior relationship, 72–75
  completion, 53–55

conflict and ambivalence, 325–327
content, 16–21
and mental health, 17–19
and subjective well-being, 316–319
and contingencies, 38
desirability, 130–132
differentiation, 331
extrinsic focus, 19–20
hierarchy, 55
intentional acts of behavior
consequences of different regulatory styles, 12–14
internalization and integration, 10–12
intrinsic and extrinsic motivation, 9–10
social context and motivational orientations, 14–15
level, 373–374
and needs, 20–21
and overconfidence, 39–40
setting and meeting, 37–43
why of behavior, 8–15
without conscious consent, 473–475
goals as knowledge structures, 599–614
goal analysis, 599–600
goal setting, 603–606
goal systems, 613–614
goal-worthiness, 600–601
knowledge utilization processes, 602
goal-setting theory, 372–373
goal-worthiness, 600–601
good moods, 120–126

H

heart rate, 426
helplessness–hopelessness model of depression, 147–152
and casual uncertainty, 149–152
heuristic goal setting, 606
heuristic–systematic information processing, 553–572
absence of motivation, 555
accuracy motivation, 556–557
defense motivation, 557–563
impression motivation, 563–570
hierarchicality, implicit theories, 647–649
high-risk populations and willpower, 213–215
hopelessness model of depression, 147–152
hypnosis, feeling of doing, 486

I

ideal self-regulation, 94
ideals, 664–668
and distinct processing sensitivities, 96–98
and regulatory disorders, 95–96
vs. oughts, 93–95
images of rewards and willpower, 203–204
imagination hypothesis, feeling of doing, 487–490
implemental intentions and mental simulation, 229–230
implemental mind-set, 300–307
implementation intention concept, 292
implicit theories, 69–88, 646–650
disengagement, 649–650
domain-specific, 70–71
hierarchicality, 647–649
and individual-difference variables, 87–88
of intelligence, 72–75
measurement of, 70–72
model, 69–70
implicit theories of personality and character, 75–87
consequences of wrongdoing, 83–87
encoding information, 81–83
intention information providing, 79–80
providing contextual information, 78–79
trait judgments, 80–81
trait vs. state social judgments, 75–78
impression motivation, 554
heuristic–systematic information processing, 563–570
incremental theories of personality, 70–75
individual-difference variables and implicit theories, 87–88

inference characteristics
  person perception, 515–516
  via person perception, 512–514
information processing
  moods and strategies of information processing, 120–126
  and uncertainty orientation, 626–630
inner state cues, person perception, 519–523
instability and low-level understanding, 264–266
instrumental activity in delayed gratification, 207–209
integrated regulation, 11–12
integrated resource allocation model, skill acquisition, 406–420
integration, 10–12
intention information, implicit theories of personality and character, 79–80
intentional acts of behavior, 8–15
internalization and integration, 10–12
interpersonal matters and positive fantasy, 248–249
interpretive defenses and defensive responses, 34–36
intrinsic motivation, 9–10
introjected regulation, 11
ironic process theory, feeling of doing, 493–496
ironic processes and automatisms, 499–502

J

junk mail theory of self-deception, 30

K

knowledge utilization processes, 602

L

latent state of organism, 170
learning goals and entity theory of intelligence, 72–73
life task interrelations and spillover, 349–352
life task pursuit, 352–353
low-level understanding, 264–266

M

means–ends relations, goal execution, 608–610
measurement of implicit theories, 70–72
mental dynamics state, action identification, 274–276
mental simulation, 219–232
  and action, 228–229
  and coping, 223–224
  and emotional regulation, 221
  evaluation, 227–228
  and exam study, 224–227
  and implemental intentions, 229–230
  intervention implications, 230–231
  making events seem true, 220
  outcome simulation, 222, 224–227
  and planning, 220–221
  and problem-solving, 221–222
  process simulation, 222–227
  process–outcome simulation, 223–227
mind-sets
  of action sequence, 129
  planning, 291–292
MODE model vs. planned behavior theory, 392–396
  mood-incongruent memory effects, 33
moods
  and action sequence, 126–138
    steps in, 128–130
  and motivational implications of moods
    feelings, 119–141
  and self-discrepancies, 97–98
  and strategies of information processing, 120–126
moral character judgments, 81
motile strategy of survival, 168

motivation, 27–29, 168–169
  and cognitive processing, 170–174
  correctional goals, 579–580
  and feelings, 119–141
  heuristic–systematic information processing, 555
  intrinsic and extrinsic, 9–10
  optimistic thinking, 238–239
    benefits, 236–237
    perils, 237–238
  and positive fantasy, 236–255
    vs. positive expectations, 239–243
  and regulatory focus, 108–109
  unconscious sources of, 460–475
motivation theory
  Brehm's, 424–449
  and cardiovascular response, 424–449
motivational orientations, 14–15
motor automatisms
  feeling of doing, 486–487
multiple pursuits
  effortful pursuits, 345–352

N

needs, 16
  goals, 20–21
negative affect and depression, 161–162
negative outcome focus regulatory system, 92
negative reality and positive fantasy, 247–252
nonattainment and goal strivings, 610–611
nonmatching priming, 94

O

optimistic expectations and chronic illness recovery, 240–241
optimistic thinking
  benefits of, 236–237
  and motivation, 237–239
  and perils of, 237–238
organismic integration, 10–11
ought self-concept, 664–668
  and distinct processing sensitivities, 96–98
  and regulatory disorders, 95–96
  vs. ideals, 93–95
ought self-regulation, 94
outcome simulation and mental simulation, 222, 224–227
overconfidence and goals, 39–40

P

pain
  regulatory focus, 92
  vs. pleasure, 91
paradigms and affect hypothesis, 63
patterned behavior, effortful pursuit as, 343–345
pendulum illusion, feeling of doing, 483, 496–499
perceiver and target goals, 542–543
perceiver behaviors
  social expectations, 532–533
  target responses to, 532–533
perceiver cognitive processes, 534–535
perceiver impression formation goals, 536–539
perceiver self-presentation goals, 539–541
perceptual readiness, planning, 294–296
perceptual reduction, person perception, 517
performance goals and entity theory of intelligence, 72–73
performance in regulatory focus, 108–109
performance standards
  setting, 132–133
person perception, 511–525, 654–656
  construct building, 515–516
    to egocentrism, 518
  constructs, 513–514
    motive for, 514–515
  cultural context, 523–525
  inference characteristics, 515–516
  inner state cues, 519–523
  perceptual reduction, 517

person perception (*continued*)
person in, 511–512
press, conflict, conflict motivation, 516–517
psychologists in, 512–513
via inferences, 512–514
personal constructs, 96
personal goals, 314–316
and personal strivings as goal units, 315–316
personality
implicit theories of personality and character, 75–87
and subjective well-being, 331–332
phenomenal will. *See* Feeling of doing
planned behavior theory
from attitudes to behavior, 395–396
from attitudes to intentions, 393–395
belief equivalence vs. mode congruence, 393
vs. mode model, 392–396
planning, 287–309
actional phase, 290
goal execution, 607
implemental mind-set, 300–307
implementation intention concept, 292
and mental simulation, 220–221
mind-set concept, 291–292
model of action phases, 288–294
postactional phase, 290
preactional phase, 290
predecisional phase, 289
structure and functions of, 287–288
volitional problems of goal achievement, 294–307
behavior orientation, 302–303
behavioral readiness, 297–300
disrupted goal pursuits, 306–307
distractions, 304–305
effort mobilization, 303–304
focused attention disruption, 296–297
illusionary optimism, 301–302
perceptual readiness, 294–296
pleasure
regulatory focus, 92
vs. pain, 91
positive expectations
vs. positive fantasies, 239–243
and weight loss, 239–240
positive fantasies
and acute illness recovery, 241–242
and chronic illness recovery, 240–241
harmfulness of, 247
and motivation, 236–255, 656–657
and negative reality, 247–252
interpersonal matters, 248–249
work and family life, 250–251
and professional success, 243
and romantic success, 242
supportive findings, 245–247
vs. positive expectations, 239–243
and weight loss, 239–240
positive illusions, 301–302
positive outcome focus regulatory system, 92
postactional phase
of action sequence, 129, 137–138
planning, 290
preactional phase
of action sequence, 129, 134–136
planning, 290
predecisional phase
of action sequence, 129, 130–134
assessing goal desirability, 130–132
goal attainment, 132–133
setting performance standards, 132–133
planning, 289
press, in person perception, 516–517
primed goal states and unconscious intentions, 471–472
priming and remembering, correctional goals, 580–582
priming conditions, 94
problem-solving and mental simulation, 221–222
process simulation, 222–223, 224–227
processing of social information in depression, 154–155
process–outcome simulation, 223, 224–227

professional success and positive fantasies, 243
protoemotional processes and evoked potentials, 183–184
protoemotional responses, 169
psychologists in person perception, 512–513
The Psychopathology of Everyday Life, 458

R

Rand's volitional theory, 365–371
reasoned vs. spontaneous processes, 396–400
recall and emotions, 176–177
refutational defenses, 34–36
regulatory disorders, 95–96
  and ideals, 95–96
  and oughts, 95–96
regulatory focus, 91–92, 664–667
  and approach vs. avoidance, 98–108
  and motivation and performance, 108–109
  pain, 92
  pleasure, 92
  and strategic concerns, 98–108
  and valence of end-state, 98–108
relative autonomy, goal orientation, 325
remembering, correctional goals, 580–582
repressors, 31
resource limitations and role strain, effortful pursuits, 347–349
rewards and willpower, 200–202
romantic success and positive fantasies, 242

S

SAT scores and delayed gratification, 211–212
self-affirmation, 57–58
  and self-evaluation maintenance, 60
self-control and willpower, 213
self-deception, 29–30
self-defense mechanisms, 63–64
self-discrepancies and mood, 97–98
self-discrepancy theory, 92
self-distraction and willpower, 202–203
self-esteem, 27, 48–64
  maintenance, 55–64
    substitutability of self zoo, 56–58
  and self-management, 40–43
self-evaluation maintenance, 49, 56–59
  and self-affirmation, 60
self-management, 37–43
  and ego threat, 40–43
  and self-esteem, 40–43
self-oriented processes
  affect hypothesis, 62–64
  substitutability, 61–64
self-presentational goals, social expectations, 541–542
self-protective mechanisms, 48–64
  association hypothesis vs. goal tension hypothesis, 52
  and goal tension, 51–53
  task substitution and goal completion, 53–55
self-regulation, 27–29
  and defensive responses, 29–37
  and ego threat, 27–44
  theory, 28
"self-zoo," 49–50
Selves Questionnaire, 102
sensitivity to social information, depression, 152–153
sessile strategy of survival, 168
skill acquisition, 404–421
  integrated resource allocation model, 406–420
    Air Traffic Controller Task, 410–414
skills perspective, integrated resource allocation model, 414–420
social behavior and unconscious intentions, 469–475
social context
  and depression dispositional control motives, 157–159
  and motivational orientations, 14–15
social expectations, 529–547
  expectancy confirmation model, 531–535
    perceiver behaviors, 532–533
    perceiver cognitive processes, 534–535

social expectations (*continued*)
limited resources, 543–544
perceiver and target goals met, 542–543
self-presentational goals, 541–542
social goals as moderators, 535–545
perceiver impression formation goals, 536–539
perceiver self-presentation goals, 539–541
social interaction, expectancy influences in, 529–547
social pressure hypothesis, feeling of doing, 491–492
social–cognitive consequences of depression, 147–152
socialization, 95–96
spillover effects, in effortful pursuits, 349–352
spontaneous
effort experience, 353–355
reasoned vs. spontaneous processes
directive influence of attitudes on behavior, 396–400
spontaneous motivation, 339–340
state vs. trait social judgments, 75–78
stereotypes, in correctional goals, 587–589
stream of thought and fantasies, 244–245
striving and feeling, 657–660
subjective well-being, 313–333
and goal content, 316–319
and goal orientation, 319–325
and personality integration, 331–332
subjective well-being theories (SWB), 313
sublimation, 53
substitutability, 54–55
goal execution, 609–610
of "self zoo," 56–58
self-oriented processes, 61–64
sufficiency principle, 554
sufficiency threshold, 554
systolic blood pressure, 426

T

task substitution and goal completion, self-protective mechanisms, 53–55
temporal bracketing, 36
Thematic Apperception Test fantasies, 243–244
tilting, feeling of doing, 484–485
trait judgments, 80–81
vs. state social judgments, 75–78
trance states, feeling of doing, 486

U

uncertainty orientation
and action, 630–633
conscious thought, 625–633
unconscious
as routinized consciousness, 460–461
as smart or dumb, 464–465
as source of error, 458–460
unconscious intentions
and behavioral schema, 470–471
and cognitive processing goals, 467–469
and goals without conscious consent, 473–475
and primed goal states, 471–472
and social behavior, 469–475
unconscious motivations, goal setting, 601

V

valence of end-state and regulatory focus, 98–108
values
and volitional theory, 371–373
volitional theory, 365–384
and action theory, 383
commitment, 375
conflict, 375–376
empirical data, 377–378
failure and frustration, 376
and goal achievement planning, 294–307
goal level, 373–374
goal specificity, 373
Ayn Rand's, 365–371
study planning and methods, 374–375
and values, 371–373
and willpower, 382–383

W

weight loss
  and positive expectations, 239–240
  and positive fantasies, 239–240
willpower, 197–216
  and delayed gratification, 198
    instrumental activity, 207–209
  effects of cognitive focus, 204–207
  and goal-directed delayed gratification, 199
  and high-risk populations, 213–215
  and images of rewards, 203–204
  reconstruing, 209–210
  and rewards, 200–202
  and self-control, 213
  and self-distraction, 202–203
  and volitional theory, 382–383
work and family life and fantasy, 250–251
wrongdoing consequences, 83–87

Y

yoked priming, 94

Z

Zeigarnik effect, 51